ROUTLEDGE LIBRARY EDITIONS:
HISTORY OF MEDICINE

Volume 5

NOBEL LAUREATES IN MEDICINE OR PHYSIOLOGY

NOBEL LAUREATES IN MEDICINE OR PHYSIOLOGY

A Biographical Dictionary

Edited by
DANIEL M. FOX, MARCIA MELDRUM
AND IRA REZAK

Routledge
Taylor & Francis Group
LONDON AND NEW YORK

First published in 1990 by Garland Publishing, Inc.

This edition first published in 2019
by Routledge
2 Park Square, Milton Park, Abingdon, Oxon OX14 4RN

and by Routledge
52 Vanderbilt Avenue, New York, NY 10017

Routledge is an imprint of the Taylor & Francis Group, an informa business

British Library Cataloguing in Publication Data
A catalogue record for this book is available from the British Library

ISBN: 978-0-367-08576-6 (Set)
ISBN: 978-0-429-02312-5 (Set) (ebk)
ISBN: 978-0-367-07490-6 (Volume 5) (hbk)
ISBN: 978-0-367-07495-1 (Volume 5) (pbk)
ISBN: 978-0-429-02098-8 (Volume 5) (ebk)

Publisher's Note
The publisher has gone to great lengths to ensure the quality of this reprint but points out that some imperfections in the original copies may be apparent.

Disclaimer
The publisher has made every effort to trace copyright holders and would welcome correspondence from those they have been unable to trace.

Nobel Laureates in Medicine or Physiology

A Biographical Dictionary

EDITED BY *Daniel M. Fox,*
Marcia Meldrum, and Ira Rezak

Garland Publishing, Inc.
New York & London 1990

Fox, Daniel M.
Biographical dictionary of Nobel Prize laureates in medicine or physiology.

(Garland reference library of the humanities ; vol. 852)
Includes index.
1. Physicians—Biography—Dictionaries.
2. Nobel prizes. 3. Medicine—History—Dictionaries.
4. Physiologists—Biography—Dictionaries. I. Meldrum, Marcia.
II. Rezak, Ira. III. Title. IV. Series.
RI34.F69 1990 610'.92'2 [B] 90-13907
ISBN 0-8240-7892-6 (acid-free paper)

Printed on acid-free, 250-year-life paper

Manufactured in the United States of America

Contents

Preface vii

Nobel Laureates In
Medicine or Physiology xi

The Laureates 1

Index 583

PREFACE

This book is a biographical reference work about the recipients of Nobel Prizes in Medicine or Physiology from 1901 to 1989. Each article is written by an accomplished historian of medicine or science. Nevertheless, the articles are written to be accessible to students and general readers as well as to specialists in medical science and history. Each article combines personal and scientific biography, and each has an extensive bibliography to guide further reading and research.

Since the first Nobel Prizes were awarded, in December 1901, they have fascinated both scientists and the general public. The star system in modern science preceded Alfred Nobel's bequest of funds to award prizes, but the prizes increased the magnitude of the stars. The prizes captured the scientific and the popular imagination because they represented two themes that have had great appeal during the past century. The first theme is progress, the unlimited potential of science and medicine to improve the human condition. The second theme is prosperity, the power of modern industry to generate wealth beyond the expectations of previous generations and to make previously ordinary individuals unexpectedly affluent.

The awards in Alfred Nobel's will recognized what was commonly regarded as the extraordinary progress of the West in the nineteenth century. In the first decade of the twentieth century, many people congratulated themselves on the contemporary situation in the five fields in which prizes were awarded: in physics, chemistry, medicine or physiology, literature and peace. Even when peace was shattered, when physics and chemistry contributed to death and destruction and literature was bent to ideological purposes, the faith in progress remained, revitalized at the end of each year by the award of prizes.

The regular awards affirmed the belief that individuals had the power to advance the welfare of humanity by altering the future. In the early years, the money value of the prizes was especially newsworthy: from four to seventy times greater than the value of other leading scientific prizes. Even later in the century, when the relative value of the prizes declined well below the windfalls from public lotteries and other prizes, the combination of prestige and proceeds was front page (and later prime time) news. The Nobels' prestige and their recognition of work done over a lifetime has given an aura no other scientific award possesses. To the general public and many scientists the prize is a form of secular canonization, complete with elaborate ceremonies, that seems to be above politics. This idealization of the prizes contributes to the bitterness of the occasional controversies about the appropriateness of specific prizes.

The prize in medicine or physiology had, from the beginning, special public significance. For most people in the West, the twentieth century has been an era of unprecedented optimism about the potential of medical science to make life longer and more fulfilling. This optimism began in the nineteenth century, with new discoveries about the causes of infectious disease, which seemed to promise vaccines and cures. More importantly, such advances were generally believed to reveal that medical scientists had devised a method for achieving progress. This method began with laboratory experiments, continued with the trial of new vaccines and treatments on animals and human beings and the devising of new technology, and concluded with the publicizing of new diagnostic and therapeutic techniques. Even when the prize was first awarded its name was, in a sense, obsolete. Medicine *or* physiology had been alternatives before the nineteenth century; one was empirical and traditional, the other experimental. By 1900, however, physiology and medicine were increasingly seen as a continuum: Laboratory investigation was to be followed by clinical experiment and then by progress in medical care.

Each of the five Nobel prizes is awarded on the recommendation of a different committee. The prize in medicine or physiology is administered by the Karolinska Institute, a world renowned center of medical education, research and patient care in Stockholm. The committee at the Karolinska Institute solicits nominations each year from more than 1,000 individuals around the world, including previous Nobel laureates, members of the medical faculties in the five Scandinavian countries, at least six other medical faculties around the world, and individual scientists. The award is formally proposed by the fifty-member Nobel Assembly of the Karolinska Institute.

According to Alfred Nobel's will, the awards in physiology or medicine are to be made to individuals "who shall have conferred the greatest benefit on mankind" in the previous year. Even before the first prize was awarded, however, the faculty of the Karolinska Institute realized that the stipulation that the prize should be awarded for work done during the preceding year was too restrictive. Consequently, from the beginning, the rules for awarding the prize stated that the "provision in the will that the annual award of prizes shall refer to works 'during the preceding year' shall be understood in the sense that the awards shall be made for the most recent achievements in [each field] and for older works only if their significance has not become apparent until recently." This regulatory language has guaranteed that the politics of the prizes would be intense (often bitter) and would involve vigorously held convictions about what was to be considered important science and how to evaluate the contribution of particular investigators. Such a controversy became public as recently as 1989.

As a result of the politics of the Nobel prizes and their high public visibility, a great deal has been written about them, in scholarship as well as in the scientific and popular press. The history of the prizes is the story of each scientific field in this century; of factions and fashions, of enmities and enthusiasms. Some notables never received the prize in medicine or physiology, even though nominated for it (e.g., Sigmund Freud). Others received it for seriously flawed work (e.g., Johannes Fibiger on malignant tumors) or for very modest contributions to other people's scientific achievements (e.g., J. J. R. MacLeod on the therapeutic application of insulin) or belatedly after other scientists developed the potential of a research finding (e.g., Alexander Fleming and penicillin).

Nevertheless, many of the greatest names in medical science in the past century have received the prize and hence are the subject of articles in this book. The biographies, presented below in alphabetical order, can be read as a modern history of medicine. Readers will note, for example, that most of the early prizes were awarded for work bearing on infectious diseases or on surgical intervention. Later on in the century, the emphasis of medical scientists, and hence of the committee awarding the prize, shifted to chronic degenerative diseases. Bacteriology gradually gave way to molecular biology as the basic science most important to the advance of medical knowledge. But the story is more complicated: the prizes, taken as a whole, signal the enormous diversity of medical science in this century. They represent as well a human story of struggle, heroism, triumph and defeat; of generosity, arrogance and bitter controversy; of individual determination to solve problems and to alleviate suffering.

Some of the readers of the biographies in this book may want to learn more about the history of the Nobel Prizes and about the broader historical context in which they were awarded. The following books, presented in alphabetical order, are useful places to begin such inquiries: Elisabeth Crawford, *The Beginnings of the Nobel Institution: The Science Prizes, 1901–1915* (Cambridge and New York: Cambridge University Press, 1984); Carl Gustaf Berhnard et al., *Science, Technology and Society in the Time of Alfred Nobel* (Oxford and New York, Pergamon Press, 1982); W. Odelberg, ed., *Nobel: The Man and His Prizes* (New York and London: American Elsevier Publishing Company, Third Edition, 1972); and Harriet Zuckerman, *Scientific Elite: Nobel Laureates in the United States* (New York, The Free Press, 1977).

***

The editors have incurred numerous obligations in the several years since this volume was conceived. Bernard S. Katz was a buoyant general editor. At Garland, Kennie Lyman has been patient and firm. Monte Kelly, Katherine Stephani and Hope Fleischer have, in sequence, performed secretarial chores for a large and often chaotic project. Most important, the scholars who wrote the biographical articles have borne the necessary steps in the creation of the book with notable good humor, far exceeding any compensation they will receive.

Daniel M. Fox
Marcia Meldrum
Ira Rezak

Nobel Laureates in Physiology or Medicine

1901	Emil Adolf Von Behring
1902	Sir Ronald Ross
1903	Niels Ryberg Finsen
1904	Ivan Petrovich Pavlov
1905	Heinrich Hermann Robert Koch
1906	Camillo Golgi Santiago Ramón y Cajal
1907	Charles Louis Alphonse Laveran
1908	Paul Ehrlich Ilya Metchnikoff
1909	Emil Theodor Kocher
1910	Albrecht Kossel
1911	Allvar Gullstrand
1912	Alexis Carrel
1913	Charles Robert Richet
1914	Robert Bárány
1915 to 1918	Reserved
1919	Jules Bordet
1920	Schack Augustus Steenberg Krogh
1922	Archibald Vivian Hill Otto Fritz Meyerhof
1923	Sir Frederick Grant Banting John James Rickard Macleod
1924	Willem Einthoven
1925	Reserved

1926	Johannes Andreas Grib Fibiger
1927	Julius Wagner-Jauregg
1928	Charles Jules Henri Nicolle
1929	Christiaan Eijkman Sir Frederick Gowland Hopkins
1930	Karl Landsteiner
1931	Otto Heinrich Warburg
1932	Lord Edgar Douglas Adrian Sir Charles Scott Sherrington
1933	Thomas Hunt Morgan
1934	George Richards Minot William Parry Murphy George Hoyt Whipple
1935	Hans Spemann
1936	Sir Henry Hallett Dale Otto Loewi
1937	Albert Szent-Györgyi von Nagyrapolt
1938	Corneille Jean François Heymans
1939	Gerhard Johannes Paul Domagk
1940 to 1942	Reserved
1943	Carl Peter Henrik Dam Edward Adelbert Doisy
1944	Joseph Erlanger Herbert Spencer Gasser
1945	Sir Ernst Boris Chain Sir Alexander Fleming Lord Howard Walter Florey
1946	Hermann Joseph Muller
1947	Carl Ferdinand Cori Gerty Theresa Cori Bernardo Alberto Houssay
1948	Paul Hermann Müller

1949	Walter Rudolf Hess Antonio Caetano de Abreu Freire Egas Moniz
1950	Philip Showalter Hench Edward Calvin Kendall Tadeus Reichstein
1951	Max Theiler
1952	Selman Abraham Waksman
1953	Sir Hans Adolf Krebs Fritz Albert Lipmann
1954	John Franklin Enders Frederick Chapman Robbins Thomas Huckle Weller
1955	Axel Hugo Theodor Theorell
1956	André Frédéric Cournand Werner Theodor Otto Forssmann Dickinson Woodruff Richards, Jr.
1957	Daniel Bovet
1958	George Wells Beadle Joshua Lederberg Edward Lawrie Tatum
1959	Arthur Kornberg Severo Ochoa
1960	Sir Frank Macfarlane Burnet Sir Peter Brian Medawar
1961	Georg von Békésy
1962	Francis Harry Compton Crick James Dewey Watson Maurice Hugh Frederick Wilkins
1963	Sir John Carew Eccles Sir Alan Lloyd Hodgkin Sir Andrew Fielding Huxley
1964	Konrad Bloch Feodor Lynen

1965	François Jacob André Michel Lwoff Jacques Lucien Monod
1966	Charles Brenton Huggins Francis Peyton Rous
1967	Ragnar Arthur Granit Haldan Keffer Hartline George Wald
1968	Robert W. Holley Har Gobind Khorana Marshall Warren Nirenberg
1969	Max Delbrück Alfred Day Hershey Salvador E. Luria
1970	Julius Axelrod Sir Bernard Katz Ulf von Euler
1971	Earl Wilbur Sutherland, Jr.
1972	Gerald M. Edelman Rodney R. Porter
1973	Konrad Zacharias Lorenz Nikolaas Tinbergen Karl von Frisch
1974	Albert Claude Christian René de Duvé George Emil Palade
1975	David Baltimore Renato Dulbecco Howard Martin Temin
1976	Baruch Samuel Blumberg Daniel Carleton Gajdusek
1977	Roger Charles Louis Guillemin Andrew Victor Schally Rosalyn Yalow

1978	Werner Arber Daniel Nathans Hamilton Othaniel Smith
1979	Allan Cormack Godfrey Newbold Hounsfield
1980	Baruj Benacerraf Jean Dausset George Davis Snell
1981	David Hunter Hubel Roger Wolcott Sperry Torsten N. Wiesel
1982	Sune K. Bergström Bengt Ingemar Samuelsson John R. Vane
1983	Barbara McClintock
1984	Niels Kaj Jerne Georges J. F. Köhler Cesar Milstein
1985	Michael Stuart Brown Joseph Leonard Goldstein
1986	Stanley Cohen Rita Levi-Montalcini
1987	Susumu Tonegawa
1988	Sir James Whyte Black Gertrude Belle Elion George Herbert Hitchings
1989	J. Michael Bishop Harold Elliot Varmus

Lord Edgar Douglas Adrian *1932*

Lord Edgar Douglas Adrian was born on November 30, 1889, in London. A neurophysiologist, Adrian shared the Nobel Prize for 1932 for his description and analysis of the functioning of the neurons in stimulation of muscle and sense organs, extending and illuminating the earlier discoveries of his colaureate, Sir Charles Scott Sherrington. Adrian's research laid the groundwork for the development of electroencephalography. At the time of the award, he was lecturer in physiology at Cambridge University; he was appointed to a full professorship five years later. He was named Baron of Cambridge in 1955. Adrian married Hester Agnes Pinsent, a descendant of David Hume, in 1923; they had one son, Richard Hume, who became a biophysicist, and two daughters, Anne and Jennet. Lady Adrian was active in social work and later became a justice of the peace. Adrian died on August 4, 1977, in Cambridge, England.

Adrian was the son of Flora Lavinia Barton and Alfred Douglas Adrian, K.C., legal adviser to the British Local Government Board. He was educated at the Westminster School in London, and entered Trinity College, Cambridge, in 1908 with a science scholarship. At Cambridge he studied physiology for the natural sciences tripos, which he passed with first-class honors in five subjects (rather than the usual three) in 1911. While at Cambridge, he did his first neurological research with Keith Lucas, who was working on the neuromuscular impulses; he showed that the neural impulse stimulating muscle contraction is succeeded by a relaxation of the nerve, the "all or none" principle. This work resulted in Adrian's election as a fellow of Trinity in 1913.

He went to St. Bartholomew's in London for his medical degree, and during World War I was assigned by the British Army to the treatment of nerve injuries and disorders in invalided servicemen at the Hospital for Nervous Diseases. After Keith Lucas died in an airplane crash, Adrian acted as his literary executor, publishing Lucas's lectures in 1917 as *The Conduction of the Nervous Impulse*. He received his bachelor of medicine degree in 1915 and his doctor of medicine degree in 1919.

Also in 1919, he returned to Cambridge as lecturer on the nervous system and took over Lucas's laboratory, where he began to apply electrical methods to the study of nerve impulses. To better detect and differentiate individual impulses, he used a combination of cathode-ray tube, capillary electrometer, and thermionic valves; with this apparatus, he succeeded in amplification by a factor of five thousand the impulses of a single nerve fiber and a single end organ in a muscle of the frog. In 1926 Adrian published his first observations on the response of the sensory end organ to various natural stimuli. (Adrian and Zotterman 1926)

By 1928 he was ready to present his conclusions on the quantitative nature of the nervous impulse. He traced the pathways of the impulses from sensory organs to the central nervous system and from there to the muscles. Adrian showed that a constant stimulus results in immediate excitement of the end organ, followed by a gradual decrease. The related nerve impulses from the end organ to the central nervous system followed a similar pattern, initially very frequent, but then decreasing in frequency, while remaining constant in intensity, resulting in a gradual relaxation of the stimulus reaching the brain. However, if the external stimulus is intensified, the nerve impulses increase in frequency. Adrian's isolation of the individual impulses into functional components clarified earlier findings by Sherrington and others (Adrian 1928).

The following year he was elected Foulerton Professor of the Royal Society, of which he had been a member since 1923. He traveled to New York, where he worked with Detlev Bronk on the conversion of electrical impulses to sound. Upon his return to Cambridge, he continued his mapping of the sensory impulses onto the brain. He found that the nerve fibers that transmit the sensations of pain appeared to terminate in the optic thalamus. Other sensations, however, were traced to the cerebral cortex, and he determined that the area of the cortex related to various end organs varied among mammals. In man and monkeys, the area receiving impulses from the face and the hands is extensive, whereas the area receiving olfactory messages is small, compared to that of other animals. The intellectual guidelines and experimental techniques developed by Adrian in this work were later followed by Erlanger and Gasser, Hodgkin and Huxley, and other Nobel laureates in neurophysiology.

But Adrian was not content to consider the nervous system as an intellectual conundrum. Perhaps because of his early experience as a practical neurologist, he was acutely aware of the difficulties of neurological diagnosis. Consequently, he applied his basic research knowledge to the development of a practical clinical method of reading the electrical wave patterns of the brain. Although researchers had been able as early as 1875 to record nerve impulses electrically, and Antonio Egas Moniz in 1927 had used such methods to localize cerebral tumors, the results were inconsistent and the variations and abnormalities, as described by Hans Berger of Jena in 1929, difficult to interpret. Adrian's review of earlier work and his careful analysis of the variations opened the way for the successful development of clinical electroencephalography (EEG) (Adrian and Matthews 1934).

He was appointed professor of physiology in 1937 and became a member of the Medical Research Council in 1939. Much of Adrian's subsequent career was pursued in the public spotlight, as a scientific administrator and advisor to the government. From 1951 to 1965 he held the distinguished position of master of Trinity College, and from 1957 to 1959 he was vice chancellor of Cambridge University. He also served as president of the Royal Society (1950–55), president of the British Association for the Advancement of Science (1954), and president of the Royal Society of Medicine (1960–62). Adrian was active as well in international affairs, working on several committees of the World Health Organization, most notably in 1961, to study the effects of atomic radiation on the future of mankind. In 1962 he was elected a trustee of Rockefeller University in New York.

A man of considerable energy, Adrian found time for many interests outside of science. He was an accomplished fencer and enjoyed sailing and rock climbing with Lady Adrian. A patron and student of modern painting, he exhibited eighty of his works in the styles of Picasso and Matisse in the Guildhall, Cambridge. Adrian pursued these leisure activities with the same single-minded purpose he gave to his work and his fast bicycle rides through the crowded streets of Cambridge. As a lecturer, he was restrained and avoided "showman's tricks."

Among the many other awards he received for his fundamental discoveries were the Baly Medal from the Royal College of Physicians (1929), the British Order of Merit (1942), the Royal Medal (1934) and the Copley Medal from the Royal Society (1946), the Gold Medal of the Royal Society of Medicine (1950), the Albert Gold Medal of the Royal Society of Arts (1953), the Harben Medal (1955), the French Legion of Honor (1956), the Sherrington Memorial Medal (1957), the Medal for Distinguished Merit of the British Medical Association (1958), and the Jephcott Medal of the Royal Society of Medicine (1963). He retired from Trinity in 1965 and died in Cambridge in 1977, at age eighty-eight.

ESTELLE BRODMAN

Selected Bibliography

PRIMARY SOURCES

Adrian, Edgar Douglas, and Yngve Zotterman. 1926. "The Impulses Produced by Sensory Nerve-Endings. Part 2. The Response of a Single Nerve-Organ." (London) *Journal of Physiology* 61:151–71.

Adrian, Edgar Douglas. 1928. *The Basis of Sensation. The Action of the Sense Organs.* London: Christophers.

———. 1932. *The Mechanism of Nervous Action.* Philadelphia: University of Pennsylvania Press.

Adrian, Edgar Douglas, and Bryan Harold Cabot Matthews. 1934. "The Interpretation of Potential Waves in the Cortex." (London) *Journal of Physiology* 81:440–71.

Adrian, Edgar Douglas. 1947. *The Physical Basis of Perception.* Oxford: Clarendon Press.

SECONDARY SOURCES

1955. "Adrian, Edgar Douglas." In *Current Biography Yearbook,* 1–3. New York: H. W. Wilson.

Zotterman, Yngve. 1978. "Obituary. Lord Adrian." *Electroencephalography and Clinical Neurophysiology* 44:137–39.

1979. "Adrian, Edgar Douglas." In *Biographical Memoirs of Fellows of the Royal Society*, 25:1–73. London: Royal Society.

Moruzzi, G. 1980. "In Memoriam: Lord Adrian (1889–1977)." *Reviews of Physiology, Biochemistry and Pharmacology* 87:1–18.

———. 1980. "Bibliography of Lord Adrian's Publications." *Reviews of Physiology, Biochemistry and Pharmacology* 87:18–24.

Werner Arber *1978*

Werner Arber was born on June 3, 1929, in Granichen, Switzerland. A molecular biologist, Arber shared the Nobel Prize in 1978 with Daniel Nathans and Hamilton O. Smith for his description of the molecular mechanism within the host that produces variation among bacterial viruses. His work was confirmed by Smith, who was then able to isolate the first restriction enzyme (known as Hind II). Nathans used the enzyme discovered by Smith to separate and map DNA molecules. These three investigations led cumulatively to the technique of DNA recombination and the potential breakthroughs of genetic engineering. Arber has been professor of molecular biology at the University of Basel since 1970. He and his wife Antonia were married in 1966; they have two daughters, Silvia and Caroline. Arber's family is his major interest outside of his research; he credits their support and understanding as factors in his success.

Arber's parents were Julius and Maria Arber. He graduated from the Federal Institute of Technology in Zurich in 1953 and went on to study biophysics at the University of Geneva with Eduard Kellenberger and Jean J. Weigle. Weigle, Giuseppe Bertani, and Salvador E. Luria had observed and described the phenomenon of variation among bacterial viruses (bacteriophages) in the 1950s. The mechanism is host-controlled; a specific phage, which will multiply rapidly and infect a specific host bacteria, will die out with equal rapidity if injected into a different bacterial strain. However, a few survivors will successfully adapt to the new strain and will then generate a variant phage that will be able to infect the new bacteria. The implications of the phenomenon for our understanding of the incidence and spread of viral infections are clearly of great interest (Linn 1978, 1069).

While at Geneva, Arber assisted in developing techniques of electron microscopic study of bacteriophages (The electron microscope uses electron bombardment in a vacuum for high-level magnification of the smallest structures.) After receiving his doctorate in 1958, Arber spent two years in the United States at the University of Southern California; there he was able to work with Bertani, Gunther Stent, and Joshua Lederberg. He also visited Luria's laboratory at MIT. Arber returned to Geneva in 1960 and began to study host-controlled variation on the molecular level, assisted by Daisy Dussoix. His research was supported by the Swiss National Science Foundation.

By 1962 Arber and Dussoix had traced the variation mechanism to modification and degradation of the phage DNA by the infected bacterium. Modification of the DNA led to a new variant; degradation led to the "restriction," or elimination, of the phage. But some phage DNA still remained in a fragmented form in the bacterial cells. Arber later noted the presence of methionine in such modification activity. In 1966 William B. Wood, working in Arber's laboratory, established that the ability to modify or restrict DNA is a genetic property of the host bacterium and that bacteria having this property are able to act on the DNA of foreign bacteria as well as on viral DNA.

Arber and his coworkers constructed a model of DNA restriction that was based on the existence of bacterium-specific restriction enzymes or endonucleases. According to their hypothesis, the endonuclease recognizes specific sequences of nucleotides in the DNA of an invading phage and cleaves the DNA molecule at those specific sites. However, the bacterium also contains a strain-specific modification enzyme that acts to protect the bacterial DNA by methylating the identical nucleotide sequences in the host; it may also act on the foreign DNA. (Methylation is the chemical combination of the DNA with a methyl group—two carbons and three hydrogens.) The phage DNA, thus modified, eventually generates a new variant virus (Arber 1962; 1968).

Over the next several years other workers carried out research that confirmed the model, including Arber, Urs Kuhnlein, and Stuart Linn in Arber's laboratory, and John Smith of the Medical Research Council at Cambridge, who were able to isolate mutated phages and to directly correlate DNA methylase with host-controlled modification; and Japanese investigators Toshiya Takano, Tsutomu Watanabe, and Toshio Fukasawa, who observed restriction activity in vitro but were unable to isolate the nuclease involved.

In 1968, however, Arber and Linn succeeded in partially isolating and describing the restriction endonuclease of *Escherichia coli B.* Matthew Meselson and Robert Yuan had similar success with the enzyme from *E. coli K.* These enzymes, now known as Type I, do in fact recognize specific nucleotide sequences in foreign DNA, exactly as Arber's model had predicted. But they cut the DNA apparently at random, not necessarily at the recognition site (Linn 1978, 1070). The full hypothesis was later confirmed by the work of Smith, who isolated the Type II restriction enzymes, which cleave DNA at specific recognition sites. Using the enzyme as a "knife," Nathans and others were then able to dissect DNA with surgical precision for observation and study.

Smith's and Nathans's methods have been applied in several laboratories, including Herbert Boyer's and Howard Goodman's at UCSF, Paul Berg's and Stanley Cohen's at Stanford, and Kenneth and Noreen Murray's in Edinburgh, to cleave and recombine various DNA molecules, and then reproduce the resulting DNA in bacterial or other host cells. Boyer and his colleagues established that different DNA molecules cut by the same enzyme at identical sites will have "sticky edges" that "fit" with each other. The new technology makes possible the in vitro production of scarce enzymes and hormones, such as insulin.

However, experiments that combine eukaryotic with bacterial or viral DNA have created fears about the creation of dangerous new pathogens. In 1974 Nathans joined other scientists in recommending that some types of recombinant DNA research be postponed until more was understood about the risks and requesting the National Institutes of Health to establish specific guidelines for recombinant DNA research (Linn 1978, 1071).

Arber was named extraordinary professor of molecular genetics at the University of Geneva in 1965. He soon felt that academic politics and teaching demands hampered his research. In 1970–71 he spent a year as visiting professor at the University of California at Berkeley. He returned to the University of Basel which had just opened the Biozentrum, a new research institute with extensive modern laboratory space. Here he continues work with genetic systems and recombinant technology, or the reconstruction of DNA molecules that have been separated, and the transplantation of new genes.

MARCIA MELDRUM

Selected Bibliography

PRIMARY SOURCES

Arber, Werner. 1962. "Biological Specificities of Deoxyribonucleic Acid." *Pathological Microbiology* 25:668–81.

Arber, Werner, Daisy Dussoix, and S. Hattman. 1963. "On the Host-Controlled Modification of Bacteriophage Lambda." *Virology* 21 (September):30–35.

Arber, Werner. 1965. "Host Specificity of DNA Produced by *Escherichia coli*. 5. The Role of Methionone in the Production of Host Specificity." *Journal of Molecular Biology* 11 (February):247–56.

———. 1965. "Host-Controlled Modification of Bacteriophage." *Annual Review of Microbiology* 19:365–78.

———. 1968. "Host-Controlled Restriction and Modification of Bacteriophages." *Symposium of the Society of Genetic Microbiology* 18:295–314.

———. 1974. "DNA Modification and Restriction." *Progress in Nucleic Acid Research in Molecular Biology* 14:1–37.

———. 1984. *Genetic Manipulation: Impact on Men and Society*. New York: Cambridge University Press.

SECONDARY SOURCES

Sylvester, Kathy. 1978. *New York Times* (October 13):61.

Linn, Stuart. 1978. "The 1978 Nobel Prize in Physiology or Medicine." *Science* 202 (December 2):1069–71.

1980. "Arber, Werner." *Modern Scientists and Engineers*, 1:25–26. New York: McGraw-Hill.

JULIUS AXELROD *1970*

As suggested by the title of his autobiographical essay, "An Unexpected Life in Research," Julius Axelrod discovered and fulfilled his promise as a scientist later in life than many other successful investigators. Once his career had been launched, however, he made significant contributions to pharmacology and biochemistry even before initiating the research for which he received the Nobel Prize. A research biochemist and pharmacologist with special interests in biochemical mechanisms of drug and hormone actions, enzymology, the pineal gland, and membranes and transduction mechanisms of lipids, Axelrod was born May 30, 1912, in a Manhattan, New York, tenement. His parents were Isadore Axelrod, a basketmaker, and Molly Axelrod, both Jewish immigrants from Polish Galicia. In 1933, at the nadir of the Great Depression, Axelrod graduated from the College of the City of New York with a B.S. in biology and chemistry and found work as a laboratory assistant in the Department of Bacteriology at New York University Medical School. In 1935 he moved to the Laboratory of Industrial Hygiene, a nonprofit organization established by the New York City Department of Health to test vitamin supplements added to foods. Although his work there as a chemist was routine, Axelrod gained experience in modifying existing chemical, biological, and microbiological methods for the assays of vitamins in food products. In 1938, he married Sally Taub Axelrod, and they had two sons. In 1941 he obtained an M.S. degree in chemistry at New York University by taking courses at night.

Axelrod's initial venture into research, which occurred by chance, revealed his aptitude for the process of scientific discovery and redirected his own career goals. Early in 1946 the Laboratory of Industrial Hygiene was offered a small grant by the Institute for the Study of Analgesic and Sedative Drugs—an organization sponsored by the pharmaceutical industry that funded research projects of interest to its members—to determine why some people habituated to nonaspirin analgesics containing acetanilide or phenacetin developed a methemoglobinemia, a failure of hemoglobin to bind oxygen. Asked to conduct the study for the laboratory, Axelrod consulted with Bernard B. Brodie, a former member of the Department of Pharmacology at New York University then working at nearby Goldwater Memorial Hospital. Already distinguished for developing methods of biological assay for the presence of drugs in the body, Brodie found Axelrod's project intriguing. He invited Axelrod to conduct the research project at Goldwater and arranged for him to become a research associate in the Third New York University Research Division. Together they set about developing methods to measure the drugs and their physiological disposition in the human body. Axelrod and Brodie determined that different metabolic products of the drugs exerted the analgesic effect and the unwanted methemoglobinemia side effect. Their research suggested that acetanilide and phenacetin be replaced in pain relievers by their common, efficacious metabolic product, acetaminophen, the active ingredient now contained in such brand-name products as Tylenol.

In 1949 Axelrod moved to the section on chemical pharmacology of the newly established National Heart Institute in Bethesda, Maryland, as did Brodie and a number of other Goldwater investigators. Although attached to Brodie's laboratory, Axelrod soon began to work independently, rising from associate chemist to senior chemist by 1953. He became intrigued with the sympathomimetic amines, compounds whose name reflects their actions as mimics of the body's sympathetic nervous system. This system prepares the body for bouts of activity by increasing heart rate, expanding the air capacity of the lungs, and the like. Axelrod studied the metabolic fate of the sympathomimetic amines amphetamine, mescaline, and ephedrine, all of which produce unusual behavioral effects. Through a series of elegant experiments, he discovered a new class of enzymes, localized in the microsomes of liver cells and essential to the drugs' metabolism in the body. Additional research by others on these enzymes, now called cytochrome-P450 monoxygenases, exerted a profound influence in many areas of biomedical science, including studies of the metabolism of normally occurring compounds and investigations of carcinogenesis.

During the mid-1950s Axelrod established a separate research program after overcoming the major impediment to obtaining complete scientific independence: lack of a Ph.D. degree. In 1955, at age forty-two, he obtained his doctorate in the Department of Pharmacology at George Washington University. The National Institute of Mental Health

(NIMH), a federal agency whose intramural program is located at the NIH but whose grant-giving offices are associated with the U.S. Alcohol, Drug Abuse, and Mental Health Administration, invited Axelrod to create a section on pharmacology in the Laboratory of Clinical Sciences. In this new position he initiated a new research program, utilizing techniques that had proved so successful in the past. He also drew a large number of postdoctoral fellows and other collaborators, who universally described him as a kind, modest, "sweet" man whose scientific vision could perceive, according to his protégé Solomon H. Snyder, "the farthest reaching implications of apparently trivial data."

In 1957 Axelrod launched the body of work that eventually led to his Nobel Prize. He became intrigued with a report that schizophrenia might be related to abnormal metabolism of epinephrine (also known as adrenaline), which is one member of the family of compounds called catecholamines. Later, he also took up the study of norepinephrine (also known as noradrenaline), another catecholamine known to be the neurotransmitter of the sympathetic nervous system, which calms the body after the exertion has ended for which the sympathetic nervous system prepared it. In collaboration with various colleagues, visiting scientists, and postdoctoral students, Axelrod entered the largely unexplored field of brain and nervous system chemistry.

The questions Axelrod addressed concerned the biochemical mechanisms involved in quickly and repeatedly transferring an electrical impulse from one nerve to another across the tiny space, or synapse, that separated them. In 1904 T. R. Elliot, a graduate student at Cambridge University, had observed that an injection of adrenal gland extract stimulated animal tissues innervated by the sympathetic nerves. Similar reactions, he noted, were caused by injecting the hormone epinephrine, which had been isolated just before the turn of the century by Johns Hopkins University pharmacologist John J. Abel. In 1921 Austrian Otto Loewi, himself later a Nobel laureate, provided the first scientific evidence for neurochemical transmission of nerve impulses. Conducting an experiment with two frog hearts in a common chemical bath, Loewi showed clearly that stimulation of one heart's vagus nerve, which slows heart rate, also caused the other heart to slow. English investigator Henry Dale subsequently identified this chemical as acetylcholine, the neurotransmitter of the parasympathetic nervous system. In the late 1940s Swedish neuropharmacologist Ulf von Euler, who shared the 1970 Nobel Prize with Axelrod, demonstrated that norepinephrine was the neurotransmitter of the sympathetic nervous system. The mechanism by which these substances accomplished their tasks, however, remained unknown when Axelrod began his research.

Beginning as he had on other problems, Axelrod traced the physiological disposition of epinephrine and norepinephrine in the body. When these substances were released from nerves, what chemical transformations did they undergo? What enzymes were involved in this process? In clarifying these metabolic pathways, Axelrod discovered a new enzyme essential to the metabolism of catecholamines and named it catechol-ø-methyltransferase (COMT). An important additional benefit of this work was that other catecholamine metabolites identified in these studies later proved extremely useful as "markers" in biochemical research on psychiatric illnesses.

These studies also provided clues that produced yet another key discovery, for they indicated that metabolic transformation was not the only means by which the neurotransmitter norepinephrine was regulated in the body. When molecules of norepinephrine are released from one nerve fiber, some cross the synaptic cleft and bind to the postsynaptic receptor, thus transmitting the message that the nerve impulse carries. In order that this process may recur rapidly as new nerve impulses are received, excess molecules must be cleared quickly from the synaptic cleft. Axelrod had observed that even when COMT and other metabolizing enzymes were inhibited in the body, the physiological action of norepinephrine came to a stop rapidly. This indicated that a second mechanism must also be at work. Working with cats whose superior cervical ganglia had been removed on one side, Axelrod injected radioactively tagged norepinephrine and showed that it accumulated only on the innervated side. He thus concluded that norepinephrine was deactivated most commonly through "reuptake" by the nerves, in which it was stored and reused for later transmissions. With the electron microscope and other imaging techniques, he and his coworkers revealed the small, dense core vesicles into which norepinephrine was recovered.

Once the mechanism of this neurotransmitter was known, a number of observations about its role in mental and physical health followed. One hypothesis held that drugs might act on neurotransmitters by blocking their reuptake, thus permitting them to remain in the synaptic cleft longer and to continue their actions on the postsynaptic receptors. Axelrod demonstrated this conclusively for a number of compounds, including antidepressant drugs, amphetamines, and cocaine. Another line of work dealt with dopamine-β-hydroxylase, which converts dopamine into norepinephrine and is also present in the norepinephrine storage vesicles. Research suggested that the substance might be released simultaneously with norepinephrine and would therefore be measurable in the blood. Indeed, when an assay was developed, abnormal concentrations of this enzyme were noted as characteristics of several diseases. Abnormally low levels were identified in patients with familial dysautonomia and Down's syndrome while patients with torsion dystonia, neuroblastoma, and certain forms of hypertension displayed abnormally high levels.

After completing much of the neurotransmitter research, Axelrod focused his attention on another subject that had intrigued him for some time: investigation of the previously unknown biochemical activity of the pineal gland. With his colleagues, he described the biosynthesis of melatonin, a compound highly localized in the pineal gland that affects the reproductive process. Subsequently, they also showed that production of serotonin, the precursor of melatonin, was controlled by a "biological clock" in the brain, which, in turn, depended upon environmental cycles of light and darkness. The pineal gland, they suggested, thus serves as a neuroendocrine transducer, converting light signals to hormone synthesis via the brain and noradrenergic nerves.

In 1970 the Nobel Committee named Axelrod, along with Ulf von Euler and Bernard Katz, as a winner of the prize in physiology or medicine, citing Axelrod for his body of work on the chemistry of nerve transmission. Those studies had helped to launch the so-called biological revolution in psychiatry, through which the context for studying many mental illnesses shifted from the psychological construct of "mind" to the physiological concept of "brain." Before the discovery of a few highly effective psychoactive drugs and before the biochemical research of Axelrod and others, much psychiatric theory and practice had focused on the environmental experiences of patients, an approach that had little impact on the most severe psychoses. In recent years, however, physicians have come to understand schizophrenia, depression, mania, and other disorders of behavior as having a biochemical basis in the brain and nervous system. Axelrod's fundamental research on the chemistry of nerve transmission, which he has continued to pursue into retirement as a guest researcher in the Laboratory of cell biology, NIMH, helped to establish a promising new line of medical research with far-reaching implications for the understanding and treatment of these disabling conditions.

VICTORIA A. HARDIN

Selected Bibliography

PRIMARY SOURCES

Wurtman, Richard J., and Julius Axelrod. 1965. "The Pineal Gland." *Scientific American* 213:50–62. Explanation of this work for a lay audience.

Axelrod, Julius. 1970. "Noradrenaline: Fate and Control of Its Biosynthesis." Nobel Lecture, December 12. Reported in *Les Prix Nobel en 1970*, 189–208. Stockholm: Impremerieal Royal P. A. Norstedt & Söner.

———. 1974. "Neurotransmitters." *Scientific American* 230:59–71. Explanation of his work for a lay audience.

———. 1982. "The Discovery of the Microsomal Drug-Metabolizing Enzymes." *Trends in Pharmacological Science* 3:383–86. Contains bibliography of key research papers.

———. 1988. "An Unexpected Life in Research." *Annual Review of Pharmacology and Toxicology* 28:1–23. Contains bibliography of key research papers.

SECONDARY SOURCES

Snyder, Solomon H., ed. 1972. *Perspectives in Pharmacology: A Tribute to Julius Axelrod.* New York: Oxford University Press. Festschrift volume for Axelrod.

Kanigel, Robert. 1986. *Apprentice to Genius: The Making of a Scientific Dynasty.* New York: Macmillan. A journalistic study of mentor relationships in science that focuses on Axelrod's scientific "lineage." No references.

DAVID BALTIMORE *1975*

The 1975 Nobel Prize in Physiology or Medicine was awarded to David Baltimore, Howard Temin, and Renato Dulbecco for "discoveries concerning the interaction between tumor viruses and the genetic material of the cell." David Baltimore was born on March 7, 1938, in New York City. Baltimore's areas of scientific specialization are virology and molecular biology. His parents are Richard I. Baltimore and Gertrude Lipschitz Baltimore. Alice S. Huang and David Baltimore were married on October 5, 1968. Dr. Huang, a microbiologist, is a professor at Harvard Medical School and the director of the Laboratories of Infectious Diseases at the Children's Hospital Medical Center in Boston. The Baltimores have one daughter.

Baltimore became interested in biology as a high school student through a summer spent at Jackson Memorial Laboratory in Bar Harbor, Maine. Although he first majored in biology, he switched to chemistry in order to carry out a research thesis and received his B.A. in chemistry from Swarthmore College in 1960. Before his senior year at Swarthmore he spent the summer at the Cold Spring Harbor Laboratories working with George Streisinger. From 1960 to 1961 he took graduate courses at Massachusetts Institute of Technology. He planned to do his graduate work in biophysics, but became very interested in animal viruses. He left MIT to spend a summer working with Philip Marcus at the Albert Einstein College of Medicine and took the animal virus course, taught by Richard Franklin and Edward Simon, at Cold Spring Harbor. In 1961 he went to Rockefeller University in New York, to work with Franklin, and received a Ph.D. in Biology in 1964.

Baltimore did postdoctoral work with James Darnell at MIT in 1963 and 1964 and was a postdoctoral researcher at the Albert Einstein College of Medicine, in New York, with Jerard Hurwitz, from 1964 to 1965. From 1965 to 1968 he was a research associate at the Salk Institute for Biological Studies, at La Jolla, California, working in association with Renato Dulbecco. Between 1968 and 1972 he served as associate professor of microbiology at MIT. Since 1972 he has been a professor of biology at MIT. From 1973 to 1983 he was American Cancer Society Research Professor. In 1982 he became director of the Whitehead Institute for Biomedical Research, in Cambridge, Massachusetts.

In his Nobel Prize Lecture, Baltimore attributed the award to the work he, Temin, and Dulbecco had done in "bringing molecular biology to bear on the awful and awesome problem of cancer." Research performed by the three laureates had demonstrated that certain viruses could cause cancer by introducing new genes into cells. Baltimore and Temin had also challenged the "central dogma of molecular biology"—that information flows only from DNA to RNA to protein—by identifying an enzyme that allowed information to flow from RNA to DNA (Baltimore 1977, vii–ix).

Baltimore and Temin independently arrived at an explanation of DNA synthesis in RNA tumor viruses through the action of a "reverse transcriptase" enzyme that allowed DNA synthesis to proceed by copying RNA. The term "reverse transcriptase" was coined by an anonymous correspondent for the British journal *Nature*. Originally this theory was quite controversial, but by 1975 it had been thoroughly substantiated and integrated into the theoretical framework of molecular biology and cancer research. Baltimore has made many contributions to our understanding of RNA virus replication, poliovirus and leukemia virus, synthetic vaccines, and genetic control mechanisms. He has been active within the scientific community in efforts to establish responsible guidelines for research in genetic engineering and has also been a spokesperson for science on issues such as recombinant DNA research, establishing priorities for national scientific goals, and matters of international concern, such as biological warfare and the regulation of science.

Howard Temin and David Baltimore came to their simultaneous but independent discoveries of RNA-dependent DNA synthesis by RNA tumor viruses by quite different routes. Temin had proposed his controversial "provirus hypothesis" in 1964, but much of the evidence was indirect. Furthermore, the possibility that the use of various inhibitors had caused artifacts could not be ruled out unequivocally until 1970 when Temin and Satoshi Mizutani proved that virions of Rous sarcoma virus (RSV) contain an enzyme that can transcribe viral RNA into DNA. Using Rauscher murine leukemia virus and RSV, Baltimore discovered the same enzyme activity. This evidence provided a mechanism for the formation of a DNA intermediate during RNA tumor virus infection and transformation, and transformed the climate of opinion in the scientific community.

Not only was the discovery of

reverse transcriptase a major advance in understanding the replication of certain types of virus, it also provided cell biologists with a powerful new tool for dissecting out the intricate control mechanisms of more complex genetic systems at the molecular level. Reverse transcriptase can be used to prepare DNA copies of messenger RNA and highly specific probes to detect viral genetic information in normal and malignant cells. This discovery has also helped to unify the study of DNA tumor viruses and RNA tumor viruses and has opened up new approaches to the study of cell growth and differentiation.

In his Nobel Prize Lecture, Baltimore expressed his belief: "The study of biology is partly an exercise in natural esthetics. We derive much of our pleasure as biologists from the continuing realization of how economical, elegant and intelligent are the accidents of evolution that have been maintained by selection. A virologist is among the luckiest of biologists because he can see into his chosen pet down to the details of all of its molecules. The virologist sees how an extreme parasite functions using just the most fundamental aspects of biological behavior" (Baltimore 1975, 495).

However, the relationship between a virus's life-style and the disease it causes generally remains obscure, except for the case of the RNA viruses known as retroviruses (RNA viruses with a genome of double-stranded RNA), which are the only RNA viruses known to cause cancer. Although originally virologists had assumed that all RNA viruses would be similar in their basic molecular biology, in the 1960s various findings suggested that poliovirus was not a model for all RNA viruses and that a variety of viral genetic systems had to be investigated. Huang and Baltimore realized the VSV was a more complex system than they had anticipated, but the discovery of a virion polymerase in VSV (vesicular stomatitus virus) led them to search for such enzymes in other viruses. It also suggested the exciting possibility that the search for the virion polymerase could shed light on the puzzle of RNA tumor virus replication.

Baltimore noted that Howard Temin's DNA provirus hypothesis was entirely logical and convincing in retrospect, but "in 1970 there were few advocates and many skeptics." Baltimore acknowledged having "enormous respect" for Temin since his high school days when Temin had been the "guru" of the summer school Baltimore attended at the Jackson Laboratory in Maine. Having no experience in the field and no strong prejudice concerning the central dogma, Baltimore decided to hedge his bets and "look for either an RNA or a DNA polymerase in virions of RNA tumor viruses" (Baltimore 1975, 499–500). Using Rauscher mouse leukemia virus, Baltimore demonstrated that the virions of Rauscher virus contained a ribonuclease-sensitive DNA polymerase activity.

Interestingly, within a few weeks of the announcements by Baltimore and Temin of the demonstration of reverse transcriptase, Sol Spiegelman, the director of Columbia University's Institute of Cancer Research and one of Temin's main critics, confirmed the existence of reverse transcription in his own laboratories in eight additional RNA cancer viruses. Francis Crick, one of the architects of the central dogma, soon published a paper in *Nature* showing that reverse transcription could be incorporated into central dogma.

Once scientists had accepted the concept of reverse transcription in the early 1970s, speculation about the relationship between viruses and cancer, and the implications for cancer cures tended towards excessive optimism. Research evolving from the discoveries of Temin and Baltimore suggests that the retroviruses are able to cause cancer because they have incorporated a DNA intermediate into their mechanism of replication. This makes it possible for a viral gene product to effect a permanent change in the growth properties of infected cells. However, Baltimore and Temin remained cautious in their comments on progress in cancer research. Explaining what guided his career, Baltimore said: "My life is dedicated to increasing knowledge. We need no more justification for scientific research than that. My motivating force is not that I will find a 'cure' for cancer. There may never be a cure as such. I work because I want to understand" (*Current Biography Yearbook*, 25).

In 1972 Baltimore and coworkers succeeded in the partial synthesis of a mammalian hemoglobin gene. Expressing his concern for the still uncertain potential of genetic engineering, Baltimore joined other eminent scientists calling for a thorough and cautious evaluation of further development of recombinant DNA techniques. The question of the possible biohazards of genetic research led to a proposal for a temporary ban on certain areas of recombinant DNA research and the famous Asilomar Conference on Recombinant DNA Molecules in May 1975. The possibility that recombinant DNA techniques would be used to produce more effective biological warfare agents and the sociological implications of genetic engineering in human beings were especially troubling to Baltimore. Within ten years, however, Baltimore and other scientists became convinced that the advantages of recombinant DNA research clearly outweighed the threats.

Other honors awarded to David Baltimore include the Gustav Stern Award in Virology (1970), the Warren Triennial Prize, Massachusetts General Hospital (1971), the Eli Lilly Award in Microbiology and Immunology (1971), the National Academy of Sciences' United States Steel Foundation Award in Molecular Biology (1974), and the Gairdner Foundation Annual Award (1974). Baltimore was elected a member of the National Academy of Science and the American Academy of Arts and Sciences in 1974; a member of the Pontifical Academy of Sciences in 1978; a fellow of the American Association for the Advancement of Science in 1980; an honorary fellow of the American Medical Writers Association in 1985;

and a foreign member of the Royal Society in 1987.

Baltimore has been a member of the editorial board of the *Journal of Molecular Biology* (1971–73), *Journal of Virology* (1969–), and *Science* (1986–). He has served on numerous advisory panels, including the National Science Foundation Advisory Panel for Genetic Biology (1969–72), Cancer Research Center Review Committees of the National Institutes of Health (1971–73), Public Issues Committee of the American Cancer Society (1978–81), NIH Recombinant DNA Advisory Committee (1979–82), International Board of Advisors of the Basel Institute for Immunology in Switzerland (1982–), and Scientific Advisory Committee, European Molecular Biology Laboratory, Heidelberg, Germany (1982–). In 1986 he became co-chair of the Committee on a National Strategy for AIDS, National Academy of Sciences and Institute of Medicine. He is also chairman of the scientific advisory boards of two biotechnology companies, Collaborative Research and Celgene.

Between 1962 and 1988 Baltimore has been the author or coauthor of 375 scientific publications. A multiauthored paper published in *Cell* in 1986 drew Baltimore into a bitter dispute over issues of possible scientific misconduct. However, after a lengthy official investigation, the National Institutes of Health found no evidence of "fraud, misconduct, manipulation of data, or serious conceptual errors" in the controversial paper (Culliton 1989). Baltimore felt that he had been vindicated by the NIH investigation, but some of his colleagues believe that congressional interest in the case was a reflection of the deliberate and vindictive pursuit of David Baltimore by Representative John Dingell (Davis 1989).

LOIS N. MAGNER

Selected Bibliography

PRIMARY SOURCES

Baltimore, D. 1970. "An RNA-Dependent DNA Polymerase in Virions of RNA Tumor Viruses." *Nature* 226: 1209–11.

Huang, A. S., and D. Baltimore. 1970. "Defective Viral Particles and Viral Disease Processes." *Nature* 226: 325–27.

Baltimore, D. 1972. "RNA-Directed DNA Synthesis and RNA Tumor Viruses." *Advances in Virus Research* 17:51–94.

———. 1976. "The Strategy of RNA Viruses." *Harvey Lectures*, series 70, 57–74. New York: Academic Press.

———. 1975. "Viruses, Polymerases and Cancer." *Nobel Lecture*, December 12, 1975. Reproduced in *Nobel Lectures in Molecular Biology 1933–1975*, 495–508. Amsterdam: Elsevier, 1977.

———. 1977. "Foreword" to *Nobel Lectures in Molecular Biology 1933–1975*. Amsterdam: Elsevier, 1977.

Weaver, D., M. H. Reis, C. Albanese, F. Costantini, D. Baltimore, and T. Imanishi-Kari. 1986. "Altered Repertoire of Endogenous Immunoglobulin Gene Expression in Transgenic Mice Containing a Rearranged Mu Heavy Chain Gene." *Cell* 45:247–59.

SECONDARY SOURCES

Gross, L. 1972. *Oncogenic Viruses.* New York: Pergamon Press.

Smith, K. M., M. A. Lauffer, and F. B. Bang, eds. 1972. *Advances in Virus Research.* Vol. 17. New York: Academic Press.

Tooze, J., ed. 1973. *The Molecular Biology of Tumor Viruses.* New York: Cold Spring Harbor Laboratory.

Eckhart, Walter. 1975. "The 1975 Nobel Prize for Physiology or Medicine." *Science* 190:650, 712–13.

Mahy, B. W. J., and R. D. Barry, eds. 1975. *Negative Strand Viruses.* Vol. 1. New York: Academic Press.

Grobstein, Clifford. 1979. *A Double Image of the Double Helix: The Recombinant-DNA Debate.* San Francisco: W. H. Freeman and Company.

Watson, James D., and John Tooze. 1981. *The DNA Story: A Documentary History of Gene Cloning.* San Francisco: W. H. Freeman and Company.

1983. *Current Biography Yearbook,* 25–28. New York: H. W. Wilson.

Culliton, Barbara J. 1989. "Baltimore Cleared of All Fraud Charges." *Science* 243:727.

Davis, Bernard D. 1989. "Why Auditing Laboratory Records Is a Bad Idea." *The Scientist* (February 20):9.

SIR FREDERICK GRANT BANTING *1923*

Sir Frederick Grant Banting was born November 4, 1891, in Alliston, Ontario, Canada. A surgeon and physiologist, Banting shared the Nobel Prize for 1923 with John James Rickard Macleod for his work in isolating and purifying the pancreatic substance that regulates blood sugar, making possible its identification as insulin. The work was carried out in Macleod's lab and under his sponsorship. At the time of the award, Banting had just been named professor of medical research at the University of Toronto and director of the Banting-Best Department of Medical Research. He was knighted in 1934. Banting's first marriage, to Marion Robertson, ended in divorce in 1932 after eight years; the couple had one son, William Robertson Banting. In 1939 he married Henrietta Ball. Banting died on February 21, 1941, in Newfoundland.

Banting's parents, William Thompson and Margaret Grant Banting, were Ontario farmers and devout Methodists. They wanted him to study for the ministry and he entered the University of Toronto in 1910 to pursue this goal. Very soon, however, he convinced his family to let him study medicine and he entered the medical school in 1912. He was interested in anatomy; work with C. L. Starr, chief surgeon of the Toronto Hospital for Sick Children, inspired his ambition to become an orthopedic surgeon.

Banting joined the Royal Canadian Army Medical Corps in 1915; the following year, after completing his bachelor's degree in medicine, he was commissioned a lieutenant. He served in England and in France during World War I and was awarded the Military Cross for exceptional bravery under fire at Cambrai in September of 1918 (Stevenson 1970, 440; Best 1959, 54).

After the war, Banting completed a year of training with Starr and then began an independent practice in London, Ontario. He had few patients and began lecturing in anatomy and physiology at Western University to keep busy and to supplement his income. The neurophysiologist F. R. Miller also enlisted him as a research assistant.

In late October 1920 Banting was preparing a lecture on the pancreas and came across an article by Moses Barron that discussed the results of ligation of the pancreatic ducts. Experiments with several animals had shown that ligation of this digestive organ led after several weeks to almost total atrophy, leaving intact only the small section called the islets of Langerhans Blockage of the ducts also resulted in the absence of glycosuria. These findings supported the theory that the pancreas, specifically the islets of Langerhans, secreted a hormone necessary for the normal metabolism of glucose by the body; and that diabetes mellitus, a disease characterized by inadequate glucose metabolism and consequent acidosis of blood and tissues, could therefore be traced to a malfunction or disorder of the pancreas.

Diabetes had been recognized as a discrete illness for centuries, but the process of glucose synthesis and metabolism was not understood until the work of Claude Bernard and others in the mid-nineteenth century. In 1889 Joseph von Mehring and Oscar Minkowski had demonstrated that the removal of the entire pancreas from dogs resulted in death, preceded by all the symptoms of severe diabetes. Minkowski and others had speculated that pancreatic extracts could be used to treat the illness, but an extract of the entire gland proved either ineffective or toxic. Several researchers had achieved partial success but no clinically useful preparation had been found.

Lydia de Witt in 1906 had isolated and extracted only the islet tissue; this substance proved to be glycolytic (sugar producing), rather than digestive. Her findings suggested that the digestive secretions of the gland, such as the enzyme trypsin, were its major products and the special sugar metabolism hormone was generated only by the islets. However, de Witt had not been able to adapt her extract to diabetes treatment. In 1920 the secretion of a sugar-metabolizing hormone by the islets of Langerhans or any other part of the pancreas was considered to be highly questionable by many authorities, including J. J. R. Macleod of the University of Toronto.

Banting was unaware of the many attempts that had been made; he quickly saw the potential of isolating the islets by ligation of the pancreatic ducts and then extracting only this tissue for diabetic treatment. He hypothesized that extractions of the whole gland had been unsuccessful because the process would release the digestive enzymes, which would effectively destroy the glycolytic tissues. Banting was an idealistic and passionate young man, and for the next year, the idea of a successful treatment for diabetes became the driving force of his life (Stevenson 1970, 440–41; Collip 1942, 401).

Miller referred Banting to J. J. R. Macleod as a possible sponsor for his projected research. Macleod was not initially enthusiastic but Banting persisted and was finally offered use of a laboratory for eight weeks, an undergraduate assistant, and ten dogs. With this meager support, Banting left his practice and returned to Toronto in April 1921.

The undergraduate assigned was Charles H. Best, who in fact had just received his B.A. in physiology and chemistry when he began work with Banting in May, and who had already done a number of metabolism experiments. They were later assisted by C. H. Noble, another recent graduate. Macleod gave the young men some assistance in planning and designing their project and then left for a summer in Scotland.

The first stage of the work was surgical: the ligation of the pancreatic ducts in one set of dogs and pancreatectomies in another set. There were many false starts and botched attempts. The initial ligations failed to result in the expected total atrophy and they had to operate again, this time applying several ligatures at different tensions. Pancreatectomy was attempted using the Hedon technique of removal in two stages but the available operating facilities were inadequate for this lengthy procedure. Banting therefore developed his own single-stage technique.

On July 27 the researchers finally had ready a dog with the necessary degree of pancreatic atrophy and another, depancreatized, animal, who was showing the symptoms of experimental diabetes. They prepared an extract of the remaining pancreatic tissue and injected it into the diabetic dog. Within two hours they observed a significant reduction in blood sugar and clinical improvement. By September, however, when Macleod returned, they had succeeded in developing an extract that would keep a diabetic animal alive indefinitely.

Banting and Best were elated but still faced the problem of developing a feasible method of hormone production for clinical use. It was hardly possible to sacrifice a gland-atrophied animal for every administration to a diabetic patient. They therefore spent the next several months searching for a method of obtaining a reliable supply of active "isletin."

Their strategies included stimulation of the pancreas to the point of exhaustion and extraction from whole fetal calf glands obtained from a local abattoir. The theory behind the latter was that the fetal gland might contain a higher proportion of islet and a lower proportion of digestive tissue than the mature pancreas. On November 17 Banting recorded the successful use of whole fetal gland "isletin." Some time passed before he and Best were able to find the right pH solution to repeat this result and still other possibilities were tested (Stevenson 1970, 441–42; Bliss 1982, 91–92).

Neither Banting nor Best had received any stipend during the summer of 1921. When they needed more dogs, they paid for the animals themselves and Banting had to sell his car in order to continue operations. He was very attached to his animals and determined that no dog be subjected to prolonged unnecessary suffering (Best 1942, 400).

Upon his return, Macleod arranged a formal appointment for Banting in the department of pharmacology. He put his own research on hold and concentrated his attention on the further purification of "isletin." At Banting's request, he enlisted James B. Collip, a young biochemist who had come to his department the previous spring. In January of 1922 Collip developed a fractional precipitation method that produced a whole gland extract pure enough for use with human patients. Macleod also suggested the name "insulin," which was used in the formal reports of the discovery.

Banting and Best first presented their research at the Physiological Journal Club of the University of Toronto in November. The following month they made a joint report with Macleod to a meeting of the American Physiological Society, of which he was the president-elect (Stevenson 1970, 442; Collip 1942, 401; Best 1959, 54).

On January 23, 1922 the first clinical trial of Collip's extract was made on a fourteen-year-old boy in Toronto General Hospital, who improved rapidly on daily doses. Throughout that year, the two problems of commercial production and clinical guidelines were pursued simultaneously. Banting did some of the work on dosage determination. But he was neither a chemist nor a practiced clinician and was compelled to allow others to carry out most of these studies. Many researchers throughout the United States and Canada participated.

He had assigned his patent rights to the University of Toronto and the National Research Council of Canada. Collip's and Best's initial work was refined by themselves, Noble, E. L. Scott, J. Hepburn, and others in the university's Connaught Laboratories. An insulin product sufficiently concentrated to be mass-produced for clinical use was developed by the Eli Lilly Company and made commercially available by January 1923. Subsequent refinements were made by J. J. Abel of Baltimore, D. A. Scott of Toronto, and H. C. Hagedorn of Denmark.

The clinical research on insulin was begun in Toronto by W. R. Campbell and A. A. Fletcher. Banting and Best had noted in their work with dogs that a large dose of the hormone resulted in hypoglycemia, which could subsequently be readjusted by glucose injections. Building on the studies of Frederick M. Allen, Campbell, Fletcher, and others soon determined that insulin was most effectively used in combination with diet therapy and careful monitoring of blood sugar levels, the approach still in use (Stevenson 1970, 442–43; Best 1942, 399).

It was Banting, however, who was the hero of Canada. In 1922 he submitted a thesis on his work to the department of medicine for his M.D. He was awarded both the Starr Gold Medal for the thesis and the George Armstrong Peters Prize in Surgical Science. The Banting and Best Department of Medical Research was created by the Ontario provincial legislature the following year. Banting was appointed its head and received the university's Charles Mickle Fellowship; the Canadian Parliament granted him an annuity of $7,500 for life.

He was an international figure as well, but the role of others in the discovery was not clearly understood, a fact made clear when the 1923 Nobel Prize was awarded jointly to Banting and to Macleod but not to Best. Banting initially wanted to refuse the prize but was finally convinced to accept it and to divide his share with Best. Macleod gave part of his award to Collip (Stevenson 1970, 443; Best 1959, 54).

This impulsive quixoticism was characteristic of Frederick Banting, as was his determined pursuit of the problem of insulin without any financial or career prospects. He was idealistic, proud, generous, stubborn, and heedless of risk: a heroic figure who, unlike many, was early rewarded for his quest. These qualities served him well as director of a research department in which he described himself as "a catalyst which accelerates a reaction without taking part in it." He consistently encouraged and assisted his staff in their work and refused to accept credit or acknowledgment; as a member of the National Research Council, he determinedly maintained government support for medical research. In return, he was idolized by his associates and by Canadians in general.

Banting's own research interests included cancer, coronary thrombosis, adrenal deficiency, silicosis, and, particularly during World War II, aviation medicine. His experiments with the adrenal cortex attempted to replicate his success with insulin; he removed the gland from animals and then attempted treatment with an extract. These attempts were not successful but did contribute to the field. He became interested in silicosis in 1928, particularly in the possibility that another "antidotal" mineral dust might be added to the atmosphere in mines to offset the toxic effects of silica dust, but encouraged others to take on the actual experiments. For most of the thirties, he concentrated on cancer.

His wide range of scientific interests was complemented by his leisuretime pursuits of painting, sketching, and reading Canadian history. He was a member of the Royal Society of London (1935). Among the many other honors he received were the John Scott Medal of the American Philosophical Society (1924), the Flavelle Medal of the Royal Society of Canada (1931), and the F. N. G. Starr Gold Medal of the Canadian Medical Association (1936). The Banting Institute (1930), the Banting Research Foundation, and the Banting Memorial Lectureship were also established in his honor.

In 1939, with the outbreak of war, he became chairman of the Medical Research Committee of the National Research Council and also of the Aviation Medical Research Committee. The Banting Institute directed a major part of its resources to this field. Banting encouraged research throughout Canada and, heedless of risk as usual, flew to England in 1940 to establish a liaison with British investigators. It was on a second trip in 1941 that he was killed in a crash landing in Newfoundland (Stevenson 1970, 443; Best 1959, 54–55; Collip 1942, 401–3; Irwin 1942, 403–5).

MARCIA MELDRUM

Selected Bibliography

PRIMARY SOURCES

Banting, Frederick G., and C. H. Best. 1922. "Internal Secretion of Pancreas." *Journal of Laboratory and Clinical Medicine* 7 (February): 251–326.

Banting, Frederick G., C. H. Best, J. B. Collip, W. R. Campbell, and A. A. Fletcher. 1922. "Pancreatic Aspects in Diabetes." *Journal of the Canadian Medical Association* 12 (March):141–46.

Banting, Frederick G. 1922. "Effect of Pancreatic Extract (Insulin) on Normal Rabbits." *American Journal of Physiology* 62 (September): 162–76.

Banting, Frederick G., W. R. Campbell, and A. A. Fletcher. 1922. "Insulin in Treatment of Diabetes Mellitus." *Journal of Metabolic Research* 2 (November–December):547–604.

SECONDARY SOURCES

Best, C. H. 1942. "Reminiscences of the Researches Which Led to the Discovery of Insulin." *Canadian Medical Association Journal* 47 (November):398–400.

Collip, J. B. 1942. "Recollections of Sir Frederick Banting." *Canadian Medical Association Journal* 47 (November):401–3.

Irwin, D. 1942. "The Contributions of Sir Frederick Banting to Silicosis Research." *Canadian Medical Association Journal* 47 (November): 403–5.

Harris, Seale. 1946. *Banting's Miracle: The Story of the Discoverer of Insulin.* Philadelphia: Lippincott.

Stevenson, Lloyd G. 1946. *Sir Frederick Banting.* Toronto: Ryerson Press.

Best, C. H. 1959. "Sir Frederick Grant Banting." In *Dictionary of National Biography, 1941–1950*, 53–55. London: Oxford University Press.

Stevenson, Lloyd G. 1970. "Frederick Grant Banting." In *Dictionary of Scientific Biography*, 1:440–43. New York: Scribner's.

Bliss, Michael. 1982. *The Discovery of Insulin.* Chicago: University of Chicago Press.

ROBERT BÁRÁNY 1914

Robert Bárány was born on April 22, 1876, in Vienna. An otorhinolaryngologist, Bárány received the Nobel Prize in 1914 for his development of the clinical investigation of the human equilibrium system based in the vestibular apparatus of the ear; he essentially founded a new area of medical science and practice. His Swedish colleague, Gunnar Holmgren, described him as a "pathbreaker, who brought an array of known but seemingly contradictory facts together under a unitary viewpoint." At the time of his award, which was delayed until 1915 by the outbreak of World War I, he was a Russian prisoner of war. The Swedish Red Cross arranged for his release and emigration to Sweden, where he became director of the otorhinolaryngology clinic at the University of Uppsala in 1917. Bárány married Ida Berger in 1909. His three children all studied medicine: Ernst became professor of pharmacology at Uppsala; Franz taught medicine in Stockholm; the youngest, Ingrid, became a psychiatrist and eventually settled in the United States. Bárány died on April 8, 1936, in Uppsala, Sweden.

Bárány was of Hungarian Jewish descent, the son of a bank official, Ignaz Bárány, and the former Marie Hock. After receiving his medical degree from the University of Vienna in 1900, he undertook further training in internal medicine in Frankfurt under Carl von Noorden, in neurology with Emil Kraepelin in Heidelberg and Freiburg, and in surgery at the Vienna General Hospital, where he worked under Carl Gussenbauer. In October 1903 he accepted an appointment at the University of Vienna otology clinic, working under Adam Politzer, who had established this specialty in Austria. Here he began his studies of the equilibrium system of the ear and the brain (Nylen 1965, 316, 318–19; Majer 1970, 446).

The organ, or system, of equilibrium, the vestibular apparatus, consisting of three semicircular membranes within bony canals lying at right angles to each other, and filled with fluid (the endolymph), is situated within the inner ear. Various researchers, notably Pierre Flourens, had studied the system in pigeons and rabbits, and the French scientist Menière had connected it to vertigo and other equilibrium disorders. Josef Breuer had repeated Florens's work and concluded that the vestibular apparatus worked like a sense organ, reacting to rotary sensations; he believed that vertigo set in as a result of overstimulation.

In 1907 Bárány delivered a paper at the Convention of German Natural Scientists and Physicians in which he criticized existing theories of vestibular functions, singling out those of Breuer. He contended that these models clarified little for the practitioner faced with the range of clinical symptoms associated with vertigo and equilibrium disturbances. There was no functional examination for the vestibular apparatus, as there were for other sense organs. The functional tests devised by Breuer stimulated both aural canals simultaneously and thus were not useful in most clinical situations, where the demand was usually for an examination of one side only.

In the Vienna clinic, the young physician heard complaints of dizziness from his patients after he had flushed their ears with water. He examined their eyes during these spells and observed a marked spasmodic rolling of the eyeballs called nystagmus. One patient complained that the water was not warm enough and he therefore tried flushing with hot water. The patient again complained of dizziness. Examining the eyes, Bárány again saw the nystagmic reaction but in the opposite direction. From these observations he deduced that both the dizziness and the eye spasms were the result of the temperature change within the ear when the water was injected. Water at normal body temperature would have no ill effects. Moreover, people with healthy ears would have the same reactions as the clinic patients. Bárány easily verified these hypotheses.

His theory of caloric nystagmus demonstrated that the endolymph, normally at body temperature, displaced itself when it came into contact with water at another temperature, the colder fluid sinking within the system, while the warmer replaced it. The internal balance was "rocked" by the displacement as if afloat. Bárány showed further that the nystagmic reaction permitted the diagnosis of the location and extent of inner ear damage with the simple flushing technique. In patients with ears impaired by trauma or surgery, the nystagmus appeared after some delay, or not at all.

He then applied his new knowledge in the light of earlier studies by Ramón y Cajal, which had demonstrated that the vestibular nerve branches off in many directions upon entering the brain. Bárány's work led him to the conclusion that the vestibular nerve transmitted the thermal disturbance within the endolymph to the brain, where it was carried to the centers controlling the brain's "sense" of balance, the eye muscles, and the skeletal musculature.

His work led to the development of clinical techniques that remained valuable for many years, including the Bárány rotating chair and the noise apparatus. Of more lasting importance was his demonstration of the relationship between the vestibular system, the nervous system, and localized centers within the cerebellum. His clinical pointing test proved valuable for the diagnosis of cerebellar disturbances. In this simple procedure the patient closes both eyes and extends the forefinger to touch the physician's finger, then the patient drops the finger to the knee and repeats the movement. A normal person succeeds at this test very quickly, while a patient with a horizontal nystagmus will consistently miss the mark by falling wide in the opposite direction of the nystagmus. Bárány used this procedure in conjunction with other neurological tests to localize in the cortex deviations of sidelong or up-and-down directional motions.

Bárány's account of his findings, in the *Monatschrift für Ohrenheilkunde* in 1906, integrated them into a thoughtful synthesis of the earlier work of Menière, Flourens, Breuer, Cajal, Louis Bolk, Julius Ewald, and Ernst Mach. His theoretical and technical contributions made possible the differentiation between equilibrium disorders resulting from otic disease and those arising in the nervous system, and led to the development of the field of otoneurology (Nylen 1965, 316; Majer 1970; Bárány 1906).

When Austria entered World War I, Bárány, like many other neurologists, saw an opportunity to investigate his ideas with brain-injured soldiers. He volunteered for the medical service and was assigned to the fortress of Przemysl in Galicia, to provide care for 123,000 men. Here he built an otolaryngology service from nothing, with the assistance of his wife, who sent equipment from Vienna. He also developed a highly successful primary suture technique for the treatment of head wounds.

Przemysl was occupied by the Russians in April 1915; Bárány was taken prisoner and transported to a prison camp in Turkestan. Although he contracted malaria in the camp, his medical services to guards, prisoners, and Russian civilians alike quickly won him respect and generous treatment. After the announcement of the Nobel Prize, Bárány was moved to the university city of Kazan. Here the Grand Duke Konstantin Konstantinovich, president of the Russian Academy of Sciences, took up his case, and negotiated his release with the Red Cross and Prince Carl of Sweden. He arrived in his new country in July 1916. His family joined him and he accepted a post at the University of Uppsala clinic, with the title of assistant professor, the following year.

Bárány missed Vienna, particularly the musical culture of the city. However, shortly after the Nobel announcement, when he had been nominated for a professorship there, members of the Vienna medical faculty had slandered his reputation, accusing him of taking credit for the work of others and publishing it as his own. In 1917 a formal investigation was initiated at Bárány's request, who spent five years seeking exoneration through his lawyer; the case dragged on until 1922, when the authorities decided it was pointless to continue in his absence. He had meanwhile been vindicated in 1921 by the editors of the *Acta Oto-Laryngologica*, who undertook a thorough investigation of the charges. But he refused to return to Austria and became a Swedish citizen (Nylen 1965, 316–17).

He returned to his research, publishing further studies on nystagmus, and developing new operations for otosclerosis and chronic frontal sinusitis. In 1925 he received the Jubilee Medal from the Royal Swedish Society of Medicine for these new contributions, and in 1926 he was promoted to full professor. He remained active until his death from cerebral hemorrhage at the age of sixty.

Bárány was a quiet, gentle man, dedicated to his work and family, but he could be arrogant and impatient when angered. A patient teacher and loyal friend, he had little interest in social interaction. Although he suffered from ankylosis of the knee, he kept active, playing tennis and hiking in the mountains, most of his life. He was a competent pianist and devoted to music.

At his death, the University of Uppsala established the Bárány Medal, to be awarded at five-year intervals to the most outstanding scientist in the field of vestibular research. The Bárány Society was founded in his honor by C. S. Hallpike and Carl O. Nylen in 1960. Among the other honors Bárány himself received were the Politzer Prize (1912), the Belgian Academy of Sciences Prize (1913), the ERB Medal of the German Neurological Society (1913), and the Guyot Prize (1914). He was decorated with the Order of the Northern Star in 1927 (Nylen 1965).

ROBERT BRAIN
MARCIA MELDRUM

Selected Bibliography

PRIMARY SOURCES

Bárány, Robert. 1906. *Untersuchungen über den Vestibular-Apparat des Ohres.* Berlin: O. Coblentz.

———. 1907. *Physiologie und Pathologie des Bogengang-Apparatus beim Menschen.* Leipzig: F. Deuticke.

Bárány, Robert, and K. Witmaack. 1911. *Funktionelle Prüfung des Vestibular-Apparatus.* Germany: G. Fischer.

Bárány, Robert. 1915. "Primäre Wundnaht bei Schlussverletzungen, speziell des Gehirns." *Wiener Klinische Wochenschrift* 28:525.

———. 1923. *Die Radikaloperation des Ohres ohne Gehoergangsplastik.* Leipzig: F. Deutike.

SECONDARY SOURCES

Wodak, Ernst. 1927. *Der Báránysche Zeigeversuch.* Berlin: Urban and Schwarzenberg.

Nylen, Carl O. 1965. "Robert Bárány." *Archives of Otolaryngology* 82 (September):316–19.

Majer, E. H. 1970. "Bárány, Robert." In *Dictionary of Scientific Biography* 1:446–47. New York: Scribners.

Wylicky, H. 1986. "Über Bárány's Entdeckung und deren Aufnahme durch die Zeitgenossen." *Wiener Klinische Wochenschrift* 98:622–25.

GEORGE WELLS BEADLE *1958*

George Wells Beadle was born on October 22, 1903, in Wahoo, Nebraska. He was a recipient of half the Nobel Prize in Physiology or Medicine in 1958 with Edward L. Tatum for their work establishing the "one gene-one enzyme" theory that genes regulate cellular processes chemically. The other half was awarded to Joshua Lederberg. Beadle married Marion Cecil Hill on August 22, 1928; they had one son. Divorced in 1953, Beadle married Murial McClure Burnett on August 12 that same year.

George Beadle was the second of three children born to Chauncey Elmer and Hattie Albro Beadle. The Beadles owned and worked a small mixed farm. Hattie Beadle died when George was four, and he was raised by a series of housekeepers. A high school teacher convinced George Beadle to pursue higher education, and he graduated from the College of Agriculture of the University of Nebraska with a B.Sc. in 1926 and an M.Sc. the following year. F. D. Keim, professor of agronomy at Nebraska, introduced him to his love of genetics, and urged him to pursue graduate work at Cornell.

It was perhaps inevitable that on moving to Cornell in 1927 the young man would soon elect to study genetics and cytology under the supervision of Rollins A. Emerson, head of the department of plant breeding at Cornell, one of the earliest supporters of Mendelian genetics in the United States, and the leading maize geneticist in the United States by the 1920s. Emerson led his students with a robust informality and generosity of spirit that caused George Beadle to write of him later as "perfect employer, graduate advisor, and friend" (Beadle 1974, 3). The farm boy from Nebraska took part in Cornell's "golden age" of maize genetics, and he would look back on his years at Cornell—1927–1931—with considerable affection. He and such other future eminent American geneticists as Barbara McClintock, Marcus Rhoades, and George Sprague did their earliest work on the genetics of maize there, as graduate students of Emerson and the cytologist Lester W. Sharp.

After graduating from Cornell in 1931, George Beadle enjoyed an increasingly distinguished career, first in scientific research and, subsequently, in educational administration. Between 1931 and 1933 he held a National Research Council fellowship, which he used to study at the California Institute of Technology in the laboratory of T. H. Morgan, the leading geneticist in the United States. He stayed on as an instructor at Caltech for a further two years, and then spent a year doing research in Paris. In 1936 he was appointed assistant professor of genetics at Harvard University, and the following year moved to Stanford as professor of biology. When T. H. Morgan died in 1945, George Beadle replaced him as professor of biology and chairman of the Division of Biology at Caltech.

On moving to Caltech in 1931, George Beadle's attention had soon turned from corn to flies. T. H. Morgan won the Nobel Prize in Physiology or Medicine in 1933 for work done at Columbia, from 1910 to 1915, on the genetics of the *Drosophila melanogaster*, or fruit fly, which had given genetics its scientific foundation. However, by the early thirties *Drosophila* genetics had reached an intellectual plateau, locked into a self-defining "classical" concept of the gene. H. J. Muller had shown the particulate nature of the gene when he had achieved artificial mutations by irradiation in 1927. Yet the English biologist J. B. S. Haldane was among a minority who believed the gene must be explained in biochemical terms, and although by the twenties and thirties considerable work had been done on the genetics of plant and animal pigmentation, there was widespread reluctance to draw conclusions about either the physical properties of the gene or direct gene action (Sturtevant 1965, 100).

The Division of Biology at Caltech, which Morgan had created in 1926, had been designed to help break down disciplinary barriers that kept *Drosophila* genetics thus confined. During the thirties it was host to domestic and international scientists from all disciplines, funded for one or two years by the National Research Council and the Rockefeller Foundation, who were interested in learning more about *Drosophila* genetics. When, therefore, Beadle, now trained in *Drosophila* genetics, and Boris Ephrussi, an embryologist from Paris trained in tissue culture and tissue transplantation, expressed interest in a collaborative effort into a genetic explanation of development, or gene expression, Morgan made it possible for Beadle to return with Ephrussi to Paris. There they devised a difficult biochemical experiment transplanting embryonic *Drosophila* tissue, from which they concluded that the trait for eye color was controlled by a combination of separate genes controlling separate substances.

On his return to America in 1937 Beadle recruited Edward L. Tatum, a microbiologist and biochemist trained in the nutritional needs of bacteria, from the University of Wisconsin. For the next three years they worked on identifying the substances responsible for eye color trait in *Drosophila*, but eventually Beadle decided to attack the problem from another angle. Instead of trying to identify unknown substances, he realized it would be much easier to prove that known substances produced specific traits. Speculating that the development of a trait was orchestrated by enzymes, he designed experiments to isolate individual enzyme deficiencies. He chose *Neurospora*, or common bread mould, rather than *Drosophila*, because it grew faster, and had a more versatile genetic mechanism: it could reproduce both asexually and sexually. It also had a highly sophisticated nutritional mechanism, having enzyme systems that enable it to synthesize for itself most of the amino acids and vitamins needed for growth.

Irradiation would, and did, produce a large variety of nutritional mutants. From these Beadle and Tatum isolated mutants with particular amino acid and vitamin deficiencies. A mutant that grew on a medium supplemented with vitamin B_6 was shown to inherit in Mendelian sequence, and sequences in which amino acid deficiencies occurred enabled them to identify them as steps in metabolic pathways. They thus proposed the "one gene-one enzyme" theory, that genes regulate the function of enzymes catalyzing steps in metabolic pathways.

Initial scientific reaction was hostile; supporters in 1951 "could be counted on the fingers of one hand," Beadle recalled (Beadle 1966, 30). Critics quickly pointed out that technically the idea was not original—thirty-three years earlier Archibald Garrod, an English physician, had proposed that genes controlled the function of enzymes. Nor did the theory prove to be entirely accurate: a gene controls not an enzyme but one polypeptide in a protein molecule (Horowitz, 1979). However, the more fundamental point, that genes direct chemical processes, was correct. Beadle and Tatum's work, followed in 1944 by the demonstration by O. T. Avery and associates that genes are made of DNA, provided a bridge across that intellectual divide between classical genetics, which used "gene" as a concept without entering into its physical nature, and a new biology that was to concentrate on biochemical reactions and molecular structure.

In the postwar era Beadle made a considerable contribution to the administration of public health. He was chairman of the Committee on the Genetic Effects of Atomic Radiation of the National Academy of Sciences, and chairman of the Scientific Advisory Council of the American Cancer Society. In 1956–57 he was president of the American Association for the Advancement of Science. He left Caltech in 1961 to become professor of biology and president of the University of Chicago. He retired from administration in 1968, but continued his own research and served as trustee at both Caltech and Chicago. He is a member of the National Academy of Sciences, the American Academy of Arts and Sciences, and numerous foreign scientific societies, including the Royal Society. Other scientific honors he has won include the Lasker Award of the American Public Health Association (1950); the National Award of the American Cancer Society (1959); and the Kimber Genetics Award of the National Academy of Sciences (1960).

ROSALIE STOTT

Selected Bibliography

PRIMARY SOURCES

Beadle, G. W., and A. H. Sturtevant. 1939. *Introduction to Genetics.* Philadelphia: Saunders.

Beadle, G. W., and E. L. Tatum. 1941. "Genetic Control of Biochemical Reactions in Neurospora." *Proceedings of the National Academy of Science* 27:499–506. Reprinted in *Classic Papers in Genetics*, edited by James A. Peters, 166–73. Englewood Cliffs, N.J.: Prentice-Hall, 1959.

Beadle, G. W. 1945. "Biochemical Genetics." *The Chemical Review* 37: 15–96.

———. 1958. "Genes and Chemical Reactions in *Neurospora*." Nobel Lecture. Reprinted in *Nobel Lectures in Molecular Biology 1933–1974*. New York: Elsevier, 1977.

———. 1963. *Genetics and Modern Biology*. Philadelphia: American Philosophical Society.

———. 1966. "Biochemical Genetics: Some Recollections." In *Phage and the Origins of Molecular Biology*, edited by J. Cairns, G. Stent, and J. Watson, 23–32. New York: Cold Spring Harbor Laboratory of Quantitative Biology.

Beadle, G. W., and Muriel Beadle. 1966. *The Language of Life*. Garden City, NY: Doubleday.

Beadle, G. W. 1974. "Recollections." *Annual Review of Biochemistry* 43: 1–13.

SECONDARY SOURCES

Sturtevant, A. H. 1965. *A History of Genetics*. New York: Harper and Row.

Carlson, Elof A. 1966. *The Gene: A Critical History*. Philadelphia: W. B. Saunders.

Caspari, Ernest. 1968. "Haldane's Place in the Growth of Biochemical Genetics." In *Haldane and Modern Biology*, edited by K. R. Dronamraju, 43–50. Baltimore: Johns Hopkins University Press.

Olby, Robert O. 1974. *The Path to the Double Helix*. Seattle: University of Washington Press.

Portugal, F. H., and J. S. Cohen. 1977. *A Century of DNA*. Cambridge, Mass.: The MIT Press.

Horowitz, N. H. 1989. "Genetics and the Synthesis of Proteins." *Annals of the New York Academy of Science*, 253–66.

EMIL ADOLF VON BEHRING
1901

Emil Adolf von Behring was born March 15, 1854, in Hansdorf, Germany. A bacteriologist, von Behring won the first Nobel Prize for Physiology or Medicine in 1901 for his development of the techniques of serum therapy, which had been successfully applied against diphtheria and tetanus, and was to become a major tool in the new field of clinical immunology. Von Behring's therapeutic achievement was not accompanied by a theoretical advance. He completely misunderstood the mechanisms that made serum treatments effective. Although his idea of a specific therapy for every disease was long accepted, it was as much an obstacle to as a stimulus for later research discoveries. At the time of the award, von Behring was professor of hygiene at Marburg, the position he would hold until his death. In 1896 he had married Else Spinola, the eighteen-year-old daughter of the director of Berlin's Charité Hospital; they had six sons and one daughter. Von Behring died on March 31, 1917, in Marburg, Germany.

Von Behring's father, August Georg Behring (the "von" came later), taught school in Hansdorf, a remote village in West Prussia. He was a widower with four children when he married Augustine Zech; Emil was the oldest of nine children born to this second marriage. The family originally planned for him to study theology but could not afford to pay for his university education. In 1874, therefore, he entered the military medical college, the Friedrich Wilhelm Institute in Berlin, where he studied medicine on the condition that he spend several years in the army medical corps.

The institute gave priority to the study of scientific methods and of hygiene; young von Behring's interests were directed to the prevention of disease. His imagination was fired by the pioneering discoveries of Louis Pasteur and Robert Koch in bacteriology. He earned his medical degree in 1878, and passed the state medical examination in 1880. Following a year's internship at the Charité, he was assigned to duty in Poland, at Wohlau and Posen, in 1881.

Von Behring was much occupied with his clinical duties but arranged to carry out research work at the Chemical Department of the Army Experimental Station in Posen. Here, in 1881–83, he studied the problem of septicemia and experimented with Iodoform as a disinfectant. He concluded that this compound did not kill bacteria but rather neutralized their toxic effects; that is, it was an antitoxin. His findings were first published in 1882.

Von Behring was also much interested in philosophy and particularly impressed by the positivist thought of Eduard von Hartmann. He also read Nietzsche and Schopenhauer. These studies, as well as his medical research, imbued the young officer with a sense of the power of Nature and of the heroic force of the individual scientist.

Von Behring's superiors recognized his intellectual capacity and abilities and, in 1887, ordered him to study with Binz at the Pharmacological Institute at the University of Bonn. Here he improved his experimental skills and his understanding of organic chemistry and aniline dyes. In 1888 he was recalled to Berlin and seconded to Robert Koch at the Institute of Hygiene. This posting completely suited von Behring's own interests and ambitions. He remained Koch's assistant for six years, accompanying him to the new Institute for Infectious Diseases in 1891. His prizewinning work with serum therapy was carried out during this happy and productive period.

Following Koch's discovery of the tubercle bacillus, scientists began searching for similar microbial culprits in other major diseases. Edwin Klebs and Friedrich Loeffler had isolated the diphtheria bacillus in 1883–84. In 1887 Emile Roux and Alexandre Yersin at the Institut Pasteur were able to infect animals with diphtheria, using filtrated cultures, from which the bacillus itself had been eliminated. Their results appeared to indicate that the bacillus acted by releasing a poison, or toxin, into the body. In 1890 Brieger and Fraenkel had been able to immunize guinea pigs against diphtheria with injections of toxalbumin, prepared from cultures of the bacillus.

Von Behring experimented initially with iodine trichloride and zinc chloride as potential treatments for diphtheria and tetanus infections. By 1898, however, he had begun experimenting with the creation of artificial immunity. Working with Koch's Japanese student, Shibasaburo Kitasato, he injected guinea pigs with a series of graduated doses of diphtheria cultures that had been treated with disinfectants. The team drew blood from the animals and then prepared serum injections for a second group of guinea pigs. They next infected this second group with live diphtheria bacilli. Not only did these animals remain healthy, but guinea pigs that had been infected and were already showing symptoms could be cured by injections of the serum preparation. Von Behring and Kitasato then conducted a further series of serum therapy experiments with tetanus cultures and rabbits, with identical results.

Their discoveries were announced in two papers appearing in *Deutsche Medizinische Wochenschrift* in December 1890. Von Behring's theory attributed the immunizing effects to "the capacity of the blood to render harmless the poisonous substances," which he identified as a quality or power of the *serum* itself, rather than as a result of any action of the blood cells from which the serum had been derived. In a footnote, he proposed the term "antitoxisch," in analogy to "antiseptisch." This suggestion also carried the idea of a humoral pathology of natural adjustment, rather than the interaction of specific substances (Behring and Kitasato 1890).

Much work remained to be done if serum antitoxin was to be used in medical practice. Koch was preoccupied with the outbreak of cholera in Hamburg and not much impressed with von Behring's research. However, Paul Ehrlich offered to collaborate and deserves the credit for developing the laboratory compounds into an effective clinical preparation and determining the appropriate dosages. The first patient was a child treated on Christmas night, 1891. In the following year the death rate from diphtheria in the Berlin children's hospitals dropped dramatically from 48 percent to 13 percent. Roux in Paris pioneered large-scale production of serum from horses. Serum therapy for both diphtheria and tetanus was soon in worldwide use.

In 1893 von Behring published a volume of his collected papers on disinfection and serum therapy. In the introduction, "The Etiological Therapy against Infectious Diseases," he vigorously defended his "antitoxin curative method." He criticized the rationalism of Virchow's cellular pathology, proposing instead the concept of a specific vaccine or therapy, a "magic bullet," for each disease, to be discovered by the heroic scientific warriors. Science, in von Behring's philosophy, was an exciting quest, rather than a methodical discipline. He also attacked liberal reform ideas about social medicine (Behring 1893). Von Behring's humoral theory of immunity was soon directly challenged by Élie Metchinkoff's discovery of the role of the white blood cells, the "phagocytes," in defending the body against disease. Von Behring had many supporters and a protracted controversy followed.

Koch was no longer one of those supporters and it became necessary for von Behring to establish an independent laboratory. In 1894 he left the army and, with the support of the Prussian government, gained an appointment as professor of hygiene at the University of Halle. He proved a mediocre teacher, and was transferred to the University of Marburg within a year, despite the opposition of the medical faculty there.

Von Behring now turned his attention to the problem of tuberculosis. He made a major contribution by insisting on the identity of bovine and human tuberculosis, thus making clear the dangers of milk from infected cows. He also developed a widely used "bovovaccine," as well as the human vaccine, "Tulase," an extract from tubercle bacilli treated with chloral hydrate; the latter was unsuccessful.

Von Behring was awarded the Nobel Prize and elevated to the Prussian nobility in the same year, 1901. His health had begun to deteriorate and he lectured only rarely after that, devoting himself instead to research. He bought shares in a commercial pharmaceutical firm, which built and equipped a new laboratory for him in Marburg. In 1913, following up on work he had first attempted in 1898, von Behring introduced an active human vaccine of diphtheria toxin neutralized by antitoxin. The following year he founded the Behringwerke in Marburg for research and production of vaccines and sera. His toxin-antitoxin mixture was the vaccine of choice for diphtheria until the introduction of toxoid in 1924.

Von Behring ended his life financially successful and renowned. He owned a large estate in Marburg, stocked with cattle, which he used for experiments. Among the many other honors he received for his work were the Legion of Honor (1895), the Paris Académie de Médicine Prize (1895), and honorary memberships in the scientific societies of France, Italy, Turkey, Hungary, and Russia. He was elected to the Prussian Privy Council in 1903 and made an honorary freeman of Marburg.

Von Behring died in 1917 at age sixty-three. Although many of his ideas are now obsolete or disproved, he remains one of the founders of immunology and a great benefactor of the world's children, who can be easily protected against diphtheria and tetanus with a simple injection.

PAUL WEINDLING

Selected Bibliography

PRIMARY SOURCES

Behring, Emil A., and S. Kitasato. 1890. "Über das Zustandekommen der Diphtherie-Immunität und der Tetanus-Immunität bei Thieren." *Deutsche Medizinische Wochenschrift* 16:113–14.

Behring, Emil A. 1893. *Gesammelte Abhandlungen zur Ätiologischen Therapie von Ansteckenden Krankheiten.* Leipzig: Thieme.

Von Behring, Emil A. 1915. *Gesammelte Abhandlungen. Neue Folge.* Bonn: Marcus and Webers. This volume and the one above contain the bulk of Behring's published papers.

SECONDARY SOURCES

Zeiss, Heinz, and R. Bieling. 1940. *Behring. Gestalt und Werk.* Berlin: Bruno Schultz.

Unger, Hellmuth. 1948. *Emil von Behring, Sein Lebenswerk als Vovergangliches Erbe.* Hamburg: Hoffman und Campe.

Macnalty, A. S. 1954. "Emil von Behring." *British Medical Journal* 1: 668–70.

Schadewaldt, H. 1970. "Von Behring, Emil Adolf." In *Dictionary of Scientific Biography,* 1:574–78. New York: Scribners.

GEORG VON BÉKÉSY *1961*

Georg von Békésy was born on June 3, 1899, in Budapest, to Alexander and Paula von Békésy. A solitary yet amiable man devoted to the study and collection of art, Georg von Békésy maintained broad scientific interests. A physicist by training and temperament, he achieved distinction primarily for his work on physiological optics and on the role of inhibitory interactions in sensory processes. In 1961 he was awarded the Nobel Prize in Physiology or Medicine "for his discoveries concerning the physical mechanism of stimulation within the cochlea." Békésy never married; he died on June 13, 1972 in Honolulu.

Georg von Békésy was the scion of an old and distinguished Hungarian family. His father, Alexander von Békésy, was a diplomat who served in many different posts. Georg von Békésy spent his childhood in Budapest, Munich, and Constantinople. In each of these cities, the Békésy family moved among artistic and intellectual circles. Thus, the young Georg became acquainted with many painters, sculptors, musicians, and writers, who were frequent guests in the family home. No doubt because of these formative experiences, Békésy rigorously pursued the study of art and archaeology throughout his life, believing that a developed capacity to evaluate aesthetic works often carries over into the practice of evaluating scientific works.

Békésy completed his baccalaureate in chemistry at Berne, Switzerland in 1916. After World War I, he returned to Hungary with a patriotic desire to help rebuild his country. After a short military service, he resumed his studies, and in 1923 he received his doctorate in physics from the University of Budapest. His doctoral research was in a branch of optics now known as interference microscopy. Békésy tried to find a position in the field of optics, but during the depression of the post-war years this proved impossible. Instead, Békésy entered the services of the Hungarian Post and Telegraph, which maintained the only laboratory in Hungary that remained well equipped after the war. Békésy worked with the Hungarian Post Office until 1946, with the exception of one year (1926–27) which he spent at the Central Laboratory of Siemens and Halske A. G. in Berlin. In 1932 Békésy was appointed privat-dozent at the University of Budapest, and in 1940 he was elevated to professor of experimental physics. Amid the foreign occupation of Hungary after World War II, Békésy accepted an invitation to work with Yngve Zotterman at the Karolinska Institut in Stockholm. A year later he came to the United States and joined the faculty at Harvard University, where in 1949 he was given a special appointment as senior research fellow in psychophysics. After retirement from Harvard in 1966, Békésy moved to Hawaii, where he took over leadership of a newly built laboratory and assumed a chair at the University of Hawaii endowed by the Hawaiian Telephone Company.

Békésy's path from physics to physiological acoustics began with his work with the Hungarian communications system. Early in his career he devised a method that could reduce the time required to check international telephone lines from a cumbersome twenty minutes to about one second. Before Békésy's innovation, the standard method used to test a telephone line was to run a specific A.C. voltage through a line, beginning in Budapest, let the current go to another city, and then feed it back to Budapest and compare the input with the output voltage for different frequencies. Békésy recognized that the problem was theoretically analogous to a musician's technique of quickly tuning an instrument by plucking the string rather than the more time-consuming bowing. Békésy therefore transmitted a click through the line by switching in a small D.C. voltage and then listening to and observing the returning signal. Thus, Békésy had effectively "plucked" rather than "bowed" the line. Each click contained a wide spectrum of frequencies that could be rapidly analyzed to reveal the precise location of the disturbance of the lines. This click method provided a fundamental insight that eventually led Békésy to study the mechanics of the inner ear.

The next problem Békésy took up was aimed at deciding how the Hungarian telephone system could be most readily improved by determining which of the basic components of telephone communication—the earphone, the microphone, or the telephone lines—was the weakest. Békésy applied a brief mechanical click to the eardrum and the microphone, and an electrical D.C. pulse to the earphone and the telephone lines. It soon became clear that the eardrum was far superior in quality to the earphones then being used. Békésy therefore recommended that the government should focus its efforts on improving the earphones.

But Békésy pursued the mechanics of the middle ear, and, eventually, the inner ear, using the "click" method that he had developed in his two previous investigations. He proceeded methodically until the physical events at all strategically important points in the ear were accounted for. First, Békésy successfully applied this technique to the eardrum and then to the tissues that conduct the sound from the eardrum to the inner ear, showing with remarkable precision the amplitude of the oscillations, their decay, their resonant frequencies, and even the changes in their decay and resonant frequency with amplitude.

Békésy's investigations of the inner ear were facilitated by the elaborate and ingenious technique that became the hallmark of his scientific reputation. Since the time of Helmholtz and Corti, anatomical investigations had revealed the question of how we hear to be reducible to a simple mechanical problem of the inner ear, more specifically the basilar membrane of the cochlea—since it is there that the cells on which the nerve endings terminate are seated. But access to these regions of the ear was difficult to obtain without the cochlea or its component tissues drying out or otherwise becoming so disturbed that any subsequent observations were rendered invalid. Békésy overcame the problem by doing the dissection in fluids, carrying out the observations with a 200-power underwater microscope.

By gaining observational access to the inner ear, Békésy was able to experimentally establish the events that make the cochlea a tiny neuromechanical frequency analyzing system. Helmholtz had assumed that the frequency of the sound waves determines the location along the basilar membrane at which stimulation occurs. Several contradictory theories subsequently emerged to explain the vibration pattern of the waves. Emphasizing their common features rather than their differences. Békésy found that all of the major theories could be reconciled by changing the numerical value of one parameter, the volume elasticity of the membrane. He found that the movements of the stirrup footplate give rise to a wave complex in the basilar membrane, which travels from the stiffer basal part to the more flexible part in the apex of the cochlea. Békésy showed that the highest crest of the traveling wave appears near the apex of the cochlea in low-frequency tones and near its base at high-frequency tones. He concluded that the tone of the sound is characterized by the particular location of the nerve cells of the membrane that are stimulated by sufficiently large amplitudes of the traveling wave.

By establishing how the ear performs frequency analysis, Békésy solved problems of physiological acoustics that had been outstanding for nearly a century. Several advantages for clinical medicine resulted from the physicist's work. Békésy skillfully combined his knowledge of art with his work in physics by designing several clinical diagnostic instruments. The audiometer that bears his name allows the otologist to distinguish between deafness caused by functional loss in the cochlea and that caused by a defect in the auditory nerve. Békésy also developed numerous important visual techniques as heuristic aids to his research. He produced many models, films, and illustrations that testify to his refined aesthetic sensibility and his particular talent for adapting it to science.

Békésy was a very private man whose entire life revolved around the study and collection of art. He kept few intimate friends beside the works of art in his extensive collection. As a gesture of friendship, Békésy would treat his closest colleagues to a glimpse of part, but never the whole, of his collection. Upon his death, Békésy extended this gesture to a broader public when he bequeathed his large and tasteful collection to the Nobel Foundation, in gratitude for the honor it had bestowed on him.

ROBERT BRAIN

Selected Bibliography

PRIMARY SOURCES

Békésy, Georg von. 1960. *Experiments in Hearing*. Translated and ed. by E. G. Wever. New York: McGraw-Hill.

———. 1961. "Concerning the Pleasures of Observing, and the Mechanics of the Inner Ear." Nobel Lecture. *Le Prix Nobel en 1961*. Stockholm: Imprimerie Royale P.A., Norstedt & Söner, 1962, 104–208.

———. 1967. *Sensory Inhibition*. Princeton: Princeton University Press.

SECONDARY SOURCES

Wirgen, J. 1974. *The Georg von Békésy Collection*. Malmö, Sweden: AB Allhem for the Nobel Foundation.

Ratliff, Floyd. 1976. "Georg von Békésy. June 3, 1899–June 13, 1972." *Biographical Memoirs of the National Academy of Sciences* 48:25–50. Includes complete bibliography of Békésy's publications.

Tonndorf, S. 1986. "Georg von Békésy and His Work." *Hearing Research* 22:3–10.

BARUJ BENACERRAF *1980*

Baruj Benacerraf was born on October 29, 1920, in Caracas, Venezuela. An immunologist, Benacerraf received the 1980 Nobel Prize in Physiology or Medicine jointly with Jean Dausset and George D. Snell. Benacerraf was specifically cited for being "chiefly responsible for the identification of the system of genes responsible for the HLA antigens."

Benacerraf's parents were Sephardic Jews. His mother, Henriette Lasry, came from French Algiers. His father, Abraham Benacerraf, emigrated to Venezuela from Spanish Morocco at the age of fourteen. In Caracas, he and his brothers built a textile import business. His business interests grew and eventually included the Banco Union of Caracas. When young Baruj was five years old, the family moved to Paris. He received a classical French education at the Lycée Janson-de-Sailly.

Late in 1938, "fearful of the impending war," Abraham Benacerraf decided to move back to Venezuela. A few months after the family's return, Baruj left for the United States to resume his schooling. His father expected that he would join him in his business and eventually succeed him. As Benacerraf later wrote, "I made an honest but abortive attempt to comply with his wishes." He enrolled at the Textile Engineering School of the Philadelphia Museum of Art, but after only two weeks, "fled" to New York, where he entered the Lycée Français and also began studying English at Columbia. His parents and brothers came to New York later that year. (Benacerraf 1985)

After obtaining his French Baccalauréat dès Lettres in 1940, Benacerraf entered the School of General Studies at Columbia with junior standing. Here he met Annette Dreyfus, a relative of Captain Alfred Dreyfus, who had also fled France and was a student at Barnard College. They were married on March 24, 1943.

After earning his B.S. from Columbia in 1942, Benacerraf was rejected by 25 medical schools, including Columbia, Yale, and Harvard. He received one acceptance, to the Medical College of Virginia in Richmond. According to Benacerraf, "At that time, it was very hard for Jews to get into medical school. This country was strongly anti-Semitic in the 1940s. In addition, there was a tendency not to take in foreigners." (McManus 1987)

Soon after entering medical school in Richmond, Benacerraf was drafted into the United States Army but allowed to continue his studies. He became a naturalized citizen in 1943. After receiving his M.D. in 1945, he spent nine months as an intern at Queens County Hospital in New York. For the next two years, he served as an officer in the Army Medical Corps.

His father had suffered a massive stroke in 1945. After his discharge from the Army in 1947, Benacerraf agreed to manage the family's financial interests in Venezuela. For many years, his scientific work was frequently interrupted by trips to South America. It was not until the early 1960s that he managed to successfully dispose of these business responsibilities. They prevented him from seeking a permanent academic position until 1956. As Benacerraf wrote, "The necessity of attending seriously to major business interests, while working in the laboratory for many years without a salary, made me feel like a dilettante scientist. I could rationalize that, if I was not successful in my chosen profession, I could fall back on the one my father had foreseen for me. This frame of mind, however, did not alter in the least my competitiveness or my ambition as a scientist; I realized that we are sometimes capable of exerting the greatest efforts in areas where we consider ourselves amateurs." (Benacerraf 1985)

Benacerraf's childhood experience with asthmatic cough led to an interest in allergic diseases and the immunological mechanisms of hypersensitivity reactions. In 1947 he looked forward to starting research training and hoped to learn immunology. Both René Dubos and Jules Freund advised him to learn immunochemistry by working with Elvin Abraham Kabat, a disciple of Michael Heidelberg, the founder of the field. He was accepted as an unpaid research fellow in Kabat's laboratory at the Neurological Institute of Columbia University and worked there until 1950. Kabat taught Benacerraf the basics of immunology but also "the significance of experimental proof, the need for intellectual honesty and scientific integrity." (Gilson 1985). These two years were Benacerraf's only formal training as a scientist.

The research project suggested by Kabat was to establish the amounts of rabbit anti-ovalbumin antibodies required to sensitize guinea pigs passively for systemic anaphylaxis and for the Arthus reaction (the localized anaphylaxis described by Maurice Arthus, generally characterized by swelling and inflammation). Kabat and Benacerraf demonstrated that the amount of antibody required to sensitize for anaphylaxis varied inversely with the time of passive sensitization. Thus, in order to sensitize, the antibody had to be fixed to some unidentified structure. The Arthus reaction, it appeared, was caused by circulating antibodies reacting with antigen in the tissues at the level of the blood vessel.

In 1949, Benacerraf accepted an invitation to work in Paris from Bernard Halpern, the discoverer of antihistamines. From 1950 to 1956 he held the position of Chargé de Recherches at the Centre National de la Recherche Scientifique at the Hôpital Broussais. Soon after he arrived, a young Italian immunologist, Guido Biozzi, joined Halpern's laboratory. Within a few months, Benacerraf and Biozzi started "a six-year partnership in studying the phagocytic function of the reticulo-endothelial system," that is the action of the many diverse cells which remove foreign particles and cells from the body, essentially by digestion. The team developed a quantitative methodology to measure the clearance of particulate matter from the blood by the phagocytes of the liver and spleen, deriving the equations to precisely describe the clearances. Biozzi introduced Benacerraf to his Hungarian friend, Zoltan Ovary, who later would join the latter at New York University and collaborate with him on the study of the functional properties of different classes of guinea pig antibodies.

In 1956, Lewis Thomas invited Benacerraf to establish a small laboratory in his Department of Pathology at New York University School of Medicine. After two years as Assistant Professor, Benacerraf was promoted to Associate Professor of Pathology in 1958, and finally to full Professor in 1960. While working as a full-time faculty member, he also managed the Colonial Trust Company for several years. According to Benacerraf, "I learned the banking business rapidly, which I must admit is very routine and a far easier occupation and considerably less hazardous than immunological research. I spent one day a week taking care of my banking responsibilities during this period." (Benacerraf 1985)

His stay at NYU "spanned the course of twelve happy years, from 1956 to 1968 . . . a golden period for me." By the mid-1960s, he had established a well-funded and active laboratory and was surrounded by gifted colleagues and students. "I came to realize that, unbeknownst to me, I had been a professional scientist all along, and that I had been an amateur businessman, rather than the other way around, as I had fantasized earlier." (Benacerraf 1985)

Benacerraf's work in the late 1950s, in collaboration with Philip G. H. Gell, an immunologist from England, concerned the specificity of cellular immune reactions, such as tuberculin or contact hypersensitivity, and the ways in which the specificity of these reactions differed from that of antibodies for specific antigens. (Benacerraf 1985)

In 1962, Benacerraf undertook a collaborative project with Gerald M. Edelman of Rockefeller University on the analysis of antibody structures. The preparations they used consisted of heterogeneous populations of antibody molecules, making such analysis difficult. Benacerraf experimented with the possibilities of immunizing guinea pigs with simple antigens and making a pure preparation of the resultant antibody, which he hoped would consist of a single kind of molecule. He found that some animals responded to a specific antigen and some did not. This observation intrigued him and led him away from the problem of antibody structure determination, for which Edelman and Rodney Porter won the Nobel Prize in 1972. (Marx 1980).

Benacerraf discovered that the answer was genetic. He demonstrated that the antibody response in the guinea pig was controlled by genes which he called Ir, or immune response genes, within the species' major histocompatibility complex (MHC), a group of closely linked genes which determine an organism's response to foreign tissues, cells, and molecules. Hugh McDevitt of Stanford University and Michael Sela of the Weizmann Institute in Israel found similar genes in mice; McDevitt showed that the Ir genes are not located in the K or D regions of the MHC, which control the rejection of grafted tissues, but in a different area, now called the I region. The I region is believed to be analogous to the HLA-D region of the HLA system in humans.

The action of the Ir genes is still being studied but is believed to influence the "helper" activities of T lymphocytes. There are several types of T cells: some directly attack foreign cells, others, the "helpers," appear to assist the B lymphocytes, the cells which actually manufacture antibodies, while T "suppressor" cells block the production of antibodies and the other activities of the T and B cells. Benacerraf and David Katz of the Scripps Clinic and Research Foundation have shown that T and B cells in mice must carry identical genes traceable to the I region, if they are to work together to produce antibodies. Further research has shown that the Ir genes are essential to the triggering response which "turns on" the T cells, which involves interraction with a phagocyte that has found and consumed the antigen. Suppressor action is also controlled by the I region. (Marx 1980)

In 1968, Benacerraf was appointed chief of the laboratory of Immunology at the National Institute of Allergy and Infectious Diseases. After only two years, he was named Fabyan Professor of Comparative Pathology and chairman of the Department of Pathology at Harvard, a prestigious appointment for an "amateur scientist"! In 1980, he became president and chief executive officer of the Dana Farber Cancer Institute in Boston. He has also served as a scientific advisor to the World Health Organization. His daughter Beryl is also pursuing a scientific career.

Baruj Benacerraf is a member of the National Academy of Sciences, the Israel Academy of Arts and Sciences, the National Institute of Medicine, and a fellow of the American Academy of Arts and Sciences. He is an editor of several major scientific journals of pathology and immunology and has served as president of the American Association for Immunology (1973–74); the Federation of American Societies for Experimental Biology (1974–75); and the International Union of Immunological Societies (1980–83). Among the many other awards he has won have been the Rabbi Shai Shacknai Prize from the Hebrew University of Jerusalem (1974); the T. Duckett Jones Memorial Award (1976); the Waterford Biomedical Science Award (1980); the Rous-Whipple Award from the American Association of Pathologists (1985); and the Légion d'Honneur (1986).

ELIE FEUERWERKER

Selected Bibliography

PRIMARY SOURCES

Benacerraf, Baruj. No date. "Biographical Sketch." Unpublished. 3 pp.

———. 1971–72. "The Genetic Control of Specific Immune Responses." *Harvey Lectures* ser. 67:109–141. New York: Academic Press.

Benacerraf, Baruj, and Hugh O. McDevitt, 1972. "The Histocompatibility-Linked Immune Response Genes." *Science* 175:273.

Benacerraf, Baruj. 1974. "The Training Experience. Presidential Address." *Journal of Immunology* 113:431.

Benacerraf, Baruj, and R. N. Germain. 1978. "The Immune Response Genes of the Major Histocompatibility Complex." *Immunological Review* 38:70–119.

Benacerraf, Baruj. 1980. "Role of MHC Gene Products in Immune Regulation." Nobel Lecture. Reprinted in *Science* 212 (1981):1229.

———. 1985. "Reminiscences." *Immunological Review* 84:7–27.

SECONDARY SOURCES

1980. "1980 Nobel Prizes." *Nature* 287: 671.

Marx, Jean L. 1980. "1980 Nobel Prize in Physiology or Medicine." *Science* 210:621–23.

Gilson, Estelle. 1985. "Nobel Profile. Immunology's World Citizen: Baruj Benacerraf." *Columbia* (November):35–36.

McManus, Otile. 1987. "Profile. They Do Medicine in a Family Way." *Boston Globe* (September 21):33–34.

SUNE KARL BERGSTRÖM *1982*

Sune Karl Bergström was born on January 10, 1916, in Stockholm. A biochemist, Bergström shared the 1982 Nobel Prize with Bengt Samuelsson and John Robert Vane for their work in characterizing, differentiating, and describing the action of the prostaglandins, a field that Bergström pioneered. At the time of his Nobel award, Bergström, one of Sweden's leading scientists, had retired from active teaching at the Karolinska Institute in Stockholm after twenty-three years and was serving as chairman of the World Health Organization Advisory Committee on Medical Research. He was also chairman of the board of directors of the Nobel Foundation. Bergström was married to Maj Bernhardt in 1943; the couple have one son.

Bergström, the son of Sverker and Wera Wistrand Bergström, was raised in Stockholm, and began his studies in biochemistry and medicine at the Karolinska at the age of eighteen. During World War II he won a Swedish-American fellowship to study in the United States, first at Columbia University (1940–41), and then at the Squibb Institute (1941–42), where he became interested in the oxidation of certain compounds at room temperature. He continued this research upon his return to

Sweden, working in the Department of Chemistry of the Medical Nobel Institute, which is based at the Karolinska. He received doctoral degrees in both medicine and biochemistry in 1944.

Bergström pursued his interest in oxidation as a research assistant at the Karolinska. He was now working with linoleic acid, a fatty acid found normally in food, and was able to identify and isolate from soybeans the enzyme lipoxygenase, which promotes and makes possible the oxidation of this lipid at low temperatures. In 1945, he presented his findings at a meeting of the Karolinska Physiological Society. Ulf von Euler was in the audience and spoke to Bergström about his own work with some biologically highly active lipids that he thought might be products of a similar oxygenation process. These were the prostaglandins (Oates 1982, 765).

The first interest in these compounds resulted from early artificial insemination procedures performed by Raphael Kurzrok, Charles Leib, and Sarah Ratner at Columbia University in 1930. The physicians noted that the injection of seminal plasma into the uterus caused the smooth muscle to contract and then to relax. Maurice Goldblatt in England and von Euler in Sweden undertook further experiments with seminal fluid from rams before the war. They observed lowered blood pressure as well as smooth muscle responses in a number of animals. Von Euler identified the active compounds in the secretions of the prostate gland and gave them the name "prostaglandins."

Bergström's interest was immediately stirred and he eagerly accepted a small quantity of the extracts von Euler had made from ram semen in the 1930s. Using the most advanced techniques available, he further purified the compounds and was astonished to observe that "after purification essentially to weightlessness, they retained extraordinary activity." Despite his fascination, Bergström's work on prostaglandins was delayed for a decade, because of the technical difficulties involved and his own administrative commitments (Oates 1982, 765).

Following a year's fellowship at the University of Basel, Bergström accepted an appointment as professor and chairman of the Department of Chemistry of the University of Lund in southern Sweden in 1947. He spent much of the next ten years developing the faculty and laboratory facilities there. His research during this period dealt primarily with cholesterol and bile acids. To assist him in these studies, he adapted the technology of reverse phase partition chromatography. Among the medical students working with him at Lund was the young Bengt Samuelsson, who speaks of Bergström as his mentor.

In 1958 Bergström returned to the Karolinska, where he was joined by Samuelsson, Jan Sjovall, and Ragnar Ryhage. Several factors, beside's Bergström's relative freedom from other responsibilities, now made possible the isolation, analysis, and characterization of the prostaglandins. The team had collected a sufficient number of sheep seminal glands to prepare the extracts for intensive study. (Roughly 100 kilograms of sheep glands were required for each usable extract.) Bergström had developed the necessary methods of gas chromatography, and Ryhage had invented a method of interface between the chromatograph and the mass spectrometer that permitted the structural analysis of small quantities. The application of this technology to the study of the prostaglandins has now been replicated in many other scientific fields (Oates 1982, 765–66; Wilford 1982).

Bergström and his colleagues soon isolated the first two compounds, and through 1964 they continued to describe the structure and activity of the prostaglandin group, including PGE_2, $PGF_{2\alpha}$, and PGD_2. The related compounds, thromboxane A_2, prostacyclin, and the leukotrienes were discovered later. Prostaglandins are found throughout the human body. Each possesses the same twenty-carbon atom skeleton and fatty acid structure, but each is produced by different cells to perform different and highly specific functions. Thromboxane A_2, for example, is a product of platelets and stimulates platelet aggregation and vasoconstriction, whereas prostacyclin, metabolized by the endothelial cells, has the opposite action.

The new understanding of prostaglandin structure confirmed von Euler's hunch that these compounds were the result of lipid oxygenation. The logical candidate was arachidonic acid, a twenty-carbon polyunsaturated fatty acid. By 1965 Bergström, Samuelsson, and David Van Dorp at the Unilever Laboratories in Holland demonstrated that arachidonic acid was indeed the common biosynthetic origin of all prostaglandins. This finding showed the way to their in vitro synthesis for research use and solved the supply problems. Between 1962 and 1964 Samuelsson further determined and explained the intracellular biosynthesis of the compounds by enzymatic oxygenation of arachidonic acid (Oates 1982, 765–66).

The multiple functions of the prostaglandins and their powerful activity has made possible a wide range of clinical applications, many still in the experimental stage. These include pain relief, induction of labor and of abortion, prevention of ulcers, correction of birth defects, vasodilation in heart surgery, and applications in asthma, cancer, and heart disease, among others. Many well-established but poorly understood biochemical effects, including the action of acetylsalicylic acid (aspirin) and the anti-inflammatory effect of the corticosteroids, may be viewed as stimuli or inhibitors of prostaglandin synthesis (Oates 1982, 767–68; Altman 1982).

A reserved, industrious man, devoted to his research, Bergström's administrative talents have often led to his enforced absence from the laboratory. He served as dean of the Karolinska medical faculty from 1963 to 1966 and as rector, or chief administrator, of the institute from 1969 to 1977. He was appointed to the Nobel Foundation Board in 1975; despite his position, colleagues agreed that his achievements were far too important not to be recognized merely to avoid the appearance of a conflict of interest. He served as chairman of the WHO Advisory Committee on Medical Research from 1977 to 1982, supervising the construction of medical facilities around the world. He has managed to continue his prostaglandin studies, however, particularly since his retirement from teaching in 1981 (Wilford 1982).

Bergström is a member of the Swedish Medical Research Council, the Royal Swedish Academy of Science, and the American Academy of Arts and Sciences. Among the many other honors he has received are the Louisa Gross Horowitz Prize (1975) and the Albert Lasker Basic Medical Research Award (1977).

MARCIA MELDRUM

Selected Bibliography

PRIMARY SOURCES

Bergström, Sune, and Bengt Samuelsson. 1967. *Prostaglandins. Proceedings of the Second Nobel Symposium, Stockholm, June 1966.* New York: Interscience Publishers.

Bergström, Sune, K. Green, and Bengt Samuelsson. 1972. *Third Conference on Prostaglandins in Fertility Control, January 17–20, 1972.* Stockholm: Karolinska Institute.

Bergström, Sune. 1973. *Report from the Meeting of the Prostaglandin Task Force Steering Committee, Chapel Hill, June 8–10, 1972, Stockholm, October 2–3, 1972, Geneva, February 26–28, 1973.* Stockholm: Karolinska Institute.

Bergström, Sune, and John R. Vane. 1979. *Prostacyclin.* New York: Raven Press.

SECONDARY SOURCES

Altman, Lawrence K. 1982. "Two Swedes and Briton Win Nobel for Clues to Body's Chemistry." *New York Times* (October 12):1, C3.

Wilford, John Noble. 1982. "Men in the News: Sune Karl Bergström." *New York Times* (October 12):C3.

Oates, John A. 1982. "The 1982 Nobel Prize in Physiology or Medicine." *Science* 218 (November 19):765–68.

J. MICHAEL BISHOP *1989*

John Michael Bishop, biochemist, was born February 22, 1936, in York, Pennsylvania. He was awarded the 1989 Nobel Prize jointly with Harold E. Varmus for their pathbreaking discovery that growth-regulating genes in normal cells can malfunction and initiate the abnormal growth processes of cancer. Bishop is currently professor of microbiology and immunology at the University of California at San Francisco.

The son of a minister, Bishop was interested in history during his undergraduate years at Gettysburg College but chose to go to medical school "out of desperation. . . . I did not know what I wanted to do but I wanted to do something altruistic." At Harvard Medical School he was deeply attracted to research, especially molecular biology. This field, however, consisted of "a very sophisticated club" of researchers, and Bishop felt it would be difficult for him to gain recognition and establish a career. Instead, he began studying virology, working in the laboratory of Elmer Pfefferkorn. Rather than take the usual fourth year of coursework and clinical experience, he was given permission to spend the time in research, "a very enlightened act" on the part of the dean of students. In order to graduate, however, he had to spend "one hectic weekend" at Boston City Hospital, assisting to deliver fifty babies (Kolata 1989).

After receiving his M.D. in 1962, Bishop spent two years at Massachusetts General Hospital as an intern and resident in internal medicine. In 1964, however, he was appointed as a Research Associate at the National Institutes of Health, allowing him to pursue his interest in virology and the possible viral etiology of cancer. He remained at NIH for four years, the last two as a senior investigator, before joining the faculty at UCSF in 1968, as an assistant professor.

Harold Varmus came to the department of microbiology two years later as a postdoctoral fellow and "ran into Mike Bishop almost by accident. . . . Mike and I hit it off right away." The two began investigating the behavior of retroviruses, which can cause cancer to develop in animals, and oncogenes, the carcinogenic genes found in the viruses. Rous sarcoma virus, for example, produced sarcomas, or cancers of the connective tissues, in chickens, and could also "infect" cells in laboratory cultures with remarkable virulence. In the 1970s, a single gene, called *src* for sarcoma, had been identified as the oncogene in Rous sarcoma virus. However, no human cancer had ever been traced to Rous sarcoma or to any other retrovirus (Marx 1989a).

Robert Huebner and George Todaro of the National Cancer Institute had suggested that all cells might contain potential oncogenes, in the form of viral DNA left over from some ancient infection of early life forms. Through many evolutionary generations, the hypothesis said, the DNA lay dormant, merely replicating itself with the normal cellular DNA. But certain stimuli, such as radiation, would cause the viral material, which Huebner and Todaro called "proviruses," to become active and to produce malignant cell growth (Marx 1989a).

Bishop and Varmus set up a series of experiments to test this oncogene hypothesis. Their idea was to find *src* gene DNA material in normal chicken cells. Lacking the techniques of gene cleavage and sequencing that have since been developed, they found the work "brutally difficult." Bishop has said that he "personally did not think the experiments would work" (Kolata 1989).

The painstaking efforts of the UCSF team, including C. T. Deng, Ramareddy Guntaka, Deborah Spector, Dominique Stehelin and P. K. Vogt, did indeed uncover *src* gene DNA, not only in chicken cells but in those of several other birds and some mammals. The guilty gene was found not to be an ancient viral invader, however, but a normal cellular gene. This observation "turned the oncogene hypothesis on its head" and was doubted by many scientists when first reported in 1976, but since then, nearly 50 normal cellular genes have been identified as "proto-oncogenes" (Marx 1989a; Kolata 1989).

The work of Bishop, Varmus, and others has shown that these genes assist in the regulation of normal cell growth and division. Radiation, chemical toxins, or other carcinogens may produce a mutation of the gene, which will then initiate abnormal cell division, resulting in malignant growth. Carcinogenesis by a retrovirus is not caused by the viral genes; rather, the virus picks up a normal gene from a cell during infection and then carries it to another cell, where the gene becomes an abnormal component of the DNA and again triggers malignancy.

The discovery of the proto-oncogene, while overturning ideas of viral origin, strongly supported researchers' convictions that "there is a final common pathway in causing cancer," and has led to much new and creative investigation. It has been important as well for clinical diagnosis, prognosis and treatment. If particular types of oncogenes are detected in cancerous cells, the physician gains a better understanding of the history and probable course of the disease and is able to plan therapy accordingly (Marx 1989a; Kolata 1989).

Michael Bishop was promoted to full professor in 1972 and in 1981 became director of the G. W. Hooper Research Foundation at USCF. He is a member of the National Academy of Sciences, the American Society of Biological Chemists, the American Academy of Arts and Sciences, and the American Society of Microbiologists, among others. He has served on the University of California Cancer Research Coordinating Committee since 1968 and also served as a consultant for NIH and the American Cancer Society. Among the many awards he has won for his work have been the Biomedical Research Award of the American Association of Medical Colleges (1981); the Lasker Award (1982); the Armand Hammer Cancer Award (1984); the Gairdner Foundation Award (1984); and the Medal of Honor of the American Cancer Society (1985).

For Bishop, winning the Nobel Prize was a "surreal" experience, slightly marred by the protest of Dominique Stehelin, now with the Institut Pasteur in Lille, France, that the prize should have been shared with him for carrying out some of the crucial experiments. His claim was rejected, however, by the Nobel Committee, which reiterated its view that Bishop and Varmus were the "key persons in the discovery" (Marx 1989b; Kolata 1989).

MARCIA MELDRUM

Selected Bibliography

PRIMARY SOURCES

Varmus, H. E., J. M. Bishop, and P. K. Vogt. 1973. "Appearance of Virus-Specific DNA in Mammalian Cells Following Transformation by Rous Sarcoma Virus." *Journal of Molecular Biology* 74 (March 15):613–26.

Bishop, J. M., C. T. Deng, A. J. Faras, *et al.* 1975. "The Provirus of Rous Sarcoma Virus: Synthesis, Integration and Transcription." *Tumor Virus-Host Cell Interaction.* A. R. Kobler, editor. New York: Plenum Press.

Stehelin, D., H. E. Varmus, and J. M. Bishop. 1975. "Detection of Nucleotide Sequences Associated with Transformation by Avian Sarcoma Viruses." *Bibliotheca Haematologica* 43 (October):539–41.

Stehelin, D., H. E. Varmus, J. M. Bishop, *et al.* 1976. "DNA Related to the Transforming Gene(s) of Avian Sarcoma Virus is Present in Normal Avian DNA." *Nature* 260 (March 11):170–73.

Bishop, J. M., B. Baker, D. Fujita, P. McCombe, D. Sheiness, K. Smith, D. H. Spector, D. Stehelin, and H. E. Varmus. 1978. "Genesis of a Virus-Transforming Gene." *National Cancer Institute Monographs* 48 (May):219–23.

SECONDARY SOURCES

Kolata, Gina. 1989. "2 Doctors Share Nobel Prize for Work with Cancer Genes." *New York Times* (October 10):C3.

Marx, Jean L. 1989. "Cancer Gene Research Wins Medicine Nobel." *Science* 246 (October 20):326–27.

———. 1989. "Controversy Over Nobel." *Science* 246 (October 20): 326–27.

SIR JAMES WHYTE BLACK *1988*

Sir James Whyte Black was born in Uddingston, Scotland, on June 14, 1924. A pharmacologist, Black shared the Nobel Prize in 1988 with George H. Hitchings and Gertrude B. Elion for their work in developing drugs for the treatment of critical diseases. Black synthesized the first beta-blockers for the treatment of heart disease as well as the H2 antagonists for gastric ulcer. The Nobel Prize is rarely given for new drugs; its award to Black recognizes not only his contributions to therapeutics but his formulation of basic principles of "rational drug development" which will continue to provide clues to researchers. Black currently heads a small private research foundation, the James Black Foundation in London, established for him by Johnson and Johnson; he is affiliated with King's College Hospital Medical School and the Rayne Institute of the University of London. He was knighted in 1981.

Black received his medical degree from the University of St. Andrews in 1946. He taught for ten years before accepting a position at Imperial Chemical Industries as a senior pharmacologist. Black is a tenacious man, "driven by obsessive curiosity," with little interest in publicity or adulation. Rather than seek advancement in business or academia, he has always preferred to work with a small, highly motivated team and to follow his own ideas. He explained in 1988 that industry is "the only constituency" that will support research without attaching limitations on time or direction of the work. "Most revolutionary work begins by being at least mildly controversial," he observed (Schmeck 1988; Conner et al. 1988, 26).

Black's research has been characterized by the formation of physiological theories and then the creation of compounds that satisfy the parameters of the theory. His development of beta-blockers had its roots in a problem of the 1940s regarding the physiological effects of epinephrine (adrenalin) and norepinephrine. These hormones appeared to both regulate and stimulate the action of smooth muscle organs, such as the heart. In 1948 Raymond Ahlqvist of the Medical College of Georgia suggested that the organs possessed two sets of receptors, which he designated alpha and beta, that mediated the hormonal stimuli. The alpha-receptors of the heart used the hormones to contract the muscle; the beta-receptors acted in a different fashion, increasing the heart rate.

In 1956, when Black began his work at Imperial Chemical, several substances were known that could selectively stimulate the receptors; these were called agonists. Other drugs, termed antagonists, could inhibit the alpha-receptors. The standard therapy for angina pectoris and other forms of heart disease, however, was to use drugs that increased the supply of oxygen to the heart.

Black hypothesized that blocking the beta-receptors would effectively relax the heart, reducing its need for oxygen and the strain on the muscle, and thus retarding the degenerative processes. He therefore set out to design a drug that would do just that. Several analogues of norepinephrine were then available; Black and his team used one of these, isoprenaline (isoproterenol), to "build" propanolol, the first specific beta-blocker.

Propanolol occupies the beta-receptor sites, thus preventing the natural hormones from attaching themselves and acting as stimuli. Since its introduction in 1964, it has been used widely to treat angina, hypertension, and vascular headache. Several studies in the late 1970s and early 1980s established its success in improving the survival rate of heart attack patients by about 25 percent. The National Heart, Lung, and Blood Institute ended one study in advance because the data had already established the drug's efficacy and it was considered unjustifiable to withhold it from the control group any longer. "For the first time

. . . a drug given to heart attack survivors actually saves lives," one of the NHLBI scientists commented (Connor et al. 1988; Marx 1988, 517; Altman 1988).

Black then became interested in the activity of histamine, a compound found naturally in the body. This chemical both generates a response to foreign matter in the body and stimulates the secretion of gastric acid; if it does its job too well, the results are allergic reactions or gastric ulcers, respectively. Antihistamines had been developed to treat allergies but appeared to have no effect on the acid secretion. Black theorized that there might be two different histamine receptors, similar to the alpha and beta model, which he named H1 and H2, each of which mediated histamine differently.

He was working now at Smith Kline, where he was to devote fourteen years to the quest for an H2 blocker. He and his associates developed a series of histamine analogues and used these to study the process of histamine action on the stomach lining. They were able to synthesize several drugs, which appeared to block the histamine, in a similar process to the beta-blockers, but their results were indeterminate for some time because they were not using a sufficient quantity of histamine to produce a differential effect. Thus an early attempt, burimamide, is a weak H2 blocker completely ineffective for clinical use. When this error had been corrected, they finally developed and demonstrated the efficacy of cimetidine, "the salvation" of peptic ulcer patients. By its retardant effect on acid secretion, this drug, introduced in 1972, allows ulcers to heal quickly and painlessly, without surgery (Connor et al. 1988, 27; Marx 1988, 517; Altman 1988).

In each case, Black began with a known chemical substance; as he has said, "the most fruitful basis for the discovery of a new drug is to start with an old drug," whose action is known and whose composition can then be analyzed and resynthesized to form a clinically effective compound. As Paul Leff, who worked with him for several years, observed, his rigorous, rational development of this model "has become the gold standard. . . . People walk around talking about the Black Approach" (Connor et al. 1988, 26).

Sir James Black joined the faculty of Kings College Hospital Medical School in London in 1973. "A dedicated teacher," he has accepted many visiting professorships in recent years. He was head of biological research at Smith Kline and French of Welwyn Garden City and then director of the Therapeutic Research Division of the Wellcome Laboratories in Kent, before Johnson and Johnson arranged to support the James Black Foundation. The foundation is designed to maximize the effectiveness of Black's small-team approach; it will employ a maximum of twenty people but offers outstanding laboratory facilities, at a cost of ten million pounds. Although sixty-four at the time of the Nobel award, Black showed no signs of impending retirement (Schmeck 1988).

MARCIA MELDRUM

Selected Bibliography

PRIMARY SOURCES

Black, James W., A. F. Crowther, R. G. Shanks, et al. 1964. "A New Adrenergic Beta Receptor Antagonist." *Lancet* 1 (May 16):1080–81.

Black, James W., W. A. Duncan, and R. G. Shanks. 1965. "Comparison of Some Properties of Pronethalol and Propanolol." *British Journal of Pharmacology* 25 (December):577–91.

Black, James W., W. A. Duncan, C. J. Durant, et al. 1972. "Definition and Antagonism of Histamine H-2 Receptors." *Nature* 236 (April 21): 385–90.

SECONDARY SOURCES

Altman, Lawrence K. 1988. "Three Drug Pioneers Win Nobel in Medicine." *New York Times* (October 18):1, C17.

Schmeck, Harold M., Jr. 1988. "A Pharmacology Pioneer Who Avoids the Spotlight: Sir James Whyte Black." *New York Times* (October 18):C16.

Connor, Steve, Dan Charles, Sharon Kingman, and Frank Lesser. 1988. "Drug Pioneers Win Nobel Laureate." *New Scientist* (October 22): 26–27.

Marx, Jean I. 1988. "The 1988 Nobel Prize for Physiology or Medicine." *Science* 242 (October 28):516–17.

KONRAD E. BLOCH *1964*

Konrad E. Bloch was born on January 21, 1912, in Neisse, Upper Silesia, then Germany. A biochemist specializing in lipid metabolism, he received the 1964 Nobel Prize in Physiology or Medicine jointly with Feodor Lynen "for their discoveries concerning the mechanism and regulation of cholesterol and fatty acid metabolism." Bloch married Lore Teutsch, a native of Munich, on February 15, 1941. The Blochs have two children.

His father, Fritz Bloch, was a lawyer and businessman; his mother was Hedwig Streimer Bloch. Bloch attended the Technische Hochschule in Munich from 1930 to 1934 with the intention of becoming a chemical engineer. But influenced by his teacher Hans Fischer, he became interested in organic chemistry, especially the structure of natural products. His studies in Germany ended in 1934 after he had obtained the degree of diplom-ingenieur in chemistry. When Nazi racial laws were instituted in German schools, Bloch was fortunate in finding an appointment as research assistant in Switzerland, at the Schweizerische Forschungsinstitut in Davos, where he carried out his first published biochemical research. This mountainous area, with its magnificent ski slopes and numerous tuberculosis sanitaria, was the setting of Thomas Mann's novel *The Magic Mountain.* Appropriately, Bloch's research involved the phospholopids of tubercle bacilli. His work revealed that previous claims that tubercle bacteria contain cholesterol were false. His first encounter with cholesterol confirmed experiments by Erwin Chargaff, Rudolf J. Anderson, and Rudolf Schoenheimer, scientists he would later meet at Columbia. With his nonrenewable residential permit in Switzerland about to expire, Bloch was delighted to receive a letter of appointment as assistant in Biological Chemistry, School of Medicine, Yale University. However, there were actually no funds available to support such a position.

In December 1936 Bloch arrived in the United States, with "great hopes," but no money. Rudolph Anderson suggested that he pursue graduate studies with Hans Clarke at the College of Physicians and Surgeons, Columbia University, rather than at Yale. With help from Max Bergmann and support from the Wallerstein Foundation, Bloch entered the Department of Biochemistry, College of Physicians and Surgeons, at Columbia University as a student of Hans Clarke. After Bloch obtained his Ph.D. in 1938, he was asked by Rudolf Schoenheimer to join his research group at Columbia's College of Physicians and Surgeons. Later Bloch referred to these years with Schoenheimer as the most influential of his "Lehrjahre." After Schoenheimer's premature death in 1941, members of his research group were encouraged by Hans Clarke to continue to develop their own special interests. During this period Bloch's interest in intermediary metabolism and the problems of biosynthesis was keenly developed. In 1942, in collaboration with David Rittenberg, Bloch began the work on the biological synthesis of cholesterol that was to remain a fertile field of research for some twenty years.

Bloch moved to the University of Chicago in 1946 as assistant professor of biochemistry. He was promoted to associate professor in 1948 and full professor in 1950. He found the intellectual atmosphere in the Biochemistry Department, then headed by E. A. Evans, Jr., stimulating and productive. During this period he continued his studies of cholesterol biosynthesis and the enzymatic synthesis of the tripeptide glutathione. A Guggenheim Fellowship in 1953 provided a productive year at the Organisch-Chemisches Institute, Eidgenössische Technische Hochschule in Zurich with L. Ruzicka, V. Prelog, and coworkers. This period was devoted to studies of the biogenesis and biochemical relationships of the terpenes and sterols. In 1954 Bloch became Higgins Professor of Biochemistry in the Department of Chemistry at Harvard University. He served as chairman of the department from 1968 to 1978.

Bloch's early research showed that acetic acid was a major precursor of cholesterol in rats, and he continued to work on explaining the steps in the biosynthesis of sterols, from the metabolism of acetic acid to squalene, the cyclization of squalene to lanosterol, and the intermediates involved in the conversion of lanosterol to cholesterol. The biosynthetic pathway is extremely complex; the transformation of acetic acid through acetyl Coenzyme A to cholesterol involves some thirty-six steps. Bloch also made important contributions to understanding the biosynthesis of glutathione and fatty acid metabolism. His researches on glutathione provided a model for one mode of activation of amino acids to form peptide bonds. Bloch was especially interested in the biosynthesis of unsaturated fatty acids; he discovered that different biosynthetic pathways exist in aerobic and anaerobic organisms. These studies stimulated his interest in comparative and evolutionary biochemistry. The complex biosynthetic pathways for fatty acids and cholesterol are of general scientific and medical importance because of their role in illuminating intermediary metabolism and their possible therapeutic significance.

Although cholesterol had been isolated from gallstones in the 1820s, and its structure had been elucidated in the 1930s, little was known about its biosynthesis when Bloch took up the problem in the 1940s. In his Nobel Lecture, Bloch recalled how "the molecular architecture of cholesterol seemed enigmatic and devoid of any clues as to how this complex molecule might be constructed from the smaller molecules available in the cells." Surprisingly, many of the early speculations about this biosynthetic enigma came close to predicting the general principles eventually found to operate in sterol biosynthesis (Bloch 1964, 78).

Chemists thought that the tetracyclic steroidal ring system must be derived from an appropriately folded long-chain precursor. Influential and prescient hypotheses were put forth by L. Ruzick, concerning the common origin of terpenes and steroids, and Sir Robert Robinson, concerning the cyclization of squalene. In 1937 Rittenberg and Schoenheimer at Columbia began their pioneering studies of intermediary metabolism using stable istotopes. They concluded that cholesterol biosynthesis involved the coupling of smaller molecules. Bloch was introduced to the powerful new methodology of isotopic tracers and its use in the investigations of intermediary metabolism as a graduate student with Hans Clarke. Rittenberg and Bloch initiated a systematic study of the utilization of labeled acetic acid for cholesterol synthesis in animal tissues. They were able to demonstrate that acetate was important in the biosynthesis of the aliphatic side chain and the tetracyclic moiety of sterol molecules.

At the University of Chicago, Bloch's research objective became the establishment of the origin of all carbon atoms of the cholesterol skeleton. Analysis of the pattern of distribution would presumably provide clues to the biosynthetic pathway that led to cholesterol. Early evidence suggested that a two-carbon metabolite of acetate was the principal building block of cholesterol. Further experimental evidence was obtained by exploiting mutants of *Neurospora crassa* isolated by E. L. Tatum that were deficient in pyruvate metabolism and required an exogenous source of acetate. When the mutant mold was grown on labeled acetate, the labeling pattern of ergosterol provided strong evidence for Bloch's hypothesis. His general hypothesis for the biosynthesis of cholesterol began to take the general outline: acetate → isoprenoid intermediate squalene → cyclization process → cholesterol. To verify this hypothesis, he tried to demonstrate the formation of squalene from labeled acetate in the shark. This apparently peculiar choice of experimental animal was based on the fact that this species accumulates very large amounts of the hydrocarbon squalene. It also called for an excursion to the Biological Station in Bermuda. Unfortunately, the first experiments with intact sharks and shark liver presented technical difficulties and were unsuccessful. Experiments carried out with R. G. Langdon back at Chicago with the more mundane rat liver system successfully demonstrated squalene biosynthesis from radioactive acetate. Labeled squalene was then used to show that this hydrocarbon served as a precursor of cholesterol in intact animals.

Putting his many years of research into perspective, Bloch predicted that future research on terpene and sterol biosynthesis, like all biosynthetic studies, would progress from the level of intact animals or whole cells to in vitro experimentation. Biochemists had learned that it was only possible to understand reaction mechanisms by the use of isolated, purified enzymes. Understanding the enzymology of the cholesterol pathway would provide a rational approach to broader questions of metabolic regulation. Such questions transcended narrow academic curiosity because basic research was essential to an understanding of the complex environmental, dietary, and hormonal factors that influenced the rate of cholesterol synthesis and the diseases associated with lipid metabolism. Moreover, comparative biochemistry would shed light on the role sterols play as structural elements of the cell. Because the sterols were not found in bacteria or blue-green algae, it seemed that the development of the sterol biosynthetic pathway indicated an evolutionary division between primitively organized cells lacking various membrane-bound intracellular organelles and more complex, differentiated cells (Bloch 1964, 96–98).

More than twenty years after winning the Nobel Prize Bloch continues to find the question of the evolutionary relationships of anaerobic versus aerobic life-styles an intriguing area for research and speculation. He suggests that "Fitness for biological function, not chance, appears to be the driving force for structural modifications of a biomolecule." Bloch is intrigued by the concept that Darwinian evolution may be "manifest at the level of small molecules as well as at the organismic and genomic level." In the case of cholesterol, it is possible that the molecule originally served as a hormonelike signal calling for the assembly of certain cell membranes. This is a question Bloch hopes to pursue in further researches. In reflecting on the rewards and privileges of a career in science, Bloch still finds the enterprise that is science a source of "glorious entertainment" (Bloch 1987, 19).

Other honors awarded to Bloch include the Medal of the Société de Chimie Biologique (1958), the Fritzsche Award, American Chemical Society (1964), the Distinguished Service Award, University of Chicago School of Medicine (1964), the Centennial Science Award, University of Notre Dame, Indiana (1965), the Cardano Medal, Lombardy Academy of Sciences (1965), and the William Lloyd Evans Award, Ohio State University (1968). Bloch is the recipient of honorary degrees from the universities of Uruguay (1966), Brazil (1966), and Nancy (1966), Columbia University (1967), Technische Hochschule, Munich (1968), and Brandeis University (1970).

Bloch is a member of the American Chemical Society, the National Academy of Sciences, the American Academy of Arts and Sciences, the American Society of Biological Chemists, the Harvey Society, and the American Philosophical Society, an honorary member of the Lombardy Academy of Sciences, and a senior fellow of the Australian Academy of Science. He was president of the American Society of Biological Chemists (1967); chairman of the Section of Biochemistry, National Academy of Sciences (1966–69); and chairman of the National Committee for the International Union of Biochemistry (1968).

LOIS N. MAGNER

Selected Bibliography

PRIMARY SOURCES

Berg, B., D. Rittenberg, and K. Bloch. 1943. "Biological Conversion of Cholesterol to Cholic Acid." *Journal of Biological Chemistry* 149: 511–17.

Bloch, Konrad, and D. Rittenberg. 1944. "The Utilization of AcOH for Fatty Acid Synthesis." *Journal of Biological Chemistry* 154:311–12.

Langdon, R. G., and K. Bloch. 1953. "Biosynthesis of Squalene." *Journal of Biological Chemistry* 200:129–34.

Bloch, Konrad. 1960. *Lipid Metabolism.* New York: Wiley.

———. 1964. "The Biological Synthesis of Cholesterol." Nobel Lecture, December 11, 1964. Reprinted in *Nobel Lectures, Physiology or Medicine*, vol. 4 (1963–1970), 78–102. Amsterdam: Elsevier, 1972.

———. 1987. "Summing Up." *Annual Review of Biochemistry* 56:1–19.

SECONDARY SOURCES

Wolstenholme, G. E. W., and M. O'Connor, eds. 1955. *CIBA Foundation Symposium on Biosynthesis of Terpenes and Sterols.* London: Churchill.

Kennedy, E. P., and F. H. Westheimer. 1964. "Nobel Laureates: Bloch and Lynen Win Prize in Medicine and Physiology." *Science* 146:504–6.

Fruton, Joseph S. 1972. *Molecules and Life. Historical Essays on the Inter-*

play of Chemistry and Biology. New York: Wiley-Interscience.

Erwin, J. A., ed. 1973. *Lipids and Biomembranes of Eukaryotic Microorganisms.* New York: Academic Press.

Florkin, Marcel, and E. H. Stotz. 1975. *Comprehensive Biochemistry.* Vol. 31, *A History of Biochemistry*, Part 3, "History of the Identification of the Sources of Free Energy in Organisms." Amsterdam: Elsevier.

BARUCH SAMUEL BLUMBERG
1976

Baruch Samuel Blumberg was born on July 28, 1925, in New York City. A virologist, Blumberg won the Nobel Prize in 1976, jointly with D. Carleton Gajudsek, for his discovery of the Australian antigen associated with hepatitis B virus, which led to the development of successful diagnostic, vaccination, and blood screening programs for this dangerous disease. At the time of the award, Blumberg was associate director of the Institute for Cancer Research at the Fox Chase Cancer Center in Philadelphia, a position he had held since 1964. Blumberg married a fellow medical student, Jean Liebesman, in 1954; they have two sons, George Micah Connor and Noah Francis Baruch, and two daughters, Jane Emily and Anne Francesca.

The son of Meyer Blumberg, a lawyer, and Ida Simonoff, Blumberg enlisted in the navy in 1943, and was assigned to study physics at Union College in Schenectady. He received a B.S. in 1946 and entered graduate school at Columbia, again working in physics and mathematics. He had, however, become increasingly intrigued by medical and biochemical problems and, in 1947, at his father's urging, he changed course and began the study of medicine at Columbia's College of Physicians and Surgeons.

Blumberg earned his M.D. in 1951 and remained in New York to complete his internship and residency at Bellevue. In 1953 he began postdoctoral work in the Arthritis Division at Columbia-Presbyterian, where he studied hyaluronic acid, the substance responsible for the gelatious consistency of connective tissues and the vitreous humor of the eyes.

In 1955 Blumberg won a fellowship to study biochemistry at Balliol College, Oxford University, where he continued his studies of hyaluronic acid. He also became interested in the problem of ethnic variation in susceptibility and resistance to different diseases. Epidemiologists had speculated that such variation might be related to genetic protein variations (polymorphisms) of the blood, but no specific mechanism was known. Blumberg developed considerable skill in identifying and distinguishing very tiny protein variations through electrophoresis. His interest was further stimulated by a visit to Surinam, with its several ethnic populations, in 1957.

Blumberg earned a Ph.D. from Oxford in 1957. Upon returning to the United States, he became chief of the geographic medicine and genetics section of the National Institutes of Health, where he served for seven years. This position gave him access to data and specimens from genetic populations all over the world. His Balliol colleague, Anthony C. Allison, joined him in 1960.

Blumberg and Allison decided to look at blood samples from patients who had received multiple transfusions. They reasoned that these individuals would have received some blood proteins of a different phenotype, which would have generated an antibody response. They obtained the serum samples and reacted them with those from a group of nontransfused blood donors from different geographic areas. One of the transfusion samples was found to have an antibody for several of the donor sera. It appeared to react specifically with antigenic low-density beta-lipoproteins.

Blumberg continued testing serum for antigen systems, hoping to identify one or more reactions to very specific proteins. In one of these experiments in 1963, two transfusion samples from American hemophiliacs reacted against one specific sample from a donor group of twenty-four. The sample in question had been taken from an Australian aborigine; the responsible antigen was a protein combined with only a small lipid component. Blumberg gave it the name "Australia antigen" (Au). This antigen was found to be relatively rare in Europe and North America, but prevalent in Asian and African populations and in people who had received multiple transfusions.

In 1964 Blumberg left NIH to accept the position of associate director of clinical research at the Institute for Cancer Research of the Fox Chase Cancer Center in Philadelphia. Here he had the opportunity to combine his diverse talents in physics, medicine, and biochemistry.

He continued testing patients for the presence of the Au protein. It was often identified in the blood of leukemia victims and Blumberg thought it might be the basis for a diagnostic test. In 1966, however, a patient in Jeanes Hospital tested positive for Au. (Jeanes is the Fox Chase Center hospital.) The patient, who had previously tested negative, soon developed chronic anicteric hepatitis.

Blumberg, A. M. Prince at the New York Blood Center, and K. Okochi at Tokyo University Hospital embarked on a long series of carefully controlled experiments, which established the connection between Au and serum hepatitis, or hepatitis B. Au was identified in 1966 as the surface antigen of the double shelled hepatitis B virus and renamed HBsAg (hepatitis B virus antigen). This discovery led by 1969 to the development of highly specific diagnostic tests for the virus, which had previously been virtually undetectable during its long incubation period.

The identification of HBsAg also raised hopes for the conquest of this major public health problem. There are about one hundred million hepatitis B carriers in the world, perhaps one million in the United States. The virus has now been linked as well to primary carcinoma of the liver, one of the world's most common cancers. Transfusion recipients often contracted hepatitis B; after Blumberg's work, blood banks had a way to test donated blood for the virus. These tests have now virtually eliminated all but a small number of transfusion hepatitis cases, which are believed to be related to a type C virus.

In the 1970s Blumberg and his colleague Irving Millman introduced a vaccine, developed from the sera of patients with the HBsAg antigen, to prevent hepatitis B infection. The vaccine is in wide use among high risk individuals, particularly health care workers and newborn children of infected mothers. It has also been administered in mass newborn vaccinations in Taiwan, Korea, Gambia, and the People's Republic of China. These national campaigns are designed to reduce the risk of primary liver cancer.

Blumberg became professor of medicine and anthropology at the University of Pennsylvania in 1977 and subsequently was named vice president of population oncology at the Fox Chase Institute. He has continued his work on genetic polymorphisms and antigen systems, noting that the significant practical applications of HBsAg were the result of an esoteric basic research investigation. But his many interests, in physics, virology, molecular biology, anthropology, history, and philosophy, have always enabled him to grasp the broad social context of his laboratory work. He has recently applied his unique perspective to the social and scientific phenomenon of AIDS and presented insightful lectures on the disease and its implications for society.

Blumberg left Fox Chase in 1989, at the age of sixty-four, to become master of Balliol College, the first American and the first scientist to hold this ancient and prestigious title. Among the many other honors he has received for his work are the Eppger Prize from the University of Freiburg (1973), the Distinguished Achievement Award in Modern Medicine (1975), the Gairdner Foundation International Award (1975), the Karl Landsteiner Memorial Award from the American Association of Blood Banks (1975), and the Scopus Award from the American Friends of Hebrew University (1977).

JAMES POUPARD
MARCIA MELDRUM

Selected Bibliography

PRIMARY SOURCES

Blumberg, Baruch S., ed. 1962. *Conference on Genetic Polymorphisms and Geographic Variations in Disease. Proceedings.* New York: Grune & Stratton.

Blumberg, Baruch S., H. J. Alter, and S. Visnich. 1965. "A New Antigen in Leukemia Sera." *Journal of the American Medical Association* 191: 541–46.

Blumberg, Baruch S., W. T. London, and A. I. Sutnick. 1969. "Relation of Australia Antigen to Virus of Hepatitis." *Bulletin of Pathology* 10:164.

Blumberg, Baruch S. 1982. *Primary Hepatocellular Carcinoma and Hepatitis B Virus.* Chicago: Yearbook Medical Publishers.

———. 1984. "The Australia Antigen Story." In *Hepatitis B: The Virus, the Disease, and the Vaccine,* by Irving Millman, Toby Eisenstein, and Baruch S. Blumberg, 5–31. New York: Plenum Press.

———. 1988. "Hepatitis B Virus and the Carrier Problem." *Social Research* 55 (Autumn):401–12.

SECONDARY SOURCES

Rensberger, Boyce. 1976. "Baruch Samuel Blumberg." *New York Times* (October 15):13.

Sullivan, Walter. 1976. "Both Laureates Found Major Clues in Studies of Primitive Tribesmen." *New York Times* (October 15):13.

Melnick, Joseph L. 1976. "The 1976 Nobel Prize in Physiology or Medicine." *Science* 194 (November 26): 927–28.

1977. "Blumberg, Baruch Samuel." In *Current Biography Yearbook,* 72–74. New York: H. W. Wilson.

Millman, Irving. 1984. "The Development of the Hepatitis B Vaccine." In *Hepatitis B: The Virus, the Disease, and the Vaccine,* by Irving Millman, Toby Eisenstein, and Baruch S. Blumberg, 137–47. New York: Plenum Press.

JULES BORDET *1919*

Jules Jean Baptiste Vincent Bordet was born on June 13, 1870, at Soignies, a small Belgian town about twenty-five miles from Brussels. His father, Charles Bordet, had begun his career as a schoolteacher at the Ecole Moyenne at Soignies, and there married Célestine Vandenabeele. The couple had three boys: the eldest died in infancy, the second son, Charles, was born in 1868, and Jules in 1870. In 1874 the family moved to Shaerbeek, a district of Brussels, where the father had received a teaching appointment at the Ecole Moyenne. Both boys attended this school, proceeding to the Athénée royal de Bruxelles for their secondary education. In 1886 Jules Bordet entered the University of Brussels as a medical student and received his doctorate of medicine in 1892, the same year as his brother Charles. While still a student, Jules Bordet had investigated the adaptation of viruses to vaccinated organisms and for this work was awarded a scholarship by the Belgian government (Bordet 1892). This award enabled him to go to Paris in 1894 to become laboratory assistant to Élie Metchnikoff at the Pasteur Institute. Here Jules Bordet embarked upon the research that would earn him the 1919 Nobel Prize for "his discoveries in regard to immunity."

From 1894 until 1901 Bordet investigated mechanisms of immunity at the Pasteur Institute. He then moved back to Brussels to become director of the newly founded Institute Antirabique et Bactériologique (authorized by Madame Pasteur to be renamed the Institut Pasteur de Brabant in 1903). In 1899 he married Marthe Levoz, who would survive him after an exceptionally happy union of more than sixty years. The couple had three children, two daughters and a son. From 1907 until 1935 Bordet was professor of bacteriology at the University of Brussels. Endowed with unusual energy, he was able to combine teaching and administration of the Institut Pasteur de Brabant with active research not only on the antigen-antibody reaction but also on blood agglutination and coagulation, on anaphylaxis, and on the morphology of bacteria. He and Gengou discovered the whooping cough bacillus in 1906. When research became impracticable during the German occupation of Belgium in World War I, Bordet wrote his *Traité de l'Immunité dans les Maladies Infectieuses*, published in 1920, with a second edition in 1939. He continued as director of the Institut Pasteur de Brabant until 1940, when he was succeeded by his son Paul. He remained actively interested in science during his retirement and frequently visited the institute although failing eyesight now prevented active laboratory work. He and his wife lived in an apartment near the university, and he remained in good health until the last few months of his life. Bordet died peacefully, surrounded by his family, on April 6, 1961.

Debates about the mechanism of immunity had been raging since the early 1880s. One theory, the humoral one, held that immunity was due to the production in the blood plasma or other body fluids of substances inimical to the infective agent. An alternative theory, introduced by Metchnikoff, attributed immunity to cellular activity, particularly to the capacity of large white blood cells, or phagocytes, to ingest foreign bodies. When Bordet arrived at the Institute Pasteur in 1894, the German bacteriologist Richard Pfeiffer had just published findings apparently devastating to the phagocytic theory. He had demonstrated that when cholera vibrios were injected into the peritoneum of guinea pigs immunized against this microorganism, the vibrios disintegrated within about thirty minutes. No such lysis happened in unvaccinated animals unless these received cholera antiserum along with the intraperitoneal injection of cholera vibrios. Pfeiffer's experiments were confirmed at the Institut Pasteur, obliging Metchnikoff to admit that at least on some occasions the lysis of bacteria could occur in the absence of phagocytes (Delaunay 1962, 85).

The "Pfeiffer phenomenon" could be duplicated in vitro. However, if cholera antiserum was heated to 70° C for one hour, it no longer induced lysis in the test tube while continuing to do so in the living animal. Metchnikoff himself further complicated the problem by showing that lysis would occur in vitro if peritoneal fluid was added to the mixture of cholera vibrios and heated cholera antiserum (Metchnikoff 1895). He also asked his new assistant, Jules Bordet, to look further into the matter.

The same year Bordet showed that blood serum could replace peritoneal exudate, so demonstrating that the heat-sensitive substance involved in cholera vibrio lysis was nonspecific in nature (Bordet 1895). Bordet also established 55° C as the critical temperature above which the heat labile substance was destroyed. To explain the phenomena thus far uncovered, he suggested that bacteriolysis was due to the presence of two distinct substances. One, which he named "alexine" (a term originally introduced by Hans Büchner, as mentioned below), was present in the serum of all animals whether immunized or not, was inactivated by heat, and was nonspecific. The other was a specific substance, resistant to heat, responsible for the special characteristics of immune sera, and capable of acting even at a very reduced dosage level.

Now far more concerned with elucidating the mechanism of lysis than with the original humoral versus cellular argument, Bordet was inspired to find a simpler experimental model for lysis than the classical one involving suspensions of cholera vibrios whose behavior could only be studied microscopically (Collard 1976, 125). He began to study hemolysis, the destruction of red blood cells that frequently occurred when defribinated mammalian blood was transfused into another species. This reaction could be read with the naked eye in the test tube since, after standing for a while, hemolysed blood became uniformly red whereas normal blood separated into a layer of clear serum overlying the deposited red cells. In the early 1890s G. Daremberg and Hans Büchner coined the term "alexine" to designate the protective, heat-sensitive substance involved and seems to have believed that it could act on its own. Bordet developed a simple method for increasing the hemolytic power of sera and then established that, like bacteriolysis, specific hemolysis only occurred in the presence of two substances, one to be found in the heated serum of the injected animal, the other in the unheated normal serum of almost any animal. He called the first, heat-resistant component, "substance sensibilisatrice," while the heat labile one was Büchner's alexine. The specific sensibilizing substance induced red blood cells or microorganisms to absorb alexine which provoked either hemolysis or bacteriolysis, according to the system in question (Bordet 1901).

Bordet's experiments were confirmed and his explanation of bacteriolysis and hemolysis found rapid acceptance. However, already by 1900, Paul Ehrlich was proposing a slightly different model for the reaction between the two components and had renamed them. Alexine became "complement," a name that would endure, and the heat stable specific factor became the "amboreceptor," soon to be permanently labelled "antibody."

Now Bordet and Octave Gengou, his brother-in-law and frequent collaborator, demonstrated the practical importance of the theory of lysis. The first application was the development of a test for specific antibodies. Having shown that during hemolysis complement became firmly fixed to red cells sensitized with specific antibody, they used complement fixation as a means of differentiating between normal serum and that containing specific antibodies. When red blood cells were added to normal serum mixed with a suspension of cholera vibrios, the vibrios remained active while the red cells were hemolysed. But when previously sensitized animal serum was used, the vibrios were destroyed while the red cells remained intact since the complement had been "fixed" or removed during lysis of the microorganisms. Until 1901 the isolation of pathogenic microorganisms in body fluids or tissues had been the only way of establishing infection, but now Bordet and Gengou showed that their simple method of serodiagnosis (as mentioned above, the presence or absence of hemolysis could be detected with the naked eye) was effective for diseases such as cholera, anthrax, and typhoid fever (Bordet and Gengou 1901). Other researchers extended the application of the complement fixation test, the most well-known example being August von Wassermann's test for the detection of syphilis, announced in 1906.

Another application of the antibody theory was the discovery in 1906, by Bordet and Gengou, of the organism responsible for whooping cough. Thus far no pathogen had been firmly indicted because, by the time diagnosis was made, secondary infection had usually set in to confuse the bacterial picture. In 1906 Bordet isolated a coccobacillus in the sputum of his son in the early stage of pertussis. He and Gengou then found that children suffering from whooping cough developed a specific antibody to this bacillus two to three weeks after infection, good evidence that it was indeed the organism responsible (Bordet and Gengou 1906). They also extracted an endotoxin and prepared a vaccine against the whooping cough bacillus.

The above represents a mere summary of the discoveries for which Bordet was rewarded with the Nobel Prize. His active mind found other problems to investigate, including blood coagulation that he researched from 1901 until 1920, and after that date he became keenly interested in the action of recently discovered bacteriophages. However, his earlier research on lysis would remain his most important work for it not only advanced theoretical understanding of immunity but also provided the basis for simple blood tests to detect the presence of specific antibodies. Today complement fixation tests are most widely used in the diagnosis of viral diseases.

In addition to the Nobel Prize for 1919, Bordet received numerous awards and honors including election as a foreign member to the Royal Society of London, the Institut de France, the Académie de Paris, and the National Academy of Sciences in the United States. In his *History of Bacteriology*, published in 1938, William Bulloch stated that Bordet was then regarded "by common consent . . . as the greatest living exponent and worker on immunology" (Bulloch 1938, 354).

ELIZABETH LOMAX

Selected Bibliography

PRIMARY SOURCES

Bordet, Jules. 1892. "Adaption des virus aux organismes vaccinés." *Annales de l'Institut Pasteur* 6:328–34.

———. 1895. "Les leucocytes et les propriétés actives du serum chez les vaccinés." *Annales de l'Institut Pasteur* 9:462–506.

———. 1901. "Sur la mode d'action des sérums cytolytiques et sur l'unité de l'alexine dans un même sérum." *Annales de l'Institut Pasteur* 15:303–18.

Bordet, Jules, and Octave Gengou. 1901. "Sur l'existence de substances sensibilatrices dans la plupart des sérums antimicrobiens." *Annales de l'Institut Pasteur* 15:289–302.

———. 1906. "Le microbe de la coqueluche." *Annales de l'Institut Pasteur* 20:731–41.

Bordet, Jules, et al. 1909. *Studies in Immunity.* Collected and translated by Frederick P. Gay. New York: Wiley.

Bordet, Jules. 1920. *Traité de l'Immunité2 dans les Maladies Infectieuses.* Paris: Masson.

SECONDARY SOURCES

Metchnikoff, Élie. 1895. "Etudes sur l'immunitél, 6ème mém. Sur la destruction extracellulaire des bactéries dans l'organisme." *Annales de l'Institut Pasteur* 9: 369–461.

———. 1968. *Immunity in Infective Diseases.* Translated by F. G. Binnie. New York: Johnson Reprint Corporation.

Bulloch, William. 1938. *The History of Bacteriology.* London: Oxford University Press.

Dalcq, A. M. 1961. "Notice biographique sur M. Jules Bordet, Membre honoraire (13–6–1870—6–4–1961)." *Bulletin de l'Académie royale de Médecine de Belgique*, 7th ser., 1:352–65.

Beumer, Jacques. 1962. "Jules Bordet 1870–1961." *Journal of General Microbiology* 29:1–13.

Delaunay, Albert. 1962. *L'Institut Pasteur: des Origines à Aujourd'hui.* Paris: Editions France Empire.

Bordet, Paul. 1968. "Jules Bordet." In *Florilège des Sciences en Belgique pendant le XIX Siècle et le Début du XXe*, 1036–67. Brussels: Académie royale de Belgique.

Delaunay, Albert. 1971. "Jules Bordet, Prix Nobel de Médecine 1919, et l'Institut Pasteur." *Histoire de la Médecine* 21:2–45.

Collard, Patrick. 1976. *The Development of Microbiology*. Cambridge: Cambridge University Press.

DANIEL BOVET 1957

Major discoveries made by Bovet are connected with three simple substances produced in the human and mammalian body and exerting important actions on the vascular and other systems and on skeletal muscles: epinephrine (adrenaline), histamine, and acetylcholine, collectively called biogenic amines. Other fields to which Bovet decisively contributed are chemotherapeutic or anti-infectious drugs and psychobiology.

Daniel Bovet was born on March 23, 1907 in Neuchâtel, a town in the French-speaking part of Switzerland. His mother was Amy Babut, his father was the psychologist Pierre Bovet, who in 1912 was elected as professor of pedagogy in Geneva. Daniel Bovet began his education in Neuchâtel, and then pursued studies in biology at the University of Geneva, from which he graduated in 1927. He stayed on for postgraduate work in physiology with F. Battelli and in zoology with E. Guyénot. A thesis on the influence of the nervous system on organ regeneration earned him a Ph.D. in 1929. In the same year Bovet began his career in pharmacological research under the inspiring leadership of E. Fourneau at the famous Pasteur Institute in Paris, first as an assistant and from 1939 on as head of the Laboratory of Therapeutic Chemistry.

During this time he married Filomena Nitti, daughter of a former Italian prime minister and sister of Bovet's coworker, the bacteriologist Federico Nitti. Filomena Nitti has closely and continuously collaborated as a scientist with her husband. The couple had a son, Daniele, who became a professor of information science at the University of Rome.

In 1947 Bovet was given the opportunity to organize and become head of a laboratory of therapeutic chemistry at the Istituto Superiore di Sanità in Rome. He has remained in Italy ever since, adding Italian to his Swiss citizenship. In 1957 he was awarded the Nobel Prize for Physiology or Medicine. When the research climate at the Istituto Superiore di Sanità deteriorated as a consequence of political intrigues in 1964, Bovet temporarily moved to Sardinia to head the Department of Pharmacology at the University of Sassari Medical School. In 1965 he was a visiting professor at the University of California in Los Angeles. From Sassari he returned to Rome in 1969 to become director of a new laboratory of psychobiology and psychopharmacology of the National Research Council until 1976. He also held a professorship for psychobiology at the University of Rome which, when he reached age seventy-five, was transformed into an honorary professorship. Bovet and his wife retired in Rome, where they actively follow scientific, political, and other events.

As early as 1904, T. R. Elliott found that the action of epinephrine (adrenaline) mimicked a stimulation of the sympathetic nervous system. In 1910 H. H. Dale described the antiadrenergic (sympatholytic) action of ergot alkaloids. When Bovet joined Fourneau's laboratory at the Pasteur Institute in 1929, a search for antimalarial drugs was going on. It was out of this search that Bovet in 1933 happened to find the first synthetic sympatholytic or antiadrenergic drug, Prosympal. More antiadrenergic compounds were then found within other chemical series. To be sure, these early antiadrenergic drugs only found temporary use in general medicine; however, they must be seen as a first step in the development of drugs against hypertension that reached maturity some twenty years later. The most important aspect of Bovet's early studies was that the investigation of a variety of compounds from different chemical series disclosed structural requirements for molecules to act as epinephrinelike agonists or as competitive antagonists.

In 1910 H. H. Dale found that histamine mimicked an anaphylactic shock, and by 1930 the role of histamine in allergy had become generally accepted: the release of stored histamine in the body or its injection into an animal leads to a variety of allergic symptoms or even to a fatal anaphylactic shock. If ergot alkaloids or synthetic antiadrenergic agents block the effects of epinephrine, why then should it not be possible to find compounds with antihistaminic properties? With this goal in mind Bovet started a project in 1937, testing compounds originally synthesized as antiadrenergic agents for antagonism of histamine-induced intestinal contraction and prevention of anaphylactic shock. Once more, success was soon at hand: a weak antiadrenergic and antihistaminic compound, codenamed F-929. This and more encouraging results served as an igniting spark for the search in other laboratories for safe antihistamines that enabled treatment for such allergic diseases as urticaria, hay fever, and edema. The first of these drugs, Antergan, appeared in 1942 and was followed by Bovet's pyrilamine (mepyramine, Neo-antergan), which is still used. A particular aspect of this discovery was the fact that no naturally occurring prototypes with antihistaminic action existed. Thousands of antihistamines were then synthesized worldwide, of which some hundred reached the market in the 1950s. Some of them also proved useful against travel sickness, nausea, and vomiting.

In the 1920s O. Loewi obtained evidence that acetylcholine is a chemical transmitter substance at numerous nerve endings. Acetylcholine was also the transmitter substance at the neuromuscular junction where it could be blocked by the arrow poison, curare. Tubocurarine, the active principle of curare, which antagonizes acetylcholine at the neuromuscular junction, was introduced into surgical anesthesia in 1942; however, it was not an ideal muscle relaxant and it was also hard to obtain and expensive. The need for improvement was obvious. During the mid-1940s Bovet's laboratory was investigating synthetic cholinergic and anticholinergic compounds, research that resulted in diethazine (Diparkol), one of the first synthetic drugs for treating Parkinson's disease. The goal of obtaining a synthetic curarelike drug was then reached by simplifying the complex structure of tubocurarine. The first compound found to have neuromuscular blocking properties was F 3381 in 1946. Further simplification of the structure then led to gallamine, which was followed in 1949 in Rome by succinylcholine. In contrast to the naturally occurring prototype, tubocararine, the number of synthetic compounds was unlimited and would even enable the synthesis of "tailor-made" drugs. This goal was clearly reached with Bovet's curarelike agents, gallamine and succinylcholine, which became widely used as adjuvants in surgical anesthesia, in tracheal intubation, electroconvulsive therapy, and in tetanus. Bovet's elaborate studies on structure-activity relationships not only helped the development of new curarelike agents but also became an important tool to map out cholinergic receptors. In addition to his research Bovet also developed a keen interest in the historical aspects of curare, from its use by the poison-compounding Indians of the Amazon to Claude Bernard's classic experiments.

The first synthetic chemotherapeutic or anti-infectious drugs were developed by P. Ehrlich, culminating with the syphilis remedy, arsphenamine (Salvarsan), in 1910. The next milestone in antibacterial therapy was Domagk's Prontosil in 1935. Bovet's first field of research after joining Fourneau in Paris was chemotherapy and resulted in an antimalarial drug, Rhodoquine. When Domagk published his discovery of Prontosil and its action on streptococcal diseases early in 1935, hectic activity broke out at the Pasteur Institute. The result was a publication appearing in November of the same year, with Bovet, Federico Nitti, and the chemists, Tréfouël and his wife, as authors. It contained the breathtaking news that the antistreptococcal action of Prontosil is due to its colorless metabolite, sulfanilamide, and it also indicated, based on clear-cut structure-activity relationships, which kinds of sulfonamides (i.e., sulfanilamide derivatives) are active.

The consequences of this classic text of only two pages cannot be overestimated. Sulfanilamide marked the end of Ehrlich's dye theory and of the older theory of chemotherapeutics as agents that strengthen defense mechanisms of the body. Sulfanilamide, a compound first synthesized in 1908, was not patentable and went immediately into cheap mass production, thereby preventing Prontosil from becoming a commercial success for the Bayer Company in Germany. The structure-activity relationships worked out by Bovet initiated the era of sulfonamide drugs, stimulating a true therapeutic revolution that was to save lives by the millions. Sulfonamides also initiated other classes of drugs, such as drugs for leprosy, oral antidiabetic drugs, mercury-free diuretics, and drugs against gout. The isolation and early production of penicillin by Florey and Chain in the 1940s was clearly influenced by the new optimism inspired by sulfonamides (as Fleming put it, "without sulfonamides no antibiotics"). And finally, the metabolic transformation of inactive Prontosil into active sulfanilamide was a first demonstration of bioactivation of a foreign compound, which was to bring the theory of detoxication to an end. Truly, this and related work made 1935 a focal point in the history of chemotherapy.

Bovet was active in the field of sulfonamides for over ten years. An early study on these drugs' mechanism of action led to the discovery of bacteriostasis. Sulfone drugs and antidiabetic sulfonamides have also originated at his laboratory.

In the 1950s it had become clear that biogenic amines and neurotransmitters were also present and active in the central nervous system. This was the beginning of a multidisciplinary research on the central nervous system which led to a host of discoveries in neurophysiology, biochemistry, and pharmacology. When Bovet described the central effects of antihistaminic and anticholinergic phenothiazines in 1947, he made a contribution to the path that was soon to lead to chlorpromazine and other psychotropic drugs. From the late 1950s on and during much of his Italian period Bovet's main interest centered on the CNS and on research in psychobiology by pharmacological and other means. The main line of this research was the study of memory and learning and its genetic background. This required a change from classical pharmacology to methods of animal psychology, electroencephalographic and behavioral techniques, automation and electronics. Bovet was active and publishing in this field well into his seventies.

Few pharmacologists are lucky enough to develop a drug that will be introduced into therapy; fewer still will succeed in developing a prototype that will initiate a new class of drugs with a new medical indication. Bovet has created at least four such classes. One tends to forget that the early 1930s was a time without antibiotics and sulfonamides, without anticoagulants, antihistamines, antihypertensive and antitumor drugs, corticosteroids, curare-like agents, dopaminergic antiparkinsonian drugs, psychotropic drugs, and other major drug classes. There is good reason to assume that Bovet's greatest discovery was his contribution to the development of sulfonamides. Yet his Nobel Prize was conferred "for his discoveries relating to synthetic compounds that inhibit the action of certain body substances, and especially their action on the vascular system and the skeletal muscles." The omission of sulfonamides, deplorable as it is, can be explained by the fact that Domagk's 1939 Nobel Prize was given "for his discovery of the effects of the sulfonamides." Looking back from a safe historical distance, Domagk's Prontosil was a great discovery, based on Ehrlich's dye theory, a mass screening, and luck. Yet, it was the end of a development—dyes had no future. In contrast, Bovet's discovery was a new beginning, packed with future. The decisive battle against the scourge of infectious diseases was won by both Domagk and Bovet.

Even without any new drug discoveries, Bovet's contribution to pharmacology, laid down in over four hundred publications, would have been impressive. Until about 1930 pharmacology was largely oriented towards and even dominated by physiology. Bovet made "therapeutic chemistry" or "chemical pharmacology" a reality. What he wrote about Fourneau characterizes his own work to an even higher degree: "He raised therapeutical chemistry to the level of a true and great science, delivering it from empiricism and giving it a more systematic (and rational) direction."

His discoveries were recognized immediately. He was the recipient of eight awards before the Nobel Prize. After this event he was flooded with memberships in national academies and national orders as well as honorary degrees. However, overwhelming success did not corrupt the man, who remained extremely modest, gentle, and soft-spoken, yet by no means ignorant of the ways of the world, and determined in the pursuit of his scientific goals. At the zenith of his life, delivering his Nobel Lecture, he emphasized that "the work I now pursue with confidence, enthusiasm and love cannot be separated from that of my masters and colleagues." His warm enthusiasm was touching indeed. In the preface to his voluminous book on neuropharmacology he wishes that "nous voudrions pouvoir faire partager à nos lecteurs les joies, les émotions et surtout les promesses du chemin qui est le nôtre," and later in his life he muses about "la poesia della nostra ricerca."

Bovet's interests and outlook went far beyond his field of research. Looking into the future he saw pharmacology as a science in which foods, drugs, and poisons will have become integrated with the metabolism of endogenous compounds. Also, modification of physiological processes, achieved so far by pharmacologists, would in the future be done in general biology and genetics. Yet, he was fully aware that all progress involves new problems, and his keen interest in social and political aspects prevented him from believing that science would solve the major problems: "Unfortunately, in our century, two-thirds of the global population are illiterate and walk barefooted, 10 to 15 percent suffer from hunger, 33 to 40 percent do not have an adequate diet, 70 percent are not provided with sufficient water supply, and 80 percent lack adequate hygienic conveniences. Even the best drugs are ineffective for people living in very poor hygienic conditions. Our apprehension originates from the awareness that we are impotent against the priority of political and economic power."

M. H. BICKEL

Selected Bibliography

PRIMARY SOURCES

Tréfouël, J., J. Tréfouël, F. Nitti, and D. Bovet. 1935. "Activité du P-aminophénylsulfamide sur les Infections Streptococciques Expérimentales de la Souris et du Lapin." *Comptes Rendus de la Sociétié de la Biologie (Paris)* 120:756–58.

Bovet, D., and F. Bovet-Nitti. 1948. *Structure Chimique et Activité Pharmacodynamique des Médicaments du Système Nerveux Végétatif.* Basel, Switzerland: S. Karger.

Bovet, D. 1957. "The Relationships between Isosterism and Competitive Phenomena in the Field of Drug Therapy of the Autonomic Nervous System and that of the Neuromuscular Transmission." Nobel Lecture. Reprinted in *Nobel Lectures in Physiology or Medicine.* Vol. 3 (1942–1962):552–78. Amsterdam: Elsevier, 1964.

Bovet, D., F. Bovet-Nitti, and G. B. Marini-Bettòlo. 1959. *Curare and Curare-like Agents.* Amsterdam: Elsevier.

Bovet, D. 1965. *Notizie sull' operosità scientifica e elenco delle pubblicazioni.* Roma.

———. 1965. "Role of the Scientist in Modern Society." *Perspectives in Biology and Medicine* 8:533–45.

———. 1970. "Approche Biochimique et Psychobiologique de la Mémoire et de l'Apprentissage." In *La mémoire*, edited by D. Bovet *et al.*: 7–55. Paris: Presses Universitaires.

SECONDARY SOURCES

Bickel, M. H. 1988. "The Development of Sulfanomides (1932–1988) as a Focal Point in the History of Chemotherapy." *Gesnerus* (Swiss Journal of the History of Medicine and Sciences) 45:46–59.

MICHAEL STUART BROWN 1985

Michael Stuart Brown was born on April 13, 1941, in New York City. A physician, molecular geneticist, and medical educator, Brown is currently professor and director of the Center for Genetic Disease at the University of Texas Health Sciences Center. Brown's parents were Harvey and Evelyn Katz Brown. He married Alice Lapin in 1964; they have two daughters, Elizabeth Jane and Sara Ellen. Brown received the Nobel Prize jointly with Joseph L. Goldstein in 1985 for their work on the etiology of familial hypercholesterolemia and their discovery of the mechanism of receptor-mediated endocytosis, now believed to be a key process of cellular metabolism. Brown and Goldstein's work is remarkable both as a model of disease-specific research that illuminated a whole area of biologic medicine, and as one of the great creative research partnerships.

Brown received both his baccalaureate (in 1962) and his medical (in 1966) degrees from the University of Pennsylvania. As a medical student, he received the Frederick Packard Prize in Internal Medicine. He met Joseph Goldstein, a graduate of Southwestern Medical School, when both were residents at Massachusetts General Hospital from 1966 to 1968. They quickly discovered mutual interests in academic careers, molecular biology, and bridge.

In 1968 both men went to the National Institutes of Health as clinical associates. Brown worked in the digestive and hereditary disease branch, where he studied the action of enzymes in digestive metabolism. Earl R. Stadtman, chief of the Laboratory of Biochemistry in the National Heart, Lung, and Blood Institute, was one of those who directed and assisted his work (Sullivan 1985).

In 1971, at Goldstein's urging, Brown accepted a research fellowship at Southwestern University. He focused his work on cholesterol production until Goldstein rejoined him in 1972. The two men then agreed to begin collaborative research on cholesterol and cholesterol-related disease, and to focus in particular on homozygous familial hypercholesterolemia (FHC), which appeared to offer the best opportunity to isolate the crucial mechanism of cholesterol metabolism.

FHC was first identified as a hereditary disorder in 1939 by Carl Muller of Norway. Frederickson had isolated two forms: "heterozygous" and "homozygous." Heterozygous FHC is linked to a single defective gene and occurs in one of every five hundred people. Individuals with this disorder have a blood cholesterol level two to three times that of a normal person and a greatly increased risk of heart disease (75 percent in males, 45 percent in females). Homozygous FHC is far more rare (one in one million people) and more lethal. A child receiving a defective gene from both parents will develop blood cholesterol four to eight times the normal level and die of heart disease before the age of thirty.

During the period 1970–72, Goldstein had completed a two-year fellowship in medical genetics at the University of Washington in Seattle under Arno G. Motulsky, where he undertook an unselected retrospective study of five hundred heart attack survivors and their relatives. He found that 31 percent of these individuals had high blood fat level, 20 percent of which were genetically linked (Goldstein et al. 1973, 1533–43, 1544–68).

Cholesterol, the "Janus-faced molecule," is produced naturally by the liver and is essential to body functioning. Inside body cells it plays a critical role in cell growth and the production of hormones. The cholesterol gets to the cells from the bloodstream, where it is attached to water-soluble proteins, called lipoproteins, also released by the liver. As the lipoproteins circulate in the blood, cells absorb cholesterol needed to continue normal processes. However, if cholesterol is not absorbed quickly enough, or not completely, it spills into the blood tissues and attaches to the vascular walls. Now the molecules become deadly blockages in the arteries, causing angina, atherosclerosis, and coronary heart disease.

These facts were understood when Goldstein and Brown began their work. But the cell absorption process—and the reasons for its failure in hypercholesterolemia—was unknown.

The team worked with tissue cultures of the human skin cells from patients with genetic FHC defects and from normal individuals. Observing these cultured fibroblasts, they identified coated pits—the LDL receptors—on the cell surface. These pits attached LDLs—the low density lipoproteins with the highest proportion of fat—and then formed endocyte vesicles that drew the LDLs inside the cell and released the cholesterol.

In the normal cell, cholesterol intake resulted in the reduction of the number of pits and an increase in cholesterol processing with the cell. As the internal level dropped, the coated pits again appeared on the cell surface to attract LDLs. Brown and Goldstein identified and described this process—"receptor-mediated endocytosis"—in 1973 (Brown and Goldstein 1974, 5153–62).

Their work was of immediate and critical importance in our understanding of FHC. They had counted around 250,000 LDL receptors on the surface of the normal cells. FHC heterozygous cells have perhaps 40–50 percent of such receptors. FHC homozygous cells have few or none. The liver contains LDL receptors, which regulate the production of blood cholesterol, as well as the processing of dietary cholesterol. Again, FHC patients have greatly reduced numbers of liver receptors. In effect, they "overdose" on cholesterol (Brown and Goldstein 1975, 147–50).

The model of receptor-mediated endocytosis was quickly found by other researchers to be the key to more than twenty cellular mechanisms, including the processing of insulin, growth factor, and immune complexes. Thus Goldstein and Brown laid the groundwork for many future discoveries (Motulsky 1986, 127).

Their work had direct application in FHC chemotherapy. Cholestyramine had been used since the 1950s to treat hypercholesterolemia but the mechanism of its action was not understood. Moreover, the positive effects could not be sustained for long. The drug was now found to work by increasing the number of LDL receptors in the liver, enabling increased excretion of the excess cholesterol as bile acid. However, the increase in receptors naturally triggered an increase in cholesterol synthesis by the liver, which neutralized the first effect.

This led to the search for a drug that would work with cholestryamine by blocking the liver's excess production of cholesterol. An "anticholesterol enzyme" developed by Alfred W. Alberts of Merck, Sharpe and Dohme, was approved by the FDA in 1987 to be sold under the trade name Lovastatin. Goldstein and Brown conducted animal trials with Lovastatin that demonstrated its efficacy; but they have warned that its long-term effects and possible toxicity are not yet clear. Other treatment applications have included liver transplant, combined with Lovastatin therapy, in a young FHC homozygous patient; and, of course, diet therapy (Motulsky 1986, 127–28).

Blood cholesterol is internally produced, not synthesized from dietary cholesterol. The effect of high fat, high cholesterol dietary intake on internal synthesis is unclear. Goldstein and Brown contend, on the basis of their animal experiments, that high dietary cholesterol can cause the liver to reduce its internal LDL receptors, thus decreasing excretion and adding to the blood level. The National Institutes of Health recommendations for lowered fat and cholesterol in American diets (1984) are a result of their ideas and have certainly had major impact on popular understanding of heart disease, if not necessarily on popular habits.

Brown and Goldstein continue their research, working now on the complex genetic etiology of FHC. In 1985 their team succeeded in cloning and sequencing the LDL receptor gene. They also continue seeing patients and working with medical students and residents. At UTHSC, they are often referred to as "Brownstein" or "the Gemini twins." In their close partnership, they plan research jointly, publish together, and share the podium for oral presentations. Out of the hospital, they are partners at bridge.

Brown is also a sailing enthusiast. He enjoys jazz and folk music, in particular the songs of Ella Fitzgerald and Bob Dylan.

Brown was elected to the National Academy of Sciences in 1980, is a member of the board of scientific advisers of the James Coffin Clinical Fund, and a senior consultant to the Lucille P. Markey Trust. Among the many awards he and Goldstein have jointly received are the Pfizer Award (1976), the Passano Foundation Award (1978), the

Gairdner Foundation Award (1981), and the Lasker Award (1985).

MARCIA MELDRUM

Selected Bibliography

PRIMARY SOURCES

Goldstein, J. L., W. R. Hazzard, H. G. Schott, E. L. Bierman, A. G. Motulsky et al. 1973. "Hyperlipidemia in Coronary Heart Disease. 1. Lipid Levels in 500 Survivors of Myocardial Infarction." *Journal of Clinical Investigation* 52 (July):1533–43.

———. 1973. "Hyperlipidemia in Coronary Heart Disease. 2. Genetic Analysis of Lipid Levels in 176 Families and Delineation of a New Inherited Disorder, Combined Hyperlipidemia." *Journal of Clinical Investigation* 52 (July):1544–68.

Brown, Michael S., and Joseph L. Goldstein. 1973. "Familial Hypercholesteremia: Identification of a Defect in the Regulation of 3-Hydroxy-3-Methylglutary Coenzyme: A Reductase Activity Associated with Overproduction of Cholesterol." *Proceedings of the National Academy of Sciences* 70:2804–8.

———. 1974. "Binding and Degradation of Low Density Lipoproteins by Cultured Human Fibroblasts: Comparison of Cells from a Normal Subjects and from a Patient with Homozygous Familial Hypercholesterolemia." *Journal of Biological Chemistry* 249:5153–62.

———. 1974. "Development of a Cell Culture System for Study of the Basic Defect in Familial Hypercholesterolemia." In *Atherosclerosis 3: Proceedings of the Third International Symposium*, 422–25. Berlin: Springer-Verlag.

———. 1974. "Expression of the Familial Hypercholesterolemia Gene in Heterozygotes: Model for a Dominant Disorder in Man." *Transactions of the Association of American Physicians* 87:120–31.

Brown, Michael S., Joseph L. Goldstein, and M. J. E. Harrod. 1974. "Homozygous Familial Hypercholesterolemia: Specificity of the Biochemical Defect in Cultured Cells and Feasibility of Prenatal Detection." *American Journal of Human Genetics* 26:199–206.

Brown, Michael S., and Joseph L. Goldstein. 1975. "Familial Hypercholesterolemia: Biochemical, Genetic, and Pathophysiological Considerations." *Advances in Internal Medicine* 20:78–96.

———. 1975. "Familial Hypercholesterolemia: A Genetic Regulatory Defect in Cholesterol Metabolism." *American Journal of Medicine* 58: 147–50.

SECONDARY SOURCES

Sullivan, Walter. 1985. "Converging on a Nobel Prize." *New York Times* (October 15):C1.

Motulsky, Arno G. 1986. "The 1985 Nobel Prize in Physiology or Medicine." *Science* 231 (January 10): 126–29.

1987. "Goldstein, Joseph L." In *Current Biography Yearbook*, 208–11. New York: H. W. Wilson.

FRANK MACFARLANE BURNET
1960

Frank Macfarlane Burnet was the greatest biologist Australia has known, a pioneer in virology and the ecology of diseases. He proposed two key concepts in immunology; acquired immunological tolerance, for which he shared the Nobel prize in Medicine with Peter Medawar in 1960, and the clonal selection theory for antibody production.

Burnet was born in 1899 in Traralgon, a country town in the state of Victoria. He was the second of six children of Frank Burnet, a Scottish-born clerk of the Colonial Bank, and Hadassah Pollock Burnet, also from a Scottish immigrant family. Apart from two visits to London, Burnet spent his whole professional life in Australia, and he contributed greatly to establishing Australia as a top-ranked scientific country. He spent forty years developing his versatile genius at the Walter and Eliza Hall Institute, initially a modest research center at the University of Melbourne that he elevated to the level of a world-famous scientific institution. At this institute, he rose from senior resident in 1924 to assistant director in 1934 and finally to director in 1944, which he remained until his retirement in 1965.

Burnet attended Geelong College from 1913 to 1916, then went to Ormond College at the University of Melbourne. He was appointed senior resident in the Pathology Department of the Royal Melbourne Hospital, and then at the neighbouring Walter and Eliza Hall Institute, where he entered basic research just at the time when the differences between bacteria and viruses were becoming clear. He acquired his M.D. degree in 1924. In 1926 he received a Beit Fellowship for medical research and went to England to spend two years training in bacteriology at the Lister Institute. He earned his Ph.D. from the University of London in 1927.

Back from England in 1929, Burnet had to face the public emotion stirred by the death of 12 Australian children who had received diphtheria vaccinations. Burnet demonstrated that some batches had been contaminated by *Staphylococcus aureus*, which secretes a virulent toxin, and that the Bundaberg tragedy could have been easily prevented by the safe storage of vaccine stocks. Burnet's experimental approach to his examination of the tragedy showed the director of the Hall Institute that he had a great research worker in the making. For Burnet himself, the event was one of the first signals of Nature revealing its explosive power of multiplication.

Burnet's first extensive research was on bacteriophages, which he worked on from 1925 to 1937. He started by investigating poultry and cattle stools in his brother's dairy and was able to elaborate the first coherent classification of bacteriophages.

Pursuing research on viruses, Burnet returned to England in 1932 and settled with his family at Hampstead. He worked with Henry Dale at the National Institute of Medical Research at the time when influenza viruses were discovered. Burnet perfected the technique of virus culture on the membrane of the chick embryo and wrote a monograph about it. He subsequently taught generations of biologists how to passage a virus from one chick to another, and where the virus, as it grows, produces a solid focus or "pock" corresponding to one cell damaged by virus proliferation. The observation of these "pocks" stamped on Burnet's mind the image of an originally single cell that had multiplication potential—the future "clone."

When Burnet returned to Australia the study of influenza virus became the major focus of his institute. He believed that intensive teamwork was essential if the institute was to be competitive with the big scientific centers in the United States. He had always been interested in the changes in levels of virus virulence that occur after serial passages of a virus in another host. He investigated the diversity of influenza strains and their capacity for genetic recombination. He also studied their properties of agglutinating red blood cells. With memories of the scourge of World War I during the Second World War Burnet concentrated on trying to produce an effective live virus vaccine (which has yet to be produced).

Continuity was remarkable in Burnet's work, except when he had to respond to urgent biomedical problems. He took those opportunities to explore little-known diseases:
—Q (for "query") fever, a respiratory disease raging among slaughterhouse workers. Burnet isolated the causal organism, which was called *Rickettsia burneti* and was later found responsible for epidemics throughout the world.
—psittacosis, an infection of birds (captive parrots) easily transmitted to man;
—encephalitis, a mysterious epidemic of which occurred in the area surrounding the Murray River. The epidemic, as it turned out, was caused by a virus harbored by waterbirds and transmitted by mosquitoes.

In each case, Burnet accomplished a complete epidemiological study: the isolation and cultivation of virus, the ecological factors of growth and transmission, and the implementation of a preventive program including, if possible, vaccination. He encapsulated his encyclopedic knowledge in a book called *Biological Aspects of Infectious Diseases*, published in 1940. In this book, reedited in a popular version in 1972, Burnet not only provided the reader with first-hand knowledge on past and modern scourges but ventured to speculate about the future.

During the Bundaberg drama in 1929, the discovery of spontaneous bacterial multiplication had fostered Burnet's interest in the exponential rise of antibodies in rabbits immunized against staphylotoxin. His paper on this subject was rejected by the editors of a scientific journal and Burnet took a lesson from his failure (*Changing Patterns: an Atypical Autobiography*, Melbourne: Heinemann, 1968, p. 32). In 1941, while Australia was isolated from the rest of the world, Burnet published a manifesto for a new perspective on immunity, *The Production of Antibodies*. While he may have still adhered to the official goal of immunology—the study of antibodies—he urged the necessity of supplementing the exclusively chemical viewpoint with considerations of living cellular phenomena, and he went so far as to dismiss the chemical viewpoint as "a pseudochemical formulation" (Burnet 1941, 53). This monograph, published by his institute, can be viewed as a declaration of independence vis-à-vis immunochemists, whose views prevailed in the field of immunity.

In 1940, Burnet found himself unable to immunize newborn chickens against influenza viruses. He first ascribed this failure to the immaturity of the young, but later considered the phenomenon to be a positive one. Antibody production is not innate; it requires a learning process. More generally, "immunological reactions of every sort are the result of a process of 'training'" (Burnet 1941, 48).

In the 1940s, the accepted model for antibody formation was Linus Pauling's version of the "instructive" theory. Pauling postulated that the antigen impressed a specific pattern on a master antibody, a "neutral" globulin molecule; in short, the antigen acted as a "template." Burnet did not oppose the instructive view but put the emphasis on immunological memory. The antibody-producing mechanism, he said, "can be transmitted to descendant cells by some hereditary process" (Burnet 1941, 52), which was an appeal to the genetic makeup of the body.

The second edition of the book (with Frank Fenner) developed that viewpoint more forcefully. The idea was emerging of an early differentiation between "self" and "notself." Burnet not only opened a new theoretical vista, he also proposed an experimental program and ventured a prediction, "If in embryonic life expendable cells from a genetically distinct race are implanted and established, no antibody response should develop against the foreign cell antigen when the animal takes on independent existence" (Burnet and Fenner 1949, 76). Unlike Burnet, Peter Medawar was able to demonstrate experimental "tolerance" (Burnet coined the word) in animals immunized during their early life, and this coincidence brought them a joint Nobel Prize for Medicine.

The revolution in Burnet's thinking about immunology occurred around 1956. Burnet's adoption of a *selective* viewpoint illustrates his willingness to challenge the most entrenched convictions. In 1949, he had still held to the instructive theory with a new hypothesis founded on the analogy between antibody production and adaptive enzymes. In 1955, he had read a paper by Niels Jerne that developed a "selective hypothesis." Jerne postulated that every organism has a large set of natural antibodies, before immunization. The function of the antigen is only to "select" and stimulate the cell that produces the appropriate antibody. Burnet advanced this selective theory of antibody formation into a clonal selective theory. Cells bear receptors on their surface; when antigens bind to the specific receptors, cells proliferate and liberate antibodies. These proliferating cells are called clones, a term derived from the Greek word for a branching twig. In 1957, Gus Nossal of the institute furnished the experimental proof that antibody-producing cells could not make more than one kind of antibody. The new theory encountered opposition for several years, but clonal selection was finally accepted by the scientific community at the Cold Spring Harbor Symposium in 1967 and has remained the standard theory for immunologists.

The clonal theory accounted for natural tolerance. During a critical period in early life, any cell that encounters an antigen corresponding to the "self" is killed. Later in life, the failure of the mechanisms of self/notself differentiation can lead to serious disorders, the so-called autoimmune diseases, with production of antibodies directed against the organism's own constituents. The hypothesis of autoimmunity as a cause of disease, once judged obsolete, regained favor and was one of Burnet's axes of research after 1960.

Although over the years Burnet had often talked of the day when he would abandon virus research for immunity, only in 1957 did he make an official switch to immunology in his institute and deploy all his researchers in this study. He realized that he had exploited the purely biological approach to influenza virus genetics as far as it would go without adopting the methods of molecular biology, and he was very reluctant to cross the psychological barrier of "making genes."

Burnet investigated autoimmunity as the possible cause of chronic active hepatitis and a wide range of diseases of unknown causation. In 1959, he heard about an animal counterpart to human autoimmune disease in a strain of mice, New Zealand Black, which spontaneously produced autoantibodies. Although Burnet failed to throw real light on the pathological process, this animal model allowed him to test the beneficial effect of some chemotherapies and paved the way for human treatment.

The theory of clonal selection provided Burnet with a rich insight into biological phenomena. One important aspect was the notion of "forbidden clones," which he suggested as an explanation of self-tolerance. Another aspect was his idea of "immunological surveillance," or monitoring of cancer cells that might result from random mutations. These were logical extensions of his Darwinian evolutionary principle of selection to the understanding of disease and cell population interaction within the body.

Burnet's major characteristic as a scientist was curiosity and fascination for the diversity of the living world. As a schoolboy, he was a bug hunter and insect collector. He undertook all his research with tremendous enthusiasm and a desire to conquer. He was a pioneer in the true sense of the word, with a fascination for the wild and a strong attachment to the New World. He chose to be faithful to his Australian homeland, even dismissing a prestigious offer from Harvard University during his visit to America in 1959.

Burnet also displayed other characteristics in his work, such as his "ecological" mode of thought, reflecting his ability to integrate information from diverse fields in science; a broad curiosity and a holistic bent; and his remarkable capacity for theorizing, i.e., weaving various experimental data into bold syntheses. He used to say that he was interested in other people's data, but not in their theories, only his own. He thoroughly enjoyed integrating discrepant facts into imaginative constructs. He was always eager to review the literature that fed his quest for alternative views of the state of the field. Although he was a tireless bench worker, he can nonetheless be described as a theoretical biologist. Burnet saw no need to compartmentalize biology. His friend and successor as the head of the institute, Gus Nossal, has called him a "twentieth century Renaissance man" (Nossal 1987, 1).

As the years rolled by and Burnet became a world figure in biology, he made more and more pronouncements on the medical, biological and social problems confronting mankind. He tackled such formidable issues as cancer and aging, which he viewed as a failure of regulation in the organism. He discussed all popular topics such as sociobiology, eugenics, immigration, smoking and cancer, fluoride and dental decay, transplantation, and the future of science. He developed the pessimistic and controversial view that most discoveries relevant to human health had already been made—the theme of "the end of immunology" or the twilight of Science. This position may have reflected his depressive mood as he neared the end of his life. Burnet died of cancer in 1985 at Port Favrit. Happily, he was spared a long period of pre-death dependency and was mentally acute until he lost consciousness.

Burnet's marriage to Linda Druce, a graduate of Melbourne University, had been very happy. He was shy, but she is said to have stimulated his desire for communication with his fellow man. They had a son and three daughters. Burnet's first wife died in 1973 and three years later he married Hazel Jenkin.

As a medically oriented scientist, Burnet had a strong interest in public health. He worked with WHO and acted as consultant on a wide range of topics, including the dangers of nuclear and biological warfare. He was president of the Australian Academy of Science and chairman of the Commonwealth Foundation. Burnet received the Royal Medal (1947) and the Copley Medal (1959) of the Royal Society of London, which elected him a fellow in 1947. He was knighted in 1951, became a member of the Royal College of Surgeons of England in 1953 and received the Order of Merit in 1958. Looking at his unrelenting activity in numerous domains of biology leaves one with the exceptional sense of a man who knew "happiness in science."

ANNE MARIE MOULIN

Selected Bibliography

PRIMARY SOURCES

Burnet, F. Macfarlane. 1941. *The Production of Antibodies.* Melbourne: Macmillan; 2nd ed., with F. Fenner, 1949.

———. 1957. "A Modification of Jerne's Theory Using the Concept of Clonal Selection." *Australian Journal of Science* 20:67–68.

———. 1959. *The Clonal Selection Theory of Acquired Immunity.* Nashville: Vanderbilt University Press.

Burnet, F. Macfarlane, and I. R. Mackay. 1963. *Auto-immune Diseases: Pathogenesis, Chemistry and Therapy.* Springfield: Charles C. Thomas.

Burnet, F. Macfarlane. 1964. "Immunological recognition of self." Nobel Prize Lecture. Reprinted in *Nobel Lectures in Physiology or Medicine*, vol. 3 (1942–1962), 689–701. Amsterdam: Elsevier, 1964.

———. 1968. *Changing Patterns: An Atypical Autobiography.* Melbourne: Heinemann.

———. 1969. *Self and Notself.* Melbourne: Melbourne University Press.

———. 1970. *Immunological Surveillance.* Oxford: Pergamon Press.

———. 1971. *Walter and Eliza Hall Institute 1915–1970.* Melbourne: Melbourne University Press.

Burnet, F. Macfarlane, and D. O. White. 1972. *Natural History of Infectious Disease.* Cambridge: Cambridge University Press.

Burnet, F. Macfarlane. 1976. *Immunity, Aging and Cancer: Medical Aspects of Mutation and Selection.* San Francisco: Freeman.

———. 1978. "Clonal Selection and After." In *Theoretical Immunology*, G. I. Bell ed. New York: Dekker.

———. 1979. *Credo and Comment: A Scientist Reflects.* Melbourne: Melbourne University Press.

SECONDARY SOURCES

Ada, G. L. 1989. In P. M. Mazumdar, ed., *Immunology 1930–1980, Essays on the History of Immunology*, 33–40. Toronto: Wall and Thompson.

Fenner, F. 1987. "Frank Macfarlane Burnet." *Biographical Memoirs of Fellows of the Royal Society* 33: 100–162.

Moulin, A. M. 1989. In P. M. Mazumdar, ed. *Immunology 1930–1980, Essays on the History of Immunology*, 291–98. Toronto: Wall and Thompson.

Nossal, G. J. V. 1969. "Burnet and Science, An Appreciation." *Australasian Annals of Medicine* 4: 311–15.

———. 1987. "The Burnetian Legacy: Scientists as Citizens." *Immunology and Cell Biology* 65:1.

Wood, I. J. "Burnet and Medicine." *Australasian Annals of Medicine* 4: 301–9.

ALEXIS CARREL *1912*

(Marie Joseph August) Alexis Carrel was born on June 28, 1873, in Sainte-Foy-les-Lyons, France. A surgeon and experimental biologist, Carrel received the Nobel Prize in 1912 for his innovative experiments in vascular suturing, vascular and organ grafting, and cell culture. At the time of the award, he had just been appointed a full member of the staff of the Rockefeller Institute in New York, where he spent most of his productive career. Carrel married Anne Laure Gourley de la Mote de Mairie, a widow with one son, in 1913; he had no children of his own. He died on November 5, 1944, in Paris.

Carrel's father, Alexis Carrel-Billiard, a textile manufacturer, died when the boy was five years old, and he was raised by his mother, Anne-Marie Ricard. Young Alexis received a conventional schooling, at which he did not excel. He showed an early interest in science, dissecting birds and doing simple chemical experiments. He attended the University of Lyons, where he earned his baccalaureate in letters in 1889 and graduated with a bachelor of science in medicine in 1893.

From 1893 to 1900 Carrel trained in surgery, working in various Lyons hospitals and serving for a year as surgeon to the Chasseurs Alpins. His interest in vascular surgery, at that time in a very primitive stage, was allegedly sparked by the 1894 assassination of French president Carnot, who died after a bullet severed a major artery. In 1898 he secured a position as prosector in the laboratory of the great anatomist, J. L. Testut, where he further developed his operative and dissecting skills. He was awarded his M.D. from Lyons in 1900.

He continued working with Testut, teaching anatomy and operative surgery at the University of Lyons, and practicing surgery at Lyons Hospital. But he became more and more absorbed in the problem of repairing blood vessels without hemorrhage, clotting, or infection. Following the lead of Jaboulay, who headed the Department of Surgery at Lyons, he developed meticulous techniques, using strict asepsis and the finest needles. To prevent blood clotting after closure, he lubricated his instruments, needles, and silk with paraffin jelly. Using these procedures on dogs, he was able to perfect a method for end-to-end anastomosis (joining) of severed vessels, folding back the cut ends like cuffs and suturing the endothelial tissue, to further insulate the blood from possible infection. This technique, described in two articles in the *Bulletin Lyons Medicale* in 1902, has been called the starting point of the modern surgery of blood vessel and organ transplantation (Carrel 1902, 114; Corner 1971, 90–91).

Despite his obvious talents, Carrel was at odds with the medical establishment in Lyons and his applications for surgical posts proved unsuccessful. He departed the city in 1903, spent some time in advanced study in Paris, and then left for North America. After a brief stay in Montreal, he moved to the University of Chicago, where he obtained an assistantship in physiology under G. N. Stewart. Here he entered into a fruitful collaboration on experimental organ transplantation with Charles C. Guthrie. Using Carrel's pioneering surgical techniques, the team carried out a remarkable series of experimental transplants in animals in 1905 and 1906. These established that such transplants were possible, even before the introduction of anticoagulants (Carrel and Guthrie 1906, 1648–50).

In 1906 Carrel was appointed an associate member of the Rockefeller Institute for Medical Research (now Rockefeller University), where he continued experimenting with transplants of various tissues. His studies soon demonstrated that, although organ transplantation was technically feasible, the grafts would not survive in the recipient. The claims of several surgeons of regular success with skin grafts were thus disproved. With remarkable insight, Carrel reasoned that rejection was an immunological event and suggested that radiation or drugs might ensure transplant survival. He failed to pursue this line of investigation because his inventive mind now turned to the problem of availability of tissues and whole organs when needed for emergency replacement.

When Ross G. Harrison of Yale reported his successful culture of frog nerve cells outside the animal in 1908, Carrel was inspired by the idea of large cell, tissue, and organ culture "banks." He was able to preserve blood vessels in cold storage and also used Harrison's technique to grow sarcoma cells. He then began intensive work on the development of long-term in vitro culture methods of cells from warm-blooded animals. Having perfected and announced his techniques in 1911, he was challenged by skeptics and became involved in a priority dispute with Harrison. Responding to these attacks, he cultured a piece of connective tissue from the heart of a chick embryo, which he proclaimed would live indefinitely. The culture, in the hands of a colleague, did indeed live for several years and is alleged to have survived after Carrel's own death in 1944, but this claim has not been confirmed. The in vitro culture method designed by Carrel, however, is still the standard in the field. He was awarded the Nobel Prize in 1912 for his achievements. His was the first Nobel Prize in Physiology or Medicine awarded for work done in the United States (Carrel and Burrows 1911, 387; Corner 1971, 91).

With the beginning of World War I, Carrel was recalled to France for service as a major in the French Army Surgical Corps. Madame Carrel accompanied him as a surgical nurse. At his hospital in Compiegne near the front lines, he set up a research laboratory with funding from the Rockefeller Foundation. Working with chemist Henry B. Dakin, he developed an effective method for the treatment of deep wounds, irrigating the open wound with a special antiseptic solution. The Carrel-Dakin method eclipsed the more cumbersome procedures advocated by Almroth Wright and was widely used until the introduction of antibiotics.

After the war he rejoined the Rockefeller Institute, but his research lacked direction. He became involved in experimental cancer susceptibility research and was briefly caught up in large-scale animal studies based on the eugenists' claim that cancer was a hereditary disease. His interest in tissue culture and organ preservation was reawakened when the energetic aviator Charles Lindbergh arrived at the institute in 1930. Lindbergh worked out the design for a perfusion machine, a sterile glass chamber with a pump capable of circulating artificial blood through an isolated organ. Carrel succeeded in keeping certain organs, specifically kidneys and thyroid glands, "alive" in this device for extended periods, but his claims for long-term survival were again disputed (Carrel and Lindbergh 1938; Corner 1971, 91). He also during this period performed a successful series of heart valvotomies with Theodore Tuffier.

As a scientist, Carrel was remarkably insightful and energetic, but he was also impulsive, personally ambitious, and somewhat insensitive to others. He preferred to work alone and was repeatedly involved in disputes over priority or over his several exaggerated claims. He had great technical skills but also a mystical outlook that sometimes led him into questionable speculations.

His best-selling book, *Man the Unknown* (1935), was a deliberately popular work and was largely ignored by his scientific colleagues. While he offered some sensible views on preserving the environment and expressed a conventional faith in the power of science to resolve the world's problems, he also displayed a preoccupation with rather crude eugenic measures directed to the creation of an intellectual elite and the reversal of what he saw as the increasing degeneracy of the white races. He later published other works in which he discussed his religious ideas as a devout but unorthodox Roman Catholic.

Carrel retired from the Rockefeller Institute in 1938 as a member emeritus. He returned to France after the outbreak of World War II as a member of a special mission for the French Ministry of Public Health. Remaining in Paris after the Germans occupied the city, he established the Carrel Foundation for the Study of Human Problems with the backing of the Vichy government. Little is known of his work during the war except that he devised a broad program for the scientific improvement of human life through hygiene, nutrition, and eugenics. His continuing negotiations with the Nazis on behalf of the foundation attracted unproven allegations of collaboration. Carrel's death from heart failure soon after the liberation in 1944 probably saved him from arrest. He was buried at his country home in Brittany (Corner 1971, 91).

Among the many other awards Carrel received for his work were the French Legion d'Honneur; the Nordhoff-Jung Award for Cancer Research (1930); and the Newman Foundation Award from the University of Illinois (1937).

DAVID HAMILTON

Selected Bibliography

A full bibliography is in Robert Soupault, *Alexis Carrel, 1873–1944* (Paris: Plon, 1952).

Carrel's papers are deposited at Georgetown University School of Medicine, Washington, D.C.

PRIMARY SOURCES

Carrel, Alexis. 1902. "Anastomose Bout a Bout de la Jugulaire et de la Carotide Primitive." *Bulletin Lyons Medicale* 99:114.

Carrel, Alexis, and Charles C. Guthrie. 1906. "Anastomosis of Blood Vessels by the Patching Method and Transplantation of the Kidney." *Journal of the American Medical Association* 47:1648–50.

Carrel, Alexis. 1907. "The Surgery of Blood Vessels." *Johns Hopkins Hospital Bulletin* 18:18–28.

Carrel, Alexis, and M. T. Burrows. 1911. "Cultivation of Tissues *In Vitro* and Its Techniques." *Journal of Experimental Medicine* 13:387.

Carrel, Alexis, and George Dehelly. 1917. *The Treatment of Infected Wounds*. New York: Hoeber.

Carrel, Alexis. 1935. *Man the Unknown*. New York: Harper and Brothers.

Carrel, Alexis, and Charles A. Lindbergh. 1938. *The Culture of Organs*. New York: Hoeber.

SECONDARY SOURCES

Converse, J. M. 1981. "Alexis Carrel: The Man, the Unknown." *Plastic and Reconstructive Surgery* 68: 629–39.

Corner, George W. 1971. "Carrel, Alexis." In *Dictionary of Scientific Biography*, 3890–92. New York: Scribners.

Durkin, J. T., ed. 1973. *Papers at the Alexis Carrel Centennial Conference*. Washington: Georgetown University.

Malavin, Theodore. 1979. *Surgery and Life: The Extraordinary Career of Alexis Carrel*. New York: Harcourt Brace Jovanovich.

Witkowski, J. A. 1979. "Alexis Carrel and the Mysticism of Tissue Culture." *Medical History* 23:279–96.

Witkowski, J. A. 1980. "Dr. Carrel's Immortal Cells." *Medical History* 24: 129–42.

SIR ERNST BORIS CHAIN 1945

Sir Ernst Boris Chain was born on June 19, 1906, in Berlin, Germany. A biochemist, he shared the Nobel Prize for Physiology or Medicine with Alexander Fleming and Howard Florey in 1945 for the discovery and development of penicillin. Chain was of Russian-Jewish descent. His father, Michael, was a chemical engineer. His mother, Margarete (née Eisner), was a close relative of Kurt Eisner, the German socialist leader. Chain became a naturalized German citizen in 1928. He adopted British citizenship in 1939. In October 1948 he married Ann Beloff; they had three children: Benjamin, and twins, Judith and Daniel. Chain died on August 12, 1979, in Mulrany, County Mayo, Eire.

Chain's father developed a successful chemical company in Aldershof, a suburb of Berlin, in the years before World War I. He died in 1919 when Ernst was thirteen. The family then found itself in serious financial difficulties and Ernst's mother was forced to convert the home into a guest house in order to make ends meet. Nevertheless, Ernst was provided with an excellent education at the Luisengymnasium and the Fredrich-Wilhelm University, from which he graduated in 1930 with a concentration in chemistry and physiology. After being employed for a short time in the Kaiser Wilhelm Institute for Physical Chemistry and Electrochemistry his interest in the chemistry of biological processes led him to take a position in the chemical department of the Pathological Institute of Berlin's famous Charité Hospital, from which he received a D. Phil for his research into phospholipids and the enzymes that decompose them.

Hitler's accession to power in January 1933 led Chain to flee Germany for England, where he arrived in April with little money or prospects. In spite of immigration restrictions which forbad employment and limited his stay until the end of the year (subsequently modified and extended), Chain immediately sought a position as a biochemist. The influence of J. B. S. Haldane, newly installed head of genetics at University College, London, who was impressed with his work in Germany, brought him an appointment in that institution's Department of Chemical Pathology under Sir Charles Harington. This, however, was to be a short-lived haven. Differences both of laboratory procedure and personal temperament between Harington and Chain led to a break between the two men. Within two months Chain was once more in search of a post. It is testimony to the regard for his potential as a scientist, held by Haldane and others in the British scientific community, that in spite of this inauspicious beginning another position was found for him, this time in the Department of Biochemistry at the Sir William Dunn School at Cambridge University. There during the following two years, in addition to meeting the terms of his employment, he earned a Ph.D. under Sir Frederick Gowland Hopkins, best known for his pioneering work on vitamins.

In the spring of 1935, Howard Florey, director of the Sir William Dunn School of Pathology at Oxford University, sought Hopkins's help in securing the services of a biochemist. A pathologist himself, Florey was putting together an interdisciplinary team with which he intended to probe the boundaries between biochemistry and bacteriology. Hopkins recommended Chain and thus secured his career. Florey gave Chain a free hand in establishing a department of biochemistry at the Dunn School and their early years of collaboration were friendly and productive. In 1936 Chain was appointed university lecturer and demonstrator in chemical pathology.

Chain brought over from Cambridge a project on the toxicity of snake venom which he continued and completed. But in addition, at Florey's suggestion, he began the systematic investigation of lysozyme, an enzyme with interesting antibiotic properties which had been discovered by Alexander Fleming. It was in the course of reading the available literature on such substances that Chain came across Fleming's 1929 paper on penicillin. Fleming had discovered the penicillin mold growing on one of his culture plates and noted the destruction of staphylococci in its vicinity. In conjunction with two research associates, Stuart Craddock and Frederick Ridley, he had spent a year investigating its properties and had concluded that while the substance had some antiseptic qualities, it was extremely unstable and unlikely to be of medical significance. Subsequently, Harold Raistrick of the London School of Hygiene and Tropical Medicine had confirmed most of the work of Craddock and Ridley but had failed to overcome the technical difficulties encountered in attempting to extract the active agent in the penicillin mold juice.

Nonetheless, Florey and Chain were intrigued by this early work. By 1938, with their lysozyme project completed, they decided to focus their investigation on penicillin. Both claimed subsequently that their interest in penicillin was purely scientific and not conditioned by thoughts of its usefulness as a therapeutic agent. The technical difficulties inherent in producing purified and concentrated penicillin were very great, though Chain found this aspect of the problem a challenge. However, both he and Florey recognized that the project required more generous funding than they had been accustomed to receiving from the Medical Research Council. Toward that end they obtained from the Rockefeller Foundation a grant of some $30,000 which proved crucial to their eventual success.

By the spring of 1940, though as yet unable to define chemically the active agent in the penicillin mold juice or to obtain a wholly purified sample, Chain, aided by Norman Heatley, had succeeded in extracting a concentrate capable of destroying bacteria in dilutions of one part per million. He now began to grasp the therapeutic potential of the substance and pressed Florey to begin animal experiments. Though using a sample no more than 1 percent pure, Florey and Chain demonstrated that penicillin was not toxic, and that it protected mice from otherwise lethal doses of streptococci. From May 1940 the penicillin program achieved the highest priority and the Dunn School was rapidly turned into a small factory for the production and extraction of the material. Clinical trials on humans were conducted shortly thereafter and although not completely satisfactory owing to the tiny quantities of penicillin then available, clearly demonstrated its almost miraculous curative qualities.

Chain was among the first to understand the need to move from laboratory to industrial production of penicillin. Florey soon agreed and to that end arranged to bring American capital and enterprise into the picture via a trip to the United States. However, instead of taking Chain with him to work with the Americans on the biochemical aspects, he chose Heatley, a decision that Chain resented and which went far to worsen a relationship already under great strain. Nonetheless Florey's trip was dramatically successful. From this point onward American involvement rapidly expanded the production of penicillin so that by 1944 it was available in sufficient quantities to play a crucial role in treating Allied wounded in the closing phases of World War II.

In the years following the breakthroughs of 1939–40 Chain worked with E. P. Abraham and others on the continuing problems of purifying penicillin and defining its precise chemical nature. He became convinced of the Beta-lactam structure for penicillin, a position vindicated in 1945 by Dorothy Hodgkin through X-ray crystallography. Chain's Continental experience, where academic and industrial scientists worked more closely together than was common in Britain, prepared him to be an early advocate of the need to obtain patents on the penicillin work. But at the time the British medical community felt patenting lifesaving drugs was unethical, and his arguments fell on deaf ears. The Americans had no such qualms. The irony, that eventually Britian would be required to pay vast sums to the United States for the drug developed first at Oxford, was not lost on him.

Following the war Chain sought to forge greater cooperation between the pharmaceutical industry and research agencies. In 1948 he left Oxford for Rome to establish an international research center for chemical microbiology at the Instituto Superiore di Sanita, where he showed strong administrative leadership and earned a reputation for being an outstanding teacher and a severe taskmaster. In addition he became an active consultant for the Beecham Group and other corporate bodies. In 1961, fearing for the financial security of the institute in the wake of the retirement of its director, Domenico Marotta, and homesick for England, Chain accepted the chair of biochemistry at Imperial College, London, where his effort to establish a state-of-the-art research and training facility proved extremely expensive and involved him in renewed controversy.

Chain had an artistic temperament. He is reputed to have had musical ability of such a high order that he could have chosen the concert stage as a career. He was outspoken, animated, and, while socially engaging, was frequently embroiled in ongoing disputes with his associates. Partly this was owing to an exceptional persistence in pursuing intellectual problems. But in the early days, such qualities tended to alienate him from his very British colleagues. For example, Heatley refused to join the Oxford team until Florey made it clear he would not be responsible to Chain (Clark 1985, 40). According to Clark, Chain saw much of his opposition as some form of anti-Semitic hostility. His relationship with Florey, at first sound and extremely productive professionally for both men, deteriorated to the point that Chain claimed that Florey's behavior toward him from 1941 to 1948 was "unpardonably bad" (Clark 1985, 46). Once independently established, Chain apparently gained greater perspective on these difficult days and he and Florey reconciled.

Chain received many honors. In addition to the Nobel Prize, he was elected to the Royal Society (1949); made an honorary fellow of the Royal College of Physicians (1965); was knighted in 1969; and received many other prizes and awards.

R. D. CASSELL

Selected Bibliography

PRIMARY SOURCES

Chain, E., H. W. Florey et al. 1940. "Penicillin as a Chemotherapeutic Agent." *Lancet* 2 (August 24):226–28.

Chain, E. B., and H. W. Florey. 1944. "Penicillin." *Endeavour* 3, no. 9 (January):3–14.

Florey, H. W., E. Chain et al. 1949. *Antibiotics: A Survey of Penicillin, Streptomycin, and Other Antimicrobial Substances from Fungi, Antinomycetes, Bacteria and Plants.* London: Oxford University Press.

Chain, E. B. 1980. "A Short History of the Penicillin Discovery from Fleming's Early Observations in 1929 to the Present Time." In *The History of Antibiotics: A Symposium*, edited by J. Parascandola. 15–29. Madison, Wisconsin: American Institute of Pharmacy.

SECONDARY SOURCES

Wilson, David. 1976. *In Search of Penicillin.* New York: Alfred A. Knopf.

Macfarlane, Gwyn. 1979. *Howard Florey: The Making of a Great Scientist.* London: Oxford University Press.

Clark, Ronald W. 1985. *The Life of Ernst Chain.* New York: St. Martin's.

Hobby, Gladys L. 1985. *Penicillin: Meeting the Challenge.* New Haven: Yale University Press.

Abraham, E. P. 1983. "Ernst Boris Chain, 1906–1979." *Biographical Memoirs of Fellows of the Royal Society*, 29 (November):43–91.

ALBERT CLAUDE *1974*

Albert Claude was born on August 24, 1898, in Longlier, Belgium (now Luxembourg). A cellular biologist, Claude shared the Nobel Prize in 1974 with Christian R. de Duvé and George E. Palade for their descriptions of the fine microscopic structure and functions of the cell, which laid the foundations of modern cell biology. Claude developed the pioneering techniques of centrifugal fractionation and electron microscopy that made the work possible and carried out the initial observations. Palade and de Duvé continued and extended the investigations. Although the three men worked separately for the most part, all were Europeans based for a part of their careers at the Rockefeller Institute for Medical Research (now Rockefeller University). Claude carried out his prizewinning work in New York but returned to Belgium in 1950 to head the Institut Jules Bordet and establish cancer research at the University of Belgium. From 1972, he was associated with the Catholic University in Louvain. In 1935, Claude married Joy Gilder of New York. The couple had one daughter, Philippa, who became a neurobiologist; they were subsequently divorced. Claude died on May 22, 1983, in Brussels.

Claude's parents were Florentin Joseph Claude, a baker, and Marie-Glaudicine Wautriquant. His early education was severely limited by poverty and the outbreak of World War I. He received the British War Medal and the Interallied Medal in 1918 for his wartime services. At first his chances of going to medical school without the usual preparation looked slim; but in 1922 he was admitted to the University of Liege under a special program for veterans. He earned his M.D. in 1928, along with a government scholarship for postgraduate study.

He spent some time at the Kaiser Wilhelm Institute in Berlin, but was interested in going to the Rockefeller Institute to study tumor cells. Uninvited, he sent a proposal to Simon Flexner for the isolation of the tumor agent in Rous sarcoma. Flexner accepted the young Belgian, who came to New York in 1929 and remained for the next twenty years, becoming an American citizen in 1941 (Hicks 1974; Rensberger 1974).

Claude began his work in James B. Murphy's laboratory. His attempts to isolate the tumor agent in the cell led him to develop a workable method of centrifugal fractionation. His technique involved the fine chopping and suspension in solution of liver tissues. Centrifugation at low speed allowed the heaviest components, the cell nuclei and intact cells, to separate out and be removed; centrifugation at high speed separated the remaining material into distinct layers of particles, each layer containing a mass of cellular material concentrated enough for study and homogenous enough for some precision in characterization. The technology was primitive—the tissues had to be chopped in a meat grinder or forced through a sieve, and the centrifuges themselves were dangerously unreliable and slow by today's standards. Claude was nevertheless able to isolate a "fraction" of the cytoplasm (the cellular material outside the nucleus) with a high capability for tumor production in healthy chickens (Claude 1937; Porter 1974, 516).

He found that his tumor agent, now known as Rous sarcoma virus, had a high ribonucleic acid (RNA) content. This was not surprising, since viruses were known to contain RNA; but he was startled to find a comparable amount of the protein in normal cellular cytoplasm. He quickly recognized that the fractionation of normal cells offered unexpected opportunities for study and insights.

He began with liver cells, whose membranes were easy to rupture. Separating out the nuclei and continually improving his techniques, he began tentatively to identify large "secretory granules" and smaller "mitochondria" within the cytoplasm. In the 1940s George Hogeboom and Rollin Hotchkiss, both biochemists, joined him in the investigations, and the three came to suspect that the large "granules" were in fact made up of mitochondria. The mitochrondria fractions consistently contained high proportions of very active enzymes, primarily cytochrome oxidase and succinoxidase. By 1945, the team reported that the mitochondria are the cellular respiratory organs: they metabolize oxygen from the blood to generate energy, which they then store. Hogeboom, W. C. Schneider, and George Palade later established conclusively that the mitochondria are the basic components of the "large granule fraction" (Claude 1946).

Claude had also been able in 1943 to separate out an amorphous fraction that appeared to be the source of the RNA and to contain the very smallest particles, which Claude named "microsomes." Palade was later able to demonstrate that these particles, now called ribosomes, are the source of cellular protein (Claude 1943; Porter 1974).

In his search for a better understanding of cellular anatomy, Claude in 1942 became interested in the electron microscope. This instrument had been invented for use in metallurgy; the object to be studied is placed in a vacuum and bombarded with electrons, forming a detailed image of fine structures. It had never been used in biology, despite its visual advantage over the standard microscope, because it seemed likely that the bombarding process would destroy cells and tissues.

Claude was offered the use of the electron microscope at Interchemical Corporation, then the only such instrument in New York City. Working with Ernest Fullman, the Interchemical microscopist, and with Keith R. Porter, he developed a feasible method of cellular microphotography with the instrument. The new pictures revealed a "lacework" of strands and small pouches, now called the endoplasmic reticulum, the infrastructure that connects the various cellular particles (Porter 1974, 517).

With the end of World War II, Claude decided to return to Belgium. He established dual citizenship and accepted the position at the Institut Jules Bordet. This responsibility involved him heavily in administration and it was not until he "retired" to join the Louvain faculty that he again became active in research, which he continued until his death.

Claude was a man of stubborn independence and vision, although blessed with a quiet, self-deprecating sense of humor. Although it was left to others to carry on the studies of cellular anatomy and physiology, it was his original insight and pathbreaking methods that opened this field to researchers, a field, as he said, "with no end to it." Before his work, the cell was a nebulous mass of "stuff" surrounding the nucleus; under his gaze, the stuff resolved into highly specialized and interactive parts, replicating human functions on the most basic level (Hicks 1974; Rensberger 1974).

Among the many other awards Albert Claude received for his work were the Louisa G. Horowitz Prize (1970) and the Paul Ehrlich and Ludwig Darmstaedter Prizes (Frankfurt, 1971). In his native country, he was honored with the Grand Cordon de l'Ordre de Leopold II and the Prix Fonds National de la Recherche Scientifique (1965). He was a member of the Belgian and French Academies of Science, and an honorary member of the American Academy of Arts and Sciences.

MARCIA MELDRUM

Selected Bibliography

PRIMARY SOURCES

Claude, Albert. 1937. "Fractionation of Chicken Tumor Extracts by High Speed Centrifugation." *American Journal of Cancer* 30:742–45.

———. 1943. "Distribution of Nucleic Acids in the Cell and Morphological Constitution of Cytoplasm." *Biological Symposia* 10:111–29.

———. 1946. "Franctionation of Mammalian Liver Cells by Differential Centrifugation. I and II." *Journal of Experimental Medicine* 84:51–89.

Claude, Albert, and George Palade. 1949. "The Nature of the Golgi Apparatus. 1 and 2." *Journal of Morphology* 85:35–111.

SECONDARY SOURCES

Hicks, Nancy. 1974. "Albert Claude." *New York Times* (October 12):22.

Rensberger, Boyce. 1974. "Three Cell Biologists Get Nobel Prize." *New York Times* (October 12):22.

Porter, Keith R. 1974. "The 1974 Nobel Prize in Physiology or Medicine." *Science* 186 (November 8):516–17.

1980. "Claude, Albert." In *Modern Scientists and Engineers*, 1:205–6. New York: McGraw-Hill.

STANLEY COHEN *1986*

Stanley Cohen was born on November 17, 1922, in Brooklyn, New York. A biochemist, Cohen won the Nobel Prize in 1986 with Rita Levi-Montalcini for their isolation and description of epidermal growth factors (EGF). Also in 1986, he was appointed distinguished professor of biochemistry at Vanderbilt University, where he has done much of his pioneering research on the processes of regulation of cell growth and development. Cohen married Olivia Barbara Larson, with whom he had three children, in 1951. They were subsequently divorced, and he married Jan Elizabeth Jordan in 1981.

Cohen's parents, Louis and Fannie Feitel Cohen, were Jewish immigrants; his father worked as a tailor. He studied chemistry and zoology at Brooklyn College, receiving his B.A. in 1943; he then studied zoology at Oberlin College in Ohio, earning his M.A. in 1945. Cohen next won a teaching fellowship to complete his Ph.D. in biochemistry at the University of Michigan. He spent a great deal of time at Michigan hunting worms on the campus grounds, eventually collecting over five thousand, for his research on nitrogenous metabolism.

From 1948 to 1952 he taught biochemistry at the University of Colorado School of Medicine, where he had a joint appointment in pediatrics and developed an interest in the growth and metabolism of premature infants. He was particularly curious about the relation of normal growth to abnormal tumor growth. This work eventually gained him a postdoctoral fellowship from the American Cancer Society to pursue metabolic studies in the Department of Radiology at Washington University in St. Louis.

During his one-year fellowship (1952–53), he so impressed his Washington colleagues, particularly Dr. Viktor Hamburger, director of the Zoology Department, and Dr. Rita Levi-Montalcini, that he was offered an appointment as associate professor of zoology. Cohen and Montalcini found that certain mouse tumors, implanted into chick embryos, stimulated the growth of specific embryonic tissue by releasing an unidentified factor.

In 1959 Cohen accepted a position at Vanderbilt University, where he was successful in obtaining a Research Career Development Award, an NIH grant designed to support the research of young investigators. He was still interested in the "side effects" he and Montalcini had discovered. He injected a crude submaxillary gland preparation into newborn mice and was startled to note precocious eyelid opening and tooth eruption (Cohen 1960, 302–11). A substance that altered the timing of specific developmental processes, such as the opening of eyelids, was of major biological significance. Cohen hypothesized that the substance might be related to those extracts involved in oncogenic transformation by a particular class of retroviruses. He was able to isolate the eyelid-opening factor from mouse glands by 1962. For a period of ten years he worked on determining and describing its evolutionary origins and physiology. The name "epidermal growth factor" (EGF) was first used in reporting his work at the Istitute Superiore de Sanita in Rome with Montalcini and Domenica Attardi in the early 1960s (Cohen 1962, 1555–62; Cohen 1965, 394–407; Cohen and Savage 1947, 554–71).

Cohen was now convinced that EGF plays a normal physiological role for many species. Amino acid analysis revealed that mouse-derived EGF is a 53 residue polypeptide devoid of alanyl, phenylalanyl, or lysyl residues. It has little periodic secondary structure. Other researchers found that EGF caused fibroblasts in culture to respond with enhanced DNA synthesis.

Mouse EGF was found to be a potent mitogen for human cells, indicating that human cells have receptors for the growth factor. Therefore, a polypeptide similar to EGF might occur in human tissue. Was it in human urine? Could it be located in cultured human fibroblasts? Cohen isolated the human counterpart of murine EGF, using again the stimulation of fibroblast proliferation by in vitro corneal epithelial cells and precocious eyelid opening in newborn mice as the biological assays. H. Gregory reported in *Nature* that urogastrone, gastric antisecretory hormone, in human urine, is identical to human EGF (*Nature* 1975, 325–27).

How does EGF stimulate cell growth? Cohen found that there are specific plasma membrane receptors for EGF. He bound 125 I-EGF to fibroblasts to observe its degradation by the cell. The plasma membrane receptors bound the EGF, and the entire receptor complex was then internalized by the cell, where the growth hormone was rapidly degraded by the lysosomes.

It is still unknown whether the intracellular processing of EGF and its receptors is essential for the generation of the biological response. Cohen has compiled quantitative biological evidence for a complex mechanism through which cells interact with extracellular regulatory signals. He and his associates were able to visualize this process through biologically active EGF-ferritin conjugate (F-EGF) in 1979, most clearly with I-EGF (McKanna, Haigler, and Cohen 1979, 5689–93).

The team found that the A-131 human epidermoid cell line has a very high concentration of EGF receptors. Working with this enriched source, they added EGF prior to phosphorylation reaction of proteins associated with the endogenous cell membrane. The reaction was enhanced. Cohen hypothesizes that phosphorylation of membrane-associated components may be an initial event in the generation of the intracellular signals regulating cell growth.

Observing the phosphorylation reaction in the cell-free A-131 membrane system, the team found the EGF activated the kinase activity very rapidly; no kinase modulator or soluble protein kinase was released by the membrane; EGF receptor kinase, if affinity purified, also showed phosphorylated tyrosine residues (Carpenter and Cohen 1979, 193–216).

Further purification of the EGF receptor was attempted. It was isolated as a 170 KD protein. The kinase, binding, and substrate present in the receptor preparation seem all to be in the same molecule, a polypeptide. The EGF receptor appears to be a glycoprotein.

Cohen believes that EGF originated by evolution in ancient times and has played various functional roles in living tissues. He has investigated its functions in several types of cells. Both fetal cells and malignant cells produce an EGF-related protein that interacts with the receptor and mimics EGF activity.

Many critical questions remain regarding the EGF regulatory system. The most important concerns its normal physiological role during growth and homeostasis. Problems include the mechanism for sending signals to the nucleus; the possible unidentified regulatory role of the autophosphorylated receptors or related oncogene proteins; the physiological significance of the intracellular translation of the tyrosine kinases; and the existence of specific cellular proteins whose functions are altered by the phosphorylation.

Cohen became a full professor in 1967. He is a member of the American Society of Biological Chemists and of the International Institute of Embryology, and a fellow of the National Academy of Sciences and of the American Academy of Arts and Sciences. His many awards include the Earl Sutherland Award from Vanderbilt University (1977); the American Cancer Society Research Professorship in Biochemistry (1976–87); the Lewis S. Rosenstiel Award from Brandeis University (1982); the Louis Gross Horowitz Award from Columbia University (1983); the Gairdner Foundation International Award (1985); the Lasker Basic Medical Research Award (1986).

LESLIE FALK
MARCIA MELDRUM

Selected Bibliography

PRIMARY SOURCES

Cohen, Stanley. 1960. "Purification of a Nerve-Growth Promoting Protein from the Mouse Salivary Gland and Its Neuro-Toxic Antiserum." *Proceedings of the National Academy of Sciences* (USA) 46:302–11.

———. 1962. "Isolation of Mouse Submaxillary Gland Protein Accelerating Incisor Eruption and Eyelid Opening in the Newborn Animal." *Journal of Biological Chemistry* 237:1555–62.

———. 1965. "The Stimulating of Epidermal Proliferation by a Specific Protein (EGF)." *Developmental Biology* 12:394–407.

Cohen, Stanley, and C. R. Savage, Jr. 1974. "Part II. Recent Studies in the Chemistry and Biology of Epidermal Growth Factor." In *Recent Progress in Hormone Research*, vol. 30, edited by R. O. Greep, 554–71. New York: Academic Press.

McKanna, J. A., H. T. Haigler, and Stanley Cohen. 1979. "Hormone Reception Topology and Dynamics: Morphological Analysis Using Ferritin-Labelled Epidermal Growth Factor." *Proceedings of the National Academy of Sciences* (USA) 76:5689–93.

Carpenter, G., and S. Cohen. 1979. "Rapid Enhancement of Protein Phosphorylation in A-131 Cell Membrane Preparations by Epidermal Growth Factor." *Annual Review of Biochemistry* 48:193–216.

Cohen, Stanley. 1985. "Nobel Lecture." *Bioscience Reports* 6:1017–28. (Also published in *In Vitro Cellular and Developmental Biology* (1987):233, 239–246.)

Staros, J. V., S. Cohen, and M. W. Russo. 1985. "Epidermal Growth Factor Receptor: Characterization of Its Protein Kinase Activity." In *Molecular Mechanisms of Transmembrane Signalling*, edited by Philip Cohen and Miles D. Houlay, 253–77. Amsterdam & New York: Elsevier.

Cohen, Stanley. 1987. "Epidermal Growth Factor." In *Reimpression de les Prize Nobel*, 261–75. Nobel Foundation.

CARL FERDINAND CORI *1947*

The 1947 Nobel Prize in Physiology or Medicine was awarded to Carl F. Cori and Gerty T. Cori "for their discovery of the course of the catalytic conversion of glycogen," and to Bernardo Alberto Houssay "for his discovery of the part played by the hormone of the anterior pituitary lobe in the metabolism of sugar." Carl Cori was born on December 5, 1896, in Prague, Czechoslovakia. His areas of scientific specialization were pharmacology, biochemistry, and carbohydrate metabolism. His parents were Carl Isidor Cori and Maria Lippich Cori. His father studied medicine but later earned a Ph.D. in zoology. When Carl was two years old, his father became director of the Marine Biological Station at Trieste. His father's devotion to research and teaching inspired Carl's early interest in biology. His maternal grandfather, Ferdinand Lippich, was professor of theoretical physics at the University of Prague. Carl Cori and Gerty Theresa Radnitz were married on August 5, 1920. They had one son, Carl Thomas. Gerty Cori died on October 26, 1957. The Coris were the third married couple to share a Nobel Prize in science. After his wife's death, Carl Cori married Anne Fitzgerald Jones on March 23, 1960. Carl Cori died on October 20, 1984, in Cambridge, Massachusetts.

Cori received his M.D. in 1920 from the German University of Prague, Czechoslovakia. He held the post of instructor in the Second Medical Clinic at Prague University from 1919 to 1920. He then became an assistant in the First Medical Clinic at the University of Vienna, and a researcher at the University of Graz from 1920 to 1921. From 1922 to 1931 Cori held the post of researcher at the State Institute for the Study of Malignant Disease, in Buffalo, New York. He was an assistant professor of physiology at the University of Buffalo from 1930 to 1931. In 1931 he accepted an appointment at the School of Medicine, Washington University, in St. Louis, as professor of pharmacology and biochemistry. From 1966 to 1984 he served as director of the Enzyme Research Laboratory at Massachusetts General Hospital (affiliated with Harvard Medical School), and held a faculty appointment as full professor at Harvard University.

Ninety years after the great French physiologist Claude Bernard discovered that the liver and muscles contain a starchlike substance, which Bernard called *glycogen*, the "sugar former," the Coris revealed the metabolic relationship between glucose and glycogen. The Coris crystallized and determined the structure of a new compound, the so-called Cori ester, in which phosphoric acid was linked to the first carbon atom of the sugar instead of to the sixth. From this starting point the Coris and their coworkers unraveled the previously mysterious interplay between glucose, phosphoric acid, and glycogen. Working together, the Coris elucidated the process by which glycogen was converted into utilizable glucose. They also isolated and characterized the enzyme known as phosphorylase, which is essential to glycolysis. The Coris made many other important contributions to the understanding of carbohydrate metabolism, the effects of the hormones insulin and epinephrine on carbohydrate metabolism, tumor glycolysis, and the action of pituitary extracts.

Carl Cori's first scientific paper was an ecological study of ant species collected on an expedition to the Dalmatian Islands with his father. While still in medical school, however, he began a scientific collaboration with a fellow medical student that endured until her death. In an autobiographical review of his life and scientific career, Cori recalled how at the Carl Ferdinand University of Prague he met Gerty Theresa Radnitz, "a fellow student, a young woman who had charm, vitality, intelligence, a sense of humor, and love of the outdoors—qualities which immediately attracted me. A very pleasant period followed during which we would plan and study together, or go off on excursions to the countryside, or on a skiing expedition." The Coris' first joint publication dealt with the complement of human serum in various diseases and appeared in an immunological journal. In reflecting on their thirty-five years of collaborative research, Cori wrote that collaboration "is a delicate operation which requires much give and take on both sides and occasionally leads to friction, if both are equal partners and not willing to yield on a given point" (Cori 1969, 12).

Carl was drafted into the Austrian army during World War I and was almost killed while serving with the ski troops. Transferred to the sanitary corps, he contracted typhoid fever while working in a bacteriological laboratory and almost died because the vaccine then in use turned out to be ineffective. This episode convinced Cori that meticulous technique was essential when handling pathogens, and also aroused an interest in immunology. Near the end of the war Cori watched the army dissolve in an undisciplined retreat. Pondering the lessons of war, he found its main legacy to be a loss of confidence in other human beings. Appalled by worsening conditions in Europe, the Coris were convinced that they were lucky to have been offered an opportunity to leave Europe for the United States.

In 1922 the Coris began their research career in the United States at the State Institute for the Study of Malignant Diseases in Buffalo, New York. The title of their first paper published from Buffalo in 1923, "Free Sugar Content of the Liver and Its Relation to Glycogen Synthesis and Glycogenolysis," presaged the direction their joint research efforts would take over the next thirty-four years. These investigations on the fate of sugar in the animal body reflected Carl Cori's skill in using various types of whole animal preparations for the study of fundamental biochemical phenomena.

The State Institute for the Study of Malignant Diseases, later the Roswell Park Memorial Institute, was affiliated with a hospital for cancer patients. When Gerty Cori arrived in Buffalo a half year after her husband, she was assigned to the institute's Pathology Department. Although the Coris had already begun to establish their pattern of collaborative research, institutional constraints like this caused them unexpected difficulties. Eventually the problem was worked out so that they were again able to work together on a given problem or not as they chose. Thereafter, Carl Cori could only recall one other occasion when the question of collaboration arose again as a possible difficulty. He received an offer of a good position at a neighboring university. However, the head of the department imposed several conditions. Cori was willing to take speech lessons but refused to agree to demands that he stop his research on insulin and stop working in collaboration with Gerty Cori.

Before leaving Buffalo the Coris had begun examining the potentialities of tissue preparations as a means of investigating the underlying mechanisms of intermediary metabolism. In later work, broken cell preparations and purified enzymes were generally used, but on many occasions the Coris found the key to gaining new insight into puzzling physiological problems in a return to the study of whole animals or intact tissues. According to Cori, the use of tissue preparation led to "a most exciting period of biochemistry. . . . The exploration of the glycolytic and oxidative pathways and the concomitant study in depth of individual enzyme systems yielded such rich information about biological mechanisms that all previous expectations about the rate of development of biochemistry were surpassed. Nothing comparable to this period happened until recently when it became possible to explore the genetic apparatus of the cell and its expression in terms of protein synthesis" (Cori 1969, 14).

In 1931 the Coris moved to Washington University School of Medicine, where Carl Cori began a new phase of his career as teacher and administrator. Many bright young scientists spent their formative years as postdoctoral students in the Coris' laboratory. The Cori laboratory was the site of many exciting biochemical discoveries: the elucidation of the enzymatic pathway by which the glucose units stored as glycogen are made available for metabolism; the purification and crystallization of phosphorylase, and the discovery that this enzyme exists in two forms and contains pyridoxal phosphate; the purification of at least eight other enzymes involved in metabolic interconversions of glucose, glycogen, and glycolytic intermediates; the crystallization of five of these enzymes; and the demonstration of the enzymatic basis of several glycogen storage diseases. Cori's interest in the question of tissue permeability also led to productive investigation of the influence of insulin, somatotrophin, and adrenal corticoids on transport phenomena.

In describing Carl and Gerty Cori, Severo Ochoa wrote that "Their lives followed more than just parallel courses; they followed a single, lofty, and straight course. This course of life they shared with their students and collaborators in a spirit of friendship and understanding which, with the integrity and excellence of their scientific leadership, resulted in high accomplishment" (Ochoa and Kalckar 1958, 16).

Cori retired as head of the Department of Biological Chemistry at Washington University School of Medicine in 1966, but he accepted the opportunity to continue his scientific work at the Massachusetts General Hospital and at Harvard Medical School.

Other honors Carl Cori received included the Midwest Award, American Chemical Society (1946), the Lasker Award (1946), the Squibb Award (1947), the Sugar Research Foundation Award (1947, 1950), the Willard Gibbs Medal, American Chemical Society (1948), and election as president for the International Congress of Biochemistry, Vienna (1958).

Cori held honorary degrees from Western Reserve University (1947), Yale University (1947), Boston University (1948), Cambridge University (1949), Gustavus Adolphus College (1964), St. Louis University (1965), Brandeis University (1965), Washington University (1966), Monash University (1966), the University of Granada (1967), and University of Trieste (1972).

LOIS N. MAGNER

Selected Bibliography

PRIMARY SOURCES

Cori, C. F. and G. T. Cori. 1936. "The Formation of Hexosephosphate Esters in Frog Muscle." *Journal of Biological Chemistry* 116:119–28.

———. 1936. "Mechanism of Formation of Hexosemonophosphate in Muscle and Isolation of a New Phosphate Ester." *Proceedings of the Society for Experimental Biology and Medicine* 34:702–5.

Cori, G. T., C. F. Cori, and G. Schmidt. 1939. "The Role of Glucose-1-Phosphate in the Formation of Blood Sugar and Synthesis of Glycogen in the Liver." *Journal of Biological Chemistry* 129:629–39.

Cori, C. F., and G. T. Cori. 1945. "The Enzymatic Conversion of Phosphorylase a to b." *Journal of Biological Chemistry* 158:321–32.

Cori, C. F. 1969. "The Cell of Science." *Annual Review of Biochemistry* 38: 1–20.

SECONDARY SOURCES

1947. *Current Biography Yearbook*, 135–37. New York: H. W. Wilson.

1956. "Enzymes and Metabolism: A Collection of Papers Dedicated to Carl F. and Gerty T. Cori on the Occasion of the 60th Birthday." *Biochimica Biophysica Acta*, vol. 20.

Houssay, B. A. 1956. "Carl F. and Gerty T. Cori." *Biochimica Biophysica Acta* 20:11–16.

Kornberg, A., B. L. Horecker, L. Cornudella, and J. Oro, eds. 1956. *Reflections on Biochemistry. In Honour of Severo Ochoa.* Oxford: Pergamon Press.

Ochoa, S., and H. M. Kalckar. 1958. "Gerty T. Cori, Biochemist." *Science* 128:16–17.

1964. *Nobel Lectures, Physiology or Medicine*, vol. 3 (1942–1962). Amsterdam: Elsevier.

Fruton, Joseph S. 1972. *Molecules and Life. Historical Essays on the Interplay of Chemistry and Biology.* New York: Wiley-Interscience.

———. 1982. *A Bio-Bibliography for the History of the Biochemical Sciences since 1800.* Philadelphia: American Philosophical Society.

Florkin, M., E. H. Stotz, and Giorgio Semenza, eds. 1983. *Comprehensive Biochemistry.* Vol. 35, *Selected Topics in the History of Biochemistry. Personal Recollections*, part 1. Amsterdam: Elsevier.

GERTY THERESA RADNITZ CORI
1947

The 1947 Nobel Prize in Physiology or Medicine was awarded to Gerty T. Cori and Carl F. Cori "for their discovery of the course of the catalytic conversion of glycogen," and to Bernardo Alberto Houssay "for his discovery of the part played by the hormone of the anterior pituitary lobe in the metabolism of sugar." Gerty Theresa Radnitz Cori was born on August 15, 1896, in Prague, Czechoslovakia. She was the eldest of the three daughters of businessman Otto Radnitz and his wife Martha Neustadt Radnitz. Gerty and Carl Cori were married on August 5, 1920. Their son Carl Thomas was born in 1936. Those who knew the Coris considered their relationship "a lasting and happy one from the human point of view and, in terms of what it meant to science, one of the most fruitful and successful on records" (Ochoa and Kalckar 1958, 16). The Coris were the third married couple to share a Nobel Prize in science. Gerty Cori was the first American woman and the third woman to receive a Nobel Prize in science. She died on October 26, 1957, in St. Louis.

Before entering a lyceum for girls in 1906, Gerty Cori received her primary education at home. She prepared for the university entrance examinations as a student at the Tetschen Gymnasium. After passing the examinations in 1914, she attended the Medical School of the German University of Prague, Czechoslovakia. She received the doctorate in medicine in 1920, the same year that she married Carl F. Cori. From 1920 to 1922 she held the position of researcher at the Carolinen Children's Hospital, Vienna. In 1922 Gerty Cori joined her husband Carl Cori at the State Institute for the Study of Malignant Diseases, in Buffalo, New York, where she held the position of researcher until 1931. When Carl Cori became professor of pharmacology at Washington University, in St. Louis, Gerty Cori was appointed as a research associate in the Department of Pharmacology. She held the title of research associate in pharmacology from 1931 to 1943, when she was promoted to research associate professor in biochemistry. Antinepotism rules and institutionalized resistance to allowing women access to regular appointments kept Gerty Cori from receiving a senior faculty position until she won the Nobel Prize. In 1947 Gerty was promoted to full professor of biochemistry. It is of interest that Gerty Cori was not considered worthy of a "star" in *American Men of Science* in the 1930s (Rossiter 1982, 291).

It is essentially impossible to separate the contributions of Gerty from those of Carl Cori, because they worked in close collaboration for thirty-five years. Their medical and physiological training gave them the background needed to correlate events at the molecular level with the processes occurring in the whole animal, a level of insight fundamental to the development of "dynamic biochemistry." Their early work dealt with the fate of glucose in the animal body and the effect of hormones, such as insulin and epinephrine, on carbohydrate metabolism, a study which they would take up later with isolated enzymes following the discovery of key enzymes in the breakdown and synthesis of glycogen and utilization of glucose. Working together, the Coris elucidated the process by which glycogen was converted into utilizable glucose. The Coris made many other important contributions to the understanding of carbohydrate metabolism, the effects of the hormones insulin and epinephrine on carbohydrate metabolism, tumor glycolysis, and the action of pituitary extracts. The discovery of phosphorylase and of glucose-1-phosphate (Cori ester) and that of the branching enzyme (amylo-1, 4 → 1,6-transglucosidase) led to an understanding of the mechanism of biosynthesis of glycogen. The identification and characterization of the enzymes involved in the formation and breakdown of the highly branched glycogen molecule made it possible for the Coris to effect the first synthesis of glycogen in the test tube.

In 1951 Gerty Cori and J. Larner described a new enzyme, called "the debrancher" or amylo-1, 6-glucosidase. This enzyme catalyzes the hydrolysis on the 1,6-glucosyl linkages at the branch points and, in cooperation with phosphorylase, phosphoglucomutase, and glucose-6-phosphatase, makes the cleavage of glycogen to glucose, the process known as glycogenolysis, possible. Almost one hundred years after the discovery of glycogen by Claude Bernard, Gerty Cori succeeded in using the enzymes involved in the biological cleavage of glycogen as tools for the chemical definition of its molecular structure. These studies also made it possible for Gerty Cori to illuminate the nature of two groups of glycogen storage diseases: one form involved excessive amounts of normal glycogen and the other was the result of abnormally branched glycogen. Gerty Cori proved that these diseases were the result of deficiencies or abnormalities in particular enzymes: a deficiency of glucose-6-phosphatase in patients with the normal form of glycogen and an alteration in the branching or debranching enzymes in the other. This classic study was the first demonstration that congenital metabolic diseases can be caused by particular enzyme defects.

These studies of congenital dysfunctions in children represented a kind of return to Gerty Cori's very first research project. During her two postdoctoral years at the Children's Hospital in Vienna, Gerty Cori worked on the problem of temperature regulation in congenital myxedema before and after thyroid therapy. This problem was of considerable interest to pharmacologists such as Geza Mansfeld and Otto Loewi at the time. Later, this study was extended by work on thyroidectomized rabbits. The hospital was not well equipped for more sophisticated work, but the clinical instruction was excellent. Gerty Cori was strongly influenced by a maternal uncle who was professor of pediatrics at the University of Prague and seemed destined for a career as a pediatrician.

The Coris began their pattern of close collaboration while they were medical students. Their first joint paper, an immunological study of complement in human serum, was written when they were still medical students. The year that the Coris were married, 1920, was a time of widespread misery, malnutrition, and even near-starvation for post–World War I Europe. Gerty Cori developed xerophthalmia, but recovered after returning to Prague.

The Coris experienced some institutional resistance to collaborative research at the State Institute for the Study of Malignant Diseases, in Buffalo, New York. The institute, which later became the Roswell Park Memorial Institute, was affiliated with a hospital for cancer patients. Although Gerty Cori was assigned to work on certain aspects of cancer, she and Carl Cori were able to publish their first joint paper on the metabolism of carbohydrates in animals in 1923. However, Gerty Cori was assigned to the institute's Pathology Department to perform routine microscopic diagnostic services. The director of the institute was a strong believer in the theory of the parasitic origin of cancer. One of his researchers claimed to have found encapsulated *Amoeba histolytica* in lymph node cells from patients with Hodgkin's disease. Unfortunately, Gerty Cori was assigned to assist him in looking for amoeba in the stools of cancer patients and controls. The results accorded with the hypothesis as long as the origin of the specimens was known. When Gerty Cori said she could not identify *Amoeba histolytica*, she was told she would lose her job unless she stopped working with her husband. While continuing to stain stool specimens, Gerty Cori carried out more interesting, but inconspicuous research that required only a microscope. This strategy resulted in a paper on the influence of thyroid extract and thyroxin on the rate of multiplication of paramecia which she published in 1923. Eventually, the Coris were allowed to work together on their own research problems.

According to Carl Cori the question of collaboration only arose on one more occasion. He was offered an attractive position at a neighboring university. However, the department head demanded that he take speech lessons, stop his research on insulin, and stop working with his wife. Cori declined because of the last two requirements, but while Carl Cori was being interviewed, Gerty Cori was being told that she was standing in the way of her husband's career and that it was un-American for a man to work with his wife. Carl Cori recalled that the pressure exerted on Gerty Cori was so strong that she was reduced to tears. Carl Cori later characterized scientific collaboration as "a delicate operation which requires much give and take on both sides and occasionally leads to friction, if both are equal partners and not willing to yield on a given point" (C. F. Cori 1969, 12).

Carl Cori's invitation to join the Washington University School of Medicine included a research position with a token salary for Gerty Cori. "Anti-nepotism rules" served as an effective barrier against hiring both husband and wife. The Coris' son was born in August 1936, one of the hottest summers on record in St. Louis. Temperatures in the laboratory were so high that enzyme test solutions could be maintained at 37° C without the use of the customary water baths. In the heroic tradition expected of "Lady Laureates," Gerty Cori remained at work until the very last moment before going to the maternity hospital. During this period the Coris made the discovery of glucose 1-phosphate that they considered the transition point in solving the biochemistry of the glycogen problem. The years spent at Washington University were happy and productive until 1947, when Gerty Cori's fatal illness first appeared only a few weeks before the Coris went to Sweden to receive the Nobel Prize.

Colleagues recalled that Gerty Cori courageously fought the chronic anemia that finally took her life for almost ten years without any diminution in her research activity. Indeed, her illness seemed to intensify the demands she made on herself. During this period she began her pioneering work on the enzymatic lesions in the glycogen storage diseases and served on the first advisory board of the National Science Foundation. Both the first and the last of Gerty Cori's scientific papers deal with biochemical aspects of pediatrics and medicine.

Gerty Cori was deeply interested in the broad aspects and implications of biological science, as well as the necessity for maintaining the highest level of "craftsmanship" in scientific work. Students and colleagues understood that she had no tolerance for mediocrity and respected her as a scientist of great stature and spiritual depth. In her own statement of her system of belief she asserted that "honesty, which stands mostly for intellectual integrity, courage, and kindness, are still the virtues I admire." In "This I Believe," a series of radio broadcasts with Edward R. Murrow, she went on to say: "Contemplation of the great human achievements through the ages is helpful to me in moments of despair and doubt. Human meanness and folly then seem less important. Humanity has but a short history of civilized life and the hope for greater wisdom must resign itself to a fairly distant future" (Ochoa and Kalckar 1958, 16).

At a memorial service for Gerty Cori at Washington University Dr. Houssay offered the following tribute: "Gerty Cori's life was a noble example of dedication to an idea, to the advancement of science for the benefit of humanity. Her charming personality, so rich in human qualities, won the friendship and admiration of all who had the privilege of knowing her. Her name is engraved forever in the annals of science, and her memory will be cherished by all her many friends as long as we live" (C. F. Cori 1969, 19).

Gerty Cori received many awards, including the Midwest Award, American Chemical Society (1946), the Squibb Award in Endocrinology (1947), the Garvan Medal (1948), the St. Louis Award (1948), the Sugar Research Prize (1950), and the Borden Award, Association of Medical Colleges (1951). She received honorary Doctor of Science degrees from Boston University (1948), Smith College (1949), Yale (1951), Columbia (1954), and Rochester (1955). In 1948 she was elected a member of the National Academy of Sciences; her husband had received that honor in 1940.

Gerty Cori was a member of the American Society of Biological Chemists, the American Chemical Society, and the American Philosophical Society.

LOIS N. MAGNER

Selected Bibliography

PRIMARY SOURCES

Green, A. A., and G. T. Cori. 1943. "Crystalline Muscle Phosphorylase. 2. Prosthetic Group." *Journal of Biological Chemistry* 151:31–38.

———. 1945. "The Enzymatic Conversion of Phosphorylase a to b." *Journal of Biological Chemistry* 158: 321–332.

Larner, J., and G. T. Cori. 1951. "Action of Amylo-1,6-Glycosidase and Phosphorylase on Glycogen and Amylopectin." *Journal of Biological Chemistry* 188:17–29.

Cori, C. F., and G. T. Cori. 1952. "Glucose 6-Phosphatase of the Liver in Glycogen Storage Disease." *Journal of Biological Chemistry* 199:661–67.

Cori, G. T. 1952–53. "Glycogen Structure and Enzyme Deficiencies in Glycogen Storage Disease." *Harvey Lectures*, series 48, 145–71. New York: Academic Press.

SECONDARY SOURCES

1947. *Current Biography Yearbook*, 135–37. New York: H. W. Wilson.

1956. "Enzymes and Metabolism: A Collection of Papers Dedicated to Carl F. and Gerty T. Cori on the Occasion of the 60th Birthday." *Biochimica Biophysica Acta*, vol. 20.

Houssay, B. A. 1956. "Carl F. and Gerty T. Cori." *Biochimica Biophysica Acta* 20:11–16.

Kornberg, A., B. L. Horecker, L. Cornudella, and J. Oro, eds. 1956. *Reflections on Biochemistry. In Honour of Severo Ochoa.* Oxford: Pergamon Press.

Ochoa, S., and H. M. Kalckar. 1958. "Gerty T. Cori, Biochemist." *Science* 128:16–17.

1964. *Nobel Lectures, Physiology or Medicine*, vol. 3 (1942–62). Amsterdam: Elsevier.

Cori, C. F. 1969. "The Call of Science." *Annual Review of Biochemistry* 38: 1–20.

Fruton, Joseph S. 1971. "Cori, Gerty Theresa Radnitz." In *Dictionary of Scientific Biography* 3:415–16. New York: Scribner's.

———. 1972. *Molecules and Life. His-*

torical Essays on the Interplay of Chemistry and Biology. New York: Wiley-Interscience.

Rossiter, Margaret W. 1982. *Women Scientists in America. Struggles and Strategies to 1940*. Baltimore: Johns Hopkins University Press.

Florkin, M., E. H. Stotz, and G. Semenza, eds. 1983. *Comprehensive Biochemistry*. Vol. 35, *Selected Topics in the History of Biochemistry. Personal Recollections*, part 1. Amsterdam: Elsevier.

ALLAN MACLEOD CORMACK
1979

Allan Macleod Cormack was born on February 23, 1924, in Johannesburg, South Africa. A physicist, Cormack was awarded the 1979 Nobel Prize jointly with Sir Godfrey Hounsfield for their invention of CAT, or computer axial tomography, the radiologic diagnostic tool now in use throughout the world. Their selection was highly unusual because neither man had any background in physiology or medicine; neither held a doctorate; and their names were not well known even to radiologists. Nevertheless, their work revolutionized clinical medicine. Cormack has been a professor of physics at Tufts University since 1957. He married Barbara Jeanne Seavey in 1950. The Cormacks have two daughters, Margaret Jean and Jean Barbara, and a son, Robert Allan.

Cormack was raised in South Africa by his parents, George and Amelia Macleod Cormack. His early ambition was to become an astronomer, which led to his choice of physics and engineering as fields of study at the University of Capetown, where he earned his undergraduate degree in 1944 and his master's the following year. By then he had developed his career interest in nuclear and theoretical physics. After a year of further graduate work at Cambridge University, he joined the faculty of the University of Capetown in 1946.

Ten years passed before his interest in radiography was aroused. In 1956 the Groote Schur Hospital lost its resident physicist and was unable to replace him immediately. The law required the presence of a physicist to monitor the use of radioactive materials, so Groote Schur appealed to the university for emergency assistance. Cormack, the only nuclear physicist available, agreed to a six-month appointment, requiring him to spend a day and a half each week at the hospital (Di Chiro and Brooks 1979, 1060; *New York Times*, October 12, 1979).

While overseeing the treatment of patients with radiotherapy, Cormack became aware for the first time of the difficulties posed by the weakening of the X-ray beam when it enters the patient's body and the need to measure that differential (the attenuation coefficient) quantitatively. He realized that a series of X-ray measurements made at points outside, as well as within, the body, would solve the problem. He began to consider the possibilities of taking a series of radiographs from several different angles at once and then comparing them. The resulting composite image would offer a more accurate and detailed picture of the body and would be of greater potential value in diagnosis. Not only would the anatomical structure be more fully displayed, but the comparison of minute differences in density between images would enable fine distinctions of organic matter not possible with conventional X-ray pictures.

After finishing his Groote Schur assignment, Cormack took a planned sabbatical leave at Harvard to do research on the interactions of subatomic particles at the Cambridge Electron Accelerator. While there, he worked on a mathematical model for his total image reconstruction. Returning to Capetown in 1957, he made a prototype image of a circular symmetrical object made of wood and aluminum. The dummy was rotated through a collimated gamma ray beam in five millimeter steps. (A collimated beam is arranged in straight parallel rays to avoid the distortion of randomly scattered radiation.) Cormack ran the data through his mathematical model, doing the calculations by hand, and obtained results that produced a satisfactorily accurate internal image of his "patient."

Later that same year Cormack accepted the position at Tufts, becoming a permanent American resident and eventually a citizen. He continued to work on his composite imaging idea and developed a more workable mathematical formula. In 1963 he applied the formula to a new set of pictures taken of a nonsymmetrical construction of plastic and aluminum. The data in this instance were quite complex and extensive and he had to use a computer to complete the calculations. Although his results were again successful, he was unable to find colleagues or radiologists who would share his vision. His published reports sank without a trace (Cormack 1963; 1964; Di Chiro and Brooks 1979, 1060).

Hounsfield, a British engineer, began his explorations of the problem independently in 1967, as a result of his work in pattern recognition studies. He developed a mathematical model less elegant than Cormack's but equally accurate with sufficient computer time. His experiments with test objects attracted interest from British radiologists and the British Department of Health rather quickly and the first clinical CAT scanner was installed in a Wimbledon hospital in 1971. This machine, designed for brain scans only, rotated an X-ray tube and detector around the head one degree at a time, projecting and recording 180 images. Hounsfield presented the results obtained from this prototype in 1972.

By 1979, there were more than twelve manufacturers of CAT scanners, more than two thousand in operation, and hundreds more in production. The basic apparatus conformed to Hounsfield's design, although significantly refined and adapted for whole body scanning. The CAT has improved, in some cases made possible for the first time, accuracy of diagnosis in cancer, brain disorders, abnormalities of the spine, birth defects, and kidney diseases. It has also obviated the necessity of subjecting patients to multiple exhausting and sometimes painful tests.

The multiple installations produced considerable controversy, which continues to this day. Although a health planner or taxpayer may logically argue that only one hospital within a regional area should have such complex and expensive (well over one million dollars) equipment, the desire of individual hospitals and physicians to have a CAT readily available generally prevails. With so many scanners in operation, there is further hot debate over its increasingly routine use—not all diagnoses *require* such a perfect picture.

Hounsfield was the actual inventor of the clinical instrument, but Cormack's model, published ten years earlier, would have been equally successful had anyone acted on his proposals. Two other CAT prototypes were designed in the 1960s, by the neurologist William H. Oldendorf, and the nuclear physicist David E. Kuhl, both Americans. (Kuhl is the inventor of emission radionuclide CT, a powerful tool for obtaining internal biochemical data.) Both these men realized the potential value of image reconstruction, but neither developed a workable mathematical model that could reconstruct the composite without blurring. The mathematical equations used today, interestingly, are neither Cormack's nor Hounsfield's but the work of an Austrian mathematician, Johann Radon, first published in 1917 (Di Chiro and Brooks 1979; *New York Times* October 12, 1979).

In an area of such controversy and excitement, it is not surprising that the Nobel assembly itself was unusually exciting. After a long debate, the members rejected the recommendation of the selection committee and awarded the prize to Cormack and Hounsfield.

Cormack's work had gone almost unrecognized until the Nobel brought him into the spotlight. He had continued teaching undergraduates and experimenting with subatomic particles at Tufts, where he served for some years as chairman of the department. Gifted with a "pungent" sense of humor, he must have been amused as well as slightly frustrated when his hobby of twenty years suddenly became a medical phenomenon. Tufts honored him with the Ballou Medal in 1978; he has also received awards from the Swedish Radiological Society (1979) and the University of Capetown (1980). In his spare time, he enjoys active sports such as tennis, sailing, and rock climbing (Altman 1979, 14; *New York Times* October 12, 1979).

MARCIA MELDRUM

Selected Bibliography

PRIMARY SOURCES

Cormack, Allan M. 1963. "Representation of a Function by Its Line Integrals, with Some Radiological Applications." *Journal of Applied Physics* 34 (September):2722–27.

———. 1964. "Representation of a Function by Its Line Integrals, with Some Radiological Applications 2." *Journal of Applied Physics* 35 (October):2908–13.

SECONDARY SOURCES

1979. "Co-Winners of Nobel Prize: Allan Macleod Cormack." *New York Times* (October 12):14.

Altman, Lawrence K. 1979. "American and Briton Get Nobel Prize for X-Ray Advance." *New York Times* (October 12):1, 14.

Di Chiro, Giovanni, and Rodney A. Brooks. 1979. "The 1979 Nobel Prize in Physiology or Medicine." *Science* 206 (November 30):1060–62.

ANDRÉ FRÉDERIC COURNAND
1956

André Frédéric Cournand was born in Paris on September 24, 1895, to Jules Cournand, a dentist, and Marguérite Weber. André Cournand received the Nobel Prize in Physiology or Medicine in 1956 for his work on heart catheterization and pathological changes in the circulatory system, a prize he shared with Dickinson Woodruff Richards, Jr., and Werner Theodor Otto Forssmann. He married Sibylle Blumer in 1924. Cournand adopted her son, who was killed in action in France in 1944, and they had three daughters. Sibylle Blumer Cournand died in 1959. In 1963 Cournand married Ruth Fabian, who died in 1973. In 1975 he married Beatrice Bishop Berle. Cournand died in Great Barrington, Massachusetts, on February 19, 1988.

Cournand's formal education started at age five at the Lycée Condorcet, although he credits his mother with teaching him to read before he entered the school, as well as with instilling within him a lifelong enthusiasm for classical and modern novels. Rather than sitting through the final year of classes at the Lycée, Cournand spent the year in private studies. He received his bachelor's degree at the Sorbonne in 1913, and took the diploma of physics, chemistry, and biology of the Faculté des Sciences the following year. He interrupted his medical studies, which had begun in 1914, to serve in the French Army in World War I. He began service as a private in an infantry regiment but eventually became a batallion surgeon, and was awarded the Croix de Guerre with three bronze stars.

After the war, Cournand returned to his medical training, repeating the single year of study he had already taken. He became Interne des Hôpitaux de Paris in 1925, and was awarded an M.D. degree from the Faculté de Médecine de Paris in 1930, with a thesis on acute disseminated sclerosis. During this period Cournand became seriously interested in art and befriended a number of modernists who were later well known, such as the sculptor Jacques Lipschitz.

Cournand then went to the United States to pursue his studies, intending to return to Paris to go into private practice as a chest physician. He was first a resident, and then chief resident, on the Tuberculosis Service of the Columbia University Division of Bellevue Hospital, in New York City. There he started collaborating with Dickinson Richards, with whom Cournand shared his Nobel Prize. Cournand soon found himself in a productive research project and elected to remain in the United States. He became an American citizen in 1941.

Cournand performed his investigations on the cardiovascular system in the Bellevue Hospital Cardio-Pulmonary Laboratory. His academic appointments elevated him from instructor (1934) to professor of medicine (1956) at Columbia University. Cournand received many honors in addition to the Nobel Prize. He was a member of the National Academy of Sciences and president of the Harvey Society. He received the Trudeau Medal and the Lasker Award.

Cournand's studies of the heart and circulation started in 1932, when he was chief resident at Bellevue Hospital. In that year he started to collaborate with Richards, then at the Columbia-Presbyterian Medical Center, on a systematic examination of cardiopulmonary function in health and disease. They started with the explicit assumption that the heart, lung, and circulation form a single system for the exchange of gases between the environment and the organism, and their early work focused on the mechanical features of the lung.

But Cournand and Richards were hindered in these early studies because they could not directly measure the gas content of blood as it was returning from the body to the lungs, after its oxygen content had been delivered to the body. If they could only obtain samples of blood from within the right auricle, the cardiac chamber that collects blood from the body before pumping the blood to the lungs, where the blood receives more oxygen, they would be able to calculate the cardiac output. That information would help them a great deal in understanding how the lungs were functioning. Forssmann had described passage of a catheter into his own right atrium in 1929, but little further investigation had been done using the technique. In 1936 Cournand returned to Paris to learn the technique of passing a tube into the right auricle. In New York, Cournand, Richards, and their colleagues practiced the technique on laboratory animals for four years, and found that the passage of catheters into animals' hearts did not significantly interfere with the functioning of these hearts.

Their first attempt to perform the procedure on a patient, in 1940, was unsuccessful. But they were encouraged to pursue this line of investigation by some senior investigators who were studying the heart's output using the ballistocardiogram, an instrument that recorded the motion of the body caused by the heart beat. These ballistocardiograph researchers wanted to compare their results with those obtained by another method of determining cardiac output. Eventually Cournand was able to insert a catheter into a human heart and measure the cardiac output. He showed that the cardiac output as measured by the ballistocardiogram was too low, but, more importantly, he also showed that it was practical and safe to routinely insert a catheter into the right side of the heart.

Over the next few years, Cournand, Richards, and their colleagues made several technical advances. A new catheter was designed that was easier to maneuver than the old one, and a measuring device was constructed that enabled simultaneous recording of four different pressure tracings and the electrocardiogram. In 1942 they advanced the catheter into the right ventricle, and by 1944 they had advanced it as far as the pulmonary artery, thus enabling them to measure both the hemodynamic pressure and the amount of oxygen present in the blood at each stage of the blood's passage through the right side of the heart.

Earlier investigators had encountered a great deal of opposition from other physicians to the idea of passing catheters into the heart, because the procedure was thought to be extremely dangerous. Cournand, Richards, and their coworkers encountered much less opposition, perhaps because their studies were performed as part of a study of various forms of shock, a subject of great importance for a country at war. Funded by the federal government through the Committee on Medical Research, from 1942 to 1944 Cournand, Richards, and their colleagues studied over one hundred critically ill patients suffering from all kinds of shock: traumatic shock, hemorrhagic shock, burn shock, shock caused by rupture of an internal organ. They outlined the profound effects of a reduction of circulating blood volume on cardiac output, particularly on the flow of blood to peripheral organs and to the kidney, and described how the condition could be reversed by appropriate volume replacement. Later, they applied the same technique to diagnose congenital cardiac defects, in which an abnormal opening between the cardiac chambers could be detected by means of pressure and oxygen measurements. In a similar fashion, measurement of the pressure in the cardiac chambers was found to be valuable for the diagnosis of acquired cardiac defects, particularly diseases of the heart valves. They also showed that elevated cardiac pressures could be a result of lung disease as well as of heart disease.

Cournand saw life as the opportunity for adventure, whether that adventure be modern art, mountain climbing, or science. He enjoyed gatherings of friends and lively conversation. He had a subtle sense of humor that was appreciated by those who had the opportunity to get to know him. The outpouring of sentiment on the occasion of a memorial service held for Cournand at Columbia University on March 17, 1988, demonstrated that those who knew him found him to be an inspiring person.

Cournand and Richards worked together from February 1932 until February 1973, a remarkably long period of collaboration. Together, using the insights of the third Nobel Prize winner of 1956, Werner Forssmann, Cournand and Richards demonstrated the feasibility of routinely measuring pressures and drawing blood samples from within the heart and the pulmonary circulation. Not long after the discovery that right-sided pressures could be measured, others extended the technique to measuring pressures on the left side of the heart. Today the passing of catheters into the heart for diagnosis is a routine procedure, one for which patients may not even spend the night in a hospital. But today's cardiologists do more than diagnose: they are using cardiac catheters to treat heart disease, both by instilling medicine directly into the heart and by using the catheters mechanically to expand a constricted blood vessel, or to ablate a diseased part of the heart. The techniques of Cournand, Richards, and Forssmann have become central to both the diagnosis and the treatment of almost every type of heart disease.

JOEL D. HOWELL

Selected Bibliography

PRIMARY SOURCES

Cournand, André, and A. Ranges. 1941. "Catheterization of the Right Auricle in Man." *Proceedings of the Society for Experimental Biology and Medicine* 46:462–66.

———. 1956. Biography. In *Nobel Lectures, Physiology or Medicine*, vol. 3 (1942–1962), 543–45. Amsterdam: Elsevier, 1964.

———. 1956. "Control of the Pulmonary Circulation in Man, with Some Remarks on Methodology." Nobel Lecture. Reprinted in *Nobel Lectures, Physiology or Medicine*, vol. 3 (1942–1962), 529–42. Amsterdam: Elsevier, 1964.

———. 1959. "The Historical Development of the Concepts of Pulmonary Circulation." In *Pulmonary Circulation: An International Symposium*, edited by Wright Adams and Ilza Veith, 1–19. New York: Grune and Stratton.

———. 1975. "Cardiac Catheterization: Development of the Technique, Its Contributions to Experimental Medicine, and Its Initial Applications in Man." *Acta Medica Scandinavica*, Supplementum 579:7–32.

———. 1986. *From Roots to Late Budding: The Intellectual Adventures of a Medical Scientist*. New York: Gardner Press.

SECONDARY SOURCES

Johnson, Steven L. 1970. *The History of Cardiac Surgery, 1896–1955*. Baltimore: Johns Hopkins University Press.

Weisse, Allen B. 1984. "André Cournand." In *Conversations in Medicine: The Story of Twentieth-Century American Medicine in the Words of Those Who Created It*, 112–31. New York: New York University Press.

1988. "Cournand, André." (Obituary) *Washington Post* (21 February).

Bradley, Stanley E. 1988. *André Cournand, 1895–1988: Remarks Delivered at the Memorial Service, St. Paul's Chapel, Columbia University, 17 March 1988*. New York: Meriden-Stinehour Press.

FRANCIS HARRY COMPTON CRICK *1962*

Francis Harry Compton Crick was born on June 8, 1916, in Northampton, England. His father, Harry Crick, was a manufacturer of shoes. His mother was Annie Elizabeth (née Wilkins). Crick was married twice; he had a son with his first wife, Ruth Doreen (née Dodd), and two daughters with his second, Odile (née Speed). After completing his B.S. in physics in 1937 at University College, London, Crick was soon engaged in wartime work for the Admiralty, where he worked on mine detection and development. He returned after the war to the Strangeways Laboratory (1947–49) to pursue biophysics as a career and then joined the Medical Research Council in Cambridge where, with the exception of a year at Brooklyn Polytechnical College (1953–54) he remained until 1977. Since 1977 he has been affiliated with the Salk Institute in La Jolla, California. He shared the Nobel Prize with James D. Watson and Maurice H. F. Wilkins in 1962.

Crick met Watson at Cambridge in 1951. Watson, a student of Salvador Luria at Indiana University, had switched his postdoctoral fellowship from Denmark to try a new approach for studying nucleic acids. Both Crick and Watson had been influenced by Erwin Schrödinger's *What Is Life?*, a popularization of genetics seen from a physicist's perspective. Crick's approach to biology was quite different from Schrödinger's because Crick was an atheist and Schrödinger's perception of life was vitalistic. What Crick found of value, however, was Schrödinger's recognition that many of the uniquely biological properties, such as heredity, were amenable to an analysis that physicists had successfully used for the structure of inanimate matter. Although Crick was still working on his Ph.D. dissertation project, the structure of hemoglobin molecules, he enjoyed the opportunity of working with Watson and teaching him about the X-ray diffraction analysis of molecules.

Crick and Watson proposed their "double helix" structure for the DNA molecule in 1953. Their analysis described two strands of deoxyribose phosphate, linked by the four nitrogenous bases (adenine, thymine, quanine, and cytosine), in hydrogen-bonded pairs. This innovative model made clear the process of DNA self-replication. The story of how the structure was discovered has been well documented by Watson, by Horace Freeland Judson, and by Anne Sayre, although each of the principals offers a slightly different recollection.

The consequences of the discovery were overwhelming. The DNA model pleased older geneticists like Herman J. Muller, who had long believed in the relationship of the physical and chemical structure of the gene. Scientific and popular acclaim were showered on Crick and Watson, and the double helix became the basis for the molecular outlook that has since dominated thought and experimentation in the life sciences.

Crick was never an enthusiastic or patient experimentalist. He considered himself a theoretician and often had greater influence through what he said to those working around him, than through his own published work. After he completed his Ph.D. in 1953, he directed his attention to cracking what Schrödinger referred to as the genetic "codescript." After George Gamow demonstrated that the codescript required a triplet code, Crick speculated on how such a code would work and how the "central dogma," as he called it, would transfer information from the genes (DNA) to RNA (ribonucleic acid) and then to proteins. Crick identified the first phase as a copying of RNA from DNA. The complementary pairing of bases that they had developed for the DNA molecule would apply to the RNA copied from a strand of DNA (a process later called transcription). This transcribed RNA was later called messenger RNA (mRNA). Once the mRNA was present in the cell cytoplasm, it had to be decoded (later the process was called translation). Crick predicted the existence of a new class of molecules, "adaptors," which would be composed of RNA and bring amino acids to the mRNA. Crick's hypothesis of copying and decoding of nucleic acid information was confirmed and demonstrated by several laboratories, including Watson's at Harvard, but his specific code, proposed in 1957, was shown to be wrong in 1960 when Marshall Nirenberg demonstrated by a novel approach that all the theoretical codes up to that time were incorrect and that the actual code could not be inferred from existing models of cryptography.

Crick and his colleagues used the new genetic code in many original ways. They proved that excisions of DNA from a gene, unless in multiples of three base pairs, would result in a category of mutation they called frame shifts, like the gibberish produced by a typist whose fingers wander from their normal alignment. Crick realized that the first two members of the triplet (later called a codon) had a more significant role in identifying an amino acid for the adaptor molecules (later called transfer RNA or tRNA molecules) than did the last base pair. This third base in a triplet would often be filled by either of two or more bases. Crick called this the "wobble hypothesis" and believed it represented a stage in the evolution of the genetic code as more amino acid types became incorporated into proteins.

Crick had a profound influence within the Cambridge group who were working on molecular problems. His free speculations stimulated his colleagues to put to experimental test many of the theories and models he conceived. He was an avid reader of the scientific literature and enjoyed discussing the implications of new observations and contradicting prevailing views.

Although Watson's autobiographical account of the discovery of the structure of DNA depicts Crick as immodest, loud, and socially awkward, Crick's autobiography gives the reader an impression of a reserved, thoughtful, and far from flamboyant personality. In the 1950s Crick's speeches were witty, brilliant, and delivered with excited enthusiasm. He stood out among his colleagues at meetings in Cold Spring Harbor or Brookhaven, a tall, elegant, gracious figure in Edwardian dress with long sideburns, at a time when most American scientists had closely cropped haircuts and wore undistinguished business suits.

Crick expressed his views favoring atheism and rejecting vitalistic ideas in science in his book *Of Molecules and Men.* In this work he rejected a religious interpretation of human origins and of human thought and values, advocating the worth of humanistic values and materialistic outlooks on life. He also provided in it his speculations on the relation of computers to human thought processes and how a molecular biology and physics of the nervous system might be realized in the forthcoming decades.

While Crick did not dispute the evolution of life on earth, he expressed doubt that life arose on earth from nonliving matter and the conditions that prevailed in the earth's early history. Instead, Crick revived, in *Life Itself*, the ideas of Svante Arrhenius, who thought life was scattered throughout parts of the universe by small molecules capable of germinating in an appropriate environment. Crick based these speculations on the presence of organic molecules in comets, stellar clouds, and meteors, holding that the formation of at least organic macromolecules may have arisen before the earth itself was formed.

Crick's speculative courage accelerated the deciphering of the genetic code and the understanding of its relation to protein synthesis and mutageneisis. His speculations on the nature of dreams (which he considers to be discharged noise to clear neuronal pathways for another day's behavioral activity), his "panspermic" proposal for the origin of life on earth, his theories of how nerves work, and other complex issues in the life sciences have not had the same success in leading to experimental confirmation or rejection as had his theories of gene function.

Crick married Ruth Doreen Dodd in 1940. They were divorced after seven years and one son, Michael. His second marriage was to Odile Speed in 1949; they have two daughters, Gabrielle and Jacqueline. He is a Fellow of the Royal Society, a member of the American Academy of Arts and Sciences, and a foreign member of the scientific societies of India, Germany, France, and Greece. Among the many awards he has received for his work are the Warren Triennial Prize (1959), the Lasker Award (1960), the Mayer Prize from the French Académie des Sciences (1961), the Gairdner Foundation Award (1962), the Royal Medal (1972) and the Copley Medal (1976) of the Royal Society, and the Michelson-Morley Award (1981).

ELOF AXEL CARLSON

Selected Bibliography

PRIMARY SOURCES

Watson, J. D., and F. H. C. Crick. 1953. "Molecular Structure of Nucleic Acids. A Structure for Deoxyribose Nucleic Acid." *Nature* 171: 737–38.

Watson, J. D., and F. H. C. Crick. 1953."Genetical Implications of the Structure of Deoxyribonucleic Acid." *Nature* 171:964–67.

Crick, F. H. C. 1957. "On Protein Synthesis." *Symposia for the Society of Experimental Biology 1957* 12:138–63.

———. 1966. *Of Molecules and Men.* Seattle, Wash.: University of Washington Press.

———. 1981. *Life Itself: Its Origin and Nature.* New York: Simon and Schuster.

———. 1988. *What Mad Pursuit.* New York: Basic Books.

SECONDARY SOURCES

Watson, J. D. 1968. *The Double Helix.* New York: Atheneum.

Olby, Robert. 1970. "Francis Crick, DNA, and the Central Dogma." *Daedalus* (Fall):938–41.

———. 1974. *The Path to the Double Helix.* Seattle, Wash.: University of Washington Press.

Judson, Horace Freeland. 1979. *The Eighth Day of Creation: The Makers of the Revolution in Biology.* New York: Simon and Schuster.

SIR HENRY HALLETT DALE
1936

Henry Dale was born in June 1875 in London, the second son of seven children born to Charles Dale, a businessman, and his wife Frances (née Hallett). In 1904 he married Ellen Hallett, his first cousin, and they had one son and two daughters (the eldest, Alison, married Alexander Todd, the 1957 Nobel Prize–winner in Chemistry). Dale's early independent work was performed, unusually for that time, in laboratories owned by a pharmaceutical manufacturer; later he moved to the newly created National Institute of Medical Research (NIMR). He was awarded the Nobel Prize for Physiology or Medicine in 1936, sharing the honor with Otto Loewi. Dale's researches, on the role of endogenous chemicals in the regulation of normal physiological, and abnormal pathological, functioning, were a major stimulus for, and contribution to, the development of experimental pharmacology and chemotherapeutics. Knighted in 1932, he served as president of the Royal Society during World War II, received numerous honors, awards, and distinctions from every part of the world, and died in Cambridge, England, in 1968.

Dale received his scientific training in the Physiological Laboratory at Cambridge University. He entered Trinity College in 1894, and came under the influence of W. H. Gaskell, H. K. Anderson, and J. N. Langley. He left Cambridge in 1900 to complete his medical studies at St. Bartholomew's Hospital Medical College in London. After qualifying, a rare research opportunity arose, the George Henry Lewes studentship in physiology, which Dale applied for successfully. He spent his tenure as Lewes student in Ernest Starling's laboratory at University College, London, working on histological changes in pancreatic cells evoked by secretin. Secretin, the first hormone to be identified, had just been discovered by Starling and his coworker Bayliss. Thus the concept of the chemical control of physiological function was in the forefront of research activites in the laboratory at that time. So while essentially working on morphological aspects of a physiological problem, Dale was closely associated with ideas of the chemical regulation of normal functioning. At University College Dale also met one of Starling's foreign visitors, Otto Loewi—this was the beginning of their lifelong friendship.

In 1904 Dale spent three months in Paul Ehrlich's laboratory in Frankfurt. Ehrlich, Nobel Prize winner in 1908, was the originator of the side-chain theory that suggested that the chemical structure of compounds determined their immunological activity; Ehrlich's ideas reinforced Dale's impressions of the association of chemical composition with physiological function and pharmacological effect. Back in London, Dale returned to Starling's department for a short period before being recommended to Henry Wellcome as a suitable person to work in the latter's Physiological Research Laboratories.

These laboratories had been started in 1894 for the raising of diphtheria antitoxin, although by 1904 Wellcome wanted to employ a first-rate physiologist to conduct basic scientific research. The "commercial" associations of such a venture were deeply distrusted by the medical and scientific community and Dale was warned against accepting such a position. Clearly, however, he saw the potential of working in a well-equipped laboratory, liberated from the routine demands of teaching and virtually free to choose problems for study. Wellcome suggested that he might like to study ergot, a drug much used in obstetrics to promote labor but of uncertain and even erratic properties. With no definite proposal of his own, Dale accepted the suggestion and this initial work became the basis of practically the whole of his subsequent research.

Almost immediately he discovered, quite by accident, that ergot reversed the activity of epinephrine (adrenaline), an animal-derived product whose physiological properties (pressor effects, i.e., the raising of blood pressure, etc.) were already well known. Such results anticipated the development in the 1960s of the beta-blocking group of drugs. At the same time Dale's experiments, like those of his Cambridge friend and colleague T. R. Elliott, showed that application of epinephrine by itself mimicked the effects of neural stimulation of the sympathetic branches of the autonomic nervous system. Elliott had actually proposed that epinephrine could be released by nerve terminals in the process of the transmission of impulses, but never followed up the work himself. Later Dale and the chemist George Barger identified a wide range of chemicals with such properties, to which the term "sympathomimetic" was applied. The most potent of these was norepinephrine (nor-adrenaline), many years later identified as a natural transmitter of nervous impulses. When Dale and Barger performed their analysis, norepinephrine was not known to be naturally occurring, so it was not investigated further.

Further collaborative work with Barger and with Arthur Ewins revealed that ergot contained a number of pharmacologically active compounds, including tyramine, histamine, and acetylcholine. Dale was appointed director of the Wellcome Laboratories in 1906. Inspired by his work on ergot and influenced by his approach to understanding the underlying chemical mechanisms of physiological functions, he began examining the chemical constituents of the posterior pituitary lobe, which had stimulatory effects on the uterus. One of his consistent aims was to relate such findings to the physiological mechanisms of the whole animal; many of the activities of these chemicals mimicked the normal functioning of mammalian tissue examined in the laboratory.

During World War I, as a member of staff of the recently created Medical Research Committee (MRC), he was diverted into work on shock, amoebic dysentery, gas gangrene, and deficiency diets. But even this war work reveals common themes of the relationship between chemical structure and physiological functioning. After 1919, in the new National Institute for Medical Research in London, Dale expanded his early work in physiology and pharmacology, although now he was hampered by routine duties associated with the administration of the MRC and the NIMR, where he became the first director in 1928.

In the late 1920s Dale, with H. W. Dudley, isolated acetylcholine from the mammalian spleen. His own prewar work had defined the pharmacological activities of this chemical in vitro and had shown that it closely paralleled normal responses in vivo. Now he had identified it as a normal constituent of the body and not merely a synthetic artifact. Was it possible therefore that it performed in vivo the functions that it mimicked so closely in vitro? Complementary work by Otto Loewi in Graz also emphasized the possible role of acetylcholine in neurotransmission. Work in Dale's laboratory accelerated, greatly assisted by coworkers such as G. L. Brown and the German refugees W. S. Feldberg and M. Vogt. Feldberg introduced a sensitive assay for acetylcholine (the eserinized leech muscle) that enabled the group to reliably measure the amount of acetylcholine released after nerve stimulation at various sites in the autonomic nervous system. During the 1930s a number of major papers appeared from the laboratory, each one providing more evidence that acetylcholine had an endogenous role in the transmission of nervous impulses. It was for this work that Dale was awarded the Nobel Prize in 1936. (The theory of chemical neurotransmission was not undisputed; Dale's main antagonist for many years was J. C. Eccles, Nobel Prize winner in 1963 [Dale 1937, 401–29].)

Closely associated with his overwhelming interest in "autopharmacology," the physiology and pharmacology of endogenous chemical substances, was Dale's concern with the standardization of drugs. He served on many national and international committees that established and promoted the acceptance of reliable international standards.

Not surprisingly, Dale's scientific preeminence brought numerous invitations to assume public duties. He exerted considerable influence on the development of medical research in Britain. He was elected a Fellow of the Royal Society in 1914, and served as biological secretary (1925–35) and president (1940–45). His service to the Royal Society also included writing the obituaries or biographical memoirs of fifteen fellows; his detailed and sympathetic portraits of distinguished colleagues and friends reveal much about his own generous personality. Among many more honors and distinctions, Dale was elected president of the Royal Institution (1942–46), president of the British Association for the Advancement of Science (1947), and president of the Royal Society of Medicine (1948–50).

He was a committee member of the Physiological Society for over twenty years, and one of the first trustees of the Wellcome Trust, which he served from 1936 until his death. He was awarded the Order of Merit in 1944. He maintained his scientific interests until just a few weeks before his death in 1968. The many tributes and obituaries emphasized his open, generous personality and his considerable talent for grasping the essential features of complex matters and expressing himself with elegant lucidity.

E. M. TANSEY

Selected Bibliography

PRIMARY SOURCES

Dale, H. H. 1935. "Pharmacology and Nerve Endings." *Proceedings of the Royal Society of Medicine* 28:319–32.

—. 1936. "Some Recent Extensions of the Chemical Transmission of the Effects of Nerve Impulse." Nobel Lecture. Reprinted in *Nobel Lectures in Physiology or Medicine*, vol. 2 (1922–1941), 402–15. Amsterdam: Elsevier, 1965.

———. 1937. "Acetylcholine as a Chemical Transmitter of the Effects of Nerve Impulses." *Journal of the Mount Sinai Hospital* 4:401–29.

———. 1953. *Adventures in Physiology, with Excursions into Autopharmacology*. London: Wellcome Trust. Reprinted 1965.

———. 1954. *An Autumn Gleaning: Occasional Lectures and Addresses.* London: Pergamon Press.

———. 1958. "Autobiographical Sketch." *Perspectives in Biology and Medicine* 1:125–37.

SECONDARY SOURCES

Gasser, H. S. 1955. "Sir Henry Dale: His Influence on Science." *British Medical Journal* (June 4):1359–61.

Feldberg, W. 1970. "Henry Hallett Dale." *Biographical Memoirs of Fellows of the Royal Society* 16: 77–173.

Bacq, Z. M. 1975. *Chemical Transmission of Nerve Impulses.* Oxford: Pergamon Press.

Feldberg, W. 1977. "The Early History of Synaptic and Neuromuscular Transmission by Acetylcholine: Reminiscences of an Eye Witness." In *Pursuit of Nature*, 65–83. Cambridge: Cambridge University Press for the Physiological Society.

CARL PETER HENDRIK DAM
1943

Carl Peter Hendrik Dam was born on February 21, 1895, in Copenhagen. A biochemist, Dam received the Nobel Prize in 1943 for his discovery of vitamin K, the blood coagulation factor. Edward Doisy of the United States, who identified the chemical structure of vitamin K (3-methyl-3-phytyl-1, 4-naphthoquinone), shared the award for that year. At the time of the award, Dam was senior research associate at Strong Memorial Hospital in Rochester, New York, where he lived throughout the German occupation of Denmark. He returned to Copenhagen in 1946 to become professor of biochemistry at the Polytechnic Institute, a position he held until his retirement. Dam was married to Inger Olsen in July 1924; they had no children. He died on April 18, 1976, in Copenhagen.

Dam was the son of Emilie Peterson Dam, a teacher, and Emil Dam, a pharmaceutical chemist who wrote a history of Danish pharmacy. He studied chemistry at the Polytechnic Institute, receiving his master of science degree in 1920. After three years (1920–23) as a chemistry instructor at the Royal School of Agriculture and Veterinary Medicine in Copenhagen, he joined the physiological laboratory of Valdemar Henriques at the University of Copenhagen. He spent five years as an instructor and research assistant, including a year studying microchemistry with Fritz Pregl in Graz, Austria, in 1925.

Dam was appointed assistant professor of biochemistry at the university in 1928 and promoted to associate professor in 1929. He began a series of experiments to determine whether chickens, like mammals, were able to synthesize cholesterol or other sterols. (A sterol is a solid alcohol compound related to the steroids.) Earlier experiments, in 1914, had appeared to show the reverse; but the action of the fat-soluble vitamins, A and D, in sterol metabolism was not then understood. Dam therefore began raising chicks on a sterol-free diet with vitamin A and D supplements. He compared the amount of cholesterol in their bodies and waste products with that of newly hatched chicks and that of other chicks on the same diet for different lengths of time.

His findings confirmed that a newly hatched chick's body contains cholesterol from the egg yolk, which is excreted over two to three weeks; but cholesterol then continues to be produced and excreted in increasing amounts by the growing chick. He thus established that chicks could both synthesize and break down the sterol. Dam continued his research into sterol metabolism during a year's leave (1932–33) as a Rockefeller Fellow in Freiburg, where he worked with Rudolph Schoenheimer. In 1934 he presented his thesis at Copenhagen and was awarded the doctor of science degree.

In the course of these studies, however, Dam noted that the chicks that remained on the sterol-free diet for more than two weeks developed hemorrhages under the skin and in various organs. Blood samples were taken and tested; the blood was abnormally slow to coagulate. Some normal dietary ingredient that was essential to coagulation was missing from the chicks' daily intake.

The missing factor was certainly not cholesterol, which the chicks produced themselves. Dam experimented by adding fats, vitamin C, salt, and wheat germ oil to the birds' diet, without effect. He therefore determined that the coagulation factor was a dietary ingredient or vitamin previously unknown. This finding was announced in 1934 (Dam 1934). He then established that the new vitamin was fat-soluble and was obtainable from a high cereal diet, leafy greens, and pork liver. In 1935 Dam named the new vitamin "K," the next in alphabetic sequence for vitamin designation, and, by coincidence, the initial letter in the Danish word "Koagulation."

Subsequent experiments, by Dam, Paul Karrer in Zurich, Doisy in St. Louis, and others, determined that vitamin K is absorbed in the intestines and acts in the liver to assist the synthesis of prothrombin, a protein-related substance which is then released into the bloodstream. Prothrombin reacts with thromboplastin and calcium to form thrombin, which further reacts with fibrinogen to form the insoluble fibrin network that clots blood cells together and prevents uncontrolled flow. Without prothrombin, none of these reactions can take place, even though all the other elements are present. A vitamin K deficiency results in the inability to produce prothrombin (Dam 1936; 1944).

By 1938 Dam had traced the hemorrhages common in operations for gallstones or other obstructions of the bile ducts (obstructive jaundice) to the body's inability to transport vitamin K to the liver without bile. He deduced that administration of K would make such surgery possible. Dam and Karrer together isolated pure K from green leaves in 1939, almost simultaneously with the success of Doisy's team using alfalfa, and with that of several others. Doisy's further analysis determined the chemical formula and made possible laboratory synthesis of the vitamin for clinical use. (Doisy also established the difference between K_1, which is the factor present in plants, and K_2, which is produced by putrefaction. Although very similar chemically, the two substances are not identical.)

Vitamin K therapy also proved important for newborn infants, who have virtually none of this substance present in their bodies and who therefore are in great danger of hemorrhage from even mild trauma. The availability of the synthetic vitamin K has saved many infant lives. It is also effective in cases of ulcerative colitis and other intestinal diseases (Dam 1944; Illson 1976).

Dam was invited to the United States in 1940 by the American-

Scandinavian Foundation. For two years he traveled and lectured in the United States and Canada, participated in research at the Marine Biological Laboratories in Woods Hole, Massachusetts, and took part in a vitamin K symposium at the University of Chicago. He had been scheduled to return to Denmark in 1941 but decided to remain in America when the Nazis occupied his homeland. From 1942 to 1945 he worked at Strong Memorial Hospital and was affiliated with the University of Rochester and in 1945 he briefly became an associate member of the Rockefeller Institute for Medical Research. In 1944 the Nobel Committee for the first and only time held its presentation ceremonies in the United States and Dam and Doisy received their awards in New York.

In June 1946 Dam was able to return to Copenhagen and to take up the professorship at the Polytechnic Institute, which had been held open for him for five years. Soon after his departure, he commented critically that "there are few really good [hospitals] in the United States, where there is too much business in the whole system." He was nevertheless invited to return in 1949 for a three-month lecture tour on his recent work on vitamin E deficiency (Illson 1976).

Dam continued his research into fat and sterol metabolism throughout the 1950s and early 1960s, serving in addition as head of the Department of Biology at the Polytechnic, and from 1956 to 1963 as director of the Biochemical Division of the Danish Fat Research Institute. When on holiday, he enjoyed extensive travel. He retired in 1965 and died quietly at age eighty-one.

Dam was a member of the Royal Danish Academy of Sciences, the Biologisk Selskab, the American Institute of Nutrition, the Society for Experimental Biology and Medicine, and the Sociétié Chimique of Zurich. Among the many other honors he received for his work were the Christian Bohr Award in Physiology (1939) and the Norman Medal of the German Fat Research Society (1960).

MARCIA MELDRUM

Selected Bibliography

PRIMARY SOURCES

Dam, Henrik. 1934. "Hemorrhages in Chicks Reared on Artificial Diets: New Deficiency Disease." *Nature* 133 (June 16):909–10.

Dam, Henrik, and F. Schønheyder. 1936. "Occurrence and Chemical Nature of Vitamin K." *Biochemical Journal* 30 (May):897–901.

Dam, Henrick. 1941. *Some Studies on Vitamin E.* Copenhagen: Munksgaard.

———. 1942. "Vitamin K, Its Chemistry and Physiology." *Advances in Enzymology* 2:285.

———. 1943. "Medical Aspects of Vitamin K." *Lancet* 63:353.

———. 1944. "The Discovery of Vitamin K, Its Biological and Therapeutical Application." Nobel Lecture, December 12, 1944. Reprinted in *Nobel Lectures in Physiology or*

Medicine, vol. 3 (1942–1962), 8–24. Amsterdam: Elsevier, 1964.

SECONDARY SOURCES

1949. "Dam, Carl Peter Hendrik." *Current Biography Yearbook*, 134–36. New York: H. W. Wilson.

Illson, Murray. April 25, 1976. "K for Koagulation." *New York Times*: 53.

1980. "Dam, Carl Peter Hendrik." *Modern Scientists and Engineers*, 1: 258–59. New York: McGraw-Hill.

JEAN DAUSSET *1980*

The French immunologist Jean Baptiste Gabriel Joachim Dausset received the Nobel Prize in Physiology or Medicine in 1980, sharing it with Baruj Benacerraf and George D. Snell. His "chief contribution was the recognition of the human histocompatibility antigens."

Jean Baptiste Gabriel Joachim Dausset was born on October 19, 1916, in Toulouse, France. He was the son of Henri Pierre Jules Dausset, a physician who specialized in radiology and rheumatism, and Elisabeth (Brullard) Dausset. He had two other siblings. His early years were spent in Biarritz. The family moved to Paris when he was eleven. He attended the Lycée Michelet in Vanves, near Paris. After receiving his baccalauréat, he entered the University of Paris Medical School. He became an externe in 1937 and an interne in 1941 at les Hôpitaux de Paris.

When World War II broke out in 1939, Dausset was drafted into the French Medical Corps. After the German occupation, he joined the Free French Army in North Africa and participated in the Tunisian Campaign and the Normandy Campaign. Before leaving France, Dausset gave his identity papers to Elie Wollman, a Jewish colleague at the Pasteur Institute, to help him evade the Nazis (*Current Biography* 1981).

Dausset obtained his medical degree from the University of Paris in 1945. He completed his internship and residency in internal medicine and hematology at the Paris Municipal Hospitals between 1946 and 1950. In 1948 Dausset was a fellow in hematology at Harvard University. He remained at Harvard another year as a fellow in immunohematology. In 1949 he became a research fellow at the Institut d'Hygiène and an associate at the Regional Blood Transfusion Center. From 1950 to 1963 Dausset was director of the Immunohematology Laboratory, at the National Blood Transfusion Center. In 1958 he became associate professor of hematology and in 1968 was promoted to professor of immunohematology at the Faculty of Medicine, University of Paris.

During World War II Dausset had worked in the resuscitation service. This experience led to his interest in the immunological aspects of blood transfusions. In the mid-1940s he started to investigate blood replacement transfusion methods.

In a paper published in 1951, Dausset outlined the adverse reactions to transfusions caused by strong immune anti-A antibodies in the plasma of universal donors. The systematic testing of donor blood for those antibodies, he showed, helped prevent such accidents. He also pioneered a method of exchange transfusion in adults who suffer from kidney failure or from septicemia.

He became interested in autoimmune hemolytic anemia. He used the serological characteristics of the corresponding autoantibodies and classified the various forms of the disorder, caused by the destruction of red blood cells and often associated with the use of certain drugs.

Dausset's research into the causes and treatment of agranulocytosis led him to a discovery that would influence all his later work. Agranulocytosis, an acute feverish illness (usually resulting from drug hypersensitivity), manifests itself with a severe reduction in the leukocyte (white blood cell) count. He and his collaborator André-Dominique Nenna published their paper entitled "Presence of a Leucoagglutinate in the Serum of a Case of Chronic Agranulolcytosis" in 1952; it was the first description of an immunological reaction in which antibodies reacted with white blood cells in the donor's blood, but not with their own leukocytes.

George D. Snell had shown that tissue rejection in mice is controlled by a few physically linked genes, the "major histocompatibility complex (MHC)." In 1958 Dausset proved the existence in human beings of antigens that denote a genetically based histocompatibility complex. He found that patients who had received many blood transfusions—and who therefore had been exposed to many antigens from foreign tissue—made antibodies that reacted with antigens found on white blood cells from other individuals but not with those on their own cells. Several patients produced antibodies against the same antigen, the Mac (which stands for the initials of three blood donors). As stated by Fritz Bach, of the University of Minnesota Medical School, "This was the first serum to define an HLA antigen and led in part to the definition of the histocompatibility system in man" (Marx 1980).

From 1962 to 1968 Dausset was cochairman at the Institute for Research into Diseases of the Blood. From 1963 to 1978 he was biologist for the Paris municipal hospital system. In 1963 he became head of Hematology-Serology-Immunology at the Saint-Louis Hospital. From 1968 to 1984 he held the position of director of the research unit on immunogenetics of human transplantation, at the National Institute of

Health and Medical Research. He became professor of experimental medicine at the Collège de France in 1977 (until 1987). From 1978 to 1984 he was codirector of the Oncology and Immunohematology Laboratory at the French National Institute for Scientific Research.

In the 1960s and 1970s Dausset undertook to further unravel the human major histocompatibility complex. In an international workshop on histocompatibility in 1965 Dausset and Pavol Ivanyi and Dagmar Ivanyi (then both at the Czechoslovak National Academy) delivered a paper that helped to organize and clarify a mass of often conflicting information. They described a system of some ten antigens. They suggested that the genetic region responsible for the coding of the system—which they called Hu-1 [for Human No. 1 (Humain n° 1)]—included several subloci, each of which determined the appearance of a limited number of specific antigens on the surface of human cells. The system was later renamed HLA (for Human Leukocyte, locus-A).

In 1967, in collaboration with Felix Theodosius Rapaport, Dausset performed a number of skin grafts, which showed that antigen incompatibility was harmful to the skin's survival. They wanted to analyze the role of antigens in transplantation. Thus, they started a skin graft program that attracted over five hundred individual volunteers and two hundred families. These skin grafts furnished statistical evidence of the importance of tissue compatibility and helped to establish the immunogenetic law of human transplantation.

In 1967 Dausset started to study the association between HLA antigens and disease. His investigation of a possible link between acute lymphocyte leukemia and HLA antigens produced a negative result. Nevertheless, it stimulated other scientists to consider other possibilities. It led eventually to the discovery of connections between HLA antigens and juvenile diabetes, autoimmune disease, multiple sclerosis, and rheumatoid arthritis.

Jean Dausset is a member of l'Académie des Sciences de l'Institut de France, of l'Académie Nationale de Médecine, the National Academy of Sciences USA, the American Academy of Arts and Sciences, and of several other national scientific societies. He has been president of the French Society of Immunology (1978–81), the French Society of Hematology (1971), and the French Transplantation Society (1978). He has also served as a Scientific Advisory Councillor to the French Ministry of Education (1946–50), vice-president of the Scientific Council of the Institut Pasteur (1975–79), and, since 1974, as an expert consultant on immunology for the World Health Organization.

Among the many honors he has received for his work are the Grand Prix des Sciences Chimiques et Naturelles (1967); the Médaille d'Argent du Centre National de la Recherche Scientifique (1967); the Prix Cognac-Jay (1969); the Karl Landsteiner Award from the American Association of Blood Banks (1970); the Gairdner Foundation Prize

(1977); the Koch Foundation Prize (1978); the Wolf Foundation Prize (1978); the Légion d'Honneur (1981); and the Grand-Croix, Ordre National du Mérite (1987).

Since 1984, when it was created, Dausset has been involved with the new Center for the Collaborative Mapping of the Human Genome at the Collège de France.

Here follows a portrait of Dausset: "Standing about five feet eleven inches tall and weighing around 160 pounds, Jean Dausset has blue eyes and white hair that is combed straight back. Passionately interested in modern art, he was once part owner of La Galerie du Dragon, a Parisian art gallery that specialized in Impressionistic painting. Hardworking and modest, he has always followed the credo 'vouloir pour valoir.'" "It was a quote he used so often that it became our motto," Felix Rapaport, the director of the Transplantation Service at the State University of New York at Stony Brook and a longtime colleague of Dausset's, explained to a reporter for the *New York Times* (October 11, 1980). "It means, to achieve any worthy goal, you must wish it hard enough" (*Current Biography* 1981).

Dausset married Rosa Mayoral Lopez on March 17, 1962. They have two children, Henri and Irène.

ELIE FEUERWERKER

Selected Bibliography

PRIMARY SOURCES

Dausset, J., G. Malinvaud, and H. Brecy. 1956. *Immuno-Hématologie Biologique et Clinique.* Paris: Flammarion.

Dausset, J., and Felix T. Rapaport, eds. 1968. *Human Transplantation.* New York: Grune and Stratton.

Dausset, Jean. 1975. *Titres et Travaux Scientifiques.* Chatelaudren: Imprimerie de Chatelaudren.

Dausset, J., George D. Snell, and Stanley Nathenson. 1976. *Histocompatibility 1976.* New York: Academic Press.

Dausset, J., and A. Svejgaard, eds. 1977. *HLA and Diseases.* Copenhagen: Munksgaard.

Dausset, Jean, and Felix T. Rapaport. 1980. *A Modern Illustration of Experimental Medicine in Action.* New York: Elsevier/North-Holland.

Dausset, J. 1986. "Editorial. Le Centre d'Etude du Polymorphisme Humain." *Presse Médicale* 15:1801–2.

———. 1987. "HLA and Its Medical Complications." *Hematology Reviews and Communications* 1:217–24.

SECONDARY SOURCES

1980. "1980 Nobel prizes." *Nature* 287: 671.

Marx, Jean L. 1980. "1980 Nobel Prize in Physiology or Medicine." *Science* 210:621–23.

1982. "Dausset, Jean." In *Current Biography Yearbook 1981*, edited by Charles Moritz, 108–11. New York: H. W. Wilson.

1987. "Dausset, Jean." In *Nobel Prize Winners*, edited by Tyler Wasson, 245–47. New York: H. W. Wilson.

Jacob, F. 1988. *An Autobiography: The Statue Within.* New York: Basic Books.

MAX LUDWIG HENNING DELBRÜCK *1969*

Max Ludwig Henning Delbrück was awarded the Nobel Prize for Physiology or Medicine in 1969 with Salvador Luria and Alfred Hershey for his share in "discoveries concerning the replication mechanism and the genetic structure of viruses." He was born in Berlin, Germany, on September 4, 1906, the seventh and youngest child of Hans Delbrück, professor of history at the University of Berlin, and Lina Thiersch, granddaughter of the eminent nineteenth-century chemist Justus von Liebig. On August 2, 1941, he married Mary Adaline Bruce, and they had four children. He died in Pasadena, California, March 10, 1981.

Max Delbrück was born into a family of considerable eminence in Berlin's intellectual world. Not only was his father a distinguished academic, his uncle was instrumental in the establishment of the Kaiser Wilhelm Institute, the private research center in Berlin modeled after the Rockefeller and Carnegie Foundations. At an early age he began asserting his own place, rejecting his humanistic inheritance, choosing science instead.

Growing up in the twenties and thirties, he was a witness to the disintegration of his family's world. After false starts at a number of German universities, he attracted the attention of some of the most renowned theoretical physicists of his day: Max Born suggested the problem in theoretical quantum mechanics he pursued to earn his Ph.D. at Göttingen in 1930; he subsequently held Rockefeller research fellowships to work with Wolfgang Pauli in Zurich and Niels Bohr in Copenhagen; and from 1932 to 1937 he was assistant to Otto Hahn and Lise Meitner at the Kaiser Wilhelm Institute for Chemistry in Berlin, where he worked on mathematical theories of nuclear fission.

In another laboratory in that institute he found the questions that would occupy him for the rest of his life. In 1933 the Russian geneticist W. W. Timofeeff-Ressovsky was host to the American geneticist H. J. Muller, who six years before had induced genetic mutation by radiation, thus becoming the first person to deliberately alter living matter. Now, in Berlin, amid the disintegration of academic discourse in the university, Max Delbrück and others met privately to explore the suggestion by Muller and Timofeeff-Ressovsky that ionization might be responsible for gene mutation. In 1935 the biologist Timofeeff-Ressovsky and the two physicists Delbrück and K. G. Zimmer published what was then the unusual collaborative "Dreimännerwerk," in which Delbrück proposed a quantum model to explain the unique properties of stability and change in the gene (Olby 1974, 232–35).

While this bold attempt to fuse

quantum physics and biological structure would eventually be proved false, it assured Max Delbrück's scientific eminence, particularly after Schrödinger used the theory in his book *What Is Life?* (1944) as proof that biological structure could be explained in terms of physical processes. However, the pedestrian nature of a crude physical reductionism was uncongenial to the younger physicist (Fleming 1969, *passim*), who in 1932 had been greatly impressed with the "Copenhagen interpretation" of quantum physics outlined by Neils Bohr in his celebrated lecture, "Light and Life." Bohr had rejected classic scientific objective models in favor of the idea of paradox—mutually exclusive but complementary explanatory modes—as a legitimate scientific tool. "Waiting for the paradox," which would explain how the gene expressed both stability and change, became the self-conscious mission Max Delbrück believed that, as a physicist, he brought to biology (Delbrück 1966; 1977).

With the aid of another Rockefeller Foundation fellowship, he left Germany in 1937 to go to the California Institute of Technology, to explore the application of physical laws to biological structures. The outbreak of World War II prevented his return to Europe, and he would remain in the United States for the rest of his life, becoming an American citizen in 1945. He was appointed to teach physics in 1940 at Vanderbilt University, Tennessee, but he actually devoted the rest of his life to biology, becoming professor of biology at Caltech in 1947 and holding that appointment until he retired in 1975.

When he left Germany in 1937 he was already speculating on the usefulness of viruses—then considered virtually indistinguishable from molecules—for investigating the structure of the gene. At Caltech, in the laboratory of Emory Ellis, he found what he considered the ideal medium—bacteriophage (phage), a mono-reprodutive bacterial virus with an extremely brief but precise life cycle—and the two men outlined a method for analysing it statistically, known as the one-step growth experiment (Ellis and Delbrück 1939). In 1943, in collaboration with Salvador Luria, an Italian physician also interested in the physical properties of phage, and using the new technology of the electron microscope, they were able to demonstrate the genetic nature of phage, and thus its applicability for genetic research (Luria and Delbrück 1943). In 1946 Delbrück (and independently Alfred Hershey) discovered genetic recombination in phage, and Hershey and Rotman subsequently constructed a genetic linear map of phage. In 1952 Hershey and Chase used phage to confirm what the English biochemist O. T. Avery and associates had shown in 1944: that the gene is DNA.

The administration of phage research during the war was made easier in the summer of 1941 with the establishment of annual symposia on quantitative genetics at the Carnegie Institute's Cold Springs Harbor Laboratory, by its new director, Milislav Demerec. Delbrück facilitated phage research further when in

1943 he standardized the strain of phage to be used, and then in 1945 introduced a program of training in viral and bacterial genetics at Cold Springs Harbor known as the annual summer symposia for quantitative research on phage.

During his later years Delbrück turned his attention to the physical properties of the neuron, hoping to unravel the mechanism by which sensory stimuli (he chose visible light) are converted into chemical and electrical signals. The fungus he chose, *Phycomyces*, eventually proved too complex; while the "*Phycomyces* Group" shed light on the mechanism of phototropism, it made little headway in understanding the mechanisms of the conversion of light.

With the establishment of the genetic nature of phage, Max Delbrück, the theoretical physicist, had become one of the most distinguished biologists in the world. He returned to Germany for two years in 1961, to be guest lecturer at the Institute of Genetics in Cologne, which he had helped to establish. In addition to the Nobel Prize, he received many scientific honors, including the Kimber Genetics Award from the National Academy of Sciences (1964).

The development of molecular biology in the United States owed most to substantial funding provided by the Rockefeller Foundation, but this institutional history has been overshadowed by a formidable mythology surrounding significant scientific players, including Max Delbrück. He has been ranked among those émigré physicists credited with bringing intellectual self-confidence to biology during World War II by turning their aggressive intellects from the traumas of war and atomic fission to genetics (Fleming 1969). He was not merely esteemed, however, he was loved; few phage researchers retrospectively admitted sharing his theoretical assumptions, but he inspired loyalty with his spirit of camaraderie and intellectual integrity (James Watson notified Max Delbrück first when he and Francis Crick discovered the structure of DNA). He led what became known variously as the Phage Group, the phage church, and the phage renaissance, offering researchers the ultimate satisfaction of work described as combining the nice and the good. He created "a phage world populated with phage people—one of the little communities of intellectual purpose and excitement that constitute the only genuine utopias of the twentieth century" (Fleming 1969, 179).

ROSALIE STOTT

Selected Bibliography

PRIMARY SOURCES

Ellis, E. L., and M. Delbrück. 1939. "The Growth of Bacteriophage." *Journal of Genetic Physiology* 22: 365–84.

Luria, S. E., and M. Delbrück. 1943. "Mutations of Bacteria from Virus Sensitivity to Virus Resistance." *Genetics* 28:491–511.

Delbrück, Max. 1966. "A Physicist Looks at Biology." In *Phage and the Origins of Molecular Biology*, edited by J. Cairns, G. Stent, and J. Watson, 9–22. New York: Cold Spring Harbor Laboratory of Quantitative Biology.

———. 1969. "A Physicist's Renewed Look at Biology—Twenty Years Later." Nobel Lecture. Reprinted in *Nobel Lectures in Molecular Biology 1933–1974*, 363–72. New York: Elsevier, 1977.

———. 1986. *Mind from Matter: An Essay on Evolutionary Epistemology*. Edited by G. S. Stent, E. P. Fischer, S. W. Golcomb, D. Presti, and H. Seiler. Oxford: Blackwell Scientific Publishing.

SECONDARY SOURCES

Stent, G. S. 1968. "That Was the Molecular Biology That Was." *Science* 60 (April):390–95.

Fleming, D. 1969. "Emigré Physicists and the Biological Revolution." In *The Intellectual Migration: Europe and America 1930–1960*, edited by Donald Fleming and Bernard Bailyn, pp. 152–89. Cambridge: Harvard University Press.

Mullins, N. C. 1972. "The Development of a Scientific Specialty: The Phage Group and the Origins of Molecular Biology." *Minerva* 10:51–82.

Olby, R. 1974. *The Path to the Double Helix*. London: Macmillan.

Judson, H. 1979. *The Eighth Day of Creation*. New York: Simon & Schuster.

Kay, L. E. 1982. "Conceptual Models and Analytic Tools: The Biology of Physicist Max Delbrück." *Journal of the History of Biology* 18:207–46.

Stent, G. S. 1982. "Max Delbrück, 1906–1981." *Genetics* 101 (May):1–16.

Hayes, M. 1984. "Max Delbrück and the Birth of Molecular Biology." *Social Research* 51 (Autumn):641–73.

Abir-Am, P. 1985. "Themes, Genres and Orders of Legitimation in the Consolidation of New Scientific Disciplines: Deconstructing the Historiography of Molecular Biology." *History of Science* 23:73–117.

Fischer, Peter. 1985. *Licht und Leben: Ein Bericht über Max Delbrück, den Wegbereiter der Molekularbiologie*. Constance: Univertsitätsverlag.

EDWARD ADELBERT DOISY

1943

Edward A. Doisy was born in Hume, Illinois, on November 13, 1893. His parents were Edward Perez and Ada (Alley) Doisy. He married Alice Ackert on July 20, 1918, and after her death in August, 1964, married Margaret McCormick in 1965. He had four sons by his first wife: Edward A., Robert A., Philip P., and Richard J., all of whom entered either medicine or medical science (two became biochemists and two became physicians). He was trained in biochemistry and was awarded the Nobel Prize in Physiology or Medicine with Hendrik Dam in 1943. Doisy died on October 23, 1986, in St. Louis.

Doisy attended the University of Illinois, earning his B.A. degree in chemistry in 1914 and his M.S. degree in 1916. His master's dissertation dealt with lipids of the brain, a project that kindled his interest in biochemistry. He then went to Boston to study under the tutelage of Otto Folin, professor of biological chemistry at the Harvard Medical School; with Folin he worked on a variety of analytical problems in clinical chemistry. This work led to the development of new methods for the determination of a variety of biological substances of clinical importance in blood and urine, for which he received a Ph.D. degree in 1920. He served in the army for two years (1917–19) during World War I, mostly at the Walter Reed Research Institute in Washington, D.C.

He was appointed an instructor in biochemistry at Washington University School of Medicine in 1919, and attained the rank of associate professor in 1923. During this period he worked on the purification of insulin by isoelectric precipitation, but more important for his future he also developed an interest in ovarian function and the nature of the ovarian hormone through collaborative studies with the anatomist, Edgar Allen, at Washington University (Allen and Doisy 1923). In 1923 he moved across town in St. Louis to accept an appointment as professor and chairman of a new Department of Biochemistry at St. Louis University School of Medicine; he held these positions until his retirement in 1965. In 1929 he was the first to isolate an estrogenic hormone from human urine, obtaining estrone in crystalline form (Doisy et al. 1929), and a year or so later isolated the more potent ovarian hormone, estradiol, from sows' ovaries (MacCorquadale et al. 1936). These discoveries opened up the field of fertility to biochemical study, the consequences of which are still being exploited today.

In 1936, following the discovery by Hendrik Dam of vitamin K as a new fat-soluble vitamin that promoted coagulation in chicks and rats, Doisy undertook the isolation of this lipid vitamin from various sources, including alfalfa and fermented fish meal. In 1939 he succeeded in crystallizing vitamin K_1 from extracts of alfalfa meal (Binkley et al. 1939) and vitamin K_2 (now called menaquinone-7) from fermented fish meal (McKee et al. 1939). He subsequently synthesized homologues in both the vitamin K_1 and K_2 series. For this work he received the Nobel Prize in Physiology or Medicine jointly with Hendrik Dam in 1943.

I first met Doisy in 1938 at St. Louis University School of Medicine following my appointment as a graduate student in his department. At that time he had been professor and chairman of the Department of Biochemistry for fifteen years and the department was well staffed, well equipped, and well funded. In fact, it was during the academic year of 1938–1939 that Doisy's program of research into the structure and function of vitamin K came to fruition with the crystallizations of vitamin K_1 and vitamin K_2. 1938 also marked the election of Edward Doisy to the National Academy of Sciences.

The department was particularly crowded because of the addition of several chemists from the Parke-Davis Company who had been dispatched to St. Louis University to aid in the isolation and characterization of vitamin K. These included Drs. Steven Binkley, Lee Cheney, and Walter Hokum. Isolation of vitamin K both from plant and bacterial sources depended upon laborious chemical and chromatographic fractionations, followed by bioassays of each fraction in chickens. Sidney Thayer, an associate professor, was the member of the team who was responsible for carrying out the bioassays which depended on the measurement of changes in the clotting time of vitamin K-deficient chickens.

Ten years earlier Doisy had isolated estrone from urine using a similar approach; that is, purification of a natural product using various techniques available to organic chemists coupled to a reliable bioassay. In that case estrus in rats induced by extracts containing the estrogenic hormone was measured by a vaginal smear. Doisy's success in the application of this strategy for the isolation of vitamins and hormones ultimately led to his Nobel Prize in 1943.

Doisy was a no-nonsense, taciturn man, direct in speech, well-organized, physically active, whether he was running up and down the halls of his department with a towel stuffed in his back pocket or playing golf at the Algonquin Golf Club where he played to a handicap of twelve. He insisted on students preparing talks for weekly seminars and encouraged students to give short papers at national meetings. Although academically a tough task-maker, he was very sympathetic to his graduate students and socialized with them on his farm, inviting them to hunt and fish with him in the foothills of the Ozark Mountains.

Doisy's early scientific training was in the area of physiological chemistry. He worked with Professor Folin at Harvard University, studying methods of determining substances of biological importance in urine such as creatine, creatinine uric acid, and phosphate. He then worked briefly at Rockefeller University with Donald J. Van Slyke, doing gasometric measurements of oxygen and carbon dioxide, from which studies he contributed to the understanding of the isohydric shift in hemoglobin. He worked with Professor Schafer at Washington University in the early 1920s on the purification of insulin by isoelectric precipitation of the hormone, thereby greatly improving the speed and purity with which insulin could be isolated. Through contacts with Edgar Allen, an anatomist at Washington University, Doisy learned about the vaginal smear assay in immature female rats for the bioassay for estrogens and used it in the isolation of the estrogenic hormones. From that time on he concentrated on isolation of natural products, including vitamin K. At the end of his career he worked on new bile acids with several of his junior colleagues. The discoveries of the nature and structure of the estrogenic hormones led to the development of birth control methods by Pincus and others using modified estrogens and progesterones which are now used by eighteen million women in the United States alone who take oral contraceptives to prevent pregnancy.

Another noteworthy thing about Doisy's career is that he directed one of only three laboratories in the 1920s to develop liaison with commercial laboratories for mutual gain. These laboratories were at St. Louis University, which developed an association with Parke-Davis and Company to exploit patents on estrogens and later on vitamin K. The laboratory at Toronto, under Frederick Banting and F. F. R. McLeod developed ties with the Connaught Laboratories in Toronto and Eli Lilly Company in Indianapolis for the development of the commercial production of insulin. Finally, Harry Steenbock at the University of Wisconsin started the Wisconsin Alumni Research Foundation with funds from patents of irradiation of milk and other foods for the production of Vitamin D.

In fact, to my knowledge, Edward Doisy never applied for or received a research grant from the National Institutes of Health during his entire career. His research was funded from the proceeds of patents earned by his discoveries, held in a charitable trust at St. Louis University and administered by a "Committee on Grants." He did apply for and receive training grants from NIH for graduate biochemistry but was totally independent of government money for his outstanding discoveries in science.

Doisy received many other awards, including honorary degrees from Yale University, Washington University, University of Chicago, University of Paris, St. Louis University, and the University of Illinois. He received the Philip A. Conne Medal from the Chemists Club of New York (1935), the Willard Gibbs Medal from the American Chemical Society (1941), the American Pharmaceutical Manufacturers Association Award (1942), and the Squibb Award (1944).

He was president of the American Society of Biological Chemists in 1945, and later president of the Endocrine Society and the Society for Experimental Biology and Medicine. He was a member of the National Academy of Sciences in the United States, the Pontifical Academy of Rome, the American Philosophical Association, and the Society of the American Academy of Arts and Sciences.

Doisy's scientific achievements centered around his masterful selection of methods for the isolation of vitamins and hormones. His many students, fellows, and associates remember Edward Doisy as a single-minded and astute judge of research problems that could be solved with the techniques available, and an excellent mentor who recognized scientific skills in young people and helped them to develop their full potential.

ROBERT E. OLSON

Selected Bibliography

PRIMARY SOURCES

Allen, E., and E. A. Doisy. 1923. "An Ovarian Hormone—Preliminary Report on Its Localization, Extraction and Partial Purfication, and Action in Test Animals." *Journal of the American Medical Association* 81:819–21.

Doisy, E. A., S. A. Thayer, and C. D. Veler. 1929. "The Crystals of the Follicular Ovarian Hormone." *Proceedings Society Experimental Biology and Medicine* 27:417–19.

MacCorquodale, D. W., S. A. Thayer, and E. A. Doisy. 1936. "The Isolation of the Principal Estrogenic Substance of Liquor Folliculi." *Journal of Biological Chemistry* 115:435–48.

Binkley, S. B., D. W. MacCorquodale, S. A. Thayer, and E. A. Doisy. 1939. "The Isolation of Vitamin K_1." *Journal of Biological Chemistry* 130:219–34.

McKee, R. W., S. B. Binkley, S. A. Thayer, D. W. MacCorquodale, and E. A. Doisy. 1939. "The Isolation of Vitamin K_2." *Journal of Biology and Chemistry* 131:327–44.

GERHARD JOHANNES PAUL DOMAGK *1939*

Gerhard Johannes Paul Domagk was born on October 30, 1895, in Lagow, Brandenburg, Germany. A pharmacologist, Domagk received the Nobel Prize in 1939 for his development of Prontosil, the prototype of the sulfonamide drugs, the first successful antibacterial drugs. He was then extraordinary professor of general pathology and pathological anatomy at the University of Münster, the position he held until his retirement in 1958. The Nazi regime forced him to refuse the Nobel Prize but he received formal recognition after the war. Domagk married Gertrud Strübe in 1925 and became the father of three sons and a daughter. Domagk died on April 24, 1964, in Beiburg, Baden, Germany.

Domagk's parents were Paul Domagk, a teacher, and Martha Reimer. He spent his childhood in Sommerfeld, and entered the gymnasium in Liegnitz in 1900. In 1914 he enrolled at the University of Kiel to study medicine, but his plans were immediately interrupted by the outbreak of World War I. Joining a grenadier regiment, he served with them until he was wounded in 1915. He then transferred to the army medical corps, which offered much practical experience, including assignment to lazarettos in Russia, where patients with cholera, typhus, and other infectious diseases died without hope of treatment.

At war's end Domagk returned to Kiel, where he became very interested in chemotherapy and the development of new drugs. After earning his medical degree in 1921, he spent some time as an assistant in Ernst Hoppe-Seyler's laboratory and published a paper on the reticuloendothelial system and its defenses against infection. This paper attracted the attention of the directors of the I. G. Farbenindustrie. For a year Domagk was a reader, or lecturer, in pathology at the University of Greifswald and, in 1925 he was appointed to a readership at Münster. Three years later, his appointment as extraordinary professor allowed Domagk to accept an offer from the I. G. Farbenindustrie to direct research into new antibacterial drugs at their laboratory for experimental pathology in Wuppertal-Elberfeld (Posner 1971, 153–54).

Germany had an established tradition of industrial-academic cooperation and of medical achievement. Her native scientists included Robert Koch, the founder of bacteriology, and Paul Ehrlich, whose "magic bullet" system had turned up Salvarsan in 1909 and led to the development of a variety of antiprotozoal agents. However, little progress against deadly bacterial infections had been made by any investigator and many scientists agreed with Emil Behring's lament that "inner disinfection is a vain dream." Most attempts had involved metallic compounds, which proved highly toxic and of little benefit.

I. G. Farben now proposed to launch a systematic search for antibacterial drugs, emulating Ehrlich's methods and in combination with the development of new dye products. Under Domagk's direction, compounds were screened in a laborious process that began with examination in vitro to establish their effect on various microbe genera; next, the compounds were tested in laboratory animals in order to determine what dosage could be tolerated; finally, they were tested against infections in animals. Drugs that passed all these tests would then be considered for clinical testing in humans.

Among the potential candidates for an effective antibiotic Domagk considered were the azo dyes. These dyes, first developed in 1909, had two nitrogen atoms between hydrocarbon groups. They bound effectively with the proteins in wool and were very resistant to fading. Several appeared to destroy streptococci in the test tube but this effect could not be replicated in animals. Despite the lack of success of the first several years of Domagk's work, I. G. Farben remained undaunted, building a new research institute for pathological anatomy and bacteriology in 1929.

In 1932 the Farben chemists Fritz Mietzsch and Joseph Klarer synthesized a new dye for leather by replacing a hydrogen atom in an azo compound with a sulfonamide group (SO_2NH_2). They gave their creation (4'sulfanomide-2-4-diaminoazobenzol) the name Prontosil Rubrum. Domagk's experiments on Prontosil showed virtual inertia in vitro but amazing effectiveness against streptococcal infections in mice, without toxic side effects.

He spent three years investigating the new compound before publishing his classic paper,"Ein Beitrag zur Chemotherapie der bakteriellen Infektionen," in 1935. By that time, there had been several successful treatments of humans, including thirty-five women with puerperal fever in London, and Domagk's own daughter, who contracted a severe streptococcal infection. She was given Prontosil and recovered, with one unfortunate and permanent side effect: her skin turned to a light reddish, lobster-like color (Posner 1971, 154; Domagk 1935).

Many physicians were skeptical of the report, after so many false alarms, but Domagk's work was confirmed in 1936 by L. Colebrook and M. Kenny of the British Medical Council. Contemporaries and later historians also seriously questioned Domagk's explanation of his three-year delay in publication—that more time was needed for rigorous confirmation of the results, particularly in humans—since he cited only one animal experiment in his article and the available clinical reports were sketchy. Some historians have suggested that the lag was actually due to the highly competitive conditions of the pharmaceutical industry and the demands for secrecy that accompany the race for patents.

The latter explanation would clarify why the I. G. Farbenindustrie failed to provide samples to a group of researchers at the Pasteur Institute in Paris who were interested in the inactivity of Prontosil in the laboratory. They suggested that the drug was metabolized into an antibacterial agent only within the body. The French scientists succeeded in synthesizing the compound on their own and quickly verified Domagk's results. They also established that, in fact, the active substance was a sulfanomide compound (sulfanilimide), which separated from the azo base in vivo. Since sulfanilimide had been known for nearly thirty years, there were no patent restrictions to its development and the synthesis of related compounds: excellent news for researchers and physicians, if not for I. G. Farben. It is an open question whether Domagk had recognized the active principle in 1932 and spent the intervening years seeking a patentable analogue of the substance, or whether he failed to understand the significance of his own findings.

Following the initial doubts and apathy, scientists in several countries confirmed the effectiveness of Prontosil and applied this discovery to the development of new analogues. Sulfapyridine, which proved effective in mice against bacteria other than hemolytic streptococci, was developed by L. E. H. Whitby in 1938. Many other "sulfa drugs" followed, including sulfathiazole, sulfacetamide, and sulfadiazine. The success of these agents also encouraged new attention to sulfone derivatives, leading in 1943 to a treatment for leprosy.

Although later superseded by penicillin, tetracycline, and others, the sulfanomides were the first glimmer of hope for victims of deadly infections such as pneumonia, meningitis, erysipelas, mastoiditis, and gonorrhea. For the first time, the majority of these patients survived and recovered without lasting damage. Serious side effects did appear and the sulfas were not effective against many bacterial agents. But the effects of hope and faith in medical science engendered by Gerhard Domagk's discovery reverberate to the present day (Posner 1971, 154).

Domagk was showered with honors in the late thirties, of which the Nobel Prize, in October 1939, was the logical culmination. Scientists from Britain, France, and the United States joined in his nomination. Among the many other awards he received at this time were the Emil Fischer Memorial Plaque (1937), the Gold Medal of the Paris Exposition (1938), the Paul Ehrlich Gold Medal (1939), and the Cameron Prize of the University of Edinburgh (1939). He was also elected to the Royal Society.

The National Socialist government, however, had been hostile to the Nobel Committee since 1936, when the latter had awarded the Peace Prize to the German radical pacifist writer, Carl von Ossietsky, who was at the time imprisoned in a concentration camp. After this incident the Hitler regime had established a Nazi Party Prize that could be won only by a German (of flawless ancestry) and had passed a decree forbidding the acceptance of a Nobel Prize. The Kultusministerium stated that the Nobel Prize was "completely unwanted" by loyal Germans. Notwithstanding extreme concern and the tense situation following the outbreak of war in September, the Nobel Committee regarded the situation as a test of its mandate and awarded the prize for physiology or medicine to Domagk.

He responded immediately with a letter in which he expressed his thanks but advised that he would have to inquire whether he would be allowed to accept the prize. Two weeks later he was arrested by the Gestapo and forced, during a week-long incarceration, to send a second letter refusing the prize. When he was arrested a second time while traveling to Berlin for an international medical conference, he realized that he was under constant surveillance and he thereafter acted cautiously to protect himself and his family.

During World War II Domagk quietly continued his work. He became interested in tuberculosis, particularly after learning that many strains were found to be resistant to streptomycin. In 1946 he and his colleagues, Mietzsch, H. Schmidt, and R. Behnisch, developed a group of compounds known as the thiosemicarbazones, which were very active against the tubercle bacillus but also highly toxic. An attempt to combine one of these with an isonicotinic acid in 1951, however, resulted in the drug isoniazid, a safe and effective agent in the treatment of tuberculosis.

In 1947 Domagk was at last able to go to Stockholm, where he presented his Nobel Lecture and was honored with the gold medal and diploma. The prize money, however, had been returned to the foundation funds and he never received it. His curiosity and energy remained strong to the end of his life. In the 1950s he began work on anticancer agents, and in the early 1960s expressed an interest in mental illness. Although he retired to the status of ordinary professor at Münster in 1958, he remained active in the Farbenindustrie laboratory until his death at the age of sixty-eight (Posner 1971, 155–56).

ROBERT BRAIN
MARCIA MELDRUM

Selected Bibliography

PRIMARY SOURCES

Domagk, Gerhard. 1935. "Ein Beitrag zur Chemotherapie der bakteriellen Infektionen." *Deutsche Medizinische Wochenschrift* 61:250–53.

Domagk, Gerhard, and F. Hegler. 1940. *Chemotherapie bacterieller Infektionen.* Leipzig: Hirzel.

Domagk, Gerhard. 1947. *Pathologische Anatomie und Chemotherapie der Infektionenskrankenheiten.* Stuttgart: Thieme.

———. 1950. *Chemotherapie der Tuberkulose mit Thiosemikarbazonen.* Stuttgart: Theime.

———. 1950. "Investigations on the Anti-Tuberculous Activity of the Thiosemicarbazones *in vitro* and *in vivo.*" *American Review of Tuberculosis and Pulmonary Diseases* 61: 8–19.

———. 1963. "Über 30 Jahre Arzt." *Therapie der Gegenwart* 102:913–17.

SECONDARY SOURCES

Colebrook, Leonard. 1964. "Gerhard Domagk." *Biographical Memoirs of the Royal Society* 10:39–50.

Warburg, O. 1965. "Gerhard Domagk." *Deutsche Medizinische Wochenschrift* 90:34, 1484–86.

Posner, Erich. 1971. "Domagk, Gerhard." In *Dictionary of Scientific Biography*, 4:153–56. New York: Scribners.

RENATO DULBECCO *1975*

Renato Dulbecco was born on February 22, 1914, in Catanzaro, Italy. Dulbecco's areas of scientific specialization are virology and the molecular biology of tumor viruses. The 1975 Nobel Prize in Physiology or Medicine was awarded to Renato Dulbecco, Howard Temin, and David Baltimore for "discoveries concerning the interaction between tumor viruses and the genetic material of the cell." His father, Leonard Dulbecco, was a civil engineer. His mother was Maria Virdia Dulbecco. Dulbecco married Guiseppina Salvo on June 1, 1940; they divorced in 1963. They had three children. Dulbecco married Maureen Muir, who became his scientific partner and supporter of his scientific life, on July 17, 1963.

Dulbecco earned his M.D. from the University of Torino, Italy, in 1936. Although he was very interested in his father's work and considered going into physics, his mother's influence and that of an uncle who was a surgeon convinced him to study medicine. Nevertheless, some of his fondest memories of life in Imperia, Italy, concern the small meteorological observatory where he spent much of his free time and his construction of a working electronic seismograph. After excelling in his first year exams at the medical school in Torino, Dulbecco was accepted as "intern" in the Institute of Anatomy, then directed by Giuseppe Levi. Here Dulbecco began his studies of tissue culture, histology, neurology, and experimental biology. Levi's other students at the time included Salvador Luria and Rita Levi-Montalcini. Dulbecco completed his degree in morbid anatomy and pathology.

In 1936 Dulbecco was called up for military service as a medical officer. Two years later he returned to pathology, but was soon called up again because of World War II. He was sent to the French front and later to Russia. After a brush with death during a major Russian offensive in 1942, he was hospitalized for several months and sent home. With Italy occupied by the German army, Dulbecco hid in a small village and joined the Resistance as physician for the local partisan units. He also participated in the underground political activities of the Institute of Morbid Anatomy and joined the "Committee for National Liberation" of the city of Torino. He became a councilor in Torino's first postwar city council but soon abandoned politics for the laboratory. For two years he studied physics and then returned to Levi's institute. At this time Dulbecco hoped to go to the United States to study the genetics of simple organisms, like Salvador Luria who had been in the United States since the beginning of the war. In 1946 Luria came to Torino and asked Dulbecco to join his laboratory at the University of Indiana. Levi-Montalcini encouraged Dulbecco to accept Luria's offer. In 1947 both Dulbecco and Levi-Montalcini began their research careers in the United States. Working with Salvador Luria, Dulbecco performed definitive studies of the problem of multiplicity reactivation of phage irradiated with ultraviolet light. He also discovered the limited participation of several phages simultaneously infecting the same cell and the time exclusion principle. Dulbecco's studies of photoreactivation of phage attracted Max Delbrück's attention and resulted in an invitation to move to the California Institute of Technology.

From 1947 to 1949 Dulbecco was a senior research fellow at Caltech. He became an associate professor in 1952 and held a full professorship from 1954 to 1963. Dulbecco was visiting professor at the Rockefeller Institute in 1962. From 1963 to 1964 he was Royal Society Visiting Professor, resident at the University of Glasgow, Scotland. Dulbecco joined the Salk Institute as one of the original group of fellows in 1963. He was assistant director of research at the Imperial Cancer Research Fund Institution, London, from 1972 to 1977. From 1977 to 1981 he was a professor in the Departments of Pathology and Medicine, University of California San Diego Medical School. Since 1977 he has been Distinguished Research Professor and Senior Clayton Foundation Investigator at the Salk Institute.

Dulbecco developed many of the techniques used by researchers to study the molecular biology of animal viruses, including those used by his previous associates, Howard Temin and David Baltimore. Dulbecco was also a pioneer in the study of gene transformation by DNA tumor viruses.

After continuing phage work for a short period at Caltech, Dulbecco initiated his studies of animal viruses and immediately made a major contribution to the field: his development of a plaque assay for animal viruses. Subsequent work in the genetics of animal viruses and the development of Albert Sabin's attenuated poliovirus vaccine were made possible by this convenient and quantitative method. Working with polyoma virus, which causes tumors in rodents, Dulbecco demonstrated that the virus has a novel circular DNA. At this stage Dulbecco initiated studies of the mechanism by which animal viruses cause host cells to become neoplastic. Dulbecco proved that this change, known as transformation, could be obtained in cultures. This established an essential experimental system. His demonstration that some mutants block transformation proved that the process is caused by a viral gene. At the Salk Institute, Dulbecco began his investigations of the molecular aspects of transformation. He demonstrated that the viral DNA became permanently associated with transformed cells and their descendants and that viral DNA became permanently associated with cellular DNA. The integrated viral DNA still expressed some of its genes. Thus, in this experimental system, cancer was shown to be the result of an intimate interaction of cellular and viral genes. Later, while at the Imperial Institution, Dulbecco discovered that the protein responsible for transformation could be found in the membrane of transformed cells.

Never one to rest on his laurels, after receiving the Nobel Prize, Dulbecco decided to study cancers of importance to humans. In order to study breast cancer, he began work on chemically induced mammary cancers in rats. Work began with the identification of the cell types present in the normal gland at various stages of development, using monoclonal antibodies as highly selective markers. This led to the establishment of the developmental pathway of the gland and to identification of cancers derived from the stem cells that give rise to various cell types and confirmation of the hypothesis that the development of cancer is associated with the activation of oncogenes. This work has been extended to human breast cancer and the development of agents that may be useful in the diagnosis and treatment of breast cancer.

In addressing the Cold Spring Harbor Symposium on Tumor Viruses in 1974, Renato Dulbecco advised his audience not to be afraid of complexities. His pioneering work in the field of tumor virology, and the discoveries of his colaureates, made it possible for scientists to address the complexities of the interaction between tumor viruses and host cells. Dulbecco took the occasion of his Nobel Lecture to discuss prospects for cancer prevention, including the necessity of identifying mutagens and eliminating them from the environment. He stressed that this approach to cancer prevention requires immediate action "since these substances can be identified with simple bacterial tests suitable for mass screening." Moreover, some of the mutagens already identified—tobacco and some hair dyes—are obviously unnecessary for human life. Despite good evidence that tobacco smoke is the agent of human lung cancer, individuals and governments apparently do not appreciate epidemiological evidence and have not responded appropriately to the dangers of tobacco smoke. Dulbecco urged scientists to find and express a social conscience and called upon governments "to act towards severely discouraging tobacco consumption; and to act now because it will be at least thirty years before their action has its full effect." It was frustrating for scientists to spend their lives asking questions about the nature of cancer and ways to prevent or cure it, only to discover that despite existing information "society merrily produces oncogenic substances and permeates the environment with them." Biologists should surely find this situation unacceptable and must work to see it corrected. Dulbecco urged a new era of cooperation between science and society for the benefit of all mankind (Dulbecco 1975, 490).

Other honors awarded to Renato Dulbecco include the Sperino Prize, Medical Academy of Torino (1936), a Guggenheim Fellowship (1957–58), the Albert and Mary Lasker Basic Medical Research Award (1964), the Howard Taylor Ricketts Award (1965), the Paul Ehrlich–Ludwig Darmstaedter Prize (1967), the Selman A. Waksman Award, National Academy of Sciences (1974); Man of the Year, London (1975); the Grand Ufficiale of the Italian Republic (1981), Honorary Citizen of Imperia, Italy (1983), and the Gold Public Health Medal, Italian government (1985).

Dulbecco holds honorary degrees from Yale University (1968), the University of Glasgow (1970), Vrije Universiteit Brussels (1978), and Indiana University (1984). He is a member of the National Academy of Science; Academia dei Lincei; Royal Society; Academia Ligure di Scienze a Lettere; Federation of American Scientists; American Association for Cancer Research; American Academy of Arts and Sciences; International Physicians for the Prevention of Nuclear War.

LOIS N. MAGNER

Selected Bibliography

PRIMARY SOURCES

Dulbecco, Renato. 1952. "Production of Plaques in Monolayer Tissue Culture by Single Particles of an Animal Virus." *Proceedings of the National Academy of Sciences* 38: 747.

Vogt, M., and R. Dulbecco. 1960. "Virus-Cell Interaction with a Tumor-Producing Virus." *Proceedings of the National Academy of Sciences* 46:365.

Dulbecco, R. 1963. "Transformation of Cells in Vivo by Viruses." *Science* 142:932.

———. 1967. *The Induction of Cancer by Viruses.* San Francisco: W. H. Freeman.

———. 1974. *The Biology of Small DNA-Tumor Viruses.* New York: MSS Information Corp.

———. 1975. "From the Molecular Biology of Oncogenic DNA Viruses to Cancer." Nobel Lecture, December 12, 1975. Reprinted in *Nobel Lectures in Molecular Biology 1933–1975*, 483–98. Amsterdam: Elsevier, 1977.

Dulbecco, Renato, and Howard Ginsberg. 1980. *Virology.* Hagerstown, Md.: Harper and Row.

SECONDARY SOURCES

Cairns, John, Gunther S. Stent, and James D. Watson, eds. 1966. *Phage and the Origins of Molecular Biology.* New York: Cold Spring Harbor Laboratory.

Gross, L. 1972. *Oncogenic Viruses.* New York: Pergamon Press.

Tooze, J., ed. 1973. *The Molecular Biology of Tumor Viruses.* New York: Cold Spring Harbor Laboratory.

Eckhart, Walter. 1975. "The 1975 Nobel Prize for Physiology or Medicine." *Science* 190:650, 712–13.

Judson, Horace Freeland. 1979. *The Eighth Day of Creation: Makers of the Revolution in Biology.* New York: Simon and Schuster.

CHRISTIAN RENÉ DE DUVE
1974

Christian René de Duve was born on October 2, 1917, in Thames Ditton, England. A cellular biologist and biochemist, de Duve shared the Nobel Prize in 1974 with Albert Claude and George E. Palade for their descriptions of the fine microscopic structure and functions of the cell, which laid the foundations of modern cell biology. Claude developed the pioneering techniques of centrifugal fractionation and electron microscopy that made the work possible and carried out the initial observations. Palade improved upon Claude's methods and conclusively established some of Claude's ideas; he was himself responsible for drawing the map of the cell as we know it today. In particular, he described the mechanism of protein synthesis by the cellular ribosomes. De Duve used the methods developed by Claude and Palade to identify the lysosome, a particle containing a digestive enzyme, and the peroxisome, the site of multiple oxidation reactions. Although the three men worked separately for the most part, all were Europeans based for a part of their careers at the Rockefeller Institute for Medical Research (now Rockefeller University). De Duve has held joint appointments in the Department of Biochemical Cytology at Rockefeller University and the Department of Physiological Chemistry at the Catholic University of Louvain in Belgium since 1962. Currently, he is Andrew W. Mellon Professor at Rockefeller University (since 1974) and professor emeritus at Louvain (since his retirement in 1985). He married Janine Herman in 1943; the de Duves have two sons, Thierry and Alain, and two daughters, Anne and Francoise.

De Duve's parents, Alphonse and Madeleine Pungs de Duve, were refugees from the German occupation of Belgium at the time of his birth. The family returned in 1920 to Antwerp, where Christian grew up. During his medical education at Louvain he became interested in the action of insulin in the regulation of glucose metabolism. In 1941 he completed his medical degree and joined the Belgian army. He was captured, escaped, and was released from active duty, allowing him to return to postgraduate research in Louvain. By 1945 de Duve had received the degree of Agrégré de l'Enseignement Supérieur for his thesis on the mechanism of insulin action and had published a book, *Glucose, Insulin and Diabetes*; in 1946 he was awarded an M.S. in chemistry.

The end of the war made it possible for him to travel to Stockholm, where he worked under Hugo Theorell at the Nobel Medical Institute (1946–47), and to the United States, as a Rockefeller Foundation fellow at Washington University in St. Louis (1947–48). Here he continued his postdoctoral studies with Carl and Gerty Cori and with Earl W. Sutherland (Hicks 1974).

De Duve returned to Louvain as lecturer in physiological chemistry in 1947, achieving the rank of full professor in 1951. He had meanwhile begun to use the techniques of centrifugal fractionation, developed by his compatriot Albert Claude, to study the process of glucose metabolism at the cellular level. He and his associates, Gery Herz, Jacques Berthet, and Robert Wattiaux, refined the methods to include intensive biochemical analysis of the fractions. Applying the new method in a series of experiments on insulin action in 1949, they unexpectedly detected acid phosphatase in a freshly separated mitochondrial fraction of rat liver cells. More interesting, however, was the discovery that the phosphatase was much more active in the same preparation five days later. Further fractionation and analyses of the liver cells revealed the presence of five acid hydrolases and urate oxidase in the L, or light mitochondrial, cell fraction.

De Duve suggested that the hydrolases within the cell were contained within an organelle so far undetected, which he named the "lysosome." These enzyme acids might act as "stomachs," digesting nutrients for the cell's use; however, they would normally have to be contained within a strong membrane to protect the rest of the cell from their powerful action. The process of fractionation had broken the membrane and released the acids.

De Duve redirected his team to isolate and describe this new particle. The collaborative efforts of de Duve, Claude, Alex Novikoff, and others resulted by 1955 in electron micrographs of the lysosome. The morphological confirmation of a body whose existence had been predicted by biochemical analysis was at that time "a startling reversal of the usual course of events." Lysosomes were soon found to be present in nearly all animal cells and to take several different forms (De Duve 1958; 1964; Novikoff 1974, 518–19).

The urate oxidase remained puzzling, as minor differences in its action made de Duve doubt whether it, too, was contained within the lysosome. Working with Berthet, Pierre Baudhuin, and Henri Beaufay, he was eventually able to find and describe the "peroxisome," which synthesizes hydrogen peroxide, among other functions. The project required still further refinement of centrifugation methods, still used by laboratories to collect masses of the tiny particles for study (De Duve and Baudhuin 1966; De Duve 1965; Novikoff 1974, 519–20).

De Duve was invited to come to Rockefeller University in 1962 to head the Department of Biochemical Cytology. He accepted and planned to continue working at Louvain part-time, commuting via transatlantic flights, for a "transition period." The transition period has lasted twenty-six years and de Duve's presence in both laboratories is still felt, although he is now retired from active teaching in Louvain. Among other advantages, the dual appointment allowed him to put two investigative teams to work on the functions and dysfunctions of the lysosome and the peroxisome. One scientist rarely dominates a field so completely as does de Duve the study of lysosomes and peroxisomes.

Like George Palade, de Duve believes that "we are sick because our cells are sick," that complex pathologies originate at the cellular level. Gery Herz began investigation of this etiological hypothesis in the 1950s, and by 1973 some thirty "storage diseases" had been traced to deficiencies of single lysosomal enzymes. The group at Rockefeller University has tentatively linked atherosclerosis to lysosome deficiencies, based on a theory that the abnormal accumulation of fatty tissue in the arteries occurs as a result of a failure in normal fat hydrolysis in the cells. De Duve feels there may be a connection to other aging and degenerative processes as well.

He is also interested in drug action on cell particles and on the possibility of particle action on drugs. His Louvain associates carried out innovative experiments in cancer chemotherapy in which the drug was buffered with DNA to reduce its toxicity. Lysosome action then separated the DNA and the drug became fully active (Hicks 1974; Rensberger 1974; Novikoff 1974, 520; Herz and van Hoof 1973).

De Duve has always retained his Belgian citizenship and tried to spend weekends with his family. After their children were grown, Mrs. de Duve often accompanied her husband to New York. Outside of the laboratory, he enjoys a good game of bridge (Hicks 1974).

De Duve and several colleagues founded the Institute of Cellular and Molecular Biology as part of the Louvain School of Medicine, now located in Brussels. He is a member of the Royal Academy of Belgium, the European Academy of Arts, Sciences, and Humanities, and the American Academy of Arts and Sciences, and a foreign associate of the National Academy of Sciences, among other affiliations. In addition to the Nobel Prize, he has received many international honors, including the Prix Quinquennial of the Belgian Royal Academy of Medicine (1967), the Gairdner Foundation Special Award (1967), and the Dr. H. P. Heineken Prijs of the Royal Netherlands Academy of Sciences (1973).

MARCIA MELDRUM

Selected Bibliography

PRIMARY SOURCES

De Duve, Christian R. 1958. "Lysosomes, a New Group of Cytoplasmic Particles." *Woods Hole Subcellular Particles Symposium*, 128–58.

De Duve, Christian R., Robert Wattiaux, and Pierre Baudhuin. 1962. "Distribution of Enzymes between Subcellular Fractions in Animal Tissues." *Advances in Enzymology* 24:291–358.

De Duve, Christian R. 1963. "The Lysosome." *Scientific American* 208 (May):64–72.

———. 1964. "From Cytases to Lysosomes." *Federal Proceedings* 23 (September–October):1045–49.

———. 1965. "The Separation and Characterization of Subcellular Particles." *Harvey Lectures*, series 59, 49–87.

De Duve, Christian R., and Pierre Baudhuin. 1966. "Peroxisomes (Microbodies and Related Particles)." *Physiological Review* 46 (April): 323–57.

De Duve, Christian R. 1966. "The Significance of Lysosomes in Pathology and Medicine." *Proceedings of the Institute of Medicine of Chicago* 26 (July):73–76.

De Duve, Christian R., with Neil Hardy. 1984. *A Guided Tour of the Living Cell.* New York: Scientific American Books.

SECONDARY SOURCES

Herz, Gery, and François van Hoof, eds. 1973. *Lysosomes and Storage Diseases.* New York: Academic Press.

Hicks, Nancy. 1974. "Christian Rene de Duve." *New York Times* (October 11):22.

Rensberger, Boyce. 1974. "Three Cell Biologists Get Nobel Prize." *New York Times* (October 11):22.

Novikoff, Alex B. 1974. "The 1974 Nobel Prize in Physiology or Medicine." *Science* 186 (November 8): 518–20.

SIR JOHN CAREW ECCLES 1963

Sir John Carew Eccles was born on January 27, 1903, in Melbourne, Australia. A neurophysiologist, Eccles shared the Nobel Prize in 1963 with Alan Hodgkin and Andrew Huxley for his demonstration of the electrical basis of neural inhibition in the polarization of the nerve cell membrane, based on Hodgkin's and Huxley's study of the giant squid axon. At the time of the award, Eccles was professor of physiology at the Australian National University. He came to the United States in 1966 and his subsequent career has been spent here. He was knighted in 1958. Eccles married his first wife, Irene Frances Miller of New Zealand, in 1928. The couple had four sons, Peter, William, John, and Richard, and five daughters, Rosamond, Alice, Mary, Judith, and Frances. Two of the children became scientists: Peter is a radar meteorologist; and Rosamond, a Ph.D., has worked with her father on much of his research. John and Irene Eccles were divorced in 1968. Later that year he married another neurophysiologist, Helena Tabarikova, a native of Czechoslovakia, who has since been his collaborator.

Eccles's parents, William James Eccles and Mary Carew Eccles, were both teachers and they provided his early education. After graduating from Melbourne High School in 1919, he enrolled at Melbourne University to study medicine. As an undergraduate he excelled both as an athlete, in tennis, cross-country, and pole vaulting, and as a student, taking first-class honors. His medical specialty was determined when he became interested in the scientific and philosophical problem of the nature of the mind. When he received the Victorian Rhodes Scholarship at graduation in 1925, he immediately made plans to enter Magdalen College, Oxford, to study under Sir Charles Scott Sherrington.

Eccles's performance at Oxford was again outstanding, winning him first-class honors in natural sciences and a Christopher Welch Scholarship. He was appointed to a junior research fellowship at Exeter College in 1927, and the following year he became one of Sherrington's assistants. He collaborated with Sherrington on the master's last great papers on neural inhibition as a distinct phenomenon and on the "motor unit," a single spinal motoneuron that coordinates the actions of many muscle fibers. This fundamental concept represented the culmination of Sherrington's work, and probably the culmination of the knowledge possible without use of electronic instruments then just being introduced. Eccles also worked with Ragnar Granit during these years. He received his Ph.D. in 1929 for a thesis on neural excitation and inhibition.

From 1932 to 1934 Eccles was Staines Medical Fellow at Exeter, a prestigious appointment; he was then appointed to posts as a Magdalen tutor and university demonstrator in physiology. His research now involved the mechanism of synaptic transmission, contended by Sir Henry Dale to be chemical in nature. Eccles and others supported a rival theory of electrical transmission. Although chemical transmission was eventually proved, by Sir Bernard Katz and Paul Fatt, to be the predominant mechanism, electrical transmission has been identified in certain specialized synapses.

In 1937 Eccles was invited to return to Australia to become director of the Kanematsu Memorial Institute of Pathology, a small but highly regarded division of Sydney Hospital. In the years before World War II he attracted a small group of brilliant young scientists to the Kanematsu, including Katz and Stephen Kuffler. Using electronic devices to detect and study neuromuscular impulses in cats and frogs, the researchers proposed that the postsynaptic muscle response was not a simple continuation of the neural impulse; rather, the synapse stimulated a discharge along the muscle neural fiber. Eccles suggested that this discharge was the result of depolarization of the surface membranes of the fiber cells.

Eccles served as a medical adviser to the Australian army from 1941 to 1943, working on vision, hearing, and aviation medicine problems, and directing the collection and processing of blood serum. In 1944 he accepted the professorship of physiology at the University of Otago in Dunedin, New Zealand. Here he began studies using very fine glass microelectrodes to detect and localize each part of the neural transmission process.

By 1951 Eccles had isolated and recorded a fairly prolonged postsynaptic depolarization of the muscle neural cell membranes identifiable with excitatory synaptic transmission. He termed this response the excitatory postsynaptic potential (EPSP). The inverse reaction, inhibitory postsynapse, was characterized by the hyperpolarization of the membranes. His careful microstudies also established, however, that synaptic transmission was not electric, as he had long believed.

Two strong influences operated on Eccles's thought at this time. His friendship in New Zealand with the Austrian philosopher Karl Popper helped him see a scientific hypothesis not as a personal cause, but as a step to further understanding, which facilitated his conversion to the idea of chemical transmission. Meanwhile, in England, Hodgkin's and Huxley's studies of the ionic basis of membrane depolarization stimulated his further research into this phenomenon.

The new series of investigations were carried out at the Australian National University in Canberra, where Eccles arrived in 1952. Here he and his associates, J. S. Coombs and Paul Fatt, devoted intensive study to the inhibitory postsynaptic potential. Eccles as able to demonstrate the chemical mechanism when chloride ions leaking out of his microelectrodes depolarized the inhibitory membrane and reversed the response. The team identified two types of neurons, excitatory and inhibitory, and confirmed that synaptic inhibition was the exclusive function of the latter. Inhibition, in

Eccles's opinion, is essential to neural functioning, in that it prevents overload and helps to "direct traffic" for the many impulses passing through the central nervous system.

In the late 1950s and early 1960s he concentrated on tracing the patterns and organization of the neural pathways. In 1964 he identified synaptic inhibitory neurons in the brain. Two years later, however, Sir John was compelled by university policy to retire at the age of sixty-three. The American Medical Association invited him to head its Institute for Biomedical Research in Chicago. Two years later Eccles was appointed distinguished professor of physiology and medicine and Buswell Research Fellow at the State University of New York in Buffalo. A neurophysiology laboratory was built especially for him and he continued active investigation of neural transmission. His most interesting findings concerned the possible relationship of excitation/inhibition interactions to the storing and processing of information in the cerebellar cortex. He finally submitted to a less active retirement in 1975.

Sir John has followed the lead of his mentor Sherrington in writing and speaking on the philosophy of science and in pursuing a broad spectrum of interests, including art, archaeology, and classical music. He was elected a Fellow of the Royal Society of London in 1941 and is also a Fellow of the Royal Society of New Zealand, and a Foreign Member of the American Academy of Arts and Sciences. He served as president of the Australian Academy of Sciences (1957–61). The many other honors he has received include the Gotch Memorial Prize (1927); the Rolleston Memorial Prize (1932); the Baly Medal from the Royal College of Physicians (1961); the Royal Medal from the Royal Society (1962); the Cothenius Medal from the Deutsche Akademie (1963); and a Special Award from the Parkinson's Disease Foundation (1972).

MARCIA MELDRUM

Selected Bibliography

PRIMARY SOURCES

Eccles, John C. 1938. *Reflex Activity of the Spinal Cord.* London: Oxford University Press.

———. 1965. *The Neurophysiological Basis of Mind.* Oxford: Clarendon Press.

———. 1967. *The Cerebellum as a Neuronal Machine.* Berlin: Springer-Verlag.

———. 1968. *The Physiology of Nerve Cells.* Baltimore: Johns Hopkins Press.

———. 1969. *The Inhibitory Pathways of the Central Nervous System.* Liverpool: Liverpool University Press.

SECONDARY SOURCES

1972. "Eccles, Sir John Carew." In *Current Biography Yearbook*, 119–22. New York: H. W. Wilson.

Robinson, John. 1970. In *One Hundred Most Important People in the World Today*, 237–40. New York: Putnam.

GERALD MAURICE EDELMAN
1972

Gerald Maurice Edelman was born on July 1, 1929, in New York City. A biochemist, Edelman shared the 1972 Nobel Prize with Rodney R. Porter for their independent, yet complementary, research on the chemical structure of antibodies. Porter began the work with his innovative cleavage of the antibody molecule. Edelman followed this lead to generate a remarkable period of creative structural analysis, in which he and Porter were the leaders. Edelman is Vincent Astor Distinguished Professor of Biochemistry at the Rockefeller Institute, a position he has held since 1974. He married Maxine Morrison in 1950; they have two sons, Eric and David, and a daughter, Judith.

Edelman's parents were Edward and Anna Freedman Edelman. His father was a physician and he originally planned a career in internal medicine, studying chemistry at Ursinius College in Pennsylvania and then enrolling in the University of Pennsylvania Medical School, where he received the Spencer Morris Award. After receiving his medical degree in 1954, he completed a year's internship at Massachusetts General Hospital, followed by two years of military service at an army hospital in Paris.

By that time (1957), he had realized that his intensity and drive were more suited to basic research than to clinical practice. He was accepted into the doctoral program at Rockefeller University and hurried to New York as soon as he was discharged in June, arriving three months before the rest of his fellows. He put the summer to good use, reading and "virtually mastering" the intricacies of immunology (Brody 1972).

Immunoglobulins are the antibody molecules in human blood that recognize and "capture," or bind, foreign antigens, including disease agents, and then modify or degrade them. They appear to be very similar in structure, yet they vary sufficiently in the healthy body to successfully combat most of the millions of antigens encountered during a person's lifetime. Among other problems, it seemed impossible that the human genetic makeup could contain sufficient genes for each of the antibodies known to exist, each specific to a particular antigen.

Karl Landsteiner had advocated chemical analysis of antibody structure as the first step toward characterizing their action and discovering the secret of their antigenic specificity. The molecules, however, are large, complex, and cannot be purified. Rodney Porter in London had developed selective cleavage with enzymes to break the molecule into fragments for easier analysis. He obtained his first "pieces" in 1950, but it was only in 1958 that he was able, using a purified form of papain, to recover three discrete and different fragments. Two of these (Fab) were very similar and active in attacking antigens; the third (Fc) clearly had a different, undetermined, function. With this work, he revolutionized immunology.

Working with Henry Kunkel, Edelman used Porter's enzymatic cleavage techniques on human myeloma proteins to carry out further structural studies of human immunoglobulins. He completed his thesis in 1960 and was invited to join the Rockefeller staff. But he was not completely happy with his findings to this point. Porter's method essentially broke the antibodies into bits of amino acids, allowing the assumption that the molecule was a single polypeptide chain. Edelman thought a more complex structure was likely and attempted analysis using the reagent urea to reduce the disulfide bonds of the proteins. His results, published in 1959 and 1961, showed that in fact the immunoglobulin molecule consisted of at least two qualitatively different polypeptides, which he designated L (light) chains and H (heavy) chains. (The terms "light" and "heavy" refer to molecular weight.)

Edelman further demonstrated differences in L chains of guinea pig antibodies that indicated a relationship to the ability to bind different antigens. Finally, he suggested that immunoglobulin-related proteins, called Bence-Jones proteins, appeared very similar to the L chains and that the structural study of these compounds might prove fruitful.

The next step, immunologists realized, was the further detailed characterization of the antibody molecule. Porter began work on the L chains, while Edelman and his colleagues tackled "the whole molecule—a ghastly big job." Many researchers contributed, however, and this was a time of great excitement in the field. Informal meetings, called "antibody workshops," held twice a year in locations "from California to Israel" were open to anyone working in the field. Porter and Edelman were prominent at these meetings, encouraging and helping others (Altman 1972; Cebra 1972; 384–85).

In 1962–63, Porter, working with his long-term associate, Elizabeth Press, and with other colleagues, used controlled cleavage of the interchain bonds, followed by detailed molecular weight, protein, and antigenic analysis, to construct a four-chain model of immunoglobulin, which is now widely confirmed as the true picture. The model shows two pairs of H and L chains, which can be cleaved into Fab fragments; the fragments are the active antigen binding sites. These consist of a whole L chain, plus a nitrogen-hydrogen fragment (NH_2) of the H chain.

Additional discoveries were made throughout the 1960s. Edelman, supporting Frantiszek Franek of the Czech Academy of Sciences, found that the fragmented H and L chains worked together to bind antigens as effectively as the intact parent molecule. Norbert Hilschmann at Rockefeller University and Frank Putnam at the University of Florida used Bence-Jones proteins to examine the amino acid sequences of the

L chains. Their work indicated that the Ls consisted of a constant half (CL) that never varied in structured and a variable half (VL). Porter and Robert Hill further contributed to the mapping of these segments.

The segmented nature of the molecule was now apparent. Porter's group hypothesized that the H chain also contained a variable region that linked to the (VL) segment to form the active antigen binding site. They used both human myeloma proteins and normal rabbit immunoglobulin, which is a mixed "pool" of antibodies. Both studies furnished evidence for a variable portion of the H chain (VH) consisting of alternating amino acids, linked in different sequences (Cebra 1972, 385).

Edelman and his team meanwhile had pursued his quest to describe the complete molecule, using human myeloma protein. With the aid of William Konigsberg of Yale, they were able to publish complete data by 1969. These results for the first time compared the (V_L) and (V_H) segments and established that a single antigen-binding site is formed from these two different, and varying, polypeptides. The marked variation in the structure of these segments suggested a solution of the problem of antigenic specificity, which was eventually developed by Susumu Tonegawa.

The Edelman model also showed the now familiar repetition of the constant segments; Edelman suggested that each was responsible for secondary biologic functions of the molecule. Altogether, the model sequenced 1300 amino acids in the complex protein.

Further research comparing sequences and attempting to bind "affinity labels" to the active sites to study their activity identified three short "hypervariable" segments within the V segments that were considered possible determinants of specific response to given antigens. Porter worked on the further characterization of the antibodies until his death. Edelman became interested in the process of their genetic synthesis, still attempting to clarify how the body is able to manufacture sufficient antibodies to meet most antigenic challenges. These investigations eventually led him to studies of brain development and a complex theory of genetic learning and variation throughout life (Cebra 1972, 385–86).

Edelman became a full professor at Rockefeller University in 1966. He was appointed to the Astor chair in 1974. For most of his career, he has worked "endless" hours, nights and weekends, and he has a reputation for being reserved and humorless. To his family and close colleagues he presents a different side. He writes poetry; plays the violin; and is interested in literature and philosophy. For exercise, he swims regularly and walks to work and back—a mile each way (Brody 1972).

He is a trustee of the Rockefeller Brothers Fund and of the Salk Institute; a member of the advisory committee of the Carnegie Institute; a fellow of the National Academy of Sciences, and belongs to the major biochemical societies. Among the many other honors he has received are the Eli Lilly Award in Biological

Chemistry (1965), the Albert Einstein Commemorative Award from Yeshiva University (1974), and the Buchman Memorial Award from the California Institute of Technology (1975).

MARCIA MELDRUM

Selected Bibliography

PRIMARY SOURCES

Edelman, Gerald M. 1970. "The Structure and Function of Antibodies." *Scientific American* 223 (August): 34–42.

———. 1974. *Cellular Selection and Regulation in the Immune Response.* New York: Raven Press.

———. 1975. *Molecular Machinery of the Membrane.* Cambridge: MIT Press.

Edelman, Gerald M., E. Gall, and W. Cowan. 1985. *Molecular Basis of Neural Development.* New York: Wiley.

SECONDARY SOURCES

Altman, Lawrence K. 1972. "Deciphering the Structure." *New York Times* (October 13):24.

Brody, Jane E. 1972. "Pioneers in Immunology Research: Gerald M. Edelman." *New York Times* (October 13):24.

Cebra, John J. 1972. "The 1972 Nobel Prize in Physiology or Medicine." *Science* 178 (October 27):384–86.

PAUL EHRLICH 1908

Paul Ehrlich, recipient of the Nobel Prize in Physiology or Medicine in 1908 with Ilya Metchnikoff, was born on March 14, 1854, in Strehlen, Germany (now Strzelin, Poland). He was the only son and the fourth child of Ismar and Rosa Weigert Ehrlich. His father was a Jewish distiller, innkeeper, and lottery collector. In 1883 Ehrlich married Hedwig Pinkhus, the daughter of a prosperous textile industrialist. The couple had two children, Stephanie, born in 1884, and Marianne, born in 1886. Ehrlich died on August 20, 1915 in Bad Homburg, Germany, after a career in which he made important contributions to the fields of immunology, chemotherapy, histology, hematology, and oncology.

After pursuing medical studies at the universities of Breslau, Strassburg, and Leipzig, Ehrlich received his medical degree from Leipzig in 1878. Upon graduation he accepted a position in Freidrich von Frerich's clinic at the Charité Hospital in Berlin. After a decade at the Charité, he resigned in 1888 to travel to southern Europe and Egypt to recuperate from tuberculosis. When Ehrlich returned from his travels in 1889, he set up a small private laboratory in which to continue his researches. In 1891 he joined the staff of Robert Koch's newly founded Institute for Infectious Diseases in Berlin, although without salary. In the same year he received an appointment as extraordinary professor at Berlin University. The Prussian Ministry of Educational and Medical Affairs established an antitoxin control station, under Ehrlich's direction, at Koch's institute in 1895, soon after Ehrlich had assisted Emil von Behring in the development of a satisfactory diphtheria antitoxin preparation. The following year a laboratory for serum research and testing was established at Steglitz with Ehrlich as its director. A new Institute for Experimental Therapy was created especially for Ehrlich in Frankfort in 1899, and he remained as its director until his death in 1915. From 1906 he was also head of the Georg-Speyer Haus, a laboratory for experimental chemotherapy built adjacent to the institute with funds provided by the widow of a wealthy banker.

Ehrlich relished cigars, mineral water, simple music, and detective stories. Although kindly and genial, he was easily provoked by what he considered to be unfair criticisms or false claims to priority. He directed the work of his laboratory in detail, providing his collaborators each day with specific written instructions that he expected them to obey explicitly. Ehrlich had a great talent for visualizing chemical molecules and a gift for coining words and phrases.

The central theme in Ehrlich's work was the concept of selective affinity of drugs and chemicals. While still a medical student, he came across an 1871 publication on lead poisoning. The author, Emil Heubel, had estimated quantitatively the lead content of various organs in animals that had been subjected to lead poisoning. He found significant differences in the lead content of the different organs. Ehrlich became intrigued by the question of the distribution of chemical substances among the cells of the body. He began by studying the distribution of dyes in living tissues, an investigation that formed the basis of his dissertation for the medical degree, because one could more easily follow the distribution of a dye through its color. His interest in dyes was probably stimulated by his cousin, the pathologist Carl Weigert, a pioneer in the field of histological staining.

In 1885 Ehrlich published the results of his study of the ability of various tissues to reduce certain dyestuffs, *Das Sauerstoffbedürfnis des Organismus: eine farbenanalytische Studie*. This work contained the first indication of his side chain theory of cellular action, a concept that played a significant role in his later thinking about immunology and chemotherapy. Ehrlich adopted Edward Pfluger's view that protoplasm may be envisioned as a giant molecule consisting of a chemical nucleus of special structure that is responsible for the specific functions of a particular type of cell (e.g., a liver cell), with attached chemical side chains that are more involved in the processes common to all cells (e.g., cellular oxidation).

After Ehrlich became involved in immunological work in the 1890s, he developed this side chain theory more fully to explain the process of immunization. He postulated that side chains in the cell, which are normally involved in ordinary physiological processes such as oxidation, might contain chemical groups capable of combining with bacterial toxins, such as the diphtheria toxin. Combination with the toxin, however, renders the side chain incapable of performing its normal physiological function. The cell then produces more of these side chains to make up for the deficiency, but it overcompensates so that excess side chains are produced, break away from the cell, and are released into the bloodstream. These excess side chains are what we call antitoxins or antibodies. They neutralize the toxin by combining with it, thus preventing it from anchoring itself to the cell and exerting its poisonous effects.

Ehrlich went on to distinguish between what he called the *haptophore* group, which was involved in binding the toxin to the side chain, and the *toxophore* group, which was responsible for the poisonous properties of the toxin. His theory eventually became much more elaborate as he struggled to explain various immunological phenomena. Ehrlich's concepts of the toxin-antitoxin (or antigen-antibody) reaction, though significantly modified by later developments in immunology, stimulated immunological research by providing a theoretical framework for discussion of the subject and by focusing attention on antitoxins and antibodies as objects of productive investigation. He also insisted that the antigen-antibody reaction was understandable in terms of ordinary chemical interactions, again stressing the concept of selective affinity.

Aside from his contributions to immunological theory, Ehrlich established the principles of standardization of bacterial toxins and antitoxins. It was through Ehrlich's efforts in this area that Emil von Behring was able to produce a diphtheria antitoxin of high enough potency to be of clinical value. Ehrlich also developed the distinction between active and passive immunity. The Nobel Prize that he shared with Ilya Metchnikoff in 1908 was for his contributions to the subject of immunity.

Although Ehrlich carried out investigations on the therapeutic potential of chemical drugs in the 1890s, it was not until about 1903 that he began to concentrate his researches in chemotherapy, the field that was to occupy most of his time for the rest of his career. Ehrlich was the founder of modern chemotherapy. Recognizing that many infectious diseases did not seem to be amenable to antitoxin or serum therapy, Ehrlich saw a need to develop chemical agents to fight these diseases. The key was to develop chemotherapeutic drugs that were toxic to the pathogenic microorganism but not to the human host (once again invoking the concept of selective affinity). Ehrlich believed that although one could probably not hope to produce synthetic compounds as specific in their action as the antibodies, it might be possible someday to synthesize a chemotherapeutic agent close to that ideal.

Beginning with dyes and later expanding his studies to include arsenic compounds, Ehrlich and his coworkers modified the chemical structure of numerous molecules in an effort to produce effective drugs against trypanosome and later spirochete infections. They tested hundreds of compounds before they came upon one, number 606, that Ehrlich felt was the successful chemotherapeutic agent he was searching for. Clinical tests confirmed the potential of the drug in treating syphilis and trypanosomiasis. In 1910 Ehrlich announced the discovery of 606, which he named Salvarsan, to the world.

Salvarsan provided the practical success that Ehrlich needed to support his concept of chemotherapy. His work created enthusiasm for the chemotherapeutic approach, and stimulated the search for other chemical drugs effective against infectious disease. The modified version of the side chain theory that he used to explain the interaction between the drug and the cell formed the basis (along with the work of the English physiologist J. N. Langley) of the modern receptor theory of drug action. He also used this theory to explain the phenomenon of resistance to drugs, which was discovered in his laboratory around 1905.

Ehrlich was nominated again for a Nobel Prize in 1912 and 1913 for his contributions in chemotherapy. The value of Salvarsan was still in dispute at the time, however, and Ehrlich's death in 1915 ended the matter.

JOHN PARASCANDOLA

Selected Bibliography

PRIMARY SOURCES

Edited by F. Himmelweit. *The Collected Papers of Paul Ehrlich.* 3 vols. London: Pergamon Press, 1956–60.

SECONDARY SOURCES

Marquardt, Martha. 1951. *Paul Ehrlich.* New York: Henry Schuman.

Dolman, Claude. 1971. "Paul Ehrlich." In *Dictionary of Scientific Biography,* edited by Charles Gillispie, 4:295–395. New York: Charles Scribner's Sons.

Mazumdar, Pauline. 1974. "The Antigen-Antibody Reaction and the Physics and Chemistry of Life." *Bulletin of the History of Medicine* 48: 1–21.

Parascandola, John, and Ronald Jasensky. 1974. "Origins of the Receptor Theory of Drug Action." *Bulletin of the History of Medicine* 48: 199–220.

Rubin, Lewis. 1980. "Styles in Scientific Explanation: Paul Ehrlich and Svante Arrhenius on Immunochemistry." *Journal of the History of Medicine* 35: 397–425.

Parascandola, John. 1981. "The Theoretical Basis of Paul Ehrlich's Chemistry." *Journal of the History of Medicine* 36:19–43.

Bäumler, Ernst. 1984. *Paul Ehrlich: Scientist for Life.* Translated by Grant Edwards. New York: Holmes and Meier.

Parascandola, John. 1986. "The Development of Receptor Theory." In *Discoveries in Pharmacology*, edited by M. J. Parnham and J. Bruinvels, 3: 129–56. Amsterdam: Elsevier.

Silverstein, Arthur. 1986. "Anti-antibodies and Anti-idiotype Immunoregulation, 1899–1904: The Inexorable Logic of Paul Ehrlich." *Cellular Immunology* 99: 507–22.

CHRISTIAAN EIJKMAN *1929*

Through his careful study of a progressive paralytic disease that appeared in a flock of chickens kept for bacteriological work at his laboratory in Java, Christiaan Eijkman demonstrated that the disease was caused by a deficiency in the diet—in fact, by the lack of a water-soluble substance found in rice polishings. Eijkman's observations led ultimately to the isolation of vitamin B1 (thiamine) and was the starting point for the whole field of vitamin research.

Christiaan Eijkman was born at Nijkerk, a small town in Gelderland, the Netherlands, the seventh child of Christiaan Eijkman and Johanna Alida Pool. His father was the headmaster of a school at Nijkerk, but a year after his birth his family moved to Zaandam, a few miles northwest of Amsterdam, where his father became headmaster of a new school for advanced elementary education. In 1875, at the age of seventeen, the young Christiaan Eijkman entered the Military Medical School of the University of Amsterdam. In return for his medical training, he agreed to serve as a medical officer with the Netherlands Army. As a student he served for two years as an assistant to the professor of physiology, Thomas Place, with whom he wrote his thesis on polarization in the nerves. On July 13, 1883, Eijkman was graduated M.D. at Amsterdam, and about the same time he married Aaltje Wigeri van Edema. Immediately after his graduation, Eijkman, accompanied by his young wife, went to the Dutch East Indies as a medical officer of health. They were posted first at Semarang on the north coast and later at Tjilatjab on the south coast of the island of Java. At Tjilatjab Eijkman contracted malaria and was thereafter chronically ill. Later they moved to the small village of Padangsidimpuan in western Sumatra, but by November 1885 malaria had so weakened Eijkman that he had to return to Holland on sick leave. Shortly after their return home his young wife died.

When Eijkman's health permitted, he began the study of bacteriology which, in the wake of Robert Koch's discovery of the tubercle bacillus a year earlier, was a new and exciting area of medical science. After a period of study at Amsterdam under Josef Förster, Eijkman went to Berlin to work in Robert Koch's laboratory. While he was there two Dutch physicians, C. A. Pekelharing and C. Winkler, visited the laboratory and became acquainted with their fellow countryman. Pekelharing and Winkler had been appointed by the Dutch government to go to the East Indies to study beriberi, a disease that was causing increasingly serious problems in the Far East, particularly where people lived together in close quarters such as in army barracks, in labor camps, and in prisons. They appointed Eijkman and one of his colleagues as assistants to their mission, and in October 1886 Eijkman sailed once again for the East.

During its first year the Pekelharing-Winkler mission demonstrated that beriberi involved a polyneuritis, and from the blood of beriberi patients they isolated a micrococcus that, they thought, produced toxins that caused the polyneuritis. After just a year, Pekelharing and Winkler were recalled to the Netherlands, but before they left Pekelharing arranged to have their temporary laboratory in the military hospital at Batavia (now Djakarta) made permanent. On January 15, 1888, Christiaan Eijkman was appointed both director of the new laboratory and director of the Javanese medical school. For the next eight years Eijkman devoted himself to medical research. He studied the physiological effects of a tropical climate on Europeans and showed that tropical conditions themselves caused no effects. Eijkman's most important researches, however, were on beriberi.

As a result of the work of the Pekelharing-Winkler mission, of which he was a part, Eijkman believed that beriberi was caused by a bacterial infection. He concluded that outbreaks of beriberi might be prevented, or controlled, by disinfection procedures, such as those used against other infectious diseases. Nevertheless, his efforts to prevent or control outbreaks of beriberi in Java failed.

In July of perhaps 1889 or 1890 when Eijkman's laboratory was still housed in makeshift quarters at the military hospital at Batavia, a disease broke out in the flock of chickens maintained in connection with the laboratory. The chickens became restless and their gait unsteady. When a bird descended from its perch it seemed to have to make an effort not to fall down, as if its feet were not solid enough to support it. It was the victim of a progressive paralysis moving from the toes upward—within a few days it lay on its side unable to stand or move. Without help the bird could not even eat or drink. It breathed only at intervals, its beak was open, and its comb and skin turned from a normal bright red to a dark bluish color. Most strikingly, the neck was bent backwards and the head retracted. The bird became comatose, its eyes closed, and it soon died of what was clearly a progressive polyneuritis.

At first Eijkman thought that the chickens were suffering from an infectious disease, but when he conducted inoculation experiments with material from sick or dying animals, the results were confusing because both the inoculated chickens and the uninoculated controls came down with the disease. Neither could he find any microorganism or parasite associated with the disease. Then suddenly, at the end of November, almost five months after it had started, the disease stopped. Sick chickens recovered, and no more became ill.

At that point Eijkman began to suspect the chicken's food, and inquired whether there had been any change in what they were fed. He learned that for several months the laboratory attendant had been feeding the chickens on cooked rice from the hospital kitchen, but on November 27 a new cook had refused any longer to supply rice for the chickens, so they had been returned to ordinary chicken food: raw, unpolished rice. When Eijkman inquired how long the chickens had been fed cooked rice, he learned that the practice had begun on June 10, about a month before the outbreak of the disease. The epizootic, therefore, began several weeks after the chickens began to eat the cooked rice and ended promptly when they were returned to their ordinary diet of raw, unpolished rice.

After he learned that the disease had coincided with the period of feeding cooked rice, Eijkman carried out planned feeding experiments that showed that the polyneuritis appeared invariably in chickens three to four weeks after they had begun to feed upon cooked rice, even when the rice was fresh. Eijkman and his colleague Grijns found that the hull and germ of the rice contained a substance, soluble in water or alcohol, that was capable of preventing polyneuritis in chickens, pigeons, or other birds. He saw immediately that polyneuritis in birds might correspond to beriberi in humans, and that beriberi might, therefore, have a dietary cause. Throughout the East Indies the country people were accustomed to eating rough rice that they grew and shelled by their own simple methods. In contrast, white rice was processed mechanically by European methods. At Eijkman's request, the medical inspector for Java studied the rice diet in prisons where outbreaks of beriberi had occurred. He found that in prisons where beriberi occurred the staple diet was polished rice, whereas in those prisons where no beriberi occurred the normal diet was rough rice.

Ill health forced Eijkman to return to the Netherlands in 1896. Initially Eijkman thought that in the digestion of the polished rice a toxin that caused the polyneuritis was formed, but in the rough rice the supposed toxin was rendered harmless by a protective substance in the rice bran. In 1901 Eijkman's successor at Batavia, G. Grijns, demonstrated that the substance in the rice bran was used directly in the body. The polyneuritis, therefore, arose because of a deficiency of an essential nutritional factor rather than from a toxin.

In 1898 Eijkman was appointed professor of public health and forensic medicine in the University of Utrecht, where he taught and directed research during the next thirty years. In 1929, a year after his retirement at age seventy, he was awarded the Nobel Prize for Physiology or Medicine for his discovery of the role of polished rice in causing polyneuritis in chickens.

LEONARD G. WILSON

Selected Bibliography

PRIMARY SOURCES

Eijkman, Christiaan. 1897. "Eine Beriberi—ähnlike Krankheit der Hühner." *Virchows Archiv für Pathologische Anatomie und Physiologie und für Klinische Medizin* 148:523–32.

———. 1929. "Antineuritic Vitamin and Beriberi." Nobel Lecture. Reprinted in *Nobel Lectures in Physiology or Medicine.* Vol. 2 (1929–1941): 199–210. Amsterdam: Elsevier, 1965.

SECONDARY SOURCES

Lindeboom, G. A., 1971. "Eijkman, Christiaan." In *Dictionary of Scientific Biography.* Vol. 4:310–312. New York: Scribners.

WILLEM EINTHOVEN *1924*

Willem Einthoven was born on May 22, 1860, in Semarang, Dutch East Indies (now Indonesia). A physiologist, Einthoven received the Nobel Prize in 1924 for his development of electrocardiography, still the basic clinical tool for the diagnosis and monitoring of heart disease. At the time of the award, Einthoven was professor of physiology at the University of Leiden, a position he occupied for most of his career. He married his cousin, Frederique Jeanne Louise de Vogel, in 1886. They had one son, Willem, who became an electrical engineer and made important contributions to radio technology, and three daughters, Augusta, Louisa, and Johanna, who became a physician. Einthoven died on September 29, 1927, in Leiden, the Netherlands.

Willem was the eldest son of Jacob Einthoven, the town doctor of Semarang, and his wife, Louise de Vogel, daughter of the colony's director of finance. The elder Einthoven died when Willem was only six. His widow returned to Europe four years later to ensure the best education for her six children. They settled in Utrecht in the Netherlands. Here, in 1878, Willem entered the University to study medicine. He planned to specialize in ophthalmology and to follow his father into the army and colonial medical services; the Dutch army provided him with financial assistance.

At Utrecht Einthoven worked

with the anatomist W. Koster, the physicist C. H. D. Buys Ballot, and the great physiologist and pioneer of ophthalmology F. C. Donders; he was also assistant to the ophthalmologist H. Snellen, at the Gasthuis voor Doglijders, a famous eye hospital. He distinguished himself and attracted the interest of the medical community when he published two papers as a student. The first, written with Koster's guidance, was a penetrating study on the pronation and supination (rotations) of the arm, modestly entitled "Some Remarks on the Elbow Joint." Prompted by an accidental fracture of his own wrist during a gymnastics exercise, Einthoven analyzed the arm's anatomy in terms of the principles of physics and mathematics.

The second paper, "Stereoscopy by Means of Color Variation," was submitted as his doctoral thesis. Donders had earlier noted the perception of a difference in depth between red and blue letters on the same dark background. He attributed this phenomenon, which he often demonstrated in lectures, to a difference in the eye's accommodation to red and blue light. Einthoven experimented with this phenomenon, using himself and others as subjects; he employed geometric constructions, partial and complete obstructions of one eye. He was able to demonstrate different degrees of depth discrimination, and even reversal, in different subjects; that is, where most people saw the red letters in front of the blue ones, Einthoven constructed experiments where some people saw the blue letters in front of the red. He concluded that the phenomenon was in fact due to the asymmetry of the eye in relation to the center of the pupil. This paper was accepted for the Ph.D. in 1885 and highly praised.

As a result of these early achievements Einthoven was nominated to the chair of physiology at Leiden when it fell vacant in 1885. Although this involved termination of his contract with the army and repayment of the money he owed for his medical education, a heavy financial burden, Einthoven accepted the professorship and took up his new responsibilities as soon as he had received his medical degree. He was then twenty-five and would remain at Leiden for the rest of his life.

His research in the late 1880s continued his student interests in vision and respiration. He conducted a fundamental study on asthma, demonstrating its basis in bronchial spasm. Although many clinicians supported such a causation, it had been disputed by physiologists in the absence of experimental proof. Einthoven insufflated a constant but adjustable flow of air into the lungs during artificial respiration and measured the intra-pulmonary pressure. He found that the latter was correlated with intrapleural pressure and thus rose with bronchial constriction, which he evoked by stimulation of the vagal nerve with carbon dioxide. These results, published in 1892, were widely recognized for their importance (Einthoven 1892, 367).

From 1893, although he continued his studies in optics, his interest was engaged by the recording of electrical action currents, first of the eye and then particularly of the heart, and their physiological implications. Until 1887 cardiac action currents had been recorded only from the exposed or excised heart. In that year the British physiologist A. D. Waller had demonstrated the feasibility of recording cardiac current from the body surface, using the Lippmann capillary electrometer. He was unable, however, to define the shape of the current or to develop a practical clinical technique.

Einthoven recognized in 1893 that these electrical tracings made possible a new method of clinical investigation, but that they would have to be defined and standardized to allow for any meaningful conclusions. By the following year, applying his knowledge of physics, he had calculated the true curve of the action current, which he called the electrocardiogram. He then used the Lippmann device to make the first recordings of heart sounds in man and in animals. In 1900 he and K. de Lint described the normal and corrected electrocardiogram, as well as readings of clinical aortic insufficiency, showing the reflection of this condition in an abnormal wave, designated the "T wave" by Einthoven. De Vogel, his brother-in-law and assistant, had meanwhile written his thesis on the characteristics of the action current (Einthoven and de Lint 1900, 139–60).

The capillary electrometer was highly sensitive, but its tracings were easily distorted by inertial movement of its mercury column. Einthoven had calculated the mathematical correction necessary for arriving at the true readings, but this was a cumbersome procedure. He therefore set out to construct an instrument that would record the heart currents accurately. He used as a model the mirror galvanometer developed by Deprez-d' Arsonval, a device that recorded tracings free from inertial distortion but was not sensitive enough for electrocardiography. His calculations showed that the sensitivity could be increased by a significant increase in the internal resistance, coupled with maximal reduction of the weight of the galvanometer and of the windings on its coil. He therefore designed an instrument consisting of a thin, short wire in a strong magnetic field, illuminated and observed through microscopes.

Einthoven acknowledged in his announcement of his design an instrument devised by Ader for the reception of underwater telegraphic signals, similar in construction to the string galvanometer but much lower in sensitivity. Allegations that Einthoven copied Ader's construction surfaced immediately and continue to be made even today; however, there seems to be little foundation for these claims.

The first electrocardiograms taken with the string galvanometer were published in 1903. A comparison of one of these with a corrected tracing from the same person, taken with the Lippmann device, showed that the recordings were in fact identical. In this paper Einthoven also suggested standardized measures of voltage and speed; these were adopted and are still in use (Einthoven 1903, 472–80).

He proceeded to carry out a more or less systematic study of cardiac abnormalities with his new instrument. Ventricular extra systoles (contractions), heart block (also experimental block induced by vagal stimulation), atrial flutter, and fibrillation were successfully recorded. Einthoven's tracings also showed changes in the ventricular complex as a result of left hypertrophy from aortic stenosis (constriction) and variations in the P wave in mitral stenosis. Many of his recordings were made from hospital patients at a distance, connected by cable with the galvanometer in the laboratory a mile away, while Einthoven spoke with the attending cardiologist on the telephone. On one occasion, having observed a ventricular extrasystole, he told the physician to expect an imminent pulse intermission before it was felt at the wrist. These and other evidences of superior data irritated the physician, who finally cut the cable between Einthoven and the hospital.

By then, however, he had published two landmark accounts of abnormal electrocardiograms and completed his system of standardization. To calibrate the accuracy of different equipment, he introduced three contact combinations: both hands (I); right hand-left foot (II); and left hand-left foot (III); and their relationship: I=II-III. These guidelines remain standard in electrocardiography (Einthoven 1906, 132–65; Einthoven and Vaandrager 1908, 517–85).

In May 1908 a London physician named Thomas Lewis wrote Einthoven to ask for a reprint of his 1906 paper, "Le telecardiogramme." Thus began a correspondence that lasted until 1926 and made major contributions to the development of clinical electrocardiography. Lewis and Einthoven were almost ideal complements. Lewis's knowledge of mathematics and physics was limited and he often sought assistance from his colleague; but he displayed a great ingenuity in devising and carrying out experiments to clarify fundamental clinical problems. Einthoven, who was "in spite of his medical training and office essentially a physicist," as A. V. Hill said, had neither the interest nor the clinical experience to do such work. His grateful recognition of Lewis's work in his Nobel Prize lecture was entirely sincere.

Einthoven's own further contributions to the field were theoretical. He demonstrated conclusively that the electrical and mechanical activities of the heart muscle were inseparable. Apparent discrepancies were caused by sensitivity differences in the recording equipment. In 1912, with G. Fahr and A. de Waart, he developed the simplified scheme of the equilateral triangle with the standard contact combinations I, II, and III, as the sides and the heart as the center and source of information. The various currents generated by the heart, recorded simultaneously, could then be combined into a single potential, whose size and direction could be measured. The use of the triangular model then made possible various mathematical calculations that accurately described cardiac activity. Despite the inherent simplification of this concept in treating the heart as an undifferentiated unit, it was entirely adequate for most studies and served as the basis for standard vectorcardiography. Later research on localized anomalies within the heart found it less satisfactory (Einthoven, Fahr, and de Waart 1913, 275–315).

In Einthoven's laboratory the string galvanometer was applied to the recording of other currents, specifically the optic reaction to light and the electrical activity of vagal and sympathetic nerves. This work was carried on into the 1920s, surprising and interesting Einstein, who visited Leiden frequently during those years. Working with his son, Einthoven developed a hypersensitive galvanometer by placing the string in a vacuum; this model was initially designed for reception and recording of radio signals from Indonesia. In his last investigation, in 1927, the vacuum string galvanometer recorded the action current of the cervical sympathetic nerve, but its mapping and study awaited electronic amplification (Einthoven, Hoogerwerf, Karplus, and Kreidl 1927, 443–53).

Einthoven's lifetime work with electrocardiography and its extended applications perfectly combined his medical training with his absorption in physics and mathematics. His temperament, logical, pragmatic, meticulous, and single-minded, was also well suited to his research. Demanding in his work, he was personally modest. When he was on a lecture tour in the United States in 1924, he saw press reports of his Nobel award, but he refused to take them seriously until the official confirmation reached him.

He was a member of the Dutch Royal Academy of Sciences and rarely missed a meeting. For most of his life he was also interested in sports and physical development, including fencing and gymnastics. His death in 1927, at the age of sixty-seven, followed a long illness.

H. A. SNELLEN

Selected Bibliography

PRIMARY SOURCES

Einthoven, Willem. 1892. "Über die Wirkung der Bronchialmuskelm, Nach einer Neuen Methode Untersucht, und Über Asthma Nervosum." *Pflügers Archiv für die gesamte Physiologie des Menschen und der Tiere* 51:367.

Einthoven, Willem, and K. de Lint. 1900. "Über das Normale Menschliche Elektrocardiogram und Uber die Capillar-Elektromische Untersuchung bei einigen Herzkranken." *Pflügers Archiv für die gesamte Physiologie des Menschen und der Tiere* 80:139–60.

Einthoven, Willem. 1903. "Die Galvanometrische Registrierung des Menschlichen Elektrokardiogramms, zugleich eine Beurteilung der Anwendung des Capillar-Elektrometers in der Physiologie." *Pflügers Archiv für die gesamte Physiologie des Menschen und der Tiere* 99: 472–80.

———. 1906. "Le télécardiogramme." *Archives Internationales de Physiologie* 4:132–65. (Partial translations of this paper appear in the

American Heart Journal, 49 (1955): 132, translated by Methewson and Jackh, and 53 (1957):602, translated by Blackburn.)

Einthoven, Willem, and B. Vaandrager. 1908. "Weiteres Über das Elektrokardiogramm." *Pflügers Archiv für die gesamte Physiologie des Menschen und der Tiere* 122:517–85.

Einthoven, Willem, G. Fahr, and A. de Waart. 1913. "Über die Richtung and die Manifeste Grösse der Potential Schwankungen in Menschlichen Herzen und über den Einfluss der Herzlagen auf die Form des Electrokardiogramms." *Pflügers Archiv für die gesamte Physiologie des Menschen und der Tiere* 150: 275–315. (Translated by Hoff and Seklj as "On the Direction and Size of the Variations of Potential in the Human Heart and on the Influence of the Position of the Heart on the Form of the Electrocardiogram," *American Heart Journal*, 40 (1950): 163.)

Einthoven, Willem, S. Hoogerwerf, J. P. Karplus, and A. Kreidl. 1927. "Gehirn und Sympathicus, die Aktionsströme des Hallssyympathicus." *Pflügers Archiv für die gesamte Physiologie des Menschen und der Tiere* 215:443–53.

Waller, A. D. 1887. "A Demonstration on Man of Electromotive Changes Accompanying the Heart's Beat." *Journal of Physiology* 8:17.

Snellen, H. A. ed. 1977. *Selected Papers on Electrocardiography of Willem Einthoven*. Leiden: Leiden University Press.

SECONDARY SOURCES

Hill, Archibald V. 1927. "Professor W. Einthoven." *Nature* 120: 591–92.

Hoogerwerf, S. 1971. "Einthoven, Willem." In *Dictionary of Scientific Biography*, 4:333–35. New York: Scribners.

Lewis, Thomas. 1927. "Willem Einthoven." *British Medical Journal* 2: 664–65.

Snellen, H. A. 1983. *Two Pioneers of Electriocardiography*. Rotterdam, the Netherlands: Donker Academic Publications.

GERTRUDE BELLE ELION *1988*

Gertrude Belle Elion was born in New York City, on January 23, 1918. A biochemist, Elion received the 1988 Nobel Prize jointly with George H. Hitchings and Sir James Whyte Black for their work in developing drugs for the treatment of many critical diseases. Elion and Hitchings, long-time collaborators at Burroughs Wellcome Research Laboratories, produced compounds that inhibit DNA synthesis and thus prevent the rapid growth of cancer cells. They then used their understanding of nucleic acid synthesis to develop immunosuppressives and antibiotics. The Nobel Prize is rarely given for new drugs and its award to Elion and Hitchings recognizes not only their multiple contributions to therapeutics but their formulation of basic principles that will continue to provide clues to researchers. Elion retired from her position as head of experimental therapies at Burroughs Wellcome in 1983; she holds the title of emeritus scientist and continues to work as a consultant and to serve on the National Cancer Advisory Board. She has never married.

Elion was the daughter of a dentist, both her parents were very supportive of her decision to pursue a career. The death of her grandfather from cancer when she was fifteen led her to choose the field of biochemistry, in the hope of helping to spare the suffering of other patients. She received her bachelor's degree from Hunter College in 1937, at age nineteen and worked for the Denver Chemical Company for a short time before returning for a master's at New York University. She had difficulty obtaining a laboratory position because these positions went to male applicants. She taught high school chemistry for two years (1941–42) before World War II suddenly opened research jobs to women.

She briefly held positions at Quaker Maid and Johnson and Johnson before coming to Burroughs Wellcome in 1944 as a senior research chemist. Hitchings treated her as a colleague rather than an assistant almost from the beginning of their work together. But Elion's career as one of the few women in research biochemistry was never easy. She believed that she could not both marry and advance in her field; after some indecision, she chose to remain single. She sought to earn a Ph.D. by attending night classes at Brooklyn Polytechnic but was told she could not finish the degree unless she left her job and enrolled full time. She has achieved her considerable success and recognition without completing her doctorate (Kolata 1988).

Drug development up to that time had often followed the "magic bullet" method made famous by Paul Ehrlich in 1910. This kind of research involved the unsystematic injection of multiple compounds into research animals, to see if any of them would prove to be the "bullet" for a specific disease. Other scientists, studying the etiology and pathology of diseases, disdained any concern with clinical drug development. Hitchings and Elion hoped to find in biochemical research "a middle course . . . that would generate basic information which chemotherapy could then exploit." As Hitchings has said, the considerable autonomy given his team by Burroughs Wellcome was crucial to their many successes. "Our orientation was basic research and yet we turned out more drugs than people who were looking for them."

In the 1940s they began looking at the cellular synthesis of nucleotides. They found that bacterial cells could not produce nucleic acid (DNA)—and therefore could not divide—in the absence of certain proteins (purines) and folic acid. With this information, they were able to develop antimetabolite compounds that blocked the enzymes necessary for the formation of cellular DNA.

The antimetabolites were initially tested on leukemia patients at Sloan-Kettering Institute in the late 1940s and early 1950s. Hitchings and Elion hoped that the new drugs would inhibit the rapid formation of the white blood cells sufficiently to bring about a remission of the leukemia. The difficulty was, of course, that the formation of other cells might be inhibited and the drug would prove more toxic to the patient than to the cancer. This was indeed the case with the first compound tested; however, later trials proved the efficacy and relative safety of 6-mercaptopurine and thioguanine, which are still used today to treat leukemia (Marx 1988, 516; Kolata 1988; Altman 1988).

Hitchings's and Elion's work was notable not only for its contribution to a particular disease but for its insight into the potential applications of DNA research and its development of a method to block the "pathways" that form nucleic acids. This concept was quite revolutionary in the 1940s (Marx 1988, 516).

The team, continuing to work along these lines, synthesized azathioprine, a modified form of 6-mercaptopurine in 1957. It proved to be "unimpressive" against leukemia, but researchers at Tufts found that it effectively suppressed the immune system's production of antibodies. This kind of drug is essential in kidney and other organ transplants to prevent the body's rejection of the implanted tissues. Azathioprine is also used in the treatment of autoimmune disorders, such as rheumatoid arthritis, in which the body is believed to attack its own tissue.

Another drug developed as an enzyme inhibitor was allopurinol. Again, it was not successful against cancer. But Hitchings and Elion noted that it blocked the enzyme xanthine oxidase, which is critical to the synthesis of uric acid. Allopurinol is now used to treat gout, which is caused by uric acid deposition in the joints, and to prevent uric acid buildup as a result of cancer chemotherapy.

By the 1960s Elion and Hitchings had turned their attention to nucleic acid synthesis in lower animals and its differences from the same process in humans. The results suggested new ways of combating infectious disease by attacking bacterial and viral DNA. Among the drugs that resulted from this work are pyramethamine, used against the protozoa that causes malaria, and trimethoprim, for urinary and respiratory tract infections caused by bacteria. Trimethoprim is also used in the treatment of *Pneumocystis carinii*, a pneumonia virus that is almost harmless in healthy people but is a major killer of AIDS victims.

Most recently, in 1975, Hitchings's and Elion's team synthesized the drug acyclovir, the first compound found to be effective against herpes. Aziodothymidine (AZT), the only drug so far developed and approved for AIDS, was also produced using the principles the two had established in their early work (Marx 1988, 516–17; Altman 1988).

Despite continued professional recognition of her contributions, Elion, unlike many laureates, never expected to win a Nobel Prize. Her selection acknowledged the unheralded but important work of many women scientists whose careers, like her own, were artificially limited by their gender. Elion spoke for many of them when she said, "The Nobel Prize is fine, but the drugs I've developed are rewards in themselves" (Kolata 1988).

Elion acted as Hitchings's second in his various positions until becoming head of experimental therapies in her own right in 1967. She has served as an NIH consultant and as an adjunct professor of pharmacology at Duke University and the University of North Carolina since 1973.

Elion is a member of the major chemical and biochemical societies and served as president of the American Association for Cancer Research in 1983–84. Among the honors she has received for her work are the Garvan Medal of the American Chemical Society (1968), the Judd Award from Sloan-Kettering (1983), and the Bruce F. Cain Award from the American Association for Cancer Research (1985).

MARCIA MELDRUM

Selected Bibliography

PRIMARY SOURCES

Hitchings, George H., et al. 1950. "Antagonists of Nucleic Acid Derivatives; *Lactobacillus casei* model." *Journal of Biological Chemistry* 183 (March):1–9.

Hitchings, George H., Gertrude B. Elion, and Elvira A. Falco. 1950. "Antagonists of Nucleic Acid Derivatives: Reversal Studies with Substances Structurally Related to Thymine." *Journal of Biological Chemistry* 185 (August):643–49.

Elion, Gertrude B., George H. Hitchings, and H. Van der Werff. 1951. "Antagonists of Nucleic Acid Derivatives: Purines." *Journal of Biological Chemistry* 192 (October):505–18.

Balis, M. E., D. H. Levin, G. B. Brown, G. B. Elion, H. C. Nathan, and G. H. Hitchings. 1957. "The Effects of 6-mercaptopurine on *Lactobacillus casei*." *Archives of Biochemistry and Biophysics* 71 (October):358–66.

Elion, G. B., S. Callahan, S. Bieber, G. H. Hitchings, and R. W. Rudles. 1962. "Experimental, Clinical, and Metabolic Studies of Thiopurines." *Cancer Chemotherapy Reports* 16 (February):197–202.

Hitchings, George H., and Gertrude B. Elion. 1963. "Chemical Suppression of the Immune Response." *Pharmaological Review* 15 (June):365–405.

SECONDARY SOURCES

Altman, Lawrence K. 1988. "Three Drug Pioneers Win Nobel in Medicine." *New York Times* (October 18):1, C17.

Kolata, Gina. 1988. "A Research Collaboration Spanning Four Decades: Gertrude Belle Elion." *New York Times* (October 18):C16.

Connor, Steve, Dan Charles, Sharon Kingman, and Frank Lesser. 1988. "Drug Pioneers Win Nobel Laureate." *New Scientist* (October 22):26–27.

Marx, Jean L. 1988. "The 1988 Nobel Prize for Physiology or Medicine." *Science* 242 (October 18):516–17.

JOHN FRANKLIN ENDERS 1954

John Franklin Enders was born on February 10, 1897, in West Hartford, Connecticut. A virologist, Enders shared the 1954 Nobel Prize with Thomas Huckle Weller and Frederick Chapman Robbins for their successful culturing of poliomyelitis virus in several types of human tissues. Their breakthrough not only laid the groundwork for the development of an effective polio vaccine but was also the prototype for modern methods of viral cultivation, diagnostic testing, and vaccine development. At the time of the award Enders was director of the Infectious Disease Research Laboratory at Children's Hospital, Boston, where the team had done the prizewinning experiments. He and his first wife, Sarah Frances Bennett, whom he married in 1927, had two children, John Ostrom II, and Sarah Steffian. Sarah Enders died in 1943. In 1951 Enders married Carolyn Keane. Enders died on September 8, 1985, in Waterford, Connecticut.

John Enders did not start his career in science. The son of John Ostrom Enders, a banker, and the former Harriet Goulden Whitmore, he was interested in business, literature, and aviation. As a young man in World War I, he taught other young men to fly. Back in Connecticut, he earned a B.A. (1920) in English at Yale, sold real estate for a while, and began studying Celtic literature at Harvard, working toward a Ph.D. He hoped to become an English teacher.

His roommate, H. K. Ward, had come from Australia to study with Hans Zinsser, the famous bacteriologist. Enders often visited Zinsser's laboratory with Ward and became increasingly fascinated with microbes, antigens, and antibodies. He had already earned his M.A. (1922) and was almost finished with his Celtic research, when he finally decided to change his plans. In 1924 he started all over again as a bacteriology student and also began a fruitful fifteen-year association with Zinsser.

His initial efforts at research dealt with the antigens of the tubercle bacillus. For his Ph.D. dissertation, he carried out a classic study on the purification of a carbohydrate tubercle antigen that caused anaphylaxis. Enders received his doctorate in 1930. The year before he had been appointed to the medical school faculty at Harvard as an instructor in bacteriology and immunology. He was to remain at Harvard for the remainder of his career.

Enders next turned his attention to pneumococci and, in 1933, published his results jointly with Ward. In 1937 he turned from bacteria to viruses when cat distemper became a major problem in the animal research quarters. His 1939 publication with William Hammon on this disease is a landmark in the field. Their findings on the distemper virus laid the basis for an effective vaccine. Enders began to devote his efforts to the development of tissue culture models where viruses could be grown and studied. He successfully cultured cowpox, influenza, and measles virus.

In 1940, working with A. E. Feller and a young medical student named Thomas Weller, Enders achieved the first successful prolonged roller tube culture of a virus (Feller, Enders, and Weller 1940). During World War II he became a consultant on epidemic diseases to the secretary of war. Much of his work dealt with the mumps virus, which often broke out among recruits and draftees. He and his team developed diagnostic tests and a killed-virus vaccine for mumps.

In 1946, now a full professor, Enders left the medical school to establish a new Infectious Disease Research Laboratory at Children's Hospital. Here he was joined in 1948 by Thomas Weller as a postdoctoral fellow (later assistant director), and by Frederick Robbins, Weller's Harvard roommate (now a National Research Council senior fellow). The three began a new series of viral culture studies.

In March 1948 Weller was growing the mumps virus in human embryonic tissue cultures with the addition of antibiotics to prevent bacterial contamination. At the end of one such experiment he had a few extra tubes and decided to "try polio" to see if that virus would thrive in his system. His results with the embryo tissue encouraged him to attempt to culture poliovirus in other preparations. He was able to grow the virus in human foreskin cultures, the first time it had been successfully established in non-neural, nonembryonic cells.

Robbins, who had been working with infant epidemic diarrhea, had developed a successful system of mouse intestinal tissue cultures. He and Weller experimented with poliovirus in these cells, but without success. They then developed a culture of human intestinal tissue that proved more hospitable: the poliovirus grew and throve. This was the first demonstration that polio could survive in the intestinal walls of infected individuals. The team also observed cellular changes in the cultures that offered clear evidence of viral replication. Enders coined the term "cytopathogenic" to describe the altered cells.

Over the next few months they were able to produce large quantities of the virus by refining their culture methods and to neutralize it with specific antibodies. The definitive report of their work appeared in *Science* in January 1949, less than a year after Weller had first introduced polio into his spare tubes (Enders, Weller, and Robbins 1949). These classic experiments formed the basis for many diagnostic and vaccine applications, as well as contemporary viral culture techniques. The Nobel Committee voted to award John Enders the 1954 Prize for his significant contribution; he declined to accept unless Robbins and Weller shared the award, and the Nobel Committee complied with his wishes.

Enders could now have pursued the development of a polio vaccine but he left that task to others, while he investigated new and interesting viruses. In the 1950s he developed a successful vaccine for measles. He then turned his interest to cancer and the elucidation of the transformation mechanisms of cells infected with simian virus 40, which then became oncogenic, giving birth to tumors. By the time he retired in 1972, he was the most prominent American virologist, known throughout the world. Virologists today are finding new applications for the pioneering techniques developed by John Enders.

Although he had given up literature for science, he was also known as a humanist, characterized by his concern for others and the breadth of his interests in science, politics, history, and the arts. Among the awards he received for his multiple contributions were the Passano Foundation Award (1953), the Lasker Award (1954), the Kyer Award from the U. S. Public Health Service (1955), the Cameron Prize from the University of Edinburgh (1960), the Robert Koch Medal from Germany (1962), the Science Achievement Award from the American Medical Association (1963), and the Presidential Medal of Freedom (1963).

MARCIA MELDRUM
JAMES J. POUPARD

Selected Bibliography

PRIMARY SOURCES

Enders, John F., Leroy D. Fothergill, and Hans Zinsser. 1939. *Immunity: Principles and Applications in Medicine and Public Health*. New York: Macmillan.

Feller, A. E., J. F. Enders, and T. H. Weller. 1940. "The Prolonged Coexistence of Vaccinia Virus in High Titre and Living Cells in Roller Tube Cultures of Chick Embryonic Tissues." *Journal of Experimental Medicine* 72:367–87.

Enders, J. F., T. H. Weller, and F. C. Robbins. 1949. "Cultivation of the Lansing Strain of Poliomyelitis Virus in Cultures of Various Human Embryonic Tissues." *Science* 109 (January 28):85–87.

Weller, T. H., F. D. Robbins, and J. F. Enders. 1949. "Cultivation of Poliomyelitis Virus in Cultures of Human Foreskin and Embryonic Tissues." *Proceedings of the Society for Experimental Biology* 72:153–55.

Enders, John F. 1959. "Tissue Culture Techniques Employed in the Propagation of Viruses and Rickettsiae." In *Viral and Rickettsial Infections of Man*, edited by Thomas Rivers and Frank L. Horsfall, 209–29. Philadelphia: J. B. Lippincott.

Enders, John F. 1959. "Mumps." In *Viral and Rickettsial Infections of Man*, edited by Thomas Rivers and Frank Horsfall, 780–89. Philadelphia: J. B. Lippincott.

SECONDARY SOURCES

1955. "Enders, John Franklin." In *Current Biography Yearbook*, 182–84. New York: H. W. Wilson.

Williams, Greer. 1960. *Virus Hunters*. New York: Alfred A. Knopf.

Rosen, F. S. 1985. "John F. Enders

(1897–1985)." *Nature* 317 (October 17):575.

Weller, T. H. 1989. "As It Was and as It Is: A Half-Century of Progress." *Journal of Infectious Diseases* 159 (March):378–83.

Weller, Thomas H., and Frederick C. Robbins. (In press.) *John Franklin Enders. 1897–1985. Biographical Memoirs.* Washington: National Academy of Sciences.

JOSEPH ERLANGER *1944*

Joseph Erlanger, physiologist, was born January 5, 1874, in San Francisco, California. He died December 5, 1965, of a cerebral hemorrhage in St. Louis, Missouri. He achieved distinction as one of America's first world-class physiologists, both for his work in cardiovascular physiology and later for his more famous studies establishing the foundation of modern neurophysiology. In addition, his organizing and administrative skills helped strengthen American scientific institutions at a time when the United States was surpassing Europe as the international leader in scientific research and training.

Erlanger was the son of California pioneers. His father, Herman, had immigrated by himself to the United States in 1842 at the age of sixteen from his birthplace of Wurttenberg, Germany. After working as an itinerant peddler along the Mississippi Valley, he was drawn to California by the Gold Rush. His attempts at mining failed, but he succeeded in business and became a merchant of moderate means. In 1849 he married Sarah Galinger, the sister of his business partner and herself an immigrant from Southern Germany. They had seven children, five sons and two daughters, of whom Joseph was the sixth-born.

Erlanger was a precocious youth who early on declared his ambition to enter medicine. He spent considerable time dissecting animals and plants, which led his older sister to give him the nickname "Doc." He entered the San Francisco Boys' High School in 1889, studying the traditional classical course for two years with Latin as his major subject.

In 1891 Erlanger enrolled at the University of California, Berkeley, graduating with the B.S. degree from the College of Chemistry in 1895. At Berkeley he performed his first piece of experimental research, a study of the development of the eggs of the newt *Amblystoma.* Following the recommendation of a friend, he enrolled in The Johns Hopkins Medical School, graduating second in his class in 1899. After graduation he worked for one year at Johns Hopkins as an intern on the internal medicine service of William Osler, the most famous clinician of the day.

At Johns Hopkins Erlanger discovered that medical research, not medical practice, was his calling. He spent the summer after his first year of medical school working in Lewellys Barker's histology laboratory, where he demonstrated the location in the spinal cord of rabbits of the anterior horn cells that innervated a given striated (voluntary) muscle. The following summer he studied how much of the small intestine of dogs could be surgically removed without interfering with the process of absorption; this project led to his first publication in 1901. This work also brought him to the attention of William H. Howell, professor of physiology at Johns Hopkins, who appointed him to the department. He served at Johns Hopkins from 1901 to 1906, first as assistant professor and later as associate professor of physiology. Erlanger worked in Baltimore continously during this period, except for a six-week trip to Europe in the summer of 1902 to study the composition and metabolism of sulfur-containing protein compounds in the biochemistry laboratory of the University of Strassburg.

As a young physiologist at Johns Hopkins Erlanger undertook a number of major projects. In 1904 he designed and built an improved sphygmomanometer, an instrument used to measure blood pressure. Erlanger's sphygmomanometer was much sturdier than any existing device, and it was also much simpler to use since it could measure the blood pressure of the upper arm. That same year he performed an important study of the relationship of blood flow to orthostatic albuminuria (the appearance of protein in the urine on standing). Using his new blood pressure measuring device, he showed that the appearance of albumin (a type of protein) in the urine of patients with this condition related much more closely to the pulse pressure (the difference between the systolic and diastolic blood pressure) than to the mean arterial blood pressure.

After 1904 Erlanger's attention turned to the electrical conduction system of the heart. Using his superb technical and mechanical skills, he devised a clamp that could reversibly apply graded degrees of pressure to the Bundle of His, an anatomic pathway that connects the auricles with the ventricles of the heart. Studying dogs, he was able to produce all degrees of reversible electrical block between the auricles and the ventricles. His most important finding was that impaired conduction through the Bundle of His, or "heart block," was responsible for the clinical syndrome of Stokes-Adams attacks (fainting episodes with slow pulse). This pioneering work formed the foundation of current knowledge of the conduction system of the heart and established Erlanger as a physiologist of the first rank.

In 1906 Erlanger moved to Madison, Wisconsin, to become the first professor of physiology at the University of Wisconsin Medical School. His assignment was to equip and staff a modern laboratory of physiology, but insufficient financial resources frustrated his efforts. When the newly reorganized and well-endowed Washington University School of Medicine in St. Louis offered him the professorship of physiology in 1910, he readily accepted. In St. Louis, with strong administrative and financial backing, he built one of the greatest departments of physiology in the world. He remained as chairman of the department until his retirement in 1946.

At Washington University Erlanger continued his research in cardiovascular physiology. During World War I he developed a solution of glucose and gum acacia for the treatment of wound shock. This preparation was used by the United States Army in France and was the first example of treatment with artificial serum containing high molecular weight polymers. He also conducted very sophisticated studies that elucidated the origin of the sounds of Korotkoff, the sounds that are heard through the stethoscope in measuring blood pressure in man.

In 1921 Erlanger's interest changed from cardiovascular physiology to neurophysiology, which remained the focus of his research for the rest of his life. Much of his work in this area was done in collaboration with his colleague at Washington University (later at the Rockefeller Institute), Herbert Gasser. Prior to 1920 very little was known about the electrophysiology of nerves because the electrical impulses they carry are so weak and short-lasting that no one had been able to measure them accurately. In 1920 Gasser devised an amplifier that magnified the impulses carried by nerves by about 100,000 times. With the strength problem solved, Erlanger and Gasser collaborated in 1921 to develop a device that could record the amplified impulse: the cathode-ray oscilloscope. Using this instrument, Erlanger and Gasser made many fundamental observations concerning the conduction of impulses through peripheral nerves. Their most important discovery was the finding that the velocity of impulse conduction is directly proportional to the diameter of the nerve fiber—that is, that large nerve fibers transmit impulses more rapidly than smaller ones. For this discovery they jointly received the Nobel Prize in Physiology or Medicine in 1944.

Erlanger continued to work following retirement age. During World War II he assumed a heavy teaching load in the department of physiology so that his younger colleagues could fulfill their military duties. For many years he also continued his researches in nerve physiology. In retirement he developed an interest in the history of medicine and wrote an elegant account of William Beaumont's pioneering nineteenth-century experiments in human digestion.

Throughout his career he was the recipient of numerous honors. He was a member of the National Academy of Sciences, the American Philosophical Society, the American Physiological Society (president, 1926–29), the Association of American Physicians, and several foreign societies. He was the recipient of honorary degrees from the universities of California, Wisconsin, Pennsylvania, Michigan, Johns Hopkins University, Washington University, and the Free University of Brussels.

Erlanger enjoyed a personal life as happy and fulfilling as his professional life. On June 21, 1906, he married Aimee Hirstel of San Francisco; they had three children and a strong marriage. Her ebullient, cheerful personality complemented Erlanger's more reserved, taciturn manner. Erlanger's outward reserve did not mask his sympathy and kindness, and he and his wife were a continual source of support for numerous American and foreign physiologists. He loved the outdoors, and his greatest recreational pleasure was mountain climbing.

Erlanger's contribution to science goes far beyond the specific discovery that earned him the Nobel Prize. More important, the cathode-ray oscilloscope that he and Gasser developed created the modern field of neurophysiology, serving as the central instrument of this new discipline. Equally important, Erlanger was part of that generation of American scientists that was wresting leadership of the scientific world away from Europe. Erlanger's teachers at Johns Hopkins had to go abroad for their scientific education, but Erlanger, except for his brief work-vacation in Europe in 1902, was trained entirely in the United States. Much of Erlanger's professional activity as a leader of American physiology was aimed at garnering increased support for scientific research and education in the United States. Erlanger will be remembered not only as one of the intellectual founders of modern neurophysiology but as an institution-builder in American science.

KENNETH M. LUDMERER

Selected Bibliography

PRIMARY SOURCES

Erlanger, Joseph, and Herbert Spencer Gasser, 1937. *Electrical Signs of Nervous Activity*. Philadelphia: University of Pennsylvania Press.

Erlanger, Joseph, 1964. "A Physiologist Reminisces." *Annual Review of Physiology* 26:1–4.

SECONDARY SOURCES

Davis, Hallowell, 1970. "Joseph Erlanger." *National Academy of Sciences Biographical Memoirs*. 41:111–39.

Monnier, A. M., 1971. "Erlanger, Joseph." *Dictionary of Scientific Biography*. Vol. 4:397–99. New York: Scribners.

Frank, Robert G., Jr., 1979. "The J. H. B. Archive Report: The Joseph Erlanger Collection at Washington University School of Medicine, St. Louis." *Journal of the History of Biology* 12: 193–201. In addition to the Erlanger Papers, a series of oral history interviews with Erlanger conducted by Estelle Brodman shortly before his death is deposited at Washington University.

ULF SVANTE VON EULER 1970

Ulf Svante von Euler was born on February 7, 1905, in Stockholm. A neurophysiologist, von Euler shared the Nobel Prize in 1970 with Julius Axelrod and Sir Bernard Katz for his important work on the role of hormones in the sympathetic nervous system, specifically for his identification and characterization of norepinephrine. At the time of the award, von Euler was professor and director of physiology at the Karolinska Institute, the position he held for most of his professional life. He retired soon after. Von Euler and his first wife, Jane Sodenstierna, whom he married in 1930, had two sons, Hans Leo and Johan Christopher, and two daughters, Ursula Katrina and Marie Jane. Both sons studied medicine: Leo von Euler is a scientist at the National Institutes of Health and his brother became an anesthesiologist in Stockholm. This first marriage ended in divorce in 1957. Von Euler married the Countess Dagmar Cronstedt the following year. Euler died on March 10, 1983, in Stockholm.

Von Euler came from a family of scientists. His father, Hans von Euler-Chelpin, was a biochemist and director of the Chemical Institute at the University of Stockholm. He shared the Nobel Prize for Chemistry in 1930 for his work on plant chemistry and sugar fermentation. Von Euler's mother, Astrid Cleve von Euler, was a prominent botanist and geologist. As a boy, he knew many of Sweden's scientific elite; his godfather, Svante Arrhenius, was a 1903 Nobel laureate in Chemistry. Young Ulf's parents were divorced in 1912; von Euler-Chelpin subsequently returned to Germany, his homeland.

Ulf showed some early interest in engineering but decided, in 1922, to study medicine at the Karolinska. He quickly became interested in physiology and pharmacology and spent some time working with Robin Fahraeus, a leading hematologist and rheologist. Under Fahraeus's tutelage, he carried out his first research investigation, a study of vasoconstriction in the blood of febrile patients, for which he won a prize in 1925.

In 1926 he began a period of four years as assistant to Goran Liljestrand in the Department of Pharmacology. Von Euler submitted his thesis and received his medical degree in 1930. He was asked to join the Karolinska as assistant professor of pharmacology but first accepted a Rockefeller Fellowship for a year's study with Henry H. Dale in London, Corneille Heymans in Ghent, I. de Burgh Daly in Birmingham, and G. Embden in Frankfurt (1930–31).

In Dale's laboratory von Euler worked with John Gaddum on a study of acetylcholine, recently identified as a chemical transmitter of autonomic nervous impulses. They isolated a substance in extracts from the intestines that appeared to have the expected action in stimulating muscular tissues but was not acetylcholine. This proved to be a new factor, a polypeptide, which they named Substance P.

After his return to Stockholm, von Euler continued his pursuit of biologically active substances. In 1935 he isolated some lipids in ram semen that were amazingly active; they appeared to stimulate both contractions and relaxation in smooth muscle and also to lower blood pressure. The technology was not then available to analyze and fully describe these substances, which von Euler named "prostaglandins" since they had been found in the prostrate gland. After World War II he would bring them to the attention of Sune Bergström, who pioneered the field of prostaglandin research.

Von Euler now became interested again in neural transmitters. In 1934 he studied biophysical methods with Archibald V. Hill in London, and returned to London again in 1938 to work on neuromuscular transmission with G. L. Brown. In his laboratory at the Karolinska, meanwhile, he studied extracts from neural and organ tissues to try to identify the chemical transmitter of the sympathetic nervous system.

The autonomic, or involuntary, nervous system, has two components, the parasympathetic, which controls normal activities such as digestion, and the sympathetic, which enables the body to respond to stress or unusual exertion. The concept of chemical neurotransmission had been developed in 1904 by T. R. Elliott, who noted the action of adrenalin, a hormone of the adrenal medulla, and its similarity to neural stimulation of the sympathetic nervous system. He hypothesized that the chemical was secreted under stress and carried from the nerves to the muscles to stimulate specific responses. In 1921 Otto Loewi had demonstrated that adrenaline acts as a neural transmitter in the sympathetic system of the frog. He had subsequently identified the carrier in the parasympathetic system as acetylcholine, which Dale also traced in the transmission of voluntary impulses. However, the identity of the sympathetic neurotransmitter in humans and mammals was still an open question in the 1930s (Von Euler 1970, 470–481).

Von Euler's tissue analyses revealed the presence of something *like* adrenaline but his analysis also showed some chemical differences. He guessed that it might be noradrenaline, a nonmethylated precursor homologue of adrenaline. (That is, a compound identical in basic structure but lacking some molecules and molecular bonds, which adrenaline has acquired by combination with the methyl radical. The formula for noradrenaline is $C_8H_{11}NO_3$; that for adrenaline is $C_9H_{13}NO_3$. In the United States, these compounds are generally called epinephrine and norepinephrine.) Von Euler confirmed his hunch by 1940, and by 1946 he and his assistants were able to publish a full description of the transmitter substance. In 1939 he had been promoted to full professor of physiology at the Karolinska. His research for the next thirty years was devoted to the neurotransmitters, or catecholamines.

Von Euler first concentrated on demonstrating the presence of noradrenaline in the organs and tissues of the body in describing its action in shock and other stressful conditions. This led to an interest in aviation medicine, in which he quickly became a world-renowned expert, acting as consultant to many national air forces (Von Euler 1970, 470; Udenfriend 1970, 423).

The methodology of the late forties and early fifties was inadequate for effective tracing of neurotransmitter activity in the body. Von Euler consequently used urinary excretion to measure the secretion and activity of the compounds. In 1946–47 he studied endocrinology and renal function in Bernardo Houssay's laboratory in Buenos Aires to assist him in this research. His finding was that noradrenaline in the urine could be used to gauge neural activity, while the presence of adrenaline reflected the secretory activity of the adrenal medulla. He and his students were able to confirm, with urinary analysis, the increased secretion of noradrenaline in response to various types of stress. They also demonstrated, in 1955, that stimulation of the nerve to the adrenal gland resulted in increased secretion, establishing a further link in the sympathetic neural mechanism (Von Euler 1970, 472–74; Udenfriend 1970, 423).

While secretion increased, hormonal levels in various organs remained the same, which indicated to von Euler that there must be storage areas within the nerves. His students Nils-Åke Hillarp and B. Falck had found a way in the late 1950s of visualizing transmitter substances by the use of fluoroscopic tracers. This technique aided von Euler, Hillarp, and others on the team in finding the subcellular particles rich in noradrenaline and "apparently loaded with transmitter all along the axon." Further studies during the 1960s defined the process of synthesis, storage, release, and resynthesis, "a rapid process . . . regulated with great precision" (Von Euler 1970, 472–74; Udenfriend 1970, 423).

Von Euler was a dedicated scientist who placed his research above everything else. When honored by a banquet at the Second Catecholamine Symposium in 1959, he elected to replace the usual humorous little speech with an illustrated lecture on his recent work. His staff nevertheless idolized him and he rarely neglected to recognize their contributions (Udenfriend 1970, 423; *New York Times* October 16, 1970).

Von Euler was a member of the Nobel Committee for Physiology or Medicine from 1953 to 1965, and became chairman of the board of the Nobel Foundation in 1965, a position "more of a handicap than an asset" for gaining a Nobel Prize (Udenfriend 1970, 422). From 1965 to 1971 he served as vice-president of the International Union of Physiological Sciences. He was a member of the Swedish Royal Academy of Science, the Swedish Endocrinological Society, the Royal Society of London, the American Philosophical Society, as well as scientific societies of Denmark, Italy, Germany, and Spain. Among the many honors he received for his work are the Carl

Ludwig Medal (1953), the Gairdner Foundation Award (1961), the Andres Jahre Prize (1965), and the Stouffer Prize from the American Sociological Association (1967). He was decorated with the Swedish Order of the North Star.

Von Euler retired in 1971 and died of arterial disease at age seventy-eight.

MARCIA MELDRUM

Selected Bibliography

PRIMARY SOURCES

Von Euler, Ulf S., and E. Braun-Menendez. 1947. "Hypertension after Bilateral Nephrectomy in the Rat." *Nature* 160:905.

Von Euler, Ulf S. 1956. *Noradrenaline: Chemistry, Physiology, Pharmacology, and Clinical Aspects*. Springfield, Illinois: Thomas.

———. 1968. *Prostaglandins*. New York: Academic Press.

———. 1970. "Adrenergic Neurotransmitter Functions." Nobel Lecture, December 12, 1970. Reprinted in *Nobel Lectures in Physiology or Medicine*, vol. 4 (1963–1970), 470–81. Amsterdam: Elsevier, 1972.

———. 1982. *Release and Uptake Functions in Adrenergic Nerve Granules*. Liverpool: Liverpool University Press.

SECONDARY SOURCES

1970. "The Three Recipients of the Nobel Prize: Ulf Svante von Euler." *New York Times* (October 16):27.

Schmeck, Harold M., Jr. 1970. "Award Honors Research in Brain and Nerve Cells." *New York Times* (October 16):27.

Udenfriend, Sidney. 1970. "Nobel Prize: Three Share 1970 Award for Medical Research. 1. Von Euler and Axelrod." *Science* 170 (October 16): 422–23.

1985. "Ulf Svante von Euler." *Biographical Memoirs of Fellows of the Royal Society* 31:143–70.

JOHANNES ANDREAS GRIB FIBIGER *1926*

Johannes Andreas Grib Fibiger was born on April 23, 1867, in Silkeborg, Denmark. A pathologist and bacteriologist, Fibiger was awarded the Nobel Prize in 1926 for his investigations of the environmental etiology of cancer, and specifically for his discovery of the carcinogenic parasite *Spiroptera*. Although his ideas proved correct in many respects, they failed to lead to the breakthrough in cancer research he visualized. Fibiger was professor of pathological anatomy at the University of Copenhagen when he received the award. He married Mathilde Fibiger in 1894; they had no children. He died less than two months after the formal presentation of the Nobel Prize, on January 30, 1928, in Copenhagen.

Fibiger's early interest in medicine was stimulated by the memory of his physician father, C. E. A. Fibiger, who died when he was still a young child; his mother, Elfride Muller, was a writer. He was attracted to the new field of bacteriology during his undergraduate and medical education at the University of Copenhagen, where he earned a bachelor's degree in 1883, and a M.D. in 1890. For a year, he undertook further hospital training and traveled to Germany, where he studied briefly with Robert Koch and Emil Behring. Upon his return to Copenhagen in 1891, he secured a university position as assistant in the cramped but distinguished laboratory of Carl Julius Salmonsen, a prominent Danish bacteriologist, and began studies of the diphtheria bacterium. He entered the Danish army reserve in 1894 but was able to complete a thesis on his diphtheria work and was awarded the Ph.D. in 1895. His dissertation was notable for its concern with the uncertain effects of serum treatment and its interest in nonvirulent bacteria.

Fibiger was assigned to the Blegdams Hospital for Infectious Diseases for his initial army service. In 1897 he spent a further six months in Germany at the pathological institute of Johannes Orth. He was then appointed prosector, or dissection assistant, at the Institute of Pathological Anatomy at the University of Copenhagen; he served simultaneously as principal of the army's Clinical Bacteriology Laboratory. In 1900 Fibiger was promoted to professor and head of the institute. He remained in the army reserve, becoming in 1905 consultant physician and director of the Central Laboratory of the Army Medical Corps.

Fibiger's research for most of this period had dealt with diphtheria but, after his appointment as professor, he began studies of tuberculosis. He was particularly interested in the relationship between human and bovine tuberculosis. In this respect, he followed prevailing scientific fashions in a shift from research on epidemic and infectious diseases to chronic degenerative pathology.

Like many others, he was interested in cancer but no animal model had been found for experimental investigation of this complex pathology. Cancerous tissue transplanted into healthy animals would continue to grow; in this sense, cancer could be experimentally "induced." But no method of a priori induction was known; that is, no bacteria or other agent introduced into a healthy animal was known to cause a tumor to develop where none had existed. The isolation of an undiscovered medium of infection depended on an effective animal model.

Fibiger's only publication on cancer prior to 1907 was a statistical discussion of cancer of the uterus, which led to a pioneering campaign for early diagnosis. In that year, however, his tuberculosis research unexpectedly opened a new investigatory path. Fibiger dissected three rats that had been injected with tubercle bacilli. He found in each a fairly advanced stomach tumor and, under the microscope, was able to identify traces of eggs and worms in the cancerous tissues. Abandoning tuberculosis for cancer, Fibiger set out on the track of this new tumor. He examined great numbers of rats but found no recurrence.

In 1878 the parasitologist Galeb had described a nematode (a minute worm) that infested both rats and cockroaches. Fibiger therefore sought rats that commonly ate cockroaches and found these at a Copenhagen sugar refinery. The rats did indeed prove to be infested, as were the roaches. He successfully isolated the parasitic nematode and was able to pass it repeatedly from an infested rat to a cockroach, via eggs in the rat's feces, and then to a healthy rat that was fed the roach. The latter rat first developed an epithelial hyperplasia in its stomach, accompanied by inflammation; if it continued to feed on the parasite-carrying roaches, tumors developed, eventually destroying the gastric wall. Fibiger succeeded in producing tumors in more than one hundred rats and, in some cases, metastasis. This was the first successful induction of a cancer in a healthy experimental animal.

With the aid of Hjalmar Ditlevson of the University Zoological Museum, Fibiger established that his nematode was not the same as Galeb's but was a new species not previously identified. He gave it the name *Spiroptera neoplastica.* He announced his discovery to the Royal Danish Academy of Science in 1913 (Fibiger 1927, 122–37).

Fibiger believed that his work confirmed the earlier hypothesis of Rudolf Virchow that cancers are caused by chronic irritation from a foreign body or external toxin. This finding challenged the work of early transplantation researchers, who attempted to identify and immunize against an infectious agent. Fibiger hoped that parasites would prove a major etiological clue but realized by the time of the Nobel award that their role in the production of cancer is relatively insignificant. His own *Spiroptera* have no connection to cancer in humans. While his results with the rats appeared entirely valid, they were difficult to reproduce. Later theorists have suggested that the tumors were in fact related to a virus present in the parasite, or to a dietary deficiency brought about by the infestation.

The larger implications of the idea of exogenic carcinogenesis were soon tested by researchers, including Alexis Carrel and two Japanese scientists, Yamagiwa and Ichikawa, who produced skin cancer on rabbits' ears by monthly applications of coal tar over a period of four years (1915–18). In 1919 the Japanese Tsutsui achieved the same result with mice. After World War I Fibiger was the first European scientist to attempt to replicate these results. Working with Fridtjof Bang and Paul Moller, he succeeded in producing skin cancer in mice but not in rats; however, several rats developed primary carcinoma of the lung. He concluded that "the development of a cancer following the same exogenous influence, and under the same conditions, does not always occur within the same period of time in all animals of the same species" and "occurs with varying frequency among animals of different, though closely-related, species. . . . there may very likely be special predispositions, but no common general predisposition to all forms of cancer, to cancer in all organs or to all carcinogenic influences."

Thus Fibiger theorized that both exogenous irritants and individual or species specific, that is, genetic, predispositions are factors in the etiology of cancer. In this idea he presaged modern ideas. Moreover, his work was the essential foundation for later experiments in cancer induction and in the understanding and prevention of occupational cancers. He laid to rest as well the lingering association of cancer with old age and degeneration; rather, his success in producing the disease in quite young animals suggested that the important factor was the nature of the carcinogen and the length of exposure (Fibiger 1927, 137–48).

Fibiger throughout his life readily accepted public and professional responsibilities. He served as first secretary and president of the Danish Medical Society, and as president of the Danish Cancer Commission; he assisted in the planning of medical facilities; he represented Denmark at the International Commission for Intellectual Cooperation with Other Countries and was elected president of Die Internationale Vereinigung fur Krebsforschung. He was a member of the Danish Royal Academy of Science and Literature, the Swedish Medical Association, the Danish Medical Association, and the Pasteur Society, and he held corresponding memberships in the professional organizations of France, Belgium, Austria, and the United States. He founded and coedited the journal *Acta Pathologica et Microbiologica Scandinavica*. In addition to the Nobel Prize, he was honored by the Nordhoff-Jung Cancer Prize (1927).

Ironically, Fibiger himself contracted cancer of the colon. Shortly after his illness was diagnosed, he was stricken by a massive heart attack with pulmonary infarction and died at age sixty.

PAUL WEINDLING
MARCIA MELDRUM

Selected Bibliography

PRIMARY SOURCES

Fibiger, Johannes. 1918–19. *Investigations on the Spiroptera Cancer*. Copenhagen: Host and Son.

———. 1919. "On *Spiroptera* Carcinomata and Their Relation to True Malignant Tumors; with Some Remarks on Cancer Age." *Journal of Cancer Research* 4:367–387.

Fibiger, Johannes, and Fridtjof Bang. 1921. *Experimental Production of Tar Cancer in White Mice*. Copenhagen: Host and Son.

Fibiger, Johannes. 1927. "Investigations on *Spiroptera carcinoma* and the Experimental Induction of Cancer." Nobel Lecture, December 12, 1927. Reprinted in *Nobel Lectures in Physiology or Medicine*, vol. 2 (1922–1941), 122–52. Amsterdam: Elsevier, 1965.

SECONDARY SOURCES

1932. "Johannes Fibiger." In *Biographisches Lexikon der hervorragenden Arzte der letzten funfzig Jahre*, edited by I. Fischer, 1:401–2. Vienna: Urban und Schwarzenberg.

Secher, K. 1947. *The Danish Cancer Researcher Johannes Fibiger*. Copenhagen: Nordisk Verlag; London: H. K. Lewis.

NIELS RYBERG FINSEN *1903*

Niels Ryberg Finsen was born in Thorshavn, in the Faeroe Islands, on December 15, 1860, the son of two natives of Iceland: Hannes Steingrim Finsen, a governor of the Faeroe Islands, and Johanne Fröman. In 1903 he received the third Nobel Prize to be awarded in physiology or medicine for his work on the treatment of diseases, particularly lupus vulgaris, by means of concentrated light radiation—known at the time as "Finsen Light Therapy." He married Ingeborg Balslev in 1892. They had four children, but the eldest died the day after he was born. Finsen died on September 24, 1904, in Copenhagen.

Finsen had a rocky childhood, suffering from jaundice, pneumonia, measles, and a poorly defined renal disorder. He spent much of his early life in Iceland, and after being dismissed from a Danish prep school for "small ability and total lack of energy," from 1876 received his schooling in Reykjavík. In 1882 Finsen moved to Copenhagen, and in 1890 he received his medical degree from the University of Copenhagen. He held a position there briefly, as a demonstrator in anatomy in the surgical division, but soon left to pursue his interests in the effects of light on living organisms, supporting himself by private tutoring of medical students. In 1896 Finsen established the first Light Institute, at Copenhagen. The institute was supported first by private funds and later by the government; when Finsen received the Nobel Prize he donated half of the prize to his Institute. In 1898 Finsen became a professor, and in 1904 he received the Cameron Prize from the University of Edinburgh.

Finsen suffered from ill health for most of his adult life. Starting at the age of twenty-three he noted a fullness after meals. In the following years his health progressively failed, and after age thirty the accumulation of generalized fluid left him an invalid. He attempted to treat himself with salt restriction, but for most of his life was confined to a wheelchair. His illness prevented Finsen from appearing for the presentation of the Nobel Prize. At the age of forty-four Finsen succumbed to what was found to be constrictive pericarditis, a disease that had prevented his heart from functioning effectively. Despite his problems with health, Finsen managed to pursue a vigorous intellectual career until the end of his short life.

Finsen's interest in the effects of light may have derived in part from his youth in Iceland, where lighting conditions are quite different from those in countries found further to the south, and from his personal experiences of the effects that light had upon his disease. Finsen noted that light gave him much relief, though he could find no clear physiological reason why this should be so. Finsen decided that he must be right, and contemporary understanding of physiology wrong, and he set out to study the effect of light on living things. He did so first by collecting observations on animals seeking the sun, then by conducting clinical experiments. He later recalled that "All that I have accomplished in my experiments with light and all that I have learned about its therapeutic value has come because I *needed* the light so much myself. I longed for it" (Moffett 1903).

Finsen's first work on the biological effects of light came in 1893. He noted that earthworms placed in a box covered with blue and red glass on either end would always move towards the end covered with red glass. He also read of soldiers who in 1832 had contracted smallpox but, confined in dark dungeons, had recovered without scarring. Finsen, who at that time had never seen a case of smallpox himself, surmised that patients suffered less scarring from smallpox when exposed to red light. He believed that red light was inherently less harmful, while other kinds of light damaged the skin, particularly light from the opposite end of the spectrum, blue and ultraviolet—or so-called chemical—rays. Finsen thought that to prevent scarring from smallpox one should filter out the ultraviolet rays with red glass or red curtains. The first trials of this treatment were carried out in Norway in August 1893; of eight patients with smallpox, none formed scars. On subsequent investigation, even small amounts of regular light were found to cause scarring, and physicians went to great lengths to make sure that only red light entered the room of a patient with smallpox.

Finsen next considered the possibility that light in some forms might have a curative element. He drew his ideas in part from his own experiences and in part from the widespread interest in bacteriology in the late-nineteenth century. Others had shown that bacteria could be killed by light. In 1895 Finsen applied light therapy to lupus vulgaris a particularly intractable form of tuberculosis of the skin that often left patients horribly disfigured and the objects of repulsion. Finsen used either sunlight or a carbon arc for the source of light, thus drawing upon a recent invention, the electric light. He filtered the light through a prism, and by applying pressure to the skin with a double layer of crystal he was able to allow the light to penetrate the skin. Cold water circulated between the layers of crystal to reduce the heat to which the patient's skin would be exposed. Finsen could thus expose the patient's skin to high concentrations of ultraviolet rays. Although the area was at first red and mildly inflamed, after a few days any skin lesions would be replaced by normal skin.

Finsen's first patient was a Dutch engineer who had suffered for eight years from a tuberculous ulcer on his face. From November 1895 through March 1896 Finsen treated the ulcer two hours each day with light therapy. The treatment was a dramatic success; the results brought Finsen widespread acclaim. The queen of England and the empress of Russia visited his new Light Institute; soon, Russia and England each had their own center for light therapy. Light therapy spread throughout the Western world, and most major hospitals developed some form of a light therapy unit by the turn of the century. In 1903, when Finsen received the Nobel Prize, some 50 percent of eight hundred cases treated at his institute were reported to be cured, a fact for which, in the words of the Nobel Prize presentation, Finsen deserved the "eternal gratitude of suffering humanity."

Finsen loved the sun. He said "Let it break through suddenly on a cloudy day, and see the change! Insects that were drowsy wake up and take wing; lizards and snakes come out to sun themselves; the birds burst into song" (Riis 1903). He was dedicated to his work, so much so that he chose to share freely the fruits of his insight, rather than going into private practice, a decision that earned him the praise and admiration not only of his countrymen, but of people throughout the world.

Despite his Nobel Prize, today Neils Ryberg Finsen and his work remain little known. Perhaps this is because his method of treatment was widely doubted, even in his own time, and is no longer held to be of much value. Perhaps this is because the use of light therapy was soon eclipsed in the public mind by a much more symbolically powerful use of electricity to produce another kind of ray, the X-ray. Nonetheless, Finsen deserves the attention of historians for the way in which his work brought together bacteriology and electricity. Ultraviolet light is now used to sterilize objects, and the importance of sunlight for health has been confirmed by studies of vitamin D. Finsen's work with light therapy also presaged the use of X-rays for therapy and more recent forms of light therapy, such as PUVA for psoriasis.

JOEL D. HOWELL

Selected Bibliography

PRIMARY SOURCES

Finsen, Neils R. 1895. "The Red Light Treatment of Smallpox." *British Medical Journal* 2:1412–14.

———. 1901. *Phototherapy*. Translated by James H. Sequeira. London: Edward Arnold.

———. 1903. "The Red Light Treatment of Smallpox." *Journal of the American Medical Association* 41:1207–08.

———. 1903. Biography. In *Nobel Lectures: Physiology or Medicine*, vol. 1 (1901–21), 123–31. Amsterdam: Elsevier, 1967.

SECONDARY SOURCES

Moffett, Cleveland. 1903. "Dr. Finsen and the Story of His Achievement." *McClure's Magazine* 20:361–68.

Riis, Jacob A. 1903. "The Surgery of Light." *McClure's Magazine* 20: 360–61.

Masters, David. 1925. *The Conquest of Disease*. London: John Lane.

DeKruif, Paul. 1932. "Finsen: The Light Hunter." In *Men Against Death*, 283–99. New York: Harcourt Brace and Company.

Roesler, Hugo. 1936. "Niels Ryberg Finsen's Disease and His Self-Instituted Treatment." *Annals of Medical History*, 353–56.

Triolo, Victor A. 1971. "Finsen, Niels Ryberg." In *Dictionary of Scientific Biography*, edited by Charles Coulston Gillispie, 4:620–21. New York: Charles Scribner's Sons.

Brodthagen, Holger. 1979. "Stamps Commemorating Medicine. 'Neils Finsen': Physician, Photobiologist, Nobel Laureate." *Journal of Dermatology and Surgical Oncology* 5:649.

SIR ALEXANDER FLEMING *1945*

Sir Alexander Fleming was born on August 6, 1881, in Lochfield, Ayrshire, Scotland. A bacteriologist, Fleming shared the Nobel Prize in 1945 with Ernst Chain and Howard Florey for his discovery of the antimicrobial effects of the *Penicillium* mold, which led to Chain and Florey's isolation and development of the highly effective antibiotic penicillin. At the time of the award, Fleming was professor of bacteriology at St. Mary's Hospital Medical School, the University of London, the institution with which he was associated throughout his career. He married Sarah Marion McElroy, an Irish nurse, in 1915; their only son, Robert, became a general practitioner. The first Lady Fleming died in 1949; four years later Fleming married his colleague, Dr. Amalia Coutsouris-Voureka, a bacteriologist from Greece. Fleming died on March 11, 1955, in London.

Alexander was the son of Hugh Fleming, a Scottish farmer, who died when the boy was seven, leaving his widow, Grace, with eight children. After a basic education in country schools, at age thirteen he joined three of his brothers in London. He enrolled at the Regent Street Polytechnic but left school in 1896 for economic reasons. Young Fleming worked for a shipping company until 1900, when he joined the London Scottish Volunteers during the Boer War. The war, however, ended before he was sent to Africa. Shortly thereafter he received a small legacy that enabled him to study medicine.

Fleming's academic career at St. Mary's Hospital School was highly successful, culminating in the baccalaureates in science and medicine with honors, the Gold Medal, and the Cheadle Medal in 1908. He had passed his qualifying examinations in 1906 and been appointed to St. Mary's Pathology Department where he worked under Sir Almroth Wright, a pioneer in vaccine therapy. Although Fleming's low-key manner and his senior's flamboyance were an odd match, they established a working relationship that would last until Wright's retirement in 1946. Wright obtained samples of Salvarsan from Paul Ehrlich, and Fleming carried out some of the early tests on the "magic bullet." In 1909 Fleming qualified as a Fellow of the Royal College of Surgeons.

He saw private patients for some years before 1914. During World War I he served in the Royal Army Medical Corps, working in a Boulogne laboratory under Wright and achieving the rank of captain. His research showed that the chemical antiseptics commonly in use actually deepened rather than retarded serious infection. He and Wright recommended the use of a saline solution to cleanse wounds. Returning to St. Mary's at war's end, Fleming demonstrated that antiseptics injected into the blood attacked white blood cells as well as bacteria. These findings supported the contention of Wright that enhancement of natural immunity with vaccines was superior to chemotherapy or Listerian methods (Fleming 1915, 638–43; 1919, 99–129; Dolman 1972, 29).

In 1921 Fleming was named assistant director of the Inoculation Department at St. Mary's. In that year he made his first identification of a true bacteriolytic substance. He had developed a cold and made a culture of his own nasal mucus. Common airborne bacteria settled on the plate and the mucus attacked and dissolved (lysed) these organisms. Fleming named his discovery lysozyme and the bacterial victim *Micrococcus lysodeikticus*. He and his colleague V. D. Allison found that many animal and plant tissues, including milk, egg white, human tears, saliva, and blood serum, were sources of lysozyme. They concluded that the substance contributed to the natural immunity of the organisms; human fluids therefore had some bacteriolytic properties. In these studies Fleming developed methods of sensitivity titration and assay that he was to use repeatedly to detect substances in fluids.

Fleming and Allison were able to raise the lytic level in rabbits without apparent damage to their immunity responses, but they could not purify the active agent sufficiently for use in humans. Moreover, in its compound state, lysozyme acted on innocuous bacteria more effectively than on known disease agents. The ensuing work on lysozyme was carried on at Oxford. Today it is used primarily in research (Fleming 1922, 306–17; Fleming and Allison 1927, 214–18; Dolman 1972, 29–30).

In 1928 Fleming, now professor of bacteriology, found another contaminated culture plate. A *Penicillium notatum* mold was growing on the plate; around it, staphyloccus colonies were becoming transparent and dissolving almost before his eyes. He made a filtered broth of the mold and found that even a diluted preparation lysed many pathogens, including the staphylococci, streptococci, and pneumococci, and the diphtheria group. Moreover, it caused no toxic effects on experimental animals and no interference with white blood cell formation. However, it was ineffective against a number of bacteria, including the coli-typhoid agents and the enteroсci. Fleming's paper announcing his findings is a classic, clear and comprehensive, with incisive observations. He limited his conclusion, however, to the suggestion that his bacteriocide, which he had named *Penicillin*, "appears to have some advantages" over the standard antiseptics in localized, nonsystemic treatment (Fleming 1929, 226–36).

Fleming's failure to proceed further has been attributed to his chief's theoretical stance, for Almroth Wright was opposed to the idea of systemic chemotherapy on principle. Probably a more important hindrance to Fleming's development of his discovery was his inability to isolate the active agent. In its broth form, penicillin was unreliable and too risky for parenteral injection, and Fleming was no chemist. During the 1930s he did his best to find colleagues willing to work on purification. Harold Raistrick, a brilliant British biochemist, dissolved penicillin in ether, but it disappeared during evaporation. Other attempts also failed. The amazing broth was for a decade used only in Fleming's laboratory to isolate bacteria in culture and to purify the vaccines produced in the Inoculation Department. He turned to other antibacterial research, investigating the sulfonamides after their 1935 introduction (Dolman 1972, 30).

Nevertheless, he remained confident of penicillin's potential and was delighted when Florey and Chain announced their success in 1940. Working at the Dunn School of Pathology at Oxford, they had purified the antibacterial agent and used it to treat twenty-five of fifty mice infected with streptococci. The twenty-five untreated mice died, as did one of the penicillin-treated animals. But twenty-four of the latter survived. The Oxford team went on to treat and publish the results of over a thousand cases.

The Florey-Chain paper caused great interest, to no one more than to Fleming. He made a trip to Oxford in 1942 and obtained a small sample to treat a family friend who had meningitis. His use of an intrathecal injection (into the membrane surrounding the spinal cord) in this case was a clinical advance (Fleming 1943, 434–438). His success with this case converted Wright, who wrote an influential letter to the *London Times*, calling attention to Fleming's original discovery of the new antibiotic. The letter launched the "Fleming Myth," as the press and public, longing for good news in the grim war years, seized happily on the romantic story of the moldy culture plate. At first startled and shy at the adulation, Fleming soon began to enjoy it, while Florey, rejecting press interruptions, found himself almost ignored.

In his case description Fleming had emphasized the scarcity of the drug. Florey, however, had gone to the United States seeking assistance to begin mass production. Urgent wartime needs gave the problem priority. By war's end penicillin was being synthesized in quantity for Allied troops. Although it was less available to civilians, the public was already well aware of its life-saving powers. Alexander Fleming became a hero.

Honors came in rapid succession. He was elected a fellow of the Royal Society in 1943, knighted by King George VI in 1944, and elected president of the new Society for General Microbiology in 1945. Among the many other honors he received were the John Scott Medal of the City Guild of Philadelphia (1944); the Cameron Prize from the University of Edinburgh (1945); the Moxon Medal of the Royal College of Physicians (1945); the Albert Gold Medal from the Royal Society of Arts (1946); the Medal for Merit from the United States (1947); and the Louis Pasteur Prize (1947). He was made an honorary member of nearly every scientific society in the world and awarded more than twenty honorary doctorates.

The Inoculation Department, which had been merged with the University of London Institute of Pathology and Research, was renamed the Wright-Fleming Institute in 1948. Fleming had succeeded Wright as principal in 1946, and therefore became its first head under its new name.

He spent most of the postwar years on lecture tours, "travelling all over the world, making modest little speeches implying that there had been a great element of luck in his discovery," and making many friends with his laconic good humor and lack of pretension. A shrewd, observant, hard-working man, Fleming conducted his research with care and persistence; he was a very good scientist but it is unlikely that he would have become a great one if not for that "element of luck." Outside of his laboratory, his main interests included gardening, antiques, and snooker. He and his first wife were noted for their hospitality at their house in Suffolk. A sportsman all his life, he excelled as a young man at rifle shooting and water polo, in his later days at golf (Dolman 1972, 29–30; Hare 1983, 347–72).

Sir Alexander became professor emeritus in 1948, but remained principal of the Wright-Fleming Institute until 1955. Shortly after his retirement from that position, he died quietly from coronary thrombosis at his London home.

LESLIE FALK
MARCIA MELDRUM

Selected Bibliography

A complete bibliography of Fleming's publications is in Gladys H. Hobby, *Penicillin: Meeting the Challenge* (New Haven: Yale University Press, 1985).

The Fleming Papers are on deposit in the British Library in London.

PRIMARY SOURCES

Fleming, Alexander. 1915. "On the Bacteriology of Septic Wounds." *Lancet* 2:638–43.

———. 1919. "The Action of Chemical and Physiological Antiseptics in a Septic Wound." *British Journal of Surgery* 7:99–129.

———. 1922. "On a Remarkable Bacteriolytic Element Found in Tissues and Secretions." *Proceedings of the Royal Society* 93B:306–17.

Fleming, A., and V. D. Allison. 1927. "Development of Lyzosome." *British Journal of Experimental Pathology* 8:214–18.

Fleming, Alexander. 1929. "On the Antibacterial Action of Cultures of a Penicillium, with Special Reference to Their Use in the Isolation of *B. influenzae*." *British Journal of Experimental Pathology* 10:226–36.

———. 1943. "Streptococcal Meningitis Treated with Penicillin." *Lancet* 2:434–38.

SECONDARY SOURCES

Dolman, Claude E. 1972. "Fleming, Alexander." In *Dictionary of Scientific Biography*, 1:28–31. New York: Scribners.

Hare, Ronald. 1983. "The Scientific Activities of Alexander Fleming, Other than the Discovery of Penicillin." *Medical History* 27:347–72.

Maurois, André. 1959. *The Life of Sir Alexander Fleming, Discoverer of Penicillin.* New York: Dutton.

Malkin, John. 1981. *Sir Alexander Fleming, Man of Penicillin.* Ayrshire, Scotland: Alloway Publishing.

Macfarlane, Gwyn. 1984. *Alexander Fleming: The Man and the Myth.* Cambridge: Harvard University Press.

HOWARD WALTER FLOREY
1945

More than any other individual Howard Walter Florey was responsible for giving penicillin to the world. Florey directed the team of investigators who, in 1940 at Oxford University, achieved the first isolation of penicillin in relatively concentrated form, and demonstrated its previously unknown power to combat infectious microorganisms within the living body. He thereby launched a profound revolution in the treatment of infectious diseases that changed every aspect of medicine and surgery.

Howard Walter Florey was born at Adelaide, Australia, on September 24, 1898, the youngest child and first son of a successful boot manufacturer, Joseph Florey, and his wife, Bertha (née Wadham). He was educated first at private schools in Adelaide and in 1911 entered St. Peter's Collegiate School, a school similar to an English public school. In March 1916 Howard Florey entered the University of Adelaide Medical School; he completed the medical course in December 1921. The previous year he had been awarded a Rhodes scholarship for study at Oxford University, and, as soon as his medical examinations were completed, he sailed for England. In January 1922 Howard Florey entered Magdalen College, where he pursued the honors course in physiology. At Oxford he was influenced deeply by Sir Charles Sherrington, who had laid the foundation of modern neurophysiology, and he became friends with a fellow physiology student and Rhodes scholar from America, John Fulton. In 1923 he took first class honors in the physiology examination and Sherrington appointed him a demonstrator in physiology. The following year Florey was appointed to the John Lucas Walker Studentship in Pathology at Cambridge University where he carried out research on inflammation. Florey spent the year 1925 in the United States working at the University of Pennsylvania with the physiologist Alfred Newton Richards. On his return to England in 1926 Florey was appointed to the Freedom Research Fellowship in Pathology at the London Hospital. On October 19, 1926, he married a fellow Australian, Mary Ethel Hayter Reed, whom he had met while a medical student at Adelaide. He began to publish his research on the contractility of capillaries, on inflammation, and on lymph flow. In 1927 he was appointed Huddersfield Lecturer in Special Pathology at Cambridge where the professor, H. R. Dean, was encouraging the development of experimental pathology. On his return to Cambridge Florey was also elected a fellow of Gonville and Caius College.

Among various lines of experimental research, Florey worked on the secretion of mucus in the alimentary canal, and especially in the colon. In 1929 he began to study lysozyme, the antibacterial component of tears, nasal secretions, saliva, and egg albumen, discovered by Alexander Fleming in 1922. Although Fleming had developed a test for the presence of lysozyme in fluids and tissues, he had not isolated the substance nor established its chemical identity. Florey, with Neil Goldsworthy, developed a technique for measuring lysozyme activity and with it found that the production of lysozyme varied so greatly among different animal species that it could not be an important component of natural immunity to bacterial infection. In the course of their lysozyme work, Goldsworthy and Florey observed the inhibition of the growth of one bacterium by another, in the same way that lysozyme inhibited the growth of bacteria (Goldsworthy and Florey 1930; Florey 1930).

In 1929 Alexander Fleming published his observation of the remarkable power of a penicillium mold to inhibit the growth and kill cultures of pathogenic staphylococci. Fleming showed that some substance secreted by the mold could inhibit the growth of a wide range of pathogenic organisms, including streptococci, staphylococci, pneumococci, meningococci, and gonococci. Most remarkable was that the crude mold juice would inhibit pathogenic organisms even in dilutions up to 1 in 800, yet did not injure living leucocytes. When Fleming injected the mold juice, which he called *penicillin*, into a rabbit and a mouse, it proved no more toxic than the broth used as a culture medium for the mold (Fleming 1929). Fleming did not test the ability of penicillin to protect mice from lethal doses of streptococci or pneumococci. In 1932 P. W. Clutterbuck, working in Harold Raistrick's laboratory at the London School of Hygiene and Tropical Medicine, attempted to purify penicillin, but failed. Clutterbuck managed to extract penicillin into acidified ether but could find no way to remove the ether without destroying the penicillin (Clutterbuck 1932).

In March 1932 Florey moved from Cambridge to the University of Sheffield as professor of pathology. At Sheffield he continued his research on mucus secretion and the antibacterial properties of intestinal mucus. With Dr. Beatrice Pullinger, Florey also began research on the lymphocyte.

In 1935 Florey was appointed professor of pathology at Oxford University, where he was director of the large, new Sir William Dunn School of Pathology. Pullinger and Florey's technical assistant, James Kent, who had been with him since his Cambridge days, accompanied Florey to Oxford. Since the extension of his research on lysozyme would require the collaboration of a biochemist, Florey appointed to his department the young biochemist Ernst Boris Chain, a refugee from Nazi Germany, who had just completed his Ph.D. degree under Sir Frederick Gowland Hopkins at Cambridge. Chain had been working to isolate the active principle in snake venoms, research that posed problems similar to those involved in the isolation of the active principle of lysozyme. Florey's first research student at Oxford was Peter B. Medawar. The following year (1936) Dr. Margaret Jennings joined Florey's department to assist with research on mucus secretion.

At Oxford, Florey and Pullinger continued their research on lymphocytes, concentrating on the factors that influenced the production of lymphocytes in the lymph nodes. In 1936, in order to receive support from cancer research funds, Chain began to study the differences between the enzymes of normal tissues and those of malignant growths. Norman G. Heatley, who like Chain had taken his Ph.D. in biochemistry under Hopkins at Cambridge, was appointed to assist Chain in the cancer enzyme research. A year later E. P. Abraham, using material provided by Florey, was able to isolate lysozyme as a pure crystalline substance. Florey's sustained study of lysozyme reflected his deep interest in the discovery of antibacterial substances for potential clinical use. The introduction of sulfonamides in 1935, which proved clinically effective against streptococcal infections, intensified Florey's interest in antibacterial substances. During 1937 Chain and Edward Duthie described a substance secreted by pathogenic streptococci and the gas-gangrene bacillus called "spreading factor" that liquefied mucus. They ultimately found the spreading factor was an enzyme that attacked hyaluronic acid, and accordingly named it hyaluronidase. During 1938–39 Chain and Leslie A. Epstein showed that lysozyme was, as Fleming had assumed originally, an enzyme that dissolved polysaccharides. They next sought to identify the polysaccharide in the bacterial cell wall that was susceptible to lysozyme, which they found to be N-acetyl glucosamine.

As Chain's research on lysozyme proceeded, he and Florey had many discussions about the desirability of a systematic study of known antibacterial substances, and Florey referred Chain to the 1928 monograph by Papagostas and Gaté that contained a sixty-page chapter on antagonistic interactions between microorganisms entitled "Antibiosis" (Papacostas and Gaté 1928). Chain collected about two hundred references on the inhibition of the growth of one microorganism by another. Early in 1938 he came across Fleming's 1929 paper on penicillin and was immediately interested by its remarkable power to inhibit the growth of a staphylococcus upon which lysozyme exerted no effect. Chain assumed that the active principle in penicillin would be an enzyme, like lysozyme, which he could readily isolate and purify, and he was eager to do so. He believed also that the pathogenic bacteria, whose growth was inhibited by penicillin, contained in their cell walls a common substrate dissolved by the supposed enzyme, penicillin. Chain was to isolate and study the chemical properties of the enzyme, while Florey would determine its biological properties.

When they began work on penicillin in 1938, Florey and Chain thought penicillin too unstable to have potential clinical value. Using a culture of Fleming's strain of *Penicillium notatum* from the culture collection at Oxford, Chain began work. Initially he was unable to reproduce Fleming's original observations of bacterial lysis. He found that penicillin was not a protein, a fact that showed also that it was not an enzyme. His problem then became to determine the chemical nature of an extremely unstable antibacterial substance of low molecular weight. He found that penicillin was relatively stable in solution between pH 5 and 8, and that he could slow down its inactivation further by working at low temperatures. By November 1938, for reasons that remain obscure, penicillin seemed a sufficiently promising substance that Howard Florey decided to throw the resources of his department into the effort to isolate and study it. In September 1939, three days after the outbreak of war, Florey applied to Edward Mellanby at the Medical Research Council for funds to support research on penicillin because its pronounced antibacterial properties, especially against staphylococci, and its lack of toxicity suggested that penicillin might possibly be of great practical importance. In response Mellanby provided twenty-five pounds sterling to launch research on penicillin, and a three-year grant to support Chain. Early in 1940, however, the Rockefeller Foundation provided a five-year grant to support Florey's proposed penicillin research.

To study penicillin the Oxford group needed a means to detect its presence, and Dr. Norman Heatley, who had joined the project in October 1939, developed the "cylinder-plate" assay. Heatley also found that penicillin could be back-extracted out of acidified ether into slightly alkaline water, thereby overcoming the obstacle that had blocked Clutterbuck's earlier attempt to isolate penicillin. After overcoming many such difficulties, and by using freeze-drying techniques, by March 1940 Chain had obtained about 100 milligrams of penicillin concentrate in the form of a brown powder. The concentrated penicillin proved harmless when injected into mice and when tested on living leucocytes in blood, but was powerful in preventing the growth of a wide range of pathogenic microorganisms. On May 25, 1940, Florey injected lethal doses of streptococci into eight mice. Keeping four mice as controls, he injected penicillin into the other four mice. The next day all the control mice were dead, whereas three of the mice treated with penicillin were perfectly well. One mouse that received a smaller dose of penicillin was ill and died two days later. The experiment demonstrated very clearly that penicillin could combat otherwise lethal infections in living animals, and Florey proceeded to further experiments, which confirmed fully the first (Chain et al. 1940). Florey and his group then began a determined effort to produce enough penicillin for a clinical trial on human beings. By February 1941 Florey had sufficient penicillin for his first clinical trials on patients suffering from staphylococcal infections. The results were striking, but the treatment was necessarily restricted by the limited supply of penicillin (Abraham et al. 1941).

Wartime Britain lacked sufficient resources to develop large-scale production of penicillin, yet Florey saw clearly that penicillin would be immensely valuable for the treatment of soldiers wounded in battle. In June 1941 Florey and Heatley flew to the United States where Florey was able to persuade the United States Department of Agriculture Research Laboratories at Peoria, Illinois, to undertake penicillin production with Heatley's help. Later Heatley also assisted the pharmaceutical firm Merck and Company in designing large-scale production methods for penicillin. With the entry of the United States into the war in December 1941, penicillin production became a national priority. After Florey's return to Oxford in September 1941, he organized more extensive production of penicillin at the Dunn School of Pathology and during the next few months he and Ethel Florey conducted further clinical trials with more adequate supplies of penicillin. By March 1943 the results demonstrated that penicillin was astonishingly potent against a wide range of bacterial infections (Florey and Florey 1943). During the next two years penicillin proved invaluable in the treatment of soldiers wounded in the battles of World War II.

In 1942 Howard Florey was elected a Fellow of the Royal Society. Priority in the discovery of penicillin became a sensitive issue between Florey and Fleming and has remained controversial. In 1944 Florey was knighted and the following year Fleming, Chain, and Florey shared the Nobel Prize in Physiology or Medicine for the discovery of penicillin. In 1960 Florey was elected president of the Royal Society and in 1962 resigned his professorship to become provost of Queen's College, Oxford. In 1965 he was elevated to the House of Lords as Baron Florey of Adelaide and Marston. Following the death of Lady Florey in October 1966, Florey married Dr. Margaret Jennings in June 1967. On February 21, 1968, Florey died at Oxford.

LEONARD G. WILSON

Selected Bibliography

PRIMARY SOURCES

Papacostas, G., and J. Gate, 1928. *Les associations microbiennes*. Paris: Doin et Cie.

Fleming, Alexander, 1929. "On the Antibacterial Action of Cultures of a Penicillium with Special Reference to Their Use in the Isolation of *B. influenzae*." *British Journal of Experimental Pathology* 10:226–36.

Goldsworthy, Neil E., and Howard Florey, 1930. "Some Properties of Mucus with Special Reference to Its Antibacterial Functions." *British Journal of Experimental Pathology* 11:192–208.

Florey, Howard, 1930. "The Relative Amounts of Lysozyme Present in the Tissues of Some Mammals." *British Journal of Experimental Pathology* 11:251–61.

Clutterbuck, Percival Walter, Reginald Lovell, and Harold Raistrick, 1932. "CCXXVII. Studies in the Biochemistry of Microorganisms. XXVI. The Formation from Glucose by Members of the *Penicillium chrysogenum* Series of a Pigment, an Alkali-Soluble Protein, and Penicillin—the Antibacterial Substance of Fleming." *Biochemical Journal* 26:1907–18.

Chain, E. B., H. W. Florey, A. D. Gardner, N. G. Heatley, M. A. Jennings, J. Orr-Ewing, and A. G. Sanders, 1940. "Penicillin as a Chemotherapeutic Agent." *Lancet* (*London*) ii:226–28.

Abraham, E. P., E. Chain, C. M. Fletcher, A. D. Gardner, N. G. Heatley, and M. A. Jennings, 1941. "Further Observations on Penicillin." *Lancet* (*London*) ii:177–189.

Florey, M. E., and H. W. Florey, 1943. "General and Local Administration of Penicillin." *Lancet* (*London*) i:387–97.

SECONDARY SOURCES
Bickel, Lennard, 1972. *Rise Up to Life: A Biography of Howard Walter Florey who Gave Penicillin to the World.* London: Angus and Robertson.
Chain, Ernest, 1972. "Thirty Years of Penicillin Therapy." *Journal of the Royal College of Physicians of London* 6:103–31.
MacFarlane, Gwyn, 1979. *Howard Florey: the Making of a Great Scientist.* Oxford: Oxford University Press.

WERNER THEODOR OTTO FORSSMANN *1956*

Werner Theodor Otto Forssmann was born in Berlin on August 29, 1904. He was the son of Julius Forssmann, who worked for a life insurance company and who died in World War I, and Emmy Hindenberg. Werner Forssmann received the Nobel Prize for Physiology or Medicine in 1956 in honor of his contributions to knowledge about heart catheterization and pathological changes in the circulatory system, a prize he shared with Dickinson Woodruff Richards, Jr. and André Frédéric Cournand. Forssman married Elsbet Engel in 1933; the couple had six children. Forssmann died on June 1, 1979, in Schopfheim, West Germany.

Forssmann received his primary education at the Askanisches Gymnasium in Berlin, a school that emphasized a classical education. In 1922 he enrolled as a medical student at the Friedrich Wilhelm University of Berlin; he graduated in 1929. Forssmann had hoped to go on to study internal medicine, but this dream was shattered when a position originally promised to him was awarded instead to a gentleman from Moscow. Paid training positions were difficult to find, and Forssmann considered himself lucky when he was able to locate a post at a women's hospital in Spandau. After three months there, he found a better position at the August Victoria Home, a Hospital in the small town of Eberswalde, near Berlin. There, Forssmann did the experiment that was to win for him the Nobel Prize some twenty-seven years later: he inserted a catheter into a vein of his arm, passed the catheter through the vein into his heart, and walked to the X-ray department, where he had a film taken. He spent the next two years attempting, with little success, to use the cardiac catheter to produce images of the heart. After enduring severe criticism for his pioneering study, Forssmann gave up experimental medicine.

Forssmann next worked at the Charité Hospital, Berlin, and at the City Hospital in Mainz. He received special training in urology at the Rudolph Virchow Hospital in Berlin, and was named chief of the Surgical Clinic of the City Hospital at Dresden-Friedrichstadt and at the Robert Koch Hospital in Berlin. During World War II Forssmann served as an army surgeon, spending six brutal years in Germany, Norway, and Russia before he became a prisoner of war. He returned home "weary, embittered, and half-starved" (Forssmann 1974, 257).

After the war Forssmann spent some years as a country doctor in Schwarzwald, and in 1950 he returned to the practice of urology in Bad Kreuznach. There he was living quietly, with no public attention, until the 1956 Nobel Prize was awarded. The sudden change in his life made Forssmann feel as though he were "a village pastor who was suddenly informed he had been made a cardinal" (*New York Times* October 19, 1956). Forssmann was awarded the prize for work on the heart, yet he was a practicing urologist, and had done almost no work on heart disease for almost twenty-seven years. The temptation to return to cardiology must have been great, but Forssmann realized that he probably would be unable to catch up with the advances in cardiology, and he decided to content himself with the role of "leading fossil" (Forssmann 1974, 284). He took a position as chief of the Surgical Department at Evangelical Hospital, in Düsseldorf.

Forssmann received the Nobel Prize for his experiment in the spring of 1929, a spectacular self-experiment performed in the most unlikely setting of a small country hospital. The idea for this experiment came to Forssmann because he had been fascinated by diagrams illustrating the work of the nineteenth-century French physiologists Bernard, Chauveau, and Marey. Forssmann was particularly intrigued by a diagram showing an experiment in which Marey had inserted a tube into the heart of a horse and then attached the tube to a mechanism for recording the pressure within the heart. Forssmann became convinced that the same procedure could safely be performed on human beings. He wanted to perform the experiment on himself by passing a urethral catheter from the main vein in his arm up into his own heart, hoping that the procedure could provide a new, more effective means for delivering medication. Forssmann took this idea to his supervisor at Eberswalde, who refused permission in no uncertain terms.

Forsmann decided to go ahead with the experiment anyway. To do so, he needed the cooperation of the surgical nurse, who controlled access to the necessary instruments. Over several weeks, Forssmann contrived excuses to spend time with her and eventually convinced her that the experiment was a safe and important one. However, the actual experiment was complicated when she insisted that Forssmann perform the experiment on her, rather than on himself. Forssmann convinced her to lie down on a cart, and then strapped her down as a "precaution against falling off the table." With the nurse thus immobilized, Forssmann inserted the catheter into his own arm and pushed it through the veins into his heart. He then unfastened the surgical nurse. She helped him walk to the basement, where an X-ray image confirmed that the catheter was indeed within Forssmann's heart.

Although he had originally disapproved of the experiment, once Forssmann's superior heard about it he helped Forssmann obtain a position at the Charité Hospital, the mecca of German surgery, as well as helping Forssmann to publish his results in the leading German medical journal, *Klinische Wochenschrift*. However, rather than being praised once his article appeared, Forssmann was violently attacked on the grounds that his article was at once foolish and irresponsible, and that he failed to give priority for cardiac catheterization to some senior faculty members (a claim that failed to withstand even superficial scrutiny). He was driven from the sight of the leading surgeon of the day, Ferdinand Sauerbruch, with the words: "You might lecture in a circus about your little tricks, but never in a respectable German university. Get out! Leave my department immediately!"

Forssmann returned to Eberswalde, where he tried to obtain X-ray images of the heart by injecting contrast material, mainly into laboratory animals, but twice on himself. He obtained some pictures, though they were of poor quality. From leading German physicians he engendered hostility, but little serious interest in his experiments. Forssmann then left academic medicine, and did no more work on cardiac catheterization.

But others plunged ahead with Forssmann's method. In 1941 Cournand acknowledged Forssmann's priority, despite the hostilities already present between Germany and other countries. Together with Richards, Cournand used cardiac catheterization to measure pressures from within the heart, as well as to take blood samples for analysis. These methods led to an improved understanding of heart failure, shock, congenital heart disease, and a wide range of acquired cardiac diseases. As a result, Forssmann, Cournand, and Richards shared the 1956 Nobel Prize.

Forssmann never lost his love for nature, nor his sense of humor—the last sentence in his autobiography is a comment about how proud he was to have his picture on a new brand of Spanish cigars! He was able therefore to cope with the hostility that his being awarded the prize engendered in some of his colleagues. Forssmann maintained a sense of both the importance of his work and of his good fortune to have it recognized at all, albeit several decades later.

Today, cardiac catheters are used for a wide range of purposes. Tubes within the heart are used to measure pressures and to guide therapy for cardiac failure. Dye can be injected to outline anatomic structures. Lesions can be corrected by surgery, or, at times, without an operative procedure, using catheters both to ablate diseased tissue and to open obstructed arteries. Forssmann's self-experiment of 1929 thus led the way for modern cardiology and cardiac surgery.

JOEL D. HOWELL

Selected Bibliography

PRIMARY SOURCES

Forssmann, Werner. 1929. "Die Sondierung des rechten Herzens." *Klinische Wochenschrift* 45:2085–87. Translated by Robert E. Asnis and reprinted as "Catheterization of the Right Heart," in *Classics of Cardiology*, edited by John A. Callahan, Thomas E. Keys, and Jack D. Key, 3:252–55. Malabar, Florida: Drieger Publishing Company, 1983.

———. 1956. "The Role of Heart Catheterization and Angiocardiography in the Development of Modern Medicine." Nobel Lecture. Reprinted in *Nobel Lectures, Physiology or Medicine*, vol. 3 (1942–1962), 506–10. Amsterdam: Elsevier, 1964.

———. 1956. Biography. In *Nobel Lectures, Physiology or Medicine*, vol. 3 (1942–1962), 511–12. Amsterdam: Elsevier, 1964.

———. *Experiments on Myself: Memoirs of a Surgeon in Germany*. Translated by Hilary Davies. New York: Saint Martin's Press, 1974.

SECONDARY SOURCES

Johnson, Steven L. 1972. *The History of Cardiac Surgery, 1896–1955*. Baltimore: Johns Hopkins University Press.

Cournand, André. 1974. Preface to *Experiments on Myself: Memoirs of a Surgeon in Germany* by Werner Forssmann. Translated by Hilary Davies. New York: Saint Martin's Press.

———. 1975. "Cardiac Catheterization: Development of the Technique, Its Contributions to Experimental Medicine, and Its Initial Applications in Man." *Acta Medica Scandinavica*, Supplementum 579:7–32.

Steckleberg, James M., Ronald E. Vlietstra, Jurgen Ludwig, and Ruth J. Mann. 1979. "Werner Forssmann (1904–1979) and His Unusual Success Story." *Mayo Clinic Proceedings* 54:746–48.

Comroe, Julius H., Jr. 1983. *Exploring the Heart: Discoveries in Heart Disease and High Blood Pressure*. New York: W. W. Norton.

KARL VON FRISCH 1973

Karl von Frisch was born on November 20, 1886, in Vienna. A zoologist, he received the Nobel Prize in 1973, jointly with Konrad Lorenz and Nikolaas Tinbergen, for his pathbreaking observations of the sensory discrimination and communication skills of bees, which helped to establish the science of ethology (animal behavior). At the time of the award, von Frisch, eighty-six years old, was director emeritus of the Zoological Institute of the University of Munich. His wife, Marguerity Mohr, whom he married in 1917, was a nurse and artist who illustrated some of his published work. The couple had one son, Otto, who also became a zoologist, and three daughters, Johanna, Maria, and Helen. Von Frisch died in Munich on June 12, 1982, at the age of ninety-five.

The son of Anton Ritter and Marie Exner von Frisch, Karl von Frisch was born into a distinguished family of physicians and professors. His father was head of surgery at the Vienna General Polyclinic. As a boy, he did not excel at school. He was fascinated by animal behavior and played with pet animals and collected and studied birds, fish, and insects at the family's summer home in Brunnwinkl. At his father's urging he began the study of medicine in 1905 at the University of Vienna, where he did very well in anatomy and physiology, studying under his uncle Sigmund Exner. But he had no interest in clinical medicine and, in 1907, he transferred to the Zoological Institute in Munich.

Von Frisch studied zoology under Richard von Hertwig in Munich, experimental biology under Hans Przibaum in Vienna, and marine biology at the Biological Institute for Marine Research in Trieste, Italy. It was during these years that his fascination with bees began. His thesis, on the light and color perceptions of minnows, was accepted for the Ph.D. in 1910. He then took a position as von Hertwig's assistant at the Zoological Institute. Here he continued his work on the color discrimination of fishes, demonstrating that minnows could be experimentally taught to respond to color variation. After two years of this work he was appointed lecturer in zoology.

Von Frisch now began to observe and experiment with color discrimination in bees. By 1914 he had successfully used food stimuli to train bees to respond to specific colors. World War I interrupted his research at this exciting juncture. Forced to abandon his studies due to lack of facilities, supplies, and even food, he worked for much of the time as a medical assistant in a Vienna hospital.

In 1919 he returned to Munich, where he had been appointed assistant professor. His research now concentrated on the ability of bees to distinguish scents. Although his previous work had used behavioral methods, von Frisch was a dedicated Darwinian, who believed that there had to be an evolutionary link between the abilities and behaviors of bees and the colors and scents of flowers. He demonstrated that bees could discriminate among many different scents, including those of very closely related flowers, and used that ability to seek food.

In the course of these experiments he was struck by the fact that a bee discovering food was instantly able to summon other bees to the exact location. By close observation he determined that the bee reported to its fellows by means of a "round dance." In 1924, after four years of research, he presented a paper with a film accompaniment on the "language" of the bees. He had now observed two types of dances, the "round dance" which led the hive to the sugar water provided in the laboratory, and the more vigorous "waggle dance," which indicated the discovery of flower pollen. Von Frisch theorized that the dancing bee carried the distinctive scent of the flower back with him, enabling the other bees to locate the new food (Marler and Griffin 1973, 464).

His reputation was rapidly growing. He was recruited first to the University of Rostock (1921–23) and then to the University of Breslau (1923–25), but returned to Munich when offered the post of von Hertwig's successor as director of the Zoological Institute in 1925. Here he continued his bee studies and also demonstrated conclusively the hearing abilities of fish. Under his direction a new research facility with carefully designed housing for bees, ants, and other insects was built in Munich. In the 1940s his work was again interrupted by war, but he was able this time to move his research to some safety in Brunnwinkl.

In 1944 von Frisch described the findings of twenty years' work: the deciphering of the "Rossetta Stone" of the honeybee. His observations clearly showed that the "round dance" was indicative of a nearby location (within ninety yards), as well as of a type of food. The "waggle dance," on the other hand, was performed to direct the hive to food at a distance. The dancing bee would point its body in the correct direction during a portion of the dance and the duration and vigor of the dance indicated the distance and amount. Inside the dark hive, the bee pantomined direction in relation to the position of the sun, indicated by a straight vertical. As von Frisch had believed, scent and vibration are also used to pinpoint the food location for the bee audience.

Von Frisch also established that bees will dance for water as well as for food, while his student, Martin Lindauer, has since shown that bees searching for a new location for a hive will dance for each other to describe and "discuss" possible locations. Dances are genetically determined and vary among subspecies of bees. Whether these hereditary and highly stylized behaviors actually constitute language is a subject for debate. But the amazing versatility and communicative power of the bees' dancing adds new dimensions to our understanding of animal behavior (Marler and Griffin 1973, 464; Altman 1973, 49).

Von Frisch was appointed chairman of Zoology at the University of Graz in Austria in 1946, but relinquished the position four years later, and returned to Munich where the facilities were the best for the research that was most important to him. Among his other contributions was the hypothesis that bees possess an internal clock. Some of von Frisch's colleagues flamboyantly proved this contention in 1955 by flying 5,000 bees from Paris to the American Museum of Natural History in New York, where the bees, apparently unaffected by jet lag, ate and otherwise acted as if they were still on Paris time. On a more practical plane, his findings have been usefully applied in apiculture (beekeeping) and plant pollination.

Von Frisch retired in 1958, but continued to collect, observe, and write about insects. By then, many of his books were published in English and other languages, bringing him worldwide acclaim. He was honored by membership in many scientific societies, including the National Academy of Sciences and the Royal Society of London. Among the other awards he received for his work were the Orden Pour le Merite für Wissenschaften und Kunste (1952); the Magellan Prize from the American Philosophical Society (1956); the Kalinga Prize from UNESCO (1959); and the Balzan Prize (1963).

MARCIA MELDRUM

Selected Bibliography

PRIMARY SOURCES

Von Frisch, Karl. 1955. *The Dancing Bees: An Account of the Life and Senses of the Honeybee*. New York: Harcourt Brace.

———. 1963. *Man and the Living World*. New York: Harcourt Brace.

———. 1967. *A Biologist Remembers*. New York: Pergamon Press.

———. 1972. *Bees: Their Vision, Chemical Senses, and Language*. Ithaca, NY: Cornell University Press.

———. 1983. *Animal Architecture*. New York: Van Nostrand Reinhold.

SECONDARY SOURCES

Altman, Lawrence K. 1973. "Birds and Bees." *New York Times* (October 12):48.

Anonymous. 1973. "Karl von Frisch." *New York Times* (October 12):48.

———. 1974. "Frisch, Karl von." In *Current Biography Yearbook*, 130–33. New York: H. W. Wilson.

———. 1983. "Karl von Frisch." *Biographical Memoirs of the Fellows of the Royal Society* 29:197–200.

Marler, P., and D. R. Griffin. 1973. "The 1973 Nobel Prize for Physiology or Medicine." *Science* 182 (November 2):464–66.

DANIEL CARLETON GAJDUSEK
1976

Daniel Carleton Gajdusek was born on September 9, 1923, in Yonkers, New York. A pediatrician and virologist, Gajdusek shared the Nobel Prize in 1976 with Baruch S. Blumberg for his identification and description of slow virus infections in humans, based on his intensive study of kuru, a degenerative brain disease found among the primitive Fore people of New Guinea. He has been based since 1958 at the National Institute of Neurological and Communicative Disorders and Stroke, where he heads the Laboratories of Slow, Latent and Temperate Virus Infections and of Central Nervous System Studies. Described by Donald Tower, his chief at NIH, as "truly a man for all seasons," he is an acknowledged expert in comparative child behavior, genetics, anthropology, literature, and primitive art, as well as in virology and neurology; he is also a fluent linguist and is conversant in several little-known tongues of primitive tribes. He managed to combine several of these interests in his prizewinning work. Although never married, he has adopted thirty-six children (to date) from New Guinea and other Pacific islands and brought them to the United States to be educated (Rensberger 1976).

Gajdusek's parents were Karl Gajdusek, a butcher born in Slovakia, and Ottilia Dobrozcsky, a first-generation Hungarian American, whose family valued culture and education. His aunt Irene Dobrozcsky, an entomologist, encouraged his early interest in science and helped him to get a summer job at the Boyce Thompson Institute for Plant Research. He received his undergraduate degree summa cum laude from the University of Rochester in 1943 and completed the Harvard Medical School curriculum in three years, earning his M.D. in 1946.

Gajdusek had chosen pediatrics as his specialty but his interests were wide ranging. From 1946 to 1951 he completed an internship at Columbia Presbyterian in New York, and residencies at Children's Hospital in Cincinnati and Children's Medical Center in Boston. During this same period he served on a postwar medical mission to Germany, studied physical chemistry at the California Institute of Technology with Linus Pauling, and won a fellowship from the National Foundation for Infantile Paralysis to do virological research in John F. Enders's laboratory at Harvard (1949–52).

He was drafted in 1952 and assigned to the Walter Reed Army Institute for Research, where he continued his virological studies under Joseph Smadel. It was apparently Smadel who recognized the difficulties of channeling and fully utilizing Gajdusek's considerable talents in the laboratory and encouraged him to undertake field epidemiology work (Marsh 1976, 928).

Discharged from the service in 1954, he took off, initially for the Institut Pasteur in Teheran, where he worked with Marcel Baltazard on epidemic diseases of the Middle East, including rabies and plague. After two years in Iran, he traveled to Melbourne to work with Sir MacFarlane Burnet at the Walter and Eliza Hall Institute of Medical Research in Melbourne.

On a field excursion to New Guinea, Gajdusek met Vincent Zigas, district medical officer of the Public Health Department in Port Moresby, Australia. Zigas had identified an unusual neurologic disorder, called kuru, which seemed to occur only among the Fore, an isolated tribe of the eastern highlands, but was killing two hundred of these people each year, mostly women and children, and threatening their continued survival in some areas. Gajdusek went into the highlands to take a look and found himself deeply attracted and intrigued by the Fore and their strange malady. He spent the next ten months living with the tribe, studying their culture, and collecting tissues from the bodies of kuru victims for further study (Gajdusek and Zigas 1959).

In 1958 he returned to the United States, where Smadel assisted him to get the NIH appointment. He continued his laboratory studies on kuru and made repeated excursions back to New Guinea and the Pacific (Marsh 1976, 929).

Initially, the problem of kuru seemed baffling. The disease is easy to describe: a period of shaking and trembling leads to a breakdown of motor functions, dementia, and death. The brain tissue after death reveals extensive lesions and atrophy. There are no symptoms of infection, such as fever or antibody production, and attempts to culture a disease agent had failed. Gajdusek logically hypothesized a complex genetic etiology (Gajdusek 1962; Gajdusek and Gibbs 1964).

While he and his associate, Clarence J. Gibbs, were exploring the possibilities, William Hadlow of the NIH Rocky Mountain Laboratory wrote a letter to *Lancet*, outlining the similarities between kuru and scrapie, a viral infection of sheep that produced symptoms only after very long incubation periods. This suggestion directed Gajdusek back to a viral etiology. He and Gibbs inoculated a pair of chimpanzees with a preparation of brain tissue from kuru victims; after an anxious two years, the animals exhibited symptoms of the disease. They then sacrificed the infected animals and used their brain tissue in a new preparation, which was administered to a second pair of chimps. Over a period of four years, they were able to transmit kuru to three pairs of animals in succession (Gajdusek, Gibbs, and Alpers 1967; Marsh 1976, 929).

The transmission among the Fore people had depended on the custom of ritual cannibalism, in which the women and children ate the brains of the dead kuru victims, to retain their wisdom and virtue in the tribe and give them immortality. Modernization and education in New Guinea have ended this practice and, it is hoped, the epidemic of kuru (Gajdusek and Zigas 1961; Sullivan 1976).

Gajdusek and Gibbs turned their attention in 1967 to other puzzling diseases that might have a similar etiology. In 1968 they were able to transmit Creutzfeldt-Jakob dementia by the same process of brain tissue inoculation and thus identified this rare (two hundred deaths a year in the United States) but worldwide disease as a slow virus infection. Certain other progressive degenerative brain pathologies, including slow measles encephalitis and progressive multifocal leukoencephalopathy, have now been traced in the same way to a viral agent. Slow virus infections have also been implicated more recently in Lyme disease, AIDS, and other diseases. Gajdusek believes that this model may be applicable as well to disorders such as Alzheimer's, Huntington's chorea, and Parkinson's, but his ideas in this respect have not been fully corroborated. The problem of isolating and characterizing the viral agent, and the related questions of diagnosis, prevention, and treatment still remain unanswered (Gajdusek 1967; Marsh 1976, 929).

Gajdusek continues his work on slow virus infections at NIH, interspersed with frequent field trips to his beloved Pacific islands. "A gentle, likable man," he is a tireless and compulsive worker, often sustaining his energy with two-hour catnaps. He has published several articles on child psychology and ethnology, as well as his virological contributions. Gajdusek is fluent in French, German, Spanish, Slavic languages, Rumanian, and Persian, and reads widely in world literature. From his varied travels, he has brought home an impressive collection of primitive art and artifacts.

The Nobel Prize money helped to finance the education of his adopted children, many of whom have returned to share their new knowledge and skills in their home lands. Carleton Gajdusek is a member of the National Academy of Sciences, the American Pediatric Society, the American Anthropological Society, and the American Academy of Neurology. Among the many other awards he has received are the Mead Johnson Award from the American Academy of Pediatrics (1963), the Distinguished Service Award from the Department of Health, Education, and Welfare (1975), and the Cotzias Prize from the American Academy of Neurology (1978).

MARCIA MELDRUM

Selected Bibliography

PRIMARY SOURCES

Gajdusek, D. Carleton, and Vincent Zigas. 1957. "Degenerative Disease of the Central Nervous System in New Guinea: The Endemic Occurrence of Kuru in the Native Population." *New England Journal of Medicine* 257 (November 14):974–78.

———. 1959. "Kuru: Clinical, Physiological and Epidemiological Study of an Acute Progressive Degenerative Disease of the Central Nervous System among Natives of the Eastern Highlands of New Guinea." *American Journal of Medicine* 26 (March): 442–69.

———. 1961. "Studies on Kuru. 1. The Ethnologic Setting of Kuru." *American Journal of Tropical Medicine* 10 (January):80–91.

Gajdusek, D. Carleton. 1962. "Kuru: An Appraisal of Five Years of Investigation." *Eugenics Quarterly* 9 (March): 69–74.

———. 1963. *Field Journals. Study of Child Growth and Development of Disease Patterns in Primitive Cultures.* Bethesda, Maryland: National Institute of Neurological Diseases and Blindness.

———. 1963. "Ethnopediatrics as a Study of Cybernetics of Human Development. The Use of Primitive Cultures as Field Laboratories for the Study of the Programming of the Nervous System of the Child." *American Journal of Diseases of Children* 105 (June):554–59.

———.1964. "The Composition of Musics for Man or Decoding from Primitive Cultures the Sources for Human Behavior." *Pediatrics* 34 (July):84–91.

Gajdusek, D. Carleton, and Clarence J. Gibbs. 1964. "Attempts to Demonstrate a Transmissible Agent in Kuru, Amyotrophic Lateral Sclerosis, and Other Subacute and Chronic Nervous System Degenerations of Man." *Nature* 204 (October 17):257–59.

Gajdusek, D. Carleton, Clarence J. Gibbs, Jr., and M. Alpers. 1965. *Slow, Latent and Temperate Virus Infections.* Bethesda, Maryland: National Institutes of Health.

———. 1967. "Transmission and Passage of Experimental 'Kuru' to Chimpanzees." *Science* 155 (January 13):212–14.

Gajdusek, D. Carleton. 1967. "Slow Virus Infections of the Nervous System." *New England Journal of Medicine* 276 (February 16):392–400.

———. 1967. "Discussion on Kuru, Scrapie, and the Experimental Kuru-Like Syndrome in Chimpanzees." *Current Topics in Microbiology and Immunology* 40:59–63.

Gajdusek, D. Carleton, and J. Farquhar. 1981. *Kuru: Early Letters and Field Notes.* New York: Raven Press.

SECONDARY SOURCES

Rensberger, Boyce. 1976. "Daniel Carleton Gajdusek." *New York Times* (October 15):13.

Sullivan, Walter. 1976. "Both Laureates Found Major Clues in Studies of Primitive Tribesmen." *New York Times* (October 15):13.

Mims, Sir Cedric. 1976. "D. Carleton Gajdusek." *Nature* 263 (October 28):716–17.

Marsh, Richard F. 1976. "The 1976 Nobel Prize in Physiology or Medicine." *Science* 194 (November 26): 928–29.

1981. "Gajdusek, Daniel Carleton." In *Current Biography Yearbook*, 156–59. New York: H. W. Wilson.

HERBERT SPENCER GASSER
1944

Herbert Spencer Gasser was born in Platteville, Wisconsin, on July 5, 1888. A neurophysiologist, Gasser shared the 1944 Nobel Prize with his longtime friend and collaborator, Joseph Erlanger, for their discoveries concerning the highly differentiated functions and electrical characteristics of vertebrate single nerve fibers, and for their development of the multistage vacuum tube electronic amplifier and the cathode-ray oscillograph, the fundamental tools of modern neurophysiology. At the time of the award, Gasser was director of the Rockefeller Institute of Medical Research, the most prestigious position in American medical science, which he occupied from 1935 until his retirement in 1953. He never married. He died on May 11, 1963, in New York City.

Gasser was the son of Herman Gasser, an Austrian-born country doctor, and his wife, Jane Elizabeth Griswold Gasser. He received his early education at the Platteville Normal School, graduating in 1907. He had long resisted his father's urging to become a physician, but, during his subsequent three years at the University of Wisconsin at Madison, under Erlanger's tutelage he became fascinated with experimental biology. He took his A.B. in zoology in 1910 with a fledgling research effort on regeneration in the nymphs of the mayfly. He stayed at Wisconsin to earn an A.M. in anatomy in 1911, also taking courses on biochemistry and physiology with Erlanger. From 1911 to 1913 he served as Erlanger's assistant. Gasser was by then firmly set on a career in medical research, so he undertook two more years of study at the American mecca for scientific medicine, the Johns Hopkins Medical School, earning his M.D. in 1915.

He then returned to the University of Wisconsin as an instructor. After a year, however, Erlanger, who had been appointed professor of physiology at the newly reorganized Washington University School of Medicine, brought him to St. Louis. Gasser's most scientifically productive years followed, working on nerve physiology with Erlanger, George Bishop, Joseph Hinsey, and Helen Graham. In 1921 he was promoted to professor of pharmacology, although his work continued to be devoted to physiology. A grant from the Rockefeller Foundation enabled him to spend two years (1923–25) in Europe, working on muscle physiology with Archibald Hill at University College, London; on nerve physiology with Louis Lapique at the Sorbonne; and on pharmacology with Henry Dale at the National Institute for Medical Research, London, and Walter Straub at the University of Munich.

Gasser had discovered nerve physiology rather by chance in 1919. He had by then coauthored more than twenty-five papers on the heart, on blood coagulation, and on the nature and treatment of traumatic circulatory shock caused by war wounds, but he had failed to find a problem that really engaged his interest. He was well aware, as were all physiologists, that after more than a century of existence as a distinct field, neurophysiology still suffered under a crippling disability: electrical nerve impulses (action potentials) were so small they could hardly be recorded. Any attempt to do so with the available technology introduced huge distortions. Gasser's physicist colleague at Washington, A. S. Langsdorf, suggested that the newly improved vacuum tubes might offer a way around this impasse. Harry Sidney Newcomer, a Wisconsin friend and Johns Hopkins classmate of Gasser's, had considerable experience in electronics and contacts at the Western Electric Company of New York, the only manufacturing source for high-quality tubes. Together, Gasser and Newcomer developed in 1920 the first useful physiological amplifier, with three stages that magnified the electrical signal of the nerve impulse as much as five thousand times. Their design was adapted widely in the 1920s. The new amplifier made possible Edgar Adrian's Nobel Prize–winning discoveries that single nerves code their messages by the frequency of identical "all-or-none" impulses.

As his work with Newcomer was progressing, Gasser often discussed the remaining problem of distortion over lunch with Erlanger. They agreed that the cathode-ray tube, or Braun tube, in which a nearly inertialess beam of electrons is deflected by the electrical signal, offered a possible solution. But the existing cathode-ray tubes operated with potentials of 10,000 to 50,000 volts, far beyond the range of the new amplifier. In December 1920, Gasser, following a tip from a fellow physiologist, attended a presentation about a new Braun tube—designed by J. B. Johnson of Western Electric—that used a hot cathode and needed only 300–400 volts—well within the amplifier's parameters. Gasser and Erlanger immediately ordered one of the new tubes, and, by 1922, they were able to publish highly precise and practically distortionless action potentials of frog and mammalian nerves.

These experiments, like all that had been performed by neurophysiologists for over a century, used nerves such as the sciatic, that are rather like telephone trunk lines: they consist of thousands of individual nerve fibers, or axons, large and small, that carry messages in and out of the brain and spinal cord. Erlanger and Gasser's experiments with their new apparatus revealed that, when one stimulated such a nerve trunk and recorded its impulses from 5–10 centimeters away, the clean rise and fall of the action potential was stretched out, showing "humps" on the declining side. They immediately guessed the reason: different groups of axons conducted at different speeds, so that the action potentials in the slower groups gradually fell behind the faster, like the spread of runners at the end of a race. The summated reading was therefore a compound action potential. By 1924 Gasser and Erlanger had distinguished four distinct fiber groups, which they named (from fastest to slowest) alpha, beta, gamma, and delta. In other words, they could use their apparatus to "dissect" physiologically a nerve trunk whose individual axons were so small they could not be dissected anatomically.

Was there some relationship between anatomical structure, physiological function, and conduction velocity of the electrical signal? Several theories that had never been testable suggested that large axons would conduct faster. Between 1924 and 1926, Gasser, with some assistance from Erlanger, painstakingly measured microscopic cross sections of nerve trunks, plotted the distribution of axon sizes and showed that size differentials could be correlated with conduction velocity. This finding in turn led to electrophysiological investigations that defined which groups of fibers could be connected to sensory or motor functions. In addition, different groups of fibers showed different sensitivities to blocking agents, such as mechanical pressure or anesthesia. By 1929 improved techniques and higher amplification demonstrated that the four original groups identified could be grouped into a single class "A" (mammalian conduction velocities of 30 to 90 meters per second) and had discerned the presence of slower fiber groups, labelled "B" (10 to 20 meters per second) and "C" (0.3 to 1.6 meters per second).

Gasser and Erlanger's innovative technology also provided a wealth of precise information about the electrical nature of the nerve impulse itself, which the team pursued together and then separately, after Gasser accepted an appointment as professor of physiology at Cornell Medical College and set up a duplicate laboratory in New York in 1932. Erlanger concentrated especially on the conditions under which the nerve impulse was propagated, the speed of the response, and under what circumstances the nerve was completely or partially refractory to propagation. Gasser observed and tried to determine the meaning of the after-potentials; he also experimented with the effects of poisons, and rapid stimulation, on the action potential. He studied as well the unmyelinated and slow-conducting "C" fibers that appeared to be related to such sensations as pain. Erlanger and Gasser reunited briefly in 1936 to give the Eldridge Reeves Johnson Lectures at the University of Pennsylvania on "Electrical Signs of Nervous Activity"; this overview, published a year later, became the classic statement of their work.

Gasser had hardly begun his investigations at his new lab when he was recruited by the Rockefeller Institute. The administrative demands of this job, including meeting the financial crises brought on by the Great Depression, and helping to direct chemical warfare research during World War II, limited his research productivity. He returned to the laboratory briefly after his retirement, but was plagued by poor health for several years before his death at age seventy-four. He was warmly respected by such friends as

Edgar Adrian and Detlev Bronk for his modesty and probity, his wide knowledge of biology, chemistry, and physics, his open and infectious enthusiasm for scientific investigation, and his kindness in encouraging the careers of younger scientists, such as Alan Hodgkin.

The Nobel award in 1944 was applauded by physiologists in Britain and America as long overdue. Among the many other honors Gasser received were the Kober Medal of the Association of American Physicians (1954), and eleven honorary degrees, including degrees awarded by Harvard, Columbia, Pennsylvania, Oxford, and Paris. He was a member of the National Academy of Sciences, a foreign member of the Royal Society, and an editor of the *Journal of Experimental Medicine.*

Although Gasser and Erlanger received the Nobel Prize for their investigation of the differentiated functions of nerve fibers, which have found a secure place in modern physiology, in retrospect their contributions to technology appear more significant. The multistage electronic amplifier, linked to the cathode-ray oscillograph, as well as the accessories developed in their laboratories, have become the standard tools of neural physiological research. Used on single cells or axons in the 1940s and 1950s, these instruments were the basis of Nobel work by Hodgkin, Huxley, Eccles, Hartline, Katz, and others, and continue to be important to today's scientists.

ROBERT FRANK

Selected Bibliography

PRIMARY SOURCES

Gasser, H. S., and H. S. Newcomer. 1921. "Physiological Action Currents in the Phrenic Nerve: An Application of the Thermionic Vacuum Tube to Nerve Physiology." *American Journal of Physiology* 57:1–26.

Gasser, H. S., and Joseph Erlanger. 1922. "A Study of the Action Currents of Nerve with the Cathode Ray Oscillograph." *American Journal of Physiology* 62:496–524.

Erlanger, Joseph, H. S. Gasser, and George H. Bishop. 1924. "The Compound Nature of the Action Current of Nerve as Disclosed by the Cathode Ray Oscillograph." *American Journal of Physiology* 70:624–666.

Gasser, H. S., and Joseph Erlanger. 1927. "The Role Played by the Sizes of the Constituent Fibers of a Nerve Trunk in Determining the Force of Its Action Potential Wave." *American Journal of Physiology* 80:522–47.

Erlanger, Joseph, and H. S. Gasser. 1937. *Electrical Signs of Nervous Activity.* Philadelphia: University of Pennsylvania Press.

SECONDARY SOURCES

1963. "Herbert Spencer Gasser." *Lancet* (May 25):1167–68.

1964. "Herbert Spencer Gasser, 1888–1963." *Experimental Neurology* Suppl. 1:1–38.

Adrian, E. D. 1964. "Herbert Spencer Gasser, 1888–1963." *Biographical Memoirs of Fellows of the Royal Society* 10:75–82.

Frank, Robert G., Jr. 1979. "The J. H. B. Archive Report: The Joseph Erlanger Collection at Washington University School of Medicine, St. Louis." *Journal of the History of Biology* 12:193–201.

Marshall, Louise H. 1983. "The Fecundity of Aggregates: The Axonologists at Washington University, 1922–1942." *Perspectives in Biology and Medicine* 26:613–36.

JOSEPH LEONARD GOLDSTEIN
1985

Joseph Leonard Goldstein was born on April 18, 1940, in Sumter, South Carolina. A physician, medical educator, and molecular geneticist, Goldstein is currently Paul J. Thomas Professor of Medicine and Genetics at the University of Texas Health Sciences Center and chairman of the Department of Molecular Genetics. He has never married. He received the Nobel Prize jointly with Michael S. Brown in 1985 for their work on the etiology of familial hypercholesterolemia and their discovery of the mechanism of receptor-mediated endocytosis, now believed to be a key process of cellular metabolism. Brown and Goldstein's work is remarkable both as a model of disease-specific research that illuminated a whole area of biologic medicine, and as one of the great creative research partnerships.

Goldstein was brought up in Kingstree, South Carolina, where his parents, Isadore E. and Fannie A. Goldstein, ran a clothing store. He graduated summa cum laude in chemistry from Washington and Lee University in 1962, and entered medical school at Southwestern in Dallas, a branch of the University of Texas Health Sciences Center. His exceptional talents were recognized by Donald Seldin, then chairman of internal medicine. Seldin discussed with the young student the possibility of his return to Texas to create a new division of medical genetics. Goldstein received his M.D. in 1966 (Motulsky 1986).

He was accepted at Massachusetts General Hospital for his residency in internal medicine (1966–68). Here he met Michael Brown, a graduate of the University of Pennsylvania. Brown and Goldstein discovered mutual interests in academic careers, molecular biology, and bridge. From MGH, both men went to the National Institutes of Health as clinical associates (1968–70). Goldstein worked in the Laboratory of Biochemical Genetics under Marshall S. Nirenberg. Here he isolated and described several proteins involved in termination of protein synthesis. As his clinical responsibility, he was assigned to the National Heart Institute to work with Donald S. Frederickson. At NHI he encountered familial hypercholesterolemia (FHC).

FHC was first identified as a hereditary disorder in 1939 by Carl Muller of Norway. Frederickson had isolated two forms: "heterozygous" and "homozygous." Heterozygous FHC is linked to a single defective gene and occurs in one of every five hundred people. Individuals with this disorder have a blood cholesterol level two to three times that of a normal person and a greatly increased risk of heart disease (75 percent in males, 45 percent in females). Homozygous FHC is far more rare (one in one million people) and more lethal. A child receiving a defective gene from both parents will develop blood cholesterol four to eight times the normal level and die of heart disease before the age of thirty.

In 1970 Goldstein began a two-year fellowship in medical genetics at the University of Washington in Seattle under Arno G. Motulsky, where he undertook an unselected retrospective study of five hundred heart attack survivors and their relatives. He found that 31 percent of these individuals had high blood fat level, 20 percent of which were genetically linked (Goldstein et al. 1973, 1533–43, 1544–68).

Goldstein returned to Dallas as an assistant professor in 1972 to organize the long-planned division of medical genetics and to begin collaborative research with Michael Brown, who had joined the UTHSC department the year before. The team chose to investigate cholesterol and cholesterol-related disease. They agreed to concentrate their efforts on FHC, particularly the homozygous form, which appeared to offer the best opportunity to isolate the crucial mechanism of cholesterol metabolism.

Cholesterol, the "Janus-faced molecule," is produced naturally by the liver and is essential to body functioning. Inside body cells, it plays a critical role in cell growth and the production of hormones. The cholesterol gets to the cells from the bloodstream, where it is attached to water-soluble proteins, called lipoproteins, also released by the liver. As the lipoproteins circulate in the blood, cells absorb cholesterol needed to continue normal processes. However, if cholesterol is not absorbed quickly enough, or not completely, it spills into the blood tissues and attaches to the vascular walls. Now the molecules become deadly blockages in the arteries, causing angina, atherosclerosis, and coronary heart disease.

These facts were understood when Goldstein and Brown began their work. But the cell absorption process—and the reasons for its failure in hypercholesterolemia—was unknown.

The team worked with tissue cultures of the human skin cells from patients with genetic FHC defects and from normal individuals. Observing these cultured fibroblasts, they identified coated pits—

the LDL receptors—on the cell surface. These pits attached LDLs—the low density lipoproteins with the highest proportion of fat—and then formed endocyte vesicles that drew the LDLs inside the cell and released the cholesterol.

In the normal cell, cholesterol intake resulted in the reduction of the number of pits and an increase in cholesterol processing within the cell. As the internal level dropped, the coated pits again appeared on the cell surface to attract LDLs. Brown and Goldstein identified and described this process—"receptor-mediated endocytosis"—in 1973 (Brown and Goldstein 1974).

Their work was of immediate and critical importance in our understanding of FHC. They had counted around 250,000 LDL receptors on the surface of the normal cells. FHC heterozygous cells have perhaps 40–50 percent of such receptors. FHC homozygous cells have few or none. The liver contains LDL receptors, which regulate the production of blood cholesterol, as well as the processing of dietary cholesterol. Again, FHC patients have greatly reduced numbers of liver receptors. In effect, they "overdose" on cholesterol (Brown and Goldstein 1975).

The model of receptor-mediated endoyctosis was quickly found by other researchers to be the key to more than twenty cellular mechanisms, including the processing of insulin, growth factors, and immune complexes. Thus Goldstein and Brown laid the groundwork for many future discoveries (Motulsky 1986, 127).

The direct application of their work was to FHC chemotherapy. Cholestyramine had been used since the 1950s to treat hypercholesterolemia but the mechanism of its action was not understood. Moreover, the positive effects could not be sustained long-term. The drug was now found to work by increasing the number of LDL receptors in the liver, enabling increased excretion of the excess cholesterol as bile acid. However, the increase in receptors naturally triggered an increase in cholesterol synthesis by the liver, which neutralized the first effect.

This led to the search for a drug that would work with cholestyramine by blocking the liver's excess production of cholesterol. An "anti-cholesterol enzyme" developed by Alfred W. Alberts of Merck, Sharpe and Dohme was approved by the FDA in 1987 to be sold under the trade name Lovastatin. Goldstein and Brown have conducted animal trials with Lovastatin which demonstrated its efficacy; but they have warned that its long-term effects and possible toxicity are not yet clear. Other treatment applications have included liver transplant, combined with Lovastatin therapy, in a young FHC homozygous patient; and, of course, diet therapy (Motulsky 1986, 127–28).

Blood cholesterol is internally produced, not synthesized from dietary cholesterol. The effect of high fat, high cholesterol dietary intake on internal synthesis is unclear. Goldstein and Brown contend, on the basis of their animal experiments, that high dietary cholesterol can cause the liver to reduce its internal LDL receptors, thus decreasing excretion and adding to the blood level. The National Institutes of Health recommendations for lowered fat and cholesterol in American diets (1984) are a result of their ideas and have certainly had major impact on popular understanding of heart disease, if not necessarily on popular habits.

Brown and Goldstein continue their research, working now on the complex genetic etiology of FHC. In 1985, their team succeeded in cloning and sequencing the LDL receptor gene.

They also continue seeing patients and working with medical students and residents. At UTHSC, they are often referred to as "Brownstein" or "the Gemini twins." In their close partnership, they plan research jointly, publish together, and share the podium for oral presentations. Out of the hospital, they are partners at bridge.

Goldstein was elected to the National Academy of Sciences in 1980 and was president of the American Society of Clinical Investigation in 1986. He is a fellow of the American College of Physicians, a nonresident fellow of the Salk Institute, and a member of the Howard Hughes Institute Scientific Advisory Board. Among the many awards he and Brown have jointly received are the NAS Lounsbery Award (1979), the Heinrich-Wieland Prize (1974), the Lita Annenberg Hazen Award (1982), and the Louisa G. Horowitz Award (1984). For relaxation, he enjoys bridge and classical music.

MARCIA MELDRUM

Selected Bibliography

PRIMARY SOURCES

Goldstein, J. L., W. R. Hazzard, H. G. Schott, E. L. Bierman, A. G. Motulsky et al. 1973. "Hyperlipidemia in Coronary Heart Disease. 1. Lipid Levels in 500 Survivors of Myocardial Infarction." *Journal of Clinical Investigation* 52 (July):1533–43.

———. 1973. "Hyperlipidemia in Coronary Heart Disease. 2. Genetic Analysis of Lipid Levels in 176 Families and Delineation of a New Inherited Disorder, Combined Hyperlipidemia." *Journal of Clinical Investigation* 52 (July):1544–68.

Brown, Michael S., and Joseph L. Goldstein. 1973. "Familial Hypercholesteremia: Identification of a Defect in the Regulation of 3-Hydroxy-3-Methylglutary Coenzyme: A Reductase Activity Associated with Overproduction of Cholesterol." *Proceedings of the National Academy of Sciences* 70:2804–8.

———. 1974. "Binding and Degradation of Low Density Lipoproteins by Cultured Human Fibroblasts: Comparison of Cells from a Normal Subjects and From a Patient with Homozygous Familial Hypercholesterolemia." *Journal of Biological Chemistry* 249:5153–62.

———. 1974. "Development of a Cell Culture System for Study of the Basic Defect in Familial Hypercholesterolemia." *Atherosclerosis 3: Proceedings of the Third International Symposium*, 422–25. Berlin: Springer-Verlag.

———. (1974). "Expression of the Familial Hypercholesterolemia Gene in Heterozygotes: Model for a Dominant Disorder in Man." *Transactions of the Association of American Physicians* 87:130–31.

Brown, Michael S., Joseph L. Goldstein, and M. J. E. Harrod. 1974. "Homozygous Familial Hypercholesterolemia: Specificity of the Biochemical Defect in Cultured Cells and Feasibility of Prenatal Detection." *American Journal of Human Genetics* 26:199–206.

Brown, Michael S., and Joseph L. Goldstein. 1975. "Familial Hypercholesterolemia: Biochemical, Genetic, and Pathophysiological Considerations." *Advances in Internal Medicine* 208:273–96.

———. 1975. "Familial Hypercholesterolemia: A Genetic Regulatory Defect in Cholesterol Metabolism." *American Journal of Medicine* 58: 147–50.

SECONDARY SOURCES

Sullivan, Walter. 1985. "Converging on a Nobel Prize." *New York Times* (October 15):C1.

Motulsky, Arno G. 1986. "The 1985 Nobel Prize in Physiology or Medicine." *Science* 231 (January 10): 126–29.

1987. "Goldstein, Joseph L". In *Current Biography Yearbook*, 208–11. New York: H. W. Wilson.

CAMILLO GOLGI *1906*

Camillo Golgi was born in Corteno in Brescia, Italy, on July 7, 1843. Very little is known about Golgi's youth and adolescence. His father was a physician, and probably provided the stimulus that led him to seek an education in medicine. Golgi started his medical studies at the University of Pavia, graduating in 1865. Golgi continued to pursue medical research throughout his long life. He shared the Nobel Prize in Physiology or Medicine in 1906 with Santiago Ramón y Cajal. He died in 1926, age eighty-two, having earned almost every major national award.

Golgi initially began his medical studies in the field of psychiatry, working under Cesare Lombroso. During this period he started to develop his histological techniques for studying the central nervous system. His initial interest was looking at psammona bodies, or what Golgi called "dural endotheliomas"; he published work on this subject in 1869.

Golgi's early scientific efforts occurred during an exciting period of time in medicine because of the recent postulation of the cell theory by Virchow, Schwann, Schleiden, and others. At the University of

Pavia Golgi came under the influence of Bizzozero, an early and influential histologist, who was working on the structure of neuroglia. After his initial studies with Bizzozero, Golgi transferred to Abbiategrasso, a small hospital for cripples. Here, under rather primitive conditions, Golgi continued his histological studies. Bored with the hospital environs and having considerable free time, he turned his attention to developing staining techniques for examining the nervous system. Thus he developed his famous silver chromate stain for identifying neurons and their processes. Up to this time, the study of the central nervous system had been considered too difficult because of the complexity of the anatomical structure involved. Golgi introduced a tremendous technological advance by developing a histological stain using silver nitrates that made the nerves and their surrounding elements stand out. By 1883 Golgi had eloquently outlined the central nervous system cells and characterized the Golgi Type I cell (nerves with long axons), and the Golgi Type II cells (nerves with short axons).

Golgi's early studies on cerebral gliomas and neuroglia, published between 1871 and 1875, earned him appointment at age thirty-two as professor of histology and pathology at the University of Pavia. Golgi would remain there for the rest of his career. At Pavia Golgi formulated his views that the central nervous system is a "Protoplasmic continuum" or a reticular network. He postulated that the neural connections and hence communication within the central nervous system occurred via a continuous network of cells, a "rete mirabile" of sorts. He held that nerve fibers form a diffuse network, and that by breaking up into smaller secondary fibers and then anastomosing they formed a trellis system or a "reticular network." Through this network the central nervous system processes the information via parallel circuitry.

Golgi held this view to his death, but, unfortunately, he was quite wrong. A review of Golgi's work reveals that he lacked the evidence to support his continuum idea, in actual fact the reticular cell theory was really only a hypothesis, not even documented by Golgi's own histological studies. It was the work of Santiago Ramon y Cajal, also awarded the Nobel Prize in 1906, that demonstrated the correct anatomical relationship of the nerves in what we now call the "neuron doctrine." One of the few discordant speeches given by a Nobel Prize winner was given by Golgi in 1906 when he, in his Nobel Lecture, read a diatribe against Cajal's work, and reiterated his belief in the reticular cell theory. Golgi's mistaken beliefs or his attack on Cajal, however, should not discredit Golgi's classic work in the 1880s, when he described in superb detail what we now call the Golgi Type I and Type II cells.

Golgi continued to branch out using new staining techniques he developed. He described the cytoplasmic reticular substance of the nerve and other cells, what we now call the "Golgi Apparatus." Golgi is also remembered by an eponym called the Golgi Organ for his description of the muscle tendon organ responsible for part of the reflex circuit.

Golgi's work on the nervous system overshadowed his other major scientific contribution, the study of malarial parasites. In a series of papers published from 1886 to 1893, he detailed the malarial parasite cycle in blood. Golgi was able to relate the fever curves seen in malaria to the development of the parasite in the blood. The quartan and tertian malarial (life) cycles were first detailed by this great histologist.

Golgi continued his studies in histology and remained active right up to his retirement from the University of Pavia in 1918. Golgi was one of Italy's greatest scientists and truly a giant in the study of the central nervous system.

JAMES T. GOODRICH

Selected Bibliography

PRIMARY SOURCES

Golgi, C. 1873. "Sulla struttura della sostanza grigia del cervello." *Gazzetta medica italiana Lombarda* (Milan) 33:224–246.

———. 1875. "Sui gliomi del cervello." *Rivista sperimentale di freniatria e medicina legale delle* 1:66–78.

———. 1883, 1884. "Recherches l'histologie des centres nerveux." *Archives italiennes de biologie*, 3:285–317, and 4:92–123.

———. 1885–86. *Sulla fina anatomia degli organi centrali del sistema nervoso*. Milan, U. Hoepli.

———. 1886. "Sull' infezione malarica." *Archivio per le scienze mediche* (*Torino*) 10:109–135.

SECONDARY SOURCES

DaFano, C. 1926. "Camillo Golgi." *Journal of Pathology and Bacteriology* 19:500–14.

Chorobski, J. 1935. "Camillo Golgi," *Archives of Neurology and Psychiatry* 33:163–70.

Clarke, E., and C. D. O'Malley. 1968. *The Human Brain and Spinal Cord*, 91–96. Berkeley and Los Angeles: University of California Press.

McHenry, L. 1969. *Garrison's History of Neurology*, 161–64. Springfield: Thomas.

Haymaker, W., and F. Schiller. 1970. *The Founders of Neurology*, 35–39. Springfield: Thomas.

RAGNAR ARTHUR GRANIT
1967

Ragnar Arthur Granit was born on October 30, 1900, in Helsinki, Finland. A neurophysiologist, Granit won the 1967 Nobel Prize, which he shared with H. K. Hartline and George Wald, for his seminal demonstration that light both stimulates and inhibits electrical activity in the eye. At the time of the award, he had just retired from his longtime position as professor and director of neurophysiology at the Karolinska Institute and was serving as a visiting professor at St. Catherine's College, Oxford. Granit and the Baroness Marguerite (Daisy) Brunn were married in 1929; their son Michael is an architect in Stockholm.

Granit's parents, Arthur Wilhelm Granit and Albertina Helena Malmberg Granit, were of Swedish descent. The elder Granit was a government forester, and later established a business firm that sold forest products. At age eighteen, Ragnar joined the Svidja Corps to fight for Finland's independence from revolutionary Russia; he was decorated for his services. The next year he entered Helsinki University to study psychology under Eino Kaila. Here he became interested in problems of vision and perception.

Granit received a master's degree in psychology in 1923, but his uncle, Dr. Lars Ringblom, urged him to enter medical school to complete his training. As a medical student at Helsinki, he soon realized that neurophysiology offered the best possibilities for seeking solutions to the questions that interested him. In 1926 he was Carl Tigerson's student assistant at the University Physiological Institute. After earning his M.D. in 1927, he was appointed docent, or instructor, in physiology.

In 1928 Granit traveled to Oxford to study with Sir Charles Sherrington and Edgar Adrian. Sherrington had demonstrated the inhibitory activity of nerves in leg muscles, while Adrian had pioneered in electroneurophysiology, attempting to record by vacuum tube amplification the impulses of individual nerve fibers. Previously, vision had chiefly been studied by physical observation, correlated with the perceptions of human subjects, but Granit realized that Adrian's techniques could be applied to the study of the retinal response to light.

After six months in England, Granit won the first fellowship in medical physics at the Eldridge Reeves Johnson Foundation of the University of Pennsylvania. He hastened his marriage to Daisy Brunn so that she could accompany him to Philadelphia in 1929. During this two years at the Johnson Foundation he worked under Detlev W. Bronk and with H. K. Hartline and the psychologist Clarence Graham, who helped him in some of his early psychophysical studies. He also met George Wald, then at Columbia.

While in the United States, Granit demonstrated, using standard observational tools (the "flicker method"), that retinal response to the brightness of a light was inversely correlated with its response to the darkness of a neighboring area; that is, that excitation of some retinal sensors enhanced the inhibition of others and vice versa. He found he was unable, as he had hoped, to "translate" psychology into neurology in a way that both fields would readily accept and therefore settled on neurology as the most promising field for his objectives (Granit 1967, 255–57).

In 1932 he returned to Oxford for further study with Sherrington and then rejoined the physiology department at Helsinki University. Granit was promoted to professor at Helsinki in 1937. He revisited Oxford in 1938 as he pursued his researches on the action potential of the retina.

The retinal action potential, the electrical discharge in response to light, was first described by Holmgren in 1865. But the nature and sequence of the response was quite complex and poorly understood. It was, as Granit perceived, impossible to interpret the ERG, the electroretinogram, purely in photochemical terms. He began by recording and comparing the ERG and the mass discharge of the optic nerve in response to light. The results clearly showed that a portion of the retinal response was inhibited at the same time that the remainder was stimulated. The implication of this discovery was that animal vision is not a simple reaction to light but uses the interplay of light and dark to analyze and interpret what it sees. Granit then used microelectrodes to break down the mass response and to record the activity of a few retinal ganglion cells at a time. These observations bore out his original insight (Granit 1967, 257–58).

The Soviet invasion of Finland in 1939 rudely interrupted his research. Reporting for military duty, he was assigned as district physician for the garrison and civilian population of three Baltic islands. From here, he was able to leave Finland after its forced capitulation in 1940. He was recruited by Harvard but chose to join the Karolinska as professor of neurophysiology and moved to Stockholm, eventually becoming a Swedish citizen. His professorship was supported by grants from the Wallenbergs Stiftelse and the Rockefeller Foundation.

Granit continued his microelectrode studies in Stockholm, switching from glass tubes to platinum wires. The retinal responses were both photographed and recorded acoustically for many animal species, including frogs, snakes, rats, and cats. In 1945 he described his model of three separate responses, based on the sensitivity of three different nerve fibers to varying wavelengths. The two principal responses are in fact directly antagonistic, as one type of fiber responds electrically to a given wavelength, while another stops discharging in response to the same wavelength. A light stimulus of a different wavelength will have exactly the reverse effects (Granit 1946).

Granit's description served as the basis for extensive work on sensory physiology. It has also been adapted as a clinical tool in the interpretation of normal and pathological vision. His work made clear that the response of the visual receptors to light and darkness was not limited to the photochemical mechanism described by George Wald but was also electroneural. These findings led to the complex understanding of vision achieved by David Hunter and Torsten Wiesel.

Granit's microelectrode studies also elucidated the processes of color vision, which he began studying in 1937. He identified some cone receptor cells ("dominators") that respond widely to the entire human visual spectrum and others ("modulators") that are stimulated only by one of three relatively narrow bands within the spectrum, corresponding with the three groups defined by the Thomas Young-Ferdinand von Helmholtz theory of color vision (red, yellow-green, and blue-violet) (Granit 1948; 1967; Ratliff 1967, 470).

In 1945 Granit's laboratory was incorporated into the Medical Nobel Institute as the Neurophysiological Institute, of which he was named director. A new building was planned, and the Ministry of Education established for him a personal research chair. His later research focused on the spinal cord and problems of motor control. He has done significant work on the electrical activity of neurons and muscle spindles (the organs that react to muscular tension) in muscle tissue and on the neural transmission of pain and of tactile sensation.

Ragnar Granit is a member of the Royal Swedish Academy of Sciences (president, 1963–65); the American Philosophical Society (1954); the Royal Society (1960); the American National Academy of Science (1968); and professional scientific organizations of many other countries, including Denmark, France, and Italy. He was appointed a visiting professor at Rockefeller University in 1956. In his retirement, he remained active as a lecturer, visiting professor, and researcher. Granit is an expert sailor and is often found in the summer piloting his yacht in the Baltic. In addition to his scientific publications, he wrote a scholarly biography of Sherrington, which came out shortly before the Nobel announcement (Ratliff 1967, 470–71).

Among the many other awards he has received for his work are the Lundsgaard Gold Medal (1938), the Jubilee Medal of the Swedish Society of Physicians (1947), the Bjorken Prize from the University of Uppsala (1948), the Anders Retzius Gold Medal from the University of Stockholm (1957), the Third International St. Vincent Prize from the Turin Academy of Medicine in Italy (1961), the Jahre Prize from Oslo University (1961), the Sherrington Memorial Gold Medal (1967), and the Purkinje Gold Medal from Prague (1969).

MARCIA MELDRUM

Selected Bibliography

PRIMARY SOURCES

Granit, Ragnar. 1935. "Two Types of Retinae and Their Electrical Responses to Intermittent Stimuli in Light and Dark Adaptation." *Journal of Physiology* 85 (December 16):421–38.

———. 1938. *On the Correlation of Some Sensory and Physiological Phenomena of Vision*. London: George Putnam.

Granit, Ragnar, and T. Helme. 1939. "Changes in Retinal Excitability Due to Polarization and Some Observations on the Relation Between Processes in Retina and Nerve." *Journal of Neurophysiology* 96 (June 14):31–44.

Granit, Ragnar. 1941. "Isolation of Color-Sensitive Elements in Mammalian Retina." *Acta Physiologica Scandinavica* 2:93–109.

———. 1946. "Distribution of Excitation and Inhibition in Single-Fibre Responses from Polarized Retina." *Journal of Physiology* 105 (July 15):45–53.

———. 1948. "Neural Organization of Retinal Elements, as Revealed by Polarization." *Journal of Neurophysiology* 11 (May):239–51.

———. 1948. "Mammalian Colour Modulators." *Journal of Neurophysiology* 11 (May):253–59.

———. 1963. *Sensory Mechanisms of the Retina*. New York: Hafner.

———. 1967. "The Development of Retinal Neurophysiology." Nobel Lecture, December 12, 1967. Reprinted in *Nobel Lectures in Physiology or Medicine* Vol. 4 (1963–1970), 255–288. Amsterdam: Elsevier.

———. 1980. *The Purposive Brain*. Cambridge: MIT Press.

SECONDARY SOURCES

Brody, Jane E. 1967. "Work of the Laureates Has Contributed to Grasp of the Visual Process." *New York Times* (October 19):40.

Wiskari, Werner. 1967. "Three Scientists Given Nobel Prize for Research on Eye." *New York Times* (October 19):1, 40.

Ratliff, Floyd. 1967. "Nobel Prize: Three Named for Medicine, Physiology Award. Ragnar Granit." *Science* 158 (October 27):469–71.

ROGER CHARLES LOUIS GUILLEMIN *1977*

Roger Charles Louis Guillemin received the Nobel prize in 1977 jointly with Andrew V. Schally "for their discoveries concerning the peptide hormone production of the brain." Rosalyn Yalow also shared the Nobel Prize that year for her development of the radioimmunoassay. Working independently and competitively, Guillemin and Schally isolated and structurally determined several hormones of the hypothalamic region of the brain that control the secretion of hormones by the anterior pituitary gland.

Roger Guillemin was born January 11, 1924, in Dijon, France. His parents were Raymond Guillemin and Blanche Rigollot Guillemin. After education in the public school of his home city, Guillemin attended the University of Dijon and was awarded a bachelor of arts and sciences degree in 1942. During the remaining wartime years he was a medical student, a medical intern, and a member of the French Resistance. Soon after the end of World War II Guillemin attended lectures in Paris given by Hans Selye on stress and diseases of adaptation. The effect on the young doctor was magnetic. Guillemin wrote years later that "for me, just out of medical school . . . in Nazi-occupied France, with teaching entirely directed toward medical care and no laboratory opportunities whatsoever, the lectures of Selye were from a different world" (Guillemin 1978, 222). Guillemin became a research assistant at Selye's Institute of Experimental Medicine and Surgery at the University of Montreal in 1948 and received his M.D. degree from the Faculty of Medicine of Lyons in 1949. Returning that year to the Montreal Institute, Guillemin now learned the fundamentals of experimental endocrinology by engaging in work dealing with the mechanisms involved in production of hypertension and kidney lesions by the adrenal hormone desoxycorticosterone acetate. He received his Ph.D. from the University of Montreal in 1953.

Guillemin married Lucienne Jeanne Billard on March 22, 1951. They have a son and five daughters.

In 1953 Guillemin became assistant professor of physiology and teacher of endocrinology at Baylor University School of Medicine in Houston. He had previously accepted a position at Yale but "there were at Baylor space, money, and an incredibly open future, and also azaleas and live oaks. Somehow I sensed that all that meant more than the Ivy League. I never regretted that decision" (Guillemin, "Pioneering in Neuroendocrinology," 224–225). He eventually became professor of physiology at Baylor before leaving in 1970 to establish the Laboratory of Neuroendocrinology at the Salk Institute for Biological Studies in La Jolla, California. Since 1970 he has worked at the Salk Institute as a resident fellow and chairman of the neuroendocrinology laboratory.

The foundation for the isolation and determination of hypothalamic hormones was established by an international group of scientists in the years immediately after World War II. The hypothalamus lies at the base of the brain in the posterior subdivision of the forebrain. It forms the floor of the third ventricle of the brain and is attached to the pituitary gland by a stalk. The hypothalamus was long known to participate in many important body functions, among them control of body temperature, blood pressure, hunger, thirst, sexual activity, and sleep. This complex collection of nerve cells and fiber tracts also contains cells that combine neural and secretory activity. It is this area, the "endocrine hypothalamus," that appears to control pituitary function.

Foremost among the scientists who assembled the evidence that established hypothalamic control of pituitary function was Geoffrey W. Harris, a British anatomist. In 1930 two other anatomists described a portal venous system that runs along the human pituitary stalk, which connects the hypothalamus and the pituitary gland. Harris and his coworkers in a series of brilliant experiments, demonstrated hypothalamic nerve fibers ending in relation to the origin of the portal system; confirmed that the anterior pituitary was electrically inexcitable (which contradicted the conventional wisdom of the time that electrical messages from the brain controlled the anterior pituitary gland); and showed that presence of the portal vessels were essential for normal anterior pituitary function. They formulated a neurovascular hypothesis which stated that neurohormones secreted by the hypothalamus coursed through the portal vessels to regulate secretion of anterior pituitary hormones. The pituitary hormones were known to control many important functions of the body including body growth, metabolism, stress responses, blood pressure regulation, sexual development and reproduction, and production of mother's milk. The pituitary performs these functions through elaboration of hormones that traverse the circulation of the body and in some instances control the secretions of other endocrine glands. Pituitary hormones with these actions include adrenocorticotropic hormone (ACTH); thyroid stimulating hormone (TSH); and the two gonodotropins, luteinizing hormone (LH), and follicle stimulating hormone (FSH), which together act on the ovaries and testes. In other instances anterior pituitary hormones act directly on peripheral tissues to exert their effects. Growth hormone and prolactin are such hormones.

With general acceptance of the neurovascular concept of anterior pituitary control came the extraordinary challenge in the 1950s of isolating and identifying the putative hypophysiotropic hormones—the hypothalamic factors that were transported in the portal system and controlled anterior pituitary secretion. The problem was to isolate and characterize at least one of these factors. Any one would do. As Guillemin recalled, "two groups of investigators approached the problem with enough constancy and resolution to stay with it for the 10 years that it took to provide the first definitive solution, that is, the primary structure of one of the hypothalamic hypophysiotropic factors" (Guillemin 1977, 390–401).

Working with Barry Rosenberg, a young student who was culturing anterior pituitary cells, Guillemin found that these cells would release ACTH when cocultured with fragments of hypothalamic tissue. (They could not measure ACTH directly but instead monitored the effect of this pituitary hormone on the depletion of adrenal ascorbic acid in animals—a sign that the pituitary hormone was stimulating adrenal activity in animal tissues.) So excited was Guillemin by this first sign in his laboratory of the presence of a hypothalamic hypophysiotropic factor that when he came home that evening he told his wife, "I have made an observation today of such importance that you will never have to worry about our future in academic medicine" (Guillemin, "Pioneering" 1978, 227).

At the same time at McGill University in Montreal, Murray Saffran and Andrew Schally were also attempting to isolate and characterize the hypothetical hypothalamic hormone that controlled release of ACTH from the anterior pituitary. They named the first putative hormone "corticotropin releasing factor" (CRF) in 1955; the terms "releasing factor" and "inhibiting factor" have been applied to chemically undetermined hypothalamic hypophysiotropic substances since. Despite exchanging information on methodology and improving culture techniques, incubation media, and experimental design, neither group succeeded in quickly isolating the elusive "corticotropin releasing factor." In 1957 Schally received his Ph.D. from McGill and joined Guillemin in Houston. For nearly five years they worked unsuccessfully on the isolation of CRF, and then Schally left for the Veterans Administration Hospital in New Orleans to establish his own research unit. Though they had failed to make real progress toward identifying the first hypothalamic hypophysiotropic factor, in Guillemin's words they "had learned a lot about the strategy of an isolation program that would be of use to both of us in future endeavors" (Guillemin 1978, 234).

According to Guillemin's recollection, over a three-year period his group organized the collection from slaughterhouses of five million fragments of sheep hypothalamus, handling in their laboratory fifty tons of hypothalamic tissue. "I went to about every one of the largest slaughterhouses in the Midwest and Southwest," he recalls, "spending one or two days working on the floor with the local people to make clear what I wanted. There were some colorful episodes; my French accent was of little help in Paris (Texas)" (Guillemin, "Pioneering in Neuroendocrinology," 233–234). Schally and his coworkers likewise harvested huge numbers of porcine hypothalamic fragments. They turned their attention from the elusive CRF to the isolation of a possible thyrotropin releasing factor (TRF) from the hypothalamus. This was the presumed substance that controlled thyroid stimulating hormone (TSH) produced by the anterior pituitary. The anterior pituitary hormone in turn regulated the functions of the thyroid gland.

After seven more years of intense, competitive work the two laboratories separately reported success. From 300,000 sheep hypothalami, Guillemin, Roger Burgus, T. F. Dunn, Wylie Vale, and D. Desiderio isolated 1.0 milligram of thyrotropin releasing factor. Schally, working with Karl Folkers, Franz Enzmann, Jan Boler, and Cyril Y. Bowers, also found a biologically active TRF, isolating 2.8 milligrams from 100,000 pig hypothalami. Both groups determined that the compound contained just three amino acids, establishing for the first time that TRH was a peptide (small protein). Schally's group determined the correct amino acid sequence, and then both groups successfully synthesized the first hypothalamic hormone. Subsequent studies have shown that human TRH has the same structure as the porcine hormone of Schally and the ovine hormone of Guillemin.

With the isolation, characterization, and synthesis of TRH completed in 1969, new hypothalamic hormones were discovered in the laboratories of the two persistent investigators. Schally and his colleagues between 1968 and 1971 isolated porcine luteinizing hormone releasing hormone (LHRH), the peptide hormone that regulates anterior pituitary production of its gonadotropins (sex hormones). In 1973 Guillemin and his coworkers isolated, sequenced, and synthesized a large hypothalamic peptide which they named somatostatin because it inhibited the secretion of anterior pituitary growth hormone. In 1981, more than twenty years after Guillemin and Schally vainly pursued CRF, Wyle Vale and colleagues at the Salk Institute finally elucidated the structure of the hypothalamic hormone that stimulates pituitary ACTH production and release. Its large size—CRF is a 41-amino acid peptide—was likely responsible for the difficulties all earlier investigators encountered in characterizing its structure.

All these hypothalamic hormones have quickly found roles in clinical medicine, particularly in the diagnosis of states of endocrine overactivity or deficiency. Most recently, an analogue of LHRH has found use as part of the hormonal preparation for women undergoing in vitro fertilization, and an analogue of somatostatin is being employed therapeutically in some patients with acromegaly (a disease produced by chronic hypersection of growth hormone).

Guillemin's and Schally's work had validated Geoffrey Harris's proposals concerning the mechanisms involved in hypothalamic control of the anterior pituitary. It was the hard-won concrete demonstration of a single hypothalamic hypophysiotropic factor that did it. As Guillemin wrote: "I consider the isolation and characterization of TRF as the major event in modern neuroendocrinology, the inflection point that separated confusion and a great deal of doubt from real knowledge. Modern neuroendocrinology was born of that event. . . . From observation of what has happened in neuroendocrinology since 1969, the isolation of TRF was also the vindication of my early decision, as a physiologist, that the most heuristic event in neuroendocrinology would be the isolation and characterization of the first one (any one) of the then-hypothetical hypothalamic hypophysiotropic factors.

"After TRF, pioneering in neuroendocrinology ceased and became the harvesting of a new and expanding science" (Guillemin, "Pioneering in Neuroendocrinology," 239).

LAWRENCE SHERMAN

Selected Bibliography

PRIMARY SOURCES

Guillemin, Roger, and B. Rosenberg. 1955. "Humoral Hypothalamic

Control of Anterior Pituitary: A Study with Combined Tissue Cultures." *Endocrinology* 57:599–607.

Guillemin, Roger, E. Yamazaki, M. Jutisz, and E. Sakiz. 1962. "Presence dans un extrait de tissues hypothalamiques d'une substance stimulant la secretion par filtration sur gel Sephadex." *Comptes Rendus del Academie des Sciences Paris* 255: 1018–20.

Guillemin, Roger, R. Burgus, and W. Vale. 1971. "The Hypothalamic Hypophysiotropic Thyrotropin-Releasing Factor." *Vitamins and Hormones* 29:1–39.

Brazeau, P., W. Vale, R. Burgus, N. Ling, M. Butcher, J. Rivier, and R. Guillemin. 1973. "Hypothalamic Polypeptide that Inhibits the Secretion of Immunoreactive Pituitary Growth Hormone." *Science*, 179: 77–79.

Guillemin, Roger. 1977. "Peptides in the Brain: The New Endocrinology of the Neuron." Nobel Lecture. Reprinted in *Science* 202 (October 27, 1978):390–401.

Guillemin, Roger. 1978. "Pioneering in Neuroendocrinology 1952–1969." In *Pioneers in Neuroendocrinology, II*, edited by J. Meites, B. T. Donovan, and S. M. McCann, 2:221–39. New York: Plenum Press.

SECONDARY SOURCES

Meites, Joseph. 1977. "The 1977 Nobel Prize in Physiology or Medicine." *Science* 198 (November 11):594–96.

Wade, Nicholas. 1981. *The Nobel Duel: Two Scientists' Twenty-one-Year Race to Win the World's Most Coveted Research Prize.* New York: Anchor Press/Doubleday.

McCann, S. M. 1988. "Saga of the Discovery of Hypothalamic Releasing and Inhibiting Hormones." In *Endocrinology: People and Ideas*, edited by S. M. McCann, 41–62. Bethesda, Md.: American Physiological Society.

ALLVAR GULLSTRAND *1911*

Allvar Gullstrand was born on June 5, 1862, in Landskrona, Sweden. An ophthalmologist, Gullstrand was awarded the Nobel Prize in 1911 for his work on the eye as an optical system. He was the oldest son of Sofia Mathilda Korsell and Pehr Alfred Gullstrand, a prominent Landskrona physician. He married Signe Christina Breitholtz in 1885, while still a student. They had one daughter, who died of diphtheria at the age of three. Gullstrand died on July 28, 1930, in Uppsala, Sweden.

Gullstrand displayed outstanding aptitude in mathematics during his elementary and high school years in Landskrona and Jönköping. From 1880 to 1885 he studied technical and medical sciences at the University of Uppsala. After a year in Vienna, he returned to Sweden to complete his license in medicine (1888) and his doctorate (1890) at Stockholm. His thesis on astigmatism, defended in May 1890, laid the ground for his theory of physiological optics (Gullstrand 1890).

In 1891 he became a lecturer in ophthalmology at the Karolinska Institut and in the same year was appointed chief physician of the Stockholm eye clinic. After holding a number of different positions in clinical medicine, teaching, and administration, he was appointed to a newly established professorship of ophthalmology at the University of Uppsala in 1894. In 1913 that institution created a special chair for Gullstrand in physiological and physical optics, a position without teaching obligations that he held until his retirement as professor emeritus in 1927.

After his retirement, he tried to continue his research, but was hampered by slowly declining health until his death from cerebral hemorrhage. He was buried in the North Cemetery of Stockholm. His scientific papers are deposited in the archives of the University of Uppsala (file D1080 a-1).

Gullstrand's contributions to medicine were both theoretical and practical. From his student days, his career was devoted to the study of "dioptrics," that is, the study of the human eye as a transparent system of lenses for the collection and refraction of light. By comparing the images actually projected on the retina with those predicted by the theoretical model of Helmholtz, he was able to demonstrate that the eye was not a homogenous medium and that accommodation, or differential bending of rays of light, was affected not only by the varying curvature of the lens (as already described by Helmholtz), but also by factors relating to the eye's internal composition. He named these factors the "intracapsular mechanism of accommodation" (Gullstrand 1900, 240). He described his theory in the appendices he added to the third edition of Helmholtz's treatise.

Gullstrand's other theoretical contributions included a study of known inaccuracies that persisted in the teaching of physiological optics even after they had been shown to be false (Gullstrand 1907). He also demonstrated that a yellow color occasionally found in the macula (the center of the retina) in cadavers was not a disease, as had previously been thought, but a postmortem change (Gullstrand 1905).

The practical advances made by Gullstrand were diverse and long lasting. He developed photographic methods for measuring the degree of corneal astigmatism (modification in the shape of the cornea causing it to resemble a cylindrical rather than a spherical section) and discovering the precise location of a paralyzed eye muscle (1892). With the aid of M. von Rohr of the Zeiss company, he worked on the Verant magnifying glass, which gave a wider field of observation for examining photographs. The magnifier was little used, but the principles developed were applied to eyeglasses. Gullstrand also designed aspheric lenses for individuals with high refractive error, or an inability to focus light, such as occurs after the removal of the crystalline lens for cataract.

His most important technical achievement, in 1910, was the improvement of the ophthalmoscope, an instrument invented by Helmholtz in 1851 for observations of the fundus, or back of the eye, where the retina and head of the optic nerve are located. Gullstrand's "reflexless" ophthalmoscope, manufactured by Zeiss, used the optical system of the patient's own eye to focus light emanating directly from a diaphragm light source, rather than via reflection. The standing model of this ophthalmoscope was the precursor of the slit lamp (1911). This instrument is a powerful microscope that allows the examiner to make detailed, stereoscopic observations of the frontal two-thirds of the darkened eye by focussing a shaft of light at varying depths. It is still one of the most important ophthalmological tools.

Gullstrand mistrusted innovation and employed a rigorous approach to mathematics. His reservations about the theory of relativity have been held responsible for the indifference of the Nobel Committee for Physics to this aspect of Einstein's work. He was completely self-taught in the field of geometrical and physiological optics, to which he made such an important contribution. He devised his own mathematical solutions, which biographers have noted as evidence of his ingenuity and the elegance of his work. But his papers have also been criticized as long and clumsy, even opaque. These defects resulted in part from his prejudice against the "false ornaments" of certain mathematical methods and his ignorance of the work of his predecessor, the nineteenth-century Irish mathematician, William Rowan Hamilton, on geometrical optics (Herzberger 1972). Former colleagues hasten, however, to remark on the lucidity of his clinical teaching and his dedication to that work.

Gullstrand held honorary doctorates from the universities of Uppsala and Iena. He was a member (1911–22) and president 1922–25) of the Nobel Committee for Physics; he was also president of the Swedish Academy of Science (1925–26). He was awarded the von Graefe medal by the Deutsche Ophthalmologische Gesellschaft.

JACKIE DUFFIN

Selected Bibliography

PRIMARY SOURCES

Gullstrand, Allvar. 1890. "Bidrag till astigmatismens teori." M.D. Thesis. Stockholm.

———. 1900. "Allgemeine Theorie des Monochromatischen Aberrationem und ihre Nächsten Ergebnisse für die Ophthalmologie." *Nova Acta Regiae Societatis Scientarum Upsaliensis*, ser. 3, 20:240.

———. 1905. "Die Farbe der Macula Centralis Retina." *Graefes Archiv für Ophthalmologie* 62:1–72, 378.

———. 1907. "Tatsachen und Fiktionen

in der Lehre von der Optischen Abbildung." *Archiv fur Optik* 1:2–41, 81–97.

———. 1909. "Appendices I–V." In *Helmholtz' Treatise on Physiological Optics*, 3 Vols., edited and translated by James P. C. Southall, 1:261–443. New York: Dover, 1962.

———. 1911. *Einführing in die Methoden de Dioptick des Auges des Menschen*. Leipzig: HIRZEL.

———. 1911. "Opthalmoscopy (Appendix VI)." Reprinted In *Helmholtz' Treatise on Physiological Optics*, 3 vols. edited and translated by James P. C. Southall, 1:443–82. New York: Dover, 1962.

———. 1911. "How I found the Mechanism of Intracapsular Accommodation." Nobel Lecture. Reprinted in *Nobel Lectures in Physiology or Medicine*, 4 vols. vol. 1 (1901–1921), 414–31. Amsterdam: Elsevier, 1967.

SECONDARY SOURCES

Ask, F. 1930."Allvar Gullstrand." *Acta Ophthalmologica* 8:247–52.

Berg, Fredrik. 1952. "Allvar Gullstrand (1862–1930)." In *Swedish Men of Science*, edited by Sten Lindroth, 239–48. Stockholm: Almquist.

Herzberger, Maximilian, J. 1960. "Allvar Gullstrand." *Optica Acta* 3: 237–41.

Nordenson, J. W. 1962. "Allvar Gullstrand." *Documenta Ophthalmologica. Advances in Ophthalmology* 16:283–337. Contains bibliography.

Snyder, C. 1962. "Allvar Gullstrand." *Archives of Ophthalmology* 68:139.

Herzberger, Maximilian J. 1972. "Gullstrand, Allvar." In *Dictionary of Scientific Biography*, 15 vols. 5: 590–91. New York: Scribners.

HALDAN KEFFER HARTLINE

1967

Haldan Keffer Hartline was born on December 22, 1903, in Bloomsburg, Pennsylvania. A biophysicist, he received the Nobel Prize in 1967 with Ragnar Granit and George Wald for his elucidation of the electroneural mechanisms of vision. At the time of the award, Hartline was Detlev W. Bronk Professor of Biophysics at Rockefeller University. He married Elizabeth Kraus, an instructor in comparative psychology at Bryn Mawr, in 1936; they had three sons, Daniel Keffer, Peter Haldan, and Frederick Flanders, all of whom chose careers in biology or neurophysiology. He retired in 1974 to his home in Maryland, and died following a heart attack on March 17, 1983.

Hartline's parents, Daniel Schollenberger Hartline and Harriet Franklin Keffer, were teachers at the State Normal School in Bloomsburg. His father taught biology but had a wide range of scientific interests and encouraged his son's early interest in science. At Lafayette College in Easton, Pennsylvania, young Keffer studied biology with Beverly W. Kunkel, who urged him to undertake his first research project on the phototropic reactions of land isopods. During the summers he worked at the Marine Biological Laboratory in Woods Hole, Massachusetts, where his work attracted the attention of Jacques Loeb, Selig Hecht, and Merkel Jacobs. These mentors introduced him to the application of quantitative measurement and analysis, as developed in physics and chemistry, to the study of animal physiology.

After his graduation from Lafayette with a B.S. degree in 1923, Hartline entered Johns Hopkins Medical School, where he continued investigations into the physiology of vision under E. K. Marshall and C. D. Snyder. Using an Einthoven string galvanometer belonging to Snyder, he developed methods of recording electrical discharge from the retinas of frogs, cats, rabbits, and—eventually—human subjects; for this work he won the William H. Howell Award in 1927. Hartline saw that much could be learned from correlating overt visual activity with electrical recordings. He was further inspired by Edgar Adrian's work in recording electrical activity in individual neurons, reported in 1926, shortly before Hartline's completion of his medical degree. The following year Adrian recorded the electrical discharge of the optic nerve of the conger eel, but was not able to differentiate the impulses of the individual nerve fibers (Ratliff 1967).

To achieve such differentiation, Hartline knew that he would have to employ rigorous and innovative methods drawn from physics and mathematics. After earning his M.D. in 1927, therefore, he obtained a National Research Council Fellowship, allowing him to study mathematics and physics at Johns Hopkins, working under F. D. Murnaghan and A. H. Pfund. After two years of this training, he received an Eldridge Reeves Johnson Traveling Fellowship from the University of Pennsylvania, which enabled him to study physics with Werner Heisenberg in Leipzig and then to spend two semesters attending the lectures of A. Somerfeld in Munich.

Returning to the United States in 1931, he accepted a position at the Johnson Foundation for Medical Physics at the University of Pennsylvania, under the directorship of Detlev W. Bronk. Bronk and Hartline thus began a productive association that extended for many years. Hartline also met and collaborated with Ragnar Granit and Clarence W. Graham at the foundation. During another Woods Hole summer, he was introduced to the young George Wald.

Graham was enlisted in the effort to record the electrical activity of single fibers in the optic nerve. For their initial experiments, the team selected the horseshoe crab,

Limulus. The crab's large compound eyes are the receptors for very long optic nerves, making separation of the individual fibers relatively easy. In 1932 Hartline and Graham succeeded in recording impulses from a single fiber. The impulses were identical in amplitude and shape but varied in frequency with the brightness of the light source on the receptor cell, showing the most dramatic change when the source was turned off altogether. They demonstrated in this way that visual information is transmitted to the brain by the frequency of the impulses and is highly responsive to variation in intensity. Further studies with *Limulus* clarified such areas as the eye's sensitivity to the color spectrum (Hartline 1934, 1935; Ratliff 1967).

Limulus is a fairly primitive animal, with a primitive visual system, and the activity recorded from each of the many fibers was quite similar. In the late 1930s, however, Hartline turned his attention to the eyes of cold-blooded vertebrates. This research required him to develop highly precise and meticulous techniques of microdissection to separate the single fibers of the retina. The results were highly significant; unlike the fibers of *Limulus*, those of the frog, for example, were discovered to be highly differentiated. Some responded to changes in brightness, some to movement, some to removal of the light only. Hartline thus demonstrated that the single response of the optic nerve recorded by Adrian represented the end product—the "spatial summation"—of multiple complex responses to fractional stimuli, processed through the retina to form an integrated "picture" for transmission to the brain (Hartline 1938, 1940).

These findings revealed a physiology of vision far more complex than any previously hypothesized. As Hartline noted, "Individual nerve cells never act independently; it is the integrated action of all the units of the visual system that give rise to vision" (Hartline 1942). The importance of this understanding for human vision was recognized by psychologists as well as neurophysiologists. The Society of Experimental Physiologists awarded Hartline its Howard Crosby Warren Medal in 1948 (Ratliff 1967).

Except for a year as associate professor at Cornell University Medical College (1940–41), Hartline remained at the Johnson Foundation through the 1940s. For a time during World War II he studied problems of human night vision for the military. In 1949 he was appointed professor and chairman of the Biophysics Department at Johns Hopkins.

By this time, methods of microelectrode recording and vacuum-tube amplification had been developed to the point where Hartline could simultaneously record and correlate the activity of the photoreceptor cells, retinal ganglion cells, and optic fibers. For these studies he returned to the simple visual network of *Limulus*. By mapping the optic fiber response to stimuli applied to the photoreceptor cells, he demonstrated that the fiber itself receives information not just from one cell or a small group of cells but from many receptors over a variety of pathways. He also noted that excitation and inhibition of the receptors appeared to be not simply opposed states, but interactive. Excitation caused by bright lights, for example, inhibits the response of other receptors to nearby dark areas.

After joining Rockefeller University in 1953, Hartline devoted his attention to this question of excitation and inhibition in *Limulus*. With his associate Floyd Ratliff, he determined that the interaction emphasizes border, change, and pattern, enhancing the contrast between light and dark, between on and off, and deepening perceptions of contour and variation. Hartline's work with the horseshoe crab was the foundation for David Hunter and Torsten Wiesel's later research with the visual cortex of the cat, which clearly established the importance of the interaction of multiple pieces of visual information in creating the complex picture seen by the animal (Hartline and Ratliff 1958, 1959; Ratliff 1967).

A shy and unassuming man, Hartline was deeply respected by his students and colleagues. From his early dissection techniques to his creation of computer programs in his sixties, his fertile mind remained active and innovative in his "slightly disorganized but extremely fertile chaos" of a laboratory. Outside the lab he enjoyed active, even reckless sports, mountain climbing as a young man, and later flying and sailing, a passion he shared with Bronk and Granit (Ratliff 1967, 471).

He was a member of the National Academy of Science, the American Association for the Advancement of Science, the Royal Society of London, and the American Physiological Society, among others. The many awards he won included the Michelson Award from the Case Institute of Technology (1964) and the Lighthouse Award (1969).

MARCIA MELDRUM

Selected Bibliography

PRIMARY SOURCES

Hartline, H. K. 1934. "Intensity and Duration in Excitation of Single Photoreceptor Units." *Journal of Cellular and Comparative Physiology* 5 (October 20):229–47.

———. 1935. "Discharge of Nerve Impulses from Single Visual Nerve Cell." *Cold Spring Harbor Symposium on Quantitative Biology* 3:245–50.

———. 1938. "Responses of Single Optic Nerve Fibers of Vertebrate Eye to Illumination of Retina." *American Journal of Physiology* 121 (February):400–415.

———. 1940. "Effects of Spatial Summation in Retina on Excitation of Fibers of Optic Nerve." *American Journal of Physiology* 130 (October):700–711.

———. 1942. "Neural Mechanisms of Vision." *Harvey Lectures*, Series 37 (1941–42):39–68.

Hartline, H. K., and F. Ratliff. 1957. "Inhibitory Interaction of Receptor Units in the Eye of *Limulus*." *Journal of General Physiology* 40 (January 20):357–76.

———. 1958. "Spatial Summation of Inhibitory Influences in the Eye of *Limulus*, and the Mutual Interaction of Receptor Units." *Journal of General Physiology* 41 (May 20): 1049–66.

———. 1959. "The Responses of *Limulus* Optic Nerve Fibers to Patterns of Illumination on the Receptor Mosaic." *Journal of General Physiology* 42 (July 20):1241–55.

Hartline, H. K. 1974. *Studies on Excitation and Inhibition in the Retina: A Collection of Papers from the Laboratories of H. Keffer Hartline.* New York: Rockefeller University Press.

SECONDARY SOURCES

Brody, Jane E. 1967. "Work of the Laureates Has Contributed to Grasp of the Visual Process." *New York Times* (October 19):40.

Ratliff, Floyd. 1967. "Nobel Prize: Three Named for Medicine, Physiology Award. Haldan Keffer Hartline." *Science* 158 (October 27): 471–73.

Wiskari, Werner. 1967. "Three Scientists Given Nobel Prize for Research on Eye." *New York Times* (October 19)1, 40.

PHILIP S. HENCH *1950*

Philip Showalter Hench was born in Pittsburgh, Pennsylvania, on February 28, 1896, the son of Jacob B. Hench, a school administrator, and Clara Showalter Hench. He had a lifelong speech impediment due to a cleft palate. After attending local schools and spending one year at the University of Pittsburgh, he transferred to Lafayette College in Pennsylvania and graduated in 1916. He then entered the University of Pittsburgh School of Medicine, receiving the M.D. in 1920. Hench served a year of internship at the St. Francis Hospital in Pittsburgh, followed by two years of residency in internal medicine at St. Mary's Hospital in Rochester, Minnesota, the main hospital of the Mayo Clinic. In 1923 he was appointed a staff internist at the Mayo Clinic, where he remained throughout his career (Slocumb 1965; Eckman 1965).

In the 1920s interest in rheumatic diseases was largely focused on rheumatic fever. Hench's interest in the broader range of rheumatic diseases was not only unusual, but immediate and consuming. As first evidence of this, in October 1924 he presented a lecture to the Pennsylvania State Medical Society based on 320 cases of rheumatoid arthritis "Hospitalized on the combined medical and orthopedic services of the Mayo Clinic during the last two years." In 1925 this lecture became his first publication, entitled "The Systemic Nature of Chronic Infectious Arthritis" (Hench 1925). His interest was rewarded in 1926 when he was appointed to initiate a Department of Diseases of Joints and Rheumatic Diseases. In 1927 he began the first rheumatologic training program in the United States. From autumn 1928 until summer 1929 he studied laboratory medicine with Ludwig Aschoff at the University of Freiburg and clinical medicine with Friedrich von Müller at the University of Munich. Upon his return he remained the only rheumatologist at the Mayo Clinic until 1935, when he was joined by Charles H. Slocumb, whom he had trained.

Hench's scientific interests always were clinically oriented and his students became clinical rheumatologists and clinical investigators, rather than basic scientists. He was slow to publish a new observation, preferring to gather longitudinal data. In 1941 he briefly described a disease he called palindromic rheumatism (a benign intermittent polyarthritis) and three years later he reported thirty-four cases, the first of whom he had followed from 1928 until 1942 (Hench and Rosenberg 1944).

His observations on the effect of liver disease on rheumatoid arthritis, which eventually led to the clinical trial of cortisone, had a similar history. In April 1929 he observed a man whose well-established rheumatoid arthritis remitted during an episode of jaundice (presumably hepatitis). The remission lasted for several weeks after the jaundice had cleared. Hench waited four years to report this phenomenon, by which time he had observed remissions in nine cases of rheumatoid arthritis and in five other patients (Hench 1933). In 1938 he published a comprehensive review based on experience with nineteen cases of rheumatoid arthritis, nine of "primary fibrositis," and three others. He found that pain relief was not related to the etiology of the hepatogenic jaundice, but that the disease had to be severe enough to raise the serum bilirubin concentration to at least 8 mg/DL. Hench concluded: "Nature possesses a highly effective method of quickly stopping the disease (rheumatoid arthritis) for a while and of producing a dramatic remission; this phenomenon is precipitated more rapidly and more completely by jaundice than by any other known physiologic change or therapeutic method. It behooves physicians to discover this antidote and the mechanism of its action." The infusion or ingestion of bile pigments or bile acids was found to exert no antirheumatic effect, while chemical injury of the liver might be effective, but hazardous (Hench 1938).

The other physiologic antirheumatic mechanism, which Hench began to study clinically in 1931, was pregnancy. There had been a few reports of a suppressive effect of pregnancy on intermittent hydrarthrosis (possibly a variant of rheumatoid arthritis), but no investigation of the effect of pregnancy on well-documented rheumatoid arthritis. In 1938 he summarized observations on thirty-seven pregnancies in twenty-two women: fifteen with rheumatoid arthritis, two with psoriatic arthropathy and five with less certain diagnoses. Remissions were obtained by twenty women during thirty-four pregnancies. The same response occurred during repeated pregnancies, remission generally beginning during the first trimester and ending within three months of delivery. Hench concluded: "It does not seem illogical to suppose that the agents responsible for both these phenomena are closely related, perhaps identical, and if the agent is a chemical substance, it would appear that it is neither bilirubin nor a strictly female sex hormone. It is interesting to note the close chemical relationship between such diverse substances as cholesterol, ergosterol (the precursor of vitamin D), some of the sex hormones, cortin and bile acids. . . . If the potent common denominator of these two phenomena—the ameliorating effects of pregnancy and of jaundice—can be discovered, progress in treatment may be expected" (Hench 1938).

By 1938 Hench was convinced that there is a physiologic antirheumatic substance and he now consulted Edward C. Kendall, the chief biochemist of the Mayo Clinic, about what this substance might be. In 1930 Kendall had begun an effort to extract "the hormone" of the adrenal cortex. As of 1938 several closely related steroids had been isolated in his laboratory. The fifth one, designated "compound E," was identified by Kendall in 1935 and in other laboratories in the following year, but its physiologic properties were not yet recognized (Kendall 1951).

From 1938 on Hench and Kendall became collaborators, and in 1941 they decided to administer compound E to a patient with rheumatoid arthritis when enough became available. This was based on Hench's unsubstantiated impression that the fatiguability commonly associated with rheumatoid arthritis may be due to an adrenal hormone deficiency and recent experimental findings by Kendall, tangential as they may have been (Hench 1952). The latter had found that as little as 30 mcgm of compound E protects an adrenalectomized rat against the stress of typhoid vaccine. Soon thereafter he showed that an even smaller dose protects such an animal against low temperature exposure (Kendall 1941).

World War II interrupted Hench's research activities. By 1942, when he became an army medical officer, he had become a nationally recognized authority on the rheumatic diseases. In 1935 he initiated the nearly annual publication of a comprehensive review of the American and English rheumatologic literature (*Rheumatism Review*), remaining its editor through the ninth edition, in 1947 (Hench et al. 1935). In 1939–40 he was the third president of the American Rheumatism Association. He became an advisor to the surgeon general of the army with the result that military "Rheumatism Centers" were established. The first of these was activated at Hot Springs, Arkansas, in 1943 with Hench as chief of medical services (Smith 1968, 3).

Quantities of adrenal steroids sufficient for clinical trials could not be extracted from glands and required partial syntheses, which then began with desoxycholic (bile) acid. This was first achieved for desoxycorticosterone and next for corticosterone (Kendall's compound A). Trials in 1946 and 1947 showed that compound A was not adequate treatment for Addison's disease. The first clinical trial of compound E was made in early 1948 in a case of Addison's disease with a daily intramuscular dose of 20 mg. This also proved inadequate (Sprague et al. 1948; Polley 1976).

In September 1948 Hench prevailed on Merck and Company to provide several grams of compound E to try in patients with rheumatoid arthritis. Slocumb decided on a dosage of 50 mg. twice daily, which was presumed to be large enough to demonstrate whether the substance is effective. The first patient appeared dramatically more comfortable and mobile after her third injection. Treatment of additional patients soon was begun with everyone sworn to secrecy for fear that results of the unorthodox treatment would be publicized prematurely. The first report was made at the weekly staff meeting of the Mayo Clinic on April 13, 1949, and published in the next *Proceedings*. It was based on observations on fourteen patients, seven of whom had been treated for at least six weeks. Although clinical benefits were observed consistently, they dissipated rapidly after treatment was stopped. Soon thereafter Hench coined the term "cortisone" for compound E, this being a contraction of *corti*co*sterone* (Polley 1976; Hench et al. 1949).

Closely associated with the question whether there is a specific antirheumatic adrenal hormone was another. Would stimulation of the adrenal cortex exert a similar desirable effect, or might a "toxic steroid" be released? Fairly pure preparations of corticotropin (ACTH) had been produced in 1943, but Hench first obtained ACTH from the Armour Company in January 1949. It was first administered to a patient with rheumatoid arthritis in the next month and no hypothetical effect occurred (Polley 1976).

Two comprehensive reports, in February 1950 (Sprague et al. 1950) and two months later (Hench et al. 1950) cited experience with twenty-three cases of rheumatoid arthritis (six probably were ankylosing spondylitis), eight cases of acute rheumatic fever, six cases of systemic lupus erythematosus, and seven others. Three rheumatoid arthritis patients also received a course of compound A, which revealed no antirheumatic effect, and one received 75 mg. of compound F (hydrocortisone) daily for twelve days with "moderate" benefit. Eleven patients received ACTH, four of them for longer than thirty days. Potency varied, but the feared toxicity was not observed and benefit resembled that obtained with cortisone.

The first reports of the dramatic effects of compound E resulted in tremendous lay and professional publicity. As more compound E, as cortisone acetate, became available, it was evaluated in numerous diseases, with similar short-term positive results in most circumstances. In 1950, after the extraordinarily brief interval of one year since the clinical discovery, Hench, together with his colleague Kendall and the Swiss biochemist, Tadeus Reichstein, were awarded the Nobel Prize, "For their discoveries concerning the suprarenal cortex hormones, their structure and biological effects." More specifically, Hench received his award because "Your brilliant investigations in respect of the beneficial effects of pregnancy and jaundice on rheumatoid arthritis have been the starting point for the famous discovery during the preceding year that these diseases and some others are favourably influenced by hormones from the adrenal cortex. Thereby new therapeutic possibilities have been opened up, and a deeper insight into the nature of these conditions and the role of the adrenal cortex has been gained" (Liljestrand 1950, 263–69). The only possible explanation for the timing of the award was the unbridled optimism that a cure had been found for a number of common, disabling diseases. Hench considered this attitude premature and did what he could to advise of the importance of maintaining scientific objectivity.

After 1950 Hench's participation in clinical research diminished. He coauthored several reviews of the clinical effects of cortisone, hydrocortisone, and ACTH. In 1954 he wrote: "The final role of these hormones in clinical medicine must await further experience. . . . Above all else, these hormones constitute the most powerful research tool ever developed for the study of rheumatic and certain other diseases. They still belong as much, if not more, to physiologists and clinical investigators as to rheumatologists and other physicians" (Ward et al. 1954). This was Hench's attitude five years after the introduction of cortisone! The last paper of which he was a coauthor was published in November 1958: "Plasma 17-hydroxycorticosteroids in Patients with Certain Rheumatic Diseases and in Normal Persons" (Ward et al. 1958).

In 1953 Hench became a senior consultant; he retired from the Mayo Clinic and the faculty of its Graduate School of Medicine in 1957. Philip Hench had married Mary G. Kahler of Rochester, Minnesota, in 1927; the couple had two sons and two daughters, all of whom survived him. Hench, who suffered from diabetes mellitus, died of pneumonia on March 30, 1965.

THOMAS G. BENEDEK, M.D.

Selected Bibliography

PRIMARY SOURCES

Hench, Philip S. 1925. "The Systemic Nature of Chronic Infectious Arthritis." *Atlantic Medical Journal.* 28:425–36.

———. 1933. "Analgesia accompanying Hepatitis and Jaundice in Cases of Chronic Arthritis, Fibrositis, and Sciatic Pain." *Proceedings of the Staff Meetings of the Mayo Clinic.* 8:430–36.

Hench, P. S., W. Bauer, A. A. Fletcher, et al. 1935. "The Present Status of the Problem of "Rheumatism;" a Review of Recent American and English Literature on "Rheumatism" and Arthritis." *Annals of Internal Medicine.* 8:1315–74.

Hench, P. S. 1938. "Effect of Jaundice on Chronic Infectious (Atrophic) Arthritis and on Primary Fibrositis." *Archives of Internal Medicine.* 61:451–60.

———. 1938. "The Ameliorating effect of Pregnancy on Chronic Atrophic (Infectious Rheumatoid) Arthritis, Fibrositis, and Intermittent Hydrarthrosis." *Proceedings of the Staff Meetings of the Mayo Clinic.* 13:161–66.

Hench, P. S., and E. F. Rosenberg. 1944. "Palindromic Rheumatism." *Archives of Internal Medicine.* 73:293–321.

Hench, P. S., E. C. Kendall, C. H. Slocumb and H. F. Polley. 1949. "The Effect of a Hormone of the Adrenal Cortex (17-hydroxy-11-dehydrocorticosterone; Compound E) and of Pituitary Adrenocorticotropic Hormone on Rheumatoid Arthritis." *Proceedings of the Staff Meetings of the Mayo Clinic.* 24:181–97 (April 13).

Sprague, R. G., M. H. Power, H. L. Mason, et al. 1950. "Observations on the Physiologic Effects of Cortisone and ACTH in Man." *Archives of Internal Medicine.* 85:199–258.

Hench, P. S., E. C. Kendall, C. H. Slocumb, and H. F. Polley. 1950. "Effects of Cortisone Acetate and Pituitary ACTH on Rheumatoid Arthritis, Rheumatic Fever and Certain Other Conditions." *Archives of Internal Medicine.* 85:545–666.

Hench, P. S. 1952. "The Reversibility of Certain Rheumatic and Nonrheumatic Conditions by the Use of Cortisone or of the Pituitary Adrenocorticotropic Hormone." [Nobel Lecture] *Annals of Internal Medicine.* 36:1–38.

Ward, L. E., H. F. Polley, C. H. Slocumb, P. S. Hench, et al. 1954. "The Effects of Adlosterone (Electrocortin) and of 9α-fluoro-hydrocortisone Acetate on Rheumatoid Arthritis: Preliminary Report." *Proceedings of the Staff Meetings of the Mayo Clinic.* 29:649–63.

Ward, L. E., Wu C., Hench, P. S., et al. 1958. "Plasma 17-hydroxycorticosteroids in Patients with certain Rheumatic Diseases and in Normal Persons." *Proceedings of the Staff Meetings of the Mayo Clinic.* 33:611–26.

SECONDARY SOURCES

Kendall, E. C. 1941. "The Adrenal Cortex." *Archives of Pathology.* 32:474–501.

Sprague, R. G., Gastineau, C. F., Mason, H. L., Power, M. H. 1948. "Effects of Synthetic 11-dehydrocorticosterone (Compound A) in a Subject with Addison's Disease." *American Journal of Medicine.* 4:175–85.

Liljestrand, G. 1950. Presentation Speech, December 11. *Nobel Lectures. Physiology or Medicine, 1942–1962.* Pp. 263–69. Amsterdam: Elsevier, 1964.

Kendall, E. C. 1951. "The Development of Cortisone as a Therapeutic Agent." *Antibiotics and Chemotherapy.* 1:7–15.

Slocumb, C. H. 1965. "Philip Showalter Hench 1896–1965. In Memoriam."

Arthritis and Rheumatism. 8: 573–76.

Eckman, J. 1965. "Philip Showalter Hench, M.D." *Journal-Lancet*. 85:218–20.

Smith, R. T. "Rheumatic Diseases." Chapter 18 in Havens, W. P., Editor, *Internal Medicine in World War II*, Volume III. Medical Department, United States Army, Washington, D.C., 1968.

Polley, H. F., Slocumb, C. H. 1976. "Behind the Scenes with Cortisone and ACTH." *Mayo Clinic Proceedings*. 51:471–77.

ALFRED DAY HERSHEY 1969

Alfred Day Hershey was born on December 4, 1908, in Owosso, Michigan. A virologist and molecular geneticist, Hershey shared the Nobel Prize in 1969 with Salvador Luria and Max Delbrück for their "transform[ation of] the landscape of classical Mendelian genetics into the latter-day 'molecular' Crick-Watsonian scene" (Stent 1969, 479). Hershey's specific accomplishment was the experimental demonstration in 1952 that DNA, not protein, is the genetic key to cellular self-reproduction, which spurred the various efforts then in progress to determine the structure of DNA and led within a year to the discovery of the double helix. At the time of his award, Hershey was director of the Carnegie Genetics Research Unit at the Cold Spring Harbor Laboratory, the position he held until his retirement. He married a former research assistant, Harriet Davidson, in 1945; she later became an editor of the *Cold Spring Harbor Symposia on Quantitative Biology*. The Hersheys have one son, Peter Manning.

Alfred Hershey grew up in Lansing, where his father, Robert Day Hershey, worked for an auto manufacturer. His mother was the former Alma Wilbur. He became interested in bacteriology while at Michigan State College and elected to pursue a doctorate there under I. F. Huddleson. In 1934 he presented his thesis, on the chemistry of *Brucella*, the bacteria that causes brucellosis or undulant fever, and received his Ph.D. in chemistry. Hershey then accepted a position as a research assistant in the Department of Bacteriology at Washington University in St. Louis. Here he had the opportunity to work with Jacques Jacob Bronfenbrenner, who had pioneered research on bacteriophages in the United States.

A bacteriophage is a virus that infects bacteria. Like other viruses, a phage is little more than a cellular nucleus, consisting of protein and deoxyribonucleic acid, or DNA, as classically described by Albrecht Kossell in the 1880s. A part of the phage invades the bacterial host cell and combines with it in such a way that the bacterium is converted completely to the self-reproduction of the virus and the production of multiple identical viruses. After their discovery in Europe in 1915, bacteriophages became the focus of much interest on the part of virologists, who saw in them the key to understanding and combating viral diseases that infect man.

A few scientists, however, identified the problem as the process of self-replication, one of the most puzzling in biology. Although animals and plants were understood to reproduce genetically, the question of how the gene reproduced *itself* remained unanswered. Since the viral phage was believed in the 1930s to be similar in size to an ordinary gene, the observation of the process of its self-reproduction within the bacterial host could provide a clue to the genetic enigma.

One of the leading proponents of this idea was Max Delbrück, a German physicist who had come to the United States in 1937 to study genetics at Caltech. He quickly abandoned the classical school and began to study phages with Emory Ellis. In 1939 Delbrück and Ellis published a landmark paper suggesting the importance of the phage model and establishing that the process of viral reproduction and lysis (or dissolution) of the bacterial cell lasted about half an hour after infection. In this time, several hundred new phages were produced (Stent 1969, 479–80).

In 1940 Delbrück met Italian physician Salvador Luria at a meeting of the American Physical Society in Philadelphia. Luria had just fled from Paris to escape the Nazi occupation and had taken a research position at Columbia. The two immigrants quickly discovered their mutual interest and launched a collaboration that was to become known as the "American Phage Group." In 1942 Luria and Thomas Anderson managed to use the electron microscope to "photograph" phages, which proved that the invasive particle was shaped rather like a comet with a round head attached to a thin tail.

The following year Delbrück and Luria published another classic paper in *Genetics*, which dealt with the phenomenon of phage-resistant bacteria within a phage-sensitive culture. Their findings directly refuted Lamarckian theory that genetic modification, or mutation, is a gradual process occurring in response to environmental factors. The phage-resistant bacteria observed by Delbrück and Luria were spontaneous mutants. When entered by the phage, these cells resisted invasion by mutating not into a viral incubator but a variant bacteria (Delbrück and Luria 1943, Stent 1969, 480).

Hershey had meanwhile been pursuing bacteriological research in St. Louis. He was promoted to assistant professor in 1938 and associate professor four years later. That same year, Hershey visited Delbrück at Vanderbilt University, where he was working on the draft of the phage mutation paper. That conversation inspired him to become a member of the "American Phage Group" and he began a regular correspondence with Delbrück and Luria.

Hershey soon began doing significant work. In 1945 he and Luria, working independently, demonstrated the spontaneous mutation of bacteriophages: introduced into a phage-resistant culture, most of the viruses would die but some of the viral material would mutate to create a new variant virus that could then infect the host. The following year Hershey and Delbrück reported on additional phage mutations; it was Hershey who perceived that these were actually forms of genetic recombination, which conventional theory held possible only in higher forms of life. Hershey and Raquel Rotman were able to demonstrate the "exchange" of genetic material between viruses, similar to that of chromosome during reproductive meiosis of other organisms (Delbrück 1946, Stent 1969, 480).

By 1951 Hershey, Seymour Benzer, and others had applied these findings to develop a model of phage genetics, which led to a new understanding of the whole field. Moreover, the observations on mutation, and Luria's later discovery that phage mutation within a resistant culture took place within the bacterial host, led directly to the work of Werner Arber on host-controlled modification, which was the foundation for recombinant DNA research.

In 1950 Hershey was invited to join the Department of Genetics at Cold Spring Harbor. He had by then determined to prove that DNA was the catalyst and raw material of the powerful self-reproductive activity of the bacteriophage. Oswald Avery, Colin MacLeod, and Maclyn McCarty had already demonstrated in 1944 that DNA was the genetic material in bacteria. However, there was no experimental proof that the viral agent was also or only DNA, without some involvement of the protein component. Thomas Anderson's micrography had further defined the phage structure, revealing that the round head was a protein "bag," filled with DNA, and that the tail, also proteinaceous, attaches its tip to the bacterial cell wall. Studying the picture, Hershey and his assistant, Martha Chase, devised the now famous "blender experiment."

The problem was to separate and identify the genetic activity within the cell from the inactive particles. Hershey and Chase solved this problem by attaching separate radioactive markers to the protein and DNA components, allowing the phage to infect a bacterial culture, mixing the culture in a Waring blender to rupture the bacterial cell walls, and then using a centrifuge to separate the components. The resulting fractions showed the presence of the marked DNA within the cell interior, while the marked proteins remained attached to the cell walls. Moreover, the phage DNA was actively replicating, even though it was now completely separated from all, or most, of the protein component. The puzzle of self-replication could now be redefined in terms of two questions regarding DNA: how DNA first replicated itself and then catalyzed and directed protein synthesis to form new phages. The publication of the blender experiment in 1952 was the catalyst for the discovery of the double helix structure of DNA the following year, and the foundation of the newly defined discipline of molecular genetics (Hershey 1952; Stent 1969:480).

Hershey remained at Cold Spring Harbor for twenty-four years, continuing phage research and training a new generation of geneticists. Some of his studies in his old field of virology were important as well, leading to the development of vaccines for viral diseases such as measles and polio. In 1962 he was appointed director of the Genetics Research Unit.

After their first meeting, Delbrück had written about Hershey to Luria: "Drinks whiskey but not tea. Simple, to the point, likes living in a sailboat for three months; likes independence." This description surely characterized the older Hershey, who lived in a secluded Long Island home, "a five-minute walk through the woods" from the laboratory. His leisure time was spent planting trees, woodworking, and reading, as well as in his sailboat (Stent 1969, 480; *New York Times* October 17, 1969).

The Nobel Prize in 1969 was welcomed by the scientific community as richly deserved. Some agreed with the *New York Times*, who wondered in an October 20 editorial why the three pioneers had had to wait so long for the honor, while others, whose work had depended on theirs, had been recognized years earlier (notably Francis Crick and James Watson in 1962). Others noted that neither Delbrück nor Luria had been responsible for a glamorous breakthrough discovery of the type usually honored by the Nobel Committee, while Hershey's blender experiment had only confirmed a theory already held by many. As Gunther Stent noted in *Science*, "all three are widely revered, but the basis of their fame is elusive and difficult to explain to strangers (and even to molecular geneticists under 30)." That such an observation could be made about men who had literally revolutionized our understanding of genetics, replacing a rather static, mechanistic conception with a dynamic new model, sheds an interesting light on scientific progress and values. The Nobel Committee did however acknowledge the pioneers, if a little late (*New York Times* October 20, 1969, Stent 1969:479).

Hershey retired from Cold Spring Harbor in 1974. He is a member of the National Academy of Sciences, the American Academy of Arts and Sciences, and the American Society for Microbiology. Among the other awards he has won for his work are the Albert Lasker Award of the American Public Health Association (1958) and the Kimber Genetics Award of the National Academy of Sciences (1965).

MARCIA MELDRUM

Selected Bibliography

PRIMARY SOURCES

Hershey, Alfred D. 1952. "Reproduction of Bacteriophage." *International Review of Cytology* 1:119–134.

———. 1953. "Nuclear Acid Economy in Bacteria Infected with Bacteriophage T2. 2. Phage Precursor Nucleic Acid." *Journal of General Physiology* 37:1–23.

———. 1955. "Upper Limit to the Protein Content of the Germinal Substance of Bacteriophage T2." *Virology* 1:108–27.

SECONDARY SOURCES

Delbrück, Max, and Salvador E. Luria. 1943. "Mutation of Bacteria from Virus-Sensitive to Virus-Resistant." *Genetics* 28:491–511.

Delbrück, Max. 1946. "Induced Mutations in Bacterial Viruses." *Cold Spring Harbor Symposia on Quantitative Biology* 11:33–37.

Luria, Salvador, E. 1958. *The Multiplication of Viruses*. Vienna: Springer.

Altman, Lawrence, K. 1969. "The Path to the Nobel Prize Began Thirty Years Ago." *New York Times* (October 17):24.

1969. "Prize-Winning Virus Researchers: Alfred Day Hershey." *New York Times* (October 17):24.

Stent, Gunther, 1969. "The 1969 Nobel Prize for Physiology or Medicine." *Science* 166 (October 17):479–81.

"Hershey, Alfred Day." 1970. In *Current Biography Yearbook*, 175–77. New York: H. W. Wilson.

WALTER RUDOLF HESS *1949*

Walter Rudolf Hess was born on March 17, 1881, in Frauenfeld, Switzerland. A physician and neurophysiologist, Hess shared the Nobel Prize in 1949 (with Antonio Egas Moniz) for his studies of the localized functions of the interbrain, which were of crucial importance to our understanding of the autonomic nervous system. His work also introduced new techniques for the experimental study of unanesthetized live animals. At the time of the award, he was professor of physiology and director of the Physiological Institute at the University of Zurich. He retired in 1951 and held the title of professor emeritus until his death. Hess married Louise Sandmeyer in 1909; they had one son, Rudolph, and one daughter, Gertrud. Hess died on August 12, 1973, in Ascona, Switzerland.

Hess received his early education from his father, Clemen, a physics teacher, and his mother, Gertrud. He studied medicine at the Universities of Lausanne, Berne, Berlin, and Kiel, finally obtaining his degree from the University of Zurich in 1906. For seven years he was a practicing ophthalmologist in Zurich, where he developed the "Hess screen" for the study of squint. A deep interest in research led him to seek further training in physiology, first in Zurich as an assistant to J. G. Gaule, a student of Emil Ludwig. Hess then studied in Bonn from 1913 to 1917. In 1917 he was invited to return to Zurich to head the Physiology Department, a position he occupied for forty-four years.

Hess began by studying hemodynamics and blood viscosity, and later became interested in respiratory function. After World War I, however, he spent some time in England, where J. N. Langley's work turned him toward the autonomic nervous system. Hess became particularly fascinated by the diencephalon, or interbrain, the portion immediately below the cerebellum. Although previous work had established the importance of this area in autonomous body functioning, the complexity and integration of the various functions had defied the efforts of researchers to localize and describe brain activity.

Hess developed a technique for the study of awake and unrestrained cats, using fine needle electrodes—insulated except at the tip and implanted under anesthesia—to stimulate specific points of the brain. With this tool, he hoped to localize stimulation of functions and forecast the effects of brain tissue destruction. His first observations, of a dozen animals, directed him only to the conclusion that the pattern of functions must be more complicated than had been assumed and that extensive experiments would be required. Moreover, the results of each observation had to be carefully recorded and related temporally to the others. He was forced to apply for extensive financial assistance, which was provided by several Swiss foundations and the Rockefeller Foundation (Hess 1949, 249).

Hess's use of the conscious animal was unique at a time when experimental physiology had moved away from "live" studies to investigation of cells and tissue in vitro. His pioneering techniques opened new possibilities for study of the nervous system and for controlled observation of live animals (McDonald 1951).

In 1925, Hess applied his new technique to very tiny localized areas of the brain and was able to induce or restrict urination, defecation, relaxation, sleep, respiration, blood circulation and pressure, and body heat. He was able to observe that even the slightest or most specific stimulation resulted in a coordinated response of several body organs or systems, not merely a simple reflex. For example, a hunger response included licking, sniffing, and salivation. His most famous response, recorded on film, was "the angry cat"—fur bristling, pupils dilated, muscles tensed, heart rate increased. But he was also able, through diathermic destruction of hypothalamic tissue, to create an "adynamy," a total lack of animal activity resembling a coma (McDonald 1951, 628).

Following stimulation and recording of the response, Hess sacrificed the cat and dissected the brain tissue for microscopic examination. Only in this way could he determine the precise location of the electrode involved in the particular response. Painstakingly, Hess constructed a detailed map of the interbrain and of the hypothalamus, the deep inner structure of the diencephalon. He theorized that the autonomous nervous system had two parts, the sympathetic, activated in the spinal cord, and the parasympathetic, activated in the midbrain, medulla oblongata, and the sacral region, which had very different, indeed opposite, effects on body reactions. The sympathetic, which generated emotional reactions such as the angry cat, apparently assisted the animal to react to stress and to adjust to external stimuli. The parasympathetic acted conversely to relax the various responses and protect the system against "overloading." The two systems acted competitively, but also reciprocally, to produce "a dynamic equilibrium" to the animal in its ever-changing environment (Hess 1949, 252–53).

Hess determined that the sympathetic system was directly controlled by the hypothalamus and only indirectly by the conscious brain. He was also able to localize motor functions in the upper parts of the diencephalon, the thalamus, and subthalamus, and to demonstrate the brain's coordination of muscle movement and relaxation to achieve maximum efficiency of body motions. With K. Akert, he studied the forebrain and accumulated some important insights into the mechanisms of sight and vocalization (McDonald 1951, 629).

Other researchers were able to build on Hess's work to continue the mapping of the brain. In neurology, his findings were of immediate importance for determining the specific effects of brain tumors, injuries, and encephalitis. In addition, his technique suggested methods for therapeutic control of functions such as blood pressure.

Despite the importance of his work, Hess was not well known outside the Germanic countries until after the Nobel Prize and the publication of his works in English. Among his earlier awards were the Marcel Benorst Prize (Swiss, 1933) and the Ludwig Medal of the German Society for Circulation Research (1938).

After his retirement from the directorship in 1951, he was allowed to retain laboratory space at the Physiological Institute and to continue his research, although with limited space and less than adequate staff assistance. He spent several years integrating and summarizing his findings on the functions of the diencephalon, thalamus, and hypothalamus for publication. The resulting books, which appeared in English in 1954 (*Diencephalon: Autonomic and Extrapyramidal Functions*) and 1956 (*Hypothalamus and Thalamus*), increased his reputation in Britain and America.

Hess then became interested in the relationship of psychology and physiology, a subject much neglected by researchers. His animal observations had demonstrated, he believed, psychological motivations and intuitions as well as autonomic responses. His work in the late 1950s dealt with the physiological basis of psychosomatic manifestations and with the mechanism of action of the psychotropic drugs. In his final major work, *The Biology of Mind* (1981), he detailed these findings and suggested certain directions for further investigation. As a result of Hess's dedication and influence, the University of Zurich established a professorship in brain research in his honor in the early 1960s.

Away from his work, Hess enjoyed country life and gardening. He died quietly at his summer home near Locarno at age ninety-two.

MARCIA MELDRUM

Selected Bibliography

PRIMARY SOURCES

Hess, W. R. 1949. "The Central Control of the Activity of Internal Organs." Nobel Lecture, December 12, 1949. Reprinted in: *Nobel Lectures in Physiology or Medicine.* Vol. 3 (1942–1962): 247–255. Elsevier: Amsterdam (1964).

———. 1954. *Diencephalon: Autonomic and Extrapyramidal Functions.* New York: Grune and Stratton.

———. 1956. *Hypothalamus and Thalamus.* New York: Grune and Stratton.

———. 1957. *The Functional Organization of the Diencephalon.* New York: Grune and Stratton.

———. 1964. *The Biology of Mind.* 2d ed. Chicago: University of Chicago Press.

———. 1981. *Biological Order and Brain Organization: Selected Works of W. R. Hess.* New York: Springer-Verlag.

SECONDARY SOURCES

McDonald, D. A. 1951. "W. R. Hess: The Control of the Autonomic Nervous System by the Hypothalamus." *Lancet* 1 (March 17):627–29.

Asimov, Isaac. 1972. "Hess, Walter Rudolf." *Asimov's Biographical Encyclopedia of Science and Technology,* Garden City, NY: Doubleday:682.

1980. "Hess, Walter Rudolf." *Modern Scientists and Engineers,* 2:52. New York: McGraw-Hill.

CORNEILLE JEAN FRANÇOIS HEYMANS *1938*

Corneille Jean François Heymans was born in Ghent, Belgium, on March 28, 1892. His father, Jean-François Heymans, was professor of pharmacology and rector of the University of Ghent, as well as the founder and director of the Institute of Pharmacology, Pharmacodynamics and Toxicology that bears his name, also at the University of Ghent. Heymans *pére* was his son's principal teacher and, during the

1920s, his primary coresearcher in the experiment that ultimately led to the Nobel Prize in Physiology or Medicine for 1938. If the elder Heymans, who died in 1932, had lived, there is a good possibility that father and son would have shared the award. Corneille Heymans married Berthe May, an ophthalmologist, in 1921; the couple had four children: Marie-Henriette, Pierre, Joan, and Berthe. Heymans died on July 18, 1968, in Knokke, Belgium.

In 1921, the younger Heymans received his medical degree from the University of Ghent, with specialization in pathophysiology. (His training had been interrupted for four years by World War I, in which he served as an artillery officer and was awarded, among other medals, the Order of the Crown of Leopold for valor.) During the 1920s Corneille Heymans and his wife studied abroad, with Corneille working with Eugène Gley at the Collège de France, Maurice Arthus at the University of Lausanne, Hans-Horst Meyer at the University of Vienna, E. H. Sterling at University College, London, and Carl Wiggers at Western Reserve Medical School in Cleveland, Ohio. In 1922, already the author of a dozen articles, Heymans began his dual career as a researcher and teacher, becoming assistant professor of pharmacology at the University of Ghent. In 1930 he succeeded his father, both as professor and head of the Department of Pharmacology and as director of the Institute, holding these posts until he became emeritus in 1962.

Corneille Heymans received the Nobel Prize for work that contributed enormously to our current understanding of the reflex mechanisms that regulate the respiratory and cardiovascular systems in humans and other mammals. He obtained his results through experiments that were carefully conceived and scrupulously executed and which often required considerable technical ingenuity and virtuosity. In pursuing his investigations, he was as exhaustive as he was deliberate. A colleague, in characterizing Heymans's work on presso- and chemoreflexes (reflexes stimulated by blood pressure and blood chemistry, respectively), wrote that "so thoroughly has Heymans explored this new physiological territory that it is scarcely possible now to make an observation that has not already been made and recorded by him" (Schmidt 1939, 578).

When Corneille Heymans began his research in the early 1920s, it had been known for more than half a century that changes in blood pressure were associated with changes in respiration, with sudden hypertension inhibiting respiration and hypotension stimulating it. Contemporary scientific opinion held that changes in respiration were caused by the direct action of blood pressure on the respiratory center of the medulla. In a parallel fashion, blood pressure was thought to affect directly the medullary cardiovascular center, which responded to arterial hypotension by increasing the heart rate and to hypertension by producing the opposite effect. The investigations of Corneille Heymans helped to undercut this "classical theory" of the blood's direct action on the brain and developed the evidence for an alternative explanation.

Beginning in 1924, Heymans, working with his father and other colleagues, conducted a series of experiments that clearly demonstrated that local blood pressure changes in the cardio-aortic region reflexly stimulated the medullary respiratory centers. These experiments (like many that followed) depended upon the "isolated head" technique, perfected by Heymans *pére* and associates. Here the head of an anesthetized dog, B, only attached to its body by the vago-aortic nerves, was perfused by the blood of a similarly anesthetized dog, A, whose two common carotid arteries and external jugular veins were joined respectively to those of B. As a result, the dog's brain, kept alive by a separate, foreign source of blood, could be affected by its body only through the sole remaining nervous pathway. The two Heymans discerned that when they induced hyper- or hypotension in the isolated, artificially ventilated trunk of dog B, its medullary respiratory center was inhibited or stimulated, respectively. (Concomitant experiments by Corneille Heymans and Ladon, published in 1924–25, showed that the cardiovascular center of the brain was similarly affected reflexly, so that hyper- or hypotension produced a decreased or an increased heart rate respectively.) Once the vago-aortic nerves were severed, so that nerve impulses from the cardio-aortic area were interrupted, all respiratory responses to changes in the blood pressure of the trunk ended, further evidence for the existence of a reflex arc. Finally, further experiments using the "isolated head" technique allowed the Heymans to demonstrate conclusively that the vago-aortic nerves were the reflex mechanism's sole sensory pathway.

Influenced by the discovery (1923–24) of reflexes in the carotid sinus (a highly innervated swelling near the base of the internal carotid artery) by Heinrich Hering, who found that the reflexes regulated arterial pressure in unison with the aortic arch, Corneille Heymans next studied the carotid pressoreceptors. His work, and further experimentation by Hering and his associate Koch, confirmed conclusively that the carotid sinus contains pressoreceptors that reflexly modulate the medullary respiratory and cardiovascular centers, and that these brain centers are not directly affected by changes in arterial blood pressure. In 1933 Heymans reported that additional investigations showed that the carotid sinus pressoreceptors also reflexly influenced the peripheral resistance of blood vessels in other regions of the body. All these findings, together with those of other investigators like Hering and Koch, severely diminished the scientific basis for the "classical theory" of direct action.

That theory was further compromised by Corneille Heymans's work on the effect of blood chemistry on respiration. As with blood pressure, the textbooks taught that chemical components in the blood, carbon dioxide and oxygen in particular, acted directly on the medullary centers. Using the "isolated head" technique, the two Heymans observed instead that low levels of oxygen or high levels of carbon dioxide in the cardio-aortic region reflexly stimulated the respiratory center (though further work showed that carbon dioxide also acted directly on the brain). In a series of classic studies published during the early thirties, Corneille Heymans and his colleagues showed that the carotid sinus, too, had reflex chemosensitivity.

Other investigations performed during the twenties and thirties allowed Heymans to demonstrate that in addition to physiological substances, the aortic and carotid sinuses have chemoreceptors that are sensitive to a number of pharmacological chemicals. For example, nicotine, lobeline, cyanide, acetylcholine, and choline derivatives were shown to reflexly stimulate the respiratory and cardiovascular centers of the brain by acting upon the carotid sinus receptors. These same substances had either no direct effect or acted as a depressant on the medulla, or stimulated it only at high doses. Finally, work by Corneille Heymans in 1930 and 1931, and by de Castro a few years earlier, led to the discovery of the location of the carotid chemoreceptors in the carotid bodies near the carotid sinus and its pressoreceptors in the large vessels adjoining the carotid artery. Subsequent experiments by Julius Comroe and others revealed that the aortic chemoreceptors lay in the aortic glomus tissue while the aortic pressoreceptors were embedded in the wall of the aortic arch.

The thorough and laborious experimentation carried out by Heymans and his associates, in which he both made his own discoveries and extended those of other outstanding scientists, created a new explanation for the body's regulation of its respiration, blood pressure, and cardiac rhythm. In a long series of articles and monographs (Heymans published more than eight hundred scientific works during his career), written with the logic and lucidity for which he was justly well known, he marshalled the evidence in favor of reflex mechanisms over direct action. For his experimental findings and, in particular, for his part in the discovery of the aortic and carotid chemoreceptors, he was awarded the Nobel Prize in Physiology or Medicine in 1938.

Over subsequent decades, Heymans, his colleagues, and students (he collaborated with some one hundred and fifty research workers at the Institute) investigated a series of related scientific problems, among which were the pathophysiology of renal hypertension, the physiology of cerebral circulation, the physiology of blood circulation during muscular exercise, and the pathology and pharmacology of sympathectomized animals (that is, animals whose sympathetic nerves were cut). This research, combined with that of his earlier years, contributed enormously to basic scientific knowledge concerning the physiology, pathology, and pharmacology of the human cardiovascular and respiratory systems.

Corneille Heymans was awarded many honors during his long career. To the Nobel Prize must be added the Alvarenga Prize of the (Belgian) Académie Royale de Médecine and the Prix Quinquennal de Médecine of the Belgian government, the Pius XI Prize of the Pontificia Academia Scientiarum, and the Monthyon Prize of the Institut de France. Heymans held sixteen honorary degrees and was a member of more than forty scientific and medical societies. An energetic and gifted organizer in the service of physiology and pharmacology, he served as president of the International Union of Physiological Sciences, the International Council of Pharmacologists, and the International Union of Pharmacology.

In addition to his success as a research scientist, an activity he relished, Heymans was a gifted teacher and mentor. At a time when many professors regally kept students at a distance, Heymans treated them as professionals and took a serious interest in their work; he followed their careers, continued to send them relevant data, and often provided unsolicited help and support when they were in trouble. He was also an esteemed colleague. Those with whom he worked describe him as an extraordinary individual, a warm, empathic, and generous man with considerable social presence, whose personal modesty, wit, and prodigious knowledge served to make a profound impression on others.

GERALD M. OPPENHEIMER

Selected Bibliography

PRIMARY SOURCES

Heymans, Corneille, J.-J. Bouckaert, and P. Regniers. 1933. *Le Sinus Carotidien et la Zone Homologue Cardio-Aortique*. Paris: G. Doin.

Heymans, Corneille. 1950. *Introduction to the Regulation of Blood Pressure and Heart Rate*. Springfield, Ill.: Charles C. Thomas.

Heymans, Corneille, and Eric Neil. 1958. *Reflexogenic Areas of the Cardiovascular System*. Boston: Little, Brown and Company.

Heymans, Corneille, and Bjorn Folkow. 1964. "Vasomotor Control and Regulation of Blood Pressure." In *Circulation of the Blood, Men and Ideas*, edited by Alfred P. Fishman and Dickenson W. Richards, 407–87. New York: Oxford University Press.

SECONDARY SOURCES

Schmidt, Carl F. 1939. "Professor Corneille Heymans, Nobel Laureate in Physiology and Medicine for 1938." *The Scientific Monthly* 49: 576–79.

1973. "Corneille Heymans, A Collective Biography." *Archives Internationales de Pharmacodynamie et de Thérapie* Supplement 202:9–307.

ARCHIBALD VIVIAN HILL 1922

Archibald Vivian Hill, known to most of his colleagues and friends as "A. V.," occasionally as "Vivian" to his family, but never "Archibald," was born in 1886. His father, Jonathan, who left his family when A. V. was a young child, was a timber merchant in Bristol; his mother Ada (née Rumney) became the major influence in his early life. In 1913 Hill married Margaret Keynes, sister of the economist J. M. [Lord] Keynes and the surgeon and writer [Sir] Geoffrey Keynes. They had four children, two of whom, like their father, became Fellows of the Royal Society. While a student at Cambridge before World War I, Hill started the experimental work on heat production by muscle for which he shared half the 1922 Nobel Prize in Physiology or Medicine with Otto Meyerhof. For the rest of his life he continued to study problems of heat production and energy metabolism in muscle and in nerve, in addition to assuming numerous professional duties. He also served as a member of Parliament during World War II and wrote extensively on a wide variety of subjects, particularly on the social obligations of science and scientists. He died in Cambridge in 1977.

Hill's scientific education began at Blundells School in Tiverton, Devonshire, and developed further after he had gained a scholarship to Trinity College, Cambridge, to study mathematics. He was third wrangler in 1907 but, advised by his college tutor, [Sir] Walter Morley Fletcher, he decided to apply his mathematical talents to physiological problems. He remained in Cambridge until World War I, working, with the aid of the George Henry Lewes Studentship in Physiology and then a research fellowship of Trinity College, in the Physiological Laboratory on heat production in muscle. At the same time, he applied his mathematical abilities to problems such as the kinetics of drug actions and the physics of hemoglobin dissociation, and he began an important and lifelong interest in the design of new experimental techniques and equipment to make the very precise measurements that his work increasingly demanded. This detailed quantitative approach to muscle contraction, and later to neuronal activity, was a formative development in the creation of the speciality of biophysics, which Hill did much to establish.

During World War I Hill served in the army in antiaircraft research. He was elected a Fellow of the Royal Society in 1918. After demobilization he became professor of physiology at Manchester. Shortly after the award of the Nobel Prize he succeeded Ernest Starling as professor of physiology at University College, London. In 1926 he obtained a Royal Society Foulerton Research Professorship but remained in the same department until the end of his active research career in the mid-1960s.

It was in 1910 that Hill first started work on heat production by muscle; characteristically, his early papers include technical developments and modifications and improvements to equipment. In particular, he attempted to correlate the heat generated by contracting muscle with the only chemical event then known to occur in muscle: the appearance of lactic acid and its subsequent degradation to carbon dioxide and water. Hill's work showed that heat was generated not only during the active contraction of the muscle, but also during its recovery period. With his colleague William Hartree, Hill was able to determine that the heat produced by muscle was related to lactic acid production and its consequent removal; further calculations suggested that the lactic acid was being resynthesized into an unidentified compound. The slightly later work of Otto Meyerhof provided the details of these associated biochemical reactions. These two supplementary approaches resulted in the joint award of half the Nobel Prize for 1922. Hill and Meyerhof together provided evidence of the energy generating processes that underlie muscle contraction, and they also conducted the first successful attempts to correlate chemical and physical mechanisms with a physiological process in a living cell.

Also of importance was Hill's later work, particularly that on the small but significant amount of heat generated by nerve fibers and the associated physical and chemical changes that occurred during the transmission of nerve impulses. Again, such work was strongly dependent on Hill's technical modifications. While some of his quantitative assessments had to be revised later, he realized that the physiological phenomenon of propagation of the impulse could be satisfactorily explained by physicochemical equations (Hill 1933).

In the late 1930s and again after World War II he returned to the problems of heat generation by muscle, and continued to provide more detail in support of his early results, as well as reevaluating them in the light of fresh ideas and further work.

However, his intellectual activities extended beyond the research laboratory, and he accepted a wide range of responsibilities at both national and international levels. In addition to his departmental duties, he was both biological (1935–45) and foreign (1945–46) secretary of the Royal Society; he was secretary (1927–34) and foreign secretary (1935–45) of the Physiological Society; and he was an editor of the *Journal of Physiology* for many years. He also served on the boards of the International Union of Physiological Societies and the International Council of Scientific Unions, and was president of the British Association for the Advancement of Science in 1952. These latter activities give a clue to some of Hill's major contributions to science: his belief in the internationalism of science and in the right (and attendant obligations) of scientists to prosecute their research without political interference. A forcible expression of these views was his personal involvement in the founding and subsequent running of the Academic Assistance Council (later the Society for the Protection of Science and Learning), an organization that did much to help refugee scientists from Continental Europe in the 1930s. One very direct way in which he provided help in these circumstances was by finding, either in his own or in friends' laboratories, space for these researchers, as has been recalled with affectionate gratitude by another Nobel Prize winner (Katz 1986). These concerns with the wider issues of science and society were exemplified by Hill's activities as an Independent Conservative Member of Parliament for Cambridge University during World War II; his work in initiating and organizing radar in Britain; and his role as adviser to the Indian government on reconstruction in the 1940s. In addition to a prolific scientific output, Hill wrote articles and papers on a wide variety of more general scientific themes. He also prepared a lengthy autobiography which was never published, although typescripts can be consulted at the Royal Society and at Churchill College, Cambridge, where the rest of his papers are deposited.

E. M. TANSEY

Selected Bibliography

PRIMARY SOURCES

Hill, A. V. 1922. "The Mechanism of Muscular Contraction." Nobel Lecture. Reprinted in *Nobel Lectures, Physiology or Medicine, 1922–1941*, vol. 2 (1922–1941), 10–26. Amsterdam: Elsevier, 1965.

———. 1932. *Chemical Wave Transmission in Nerve*. Cambridge: Cambridge University Press.

———. 1933. "The Physical Nature of the Nerve Impulse." *Nature* 131 (April 8):501–8.

———. 1960. *The Ethical Dilemma of Science and Other Writings*. New York: Rockefeller Institute Press.

———. 1965. *Trails and Trials in Physiology*. London: Edward Arnold.

———. 1970. *First and Last Experiments in Muscle Mechanics*. Cambridge: Cambridge University Press.

———. No date. Typescript autobiography. A. V. Hill papers, Churchill College Archives, Cambridge.

SECONDARY SOURCES

Katz, B. 1978. "Archibald Vivian Hill." *Biographical Memoirs of Fellows of the Royal Society* 24:71–149.

Katz, B. 1986. "Reminiscences of a Physiologist, Fifty Years After." *Journal of Physiology* 370:1–12.

GEORGE HERBERT HITCHINGS
1988

George Herbert Hitchings was born in Hoquiam, Washington, on April 18, 1905. A biochemist, Hitchings shared the Nobel Prize in 1988 with Gertrude Elion and Sir James Whyte Black for their work in developing drugs for the treatment of many critical diseases. Hitchings and Elion, long-time collaborators at Burroughs Wellcome Research Laboratories, produced compounds that inhibit DNA synthesis and thus prevent the rapid growth of cancer cells. They then used their understanding of nucleic acid synthesis to develop immunosuppressives and antibiotics. The Nobel Prize is rarely given for new drugs and its award to Hitchings and Elion recognizes not only their multiple contributions to therapeutics but their formulation of basic principles that will continue to provide clues to researchers. Hitchings retired from his position as vice president for research at Burroughs Wellcome in 1975 but remains active as an emeritus consultant and as president of the Burroughs Wellcome Fund, the company philanthropic arm. He was married to Beverly Reimer for fifty-three years, from 1933 until her death in 1986; they had two children, a son and a daughter.

The son of a shipbuilder, Hitchings attended the University of Washington in Seattle, where he earned a bachelor's degree in 1927 and a master's in 1928. He was admitted to Harvard as a doctoral candidate in biochemistry and remained for six years as a research associate and instructor after receiving his Ph.D. in 1933. In 1939 he took a position at Case Western Reserve University in Ohio but did not advance beyond senior instructor. In 1942 he was invited to join the biochemistry department at Burroughs Wellcome in Tuckahoe, New York: "a department of one." Elion came to his laboratory in 1944 (Marx 1988; Altman 1988).

Drug development up to that time had often followed the "magic bullet" method made famous by Paul Ehrlich in 1910. This kind of research involved the unsystematic injection of multiple compounds into research animals, to see if any of them would prove to be the "bullet" for a specific disease. Other scientists, studying the etiology and pathology of diseases, disdained any concern with clinical drug development. Hitchings and Elion hoped to find "a middle course . . . that would generate basic information which chemotherapy could then exploit." As Hitchings has said, the considerable autonomy given his team by Burroughs Wellcome was crucial to their many successes: "Our orientation was basic research and yet we turned out more drugs than people who were looking for them."

In the 1940s they began looking at the cellular synthesis of nucleotides. They found that bacterial cells could not produce nucleic acid (DNA)—and therefore could not divide—in the absence of certain proteins (purines) and folic acid. Using this information, they were able to develop antimetabolite compounds that blocked the enzymes necessary for the formation of cellular DNA.

The antimetabolites were initially tested on leukemia patients at Sloan-Kettering Institute in the late 1940s and early 1950s. Hitchings and Elion hoped that the new drugs would inhibit the rapid formation of the white blood cells sufficiently to bring about a remission of the leukemia. The difficulty was, of course, that the formation of other cells might be inhibited and the drug would prove more toxic to the patient than to the cancer. This was indeed the case with the first compound tested; however, later trials proved the efficacy and relative safety of 6-mercaptopurine and thioguanine, which are still used today to treat leukemia (Marx 1988, 516; Kolata 1988; Altman 1988).

Hitchings and Elion's work was notable not only for its contribution to a particular disease but for its insight into the potential applications of DNA research and its development of a method to block the "pathways" that form nucleic acids. This concept was quite revolutionary in the 1940s (Marx 1988, 516).

The team, continuing to work along these lines, synthesized azathioprine, a modified form of 6-mercaptopurine in 1957. It proved to be "unimpressive" against leukemia, but researchers at Tufts University found that it effectively suppressed the immune system's production of antibodies. This kind of drug is essential in kidney and other organ transplants to prevent the body's rejection of the implanted tissues. Azathioprine is also used in the treatment of autoimmune disorders, such as rheumatoid arthritis, in which the body is believed to attack its own tissue.

Another drug developed as an enzyme inhibitor was allopurinol. Again, it was not successful against cancer. But Hitchings and Elion noted that it blocked the enzyme xanthine oxidase, which is critical to the synthesis of uric acid. Allopurinol is now used to treat gout, which is caused by uric acid deposition in the joints, and to prevent uric acid buildup as a result of cancer chemotherapy.

By the 1960s Elion and Hitchings had turned their attention to nucleic acid synthesis in lower animals and its differences from the same process in humans. The results suggested new ways of combating infectious disease by attacking bacterial and viral DNA. Among the drugs that resulted from this work are pyramethamine, used against the protozoa that causes malaria, and trimethoprim, for urinary and respiratory tract infections caused by bacteria. Trimethoprim is also used in the treatment of *Pneumocystis carinii*, a pneumonia virus that is almost harmless in healthy people but is a major killer of AIDS victims.

Most recently, in 1975, Hitchings and Elion's team synthesized the drug acyclovir, the first compound found to be effective against herpes. Azidothymidine (AZT), the only drug so far developed and approved for

AIDS, was also produced using the principles the two had established in their early work (Marx 1988; Altman 1988).

Hitchings became associate research director at Burroughs Wellcome in 1955, research director of chemotherapy in 1963, and vice-president in 1967. He has also served as a consultant to the National Institute of Health, the American Cancer Society, and other agencies. He is currently active in the American Red Cross and the George and Beverly Hitchings Educational Foundation, which he established in Durham, North Carolina, where he now lives. Hitchings's philanthropic work is a continuation of his lifelong devotion to service; his "real award," he has said, came from saving patients' lives through his pharmaceutical discoveries (Kolata 1988).

Among the many honors he has received are the Gairdner Award (1968), the Passano Award (1969), the Award for Scientific Achievement of the National Cancer Society (1978), and the Cain Award of the American Association for Cancer Research (1984).

MARCIA MELDRUM

Selected Bibliography

PRIMARY SOURCES

Hitchings, George H., et al. 1950. "Antagonists of Nucleic Acid Derivatives; *Lactobacillus casei* model." *Journal of Biological Chemistry* 183 (March):1–9.

Hitchings, George H., Gertrude B. Elion, and Elvira A. Falco. 1950. "Antagonists of Nucleic Acid Derivatives: Reversal Studies with Substances Structurally Related to Thymine." *Journal of Biological Chemistry* 185 (August):643–49.

Elion, Gertrude B., George H. Hitchings, and H. Van der Werff. 1951. "Antagonists of Nucleic Acid Derivatives: Purines." *Journal of Biological Chemistry* 192 (October):505–18.

Balis, M. E., D. H. Levin, G. B. Brown, G. B. Elion, H. C. Nathan, and G. H. Hitchings. 1957. "The Effects of 6-mercaptopurine on *Lactobacillus casei*." *Archives of Biochemistry and Biophysics* 71 (October): 358–66.

Elion, G. B., S. Callahan, S. Bieber, G. H. Hitchings, and R. W. Rudles. 1962. "Experimental, Clinical, and Metabolic Studies of Thiopurines." *Cancer Chemotherapy Reports* 16 (February):197–202.

Hitchings, George H., and Gertrude B. Elion. 1963. "Chemical Suppression of the Immune Response." *Pharmacological Review* 15 (June):365–405.

SECONDARY SOURCES

Altman, Lawrence K. 1988. "Three Drug Pioneers Win Nobel in Medicine." *New York Times* (October 18):1, C17.

Kolata, Gina. 1988. "A Research Collaboration Spanning Four Decades: George Herbert Hitchings." *New York Times* (October 18):C16.

Connor, Steve, Dan Charles, Sharon Kingman, and Frank Lesser. 1988. "Drug Pioneers Win Nobel Laureate." *New Scientist* (October 22):26–27.

Marx, Jean L. 1988. "The 1988 Nobel Prize for Physiology or Medicine." *Science* 242 (October 28):516–17.

SIR ALAN LLOYD HODGKIN
1963

Sir Alan Lloyd Hodgkin was born in Banbury, England, on February 5, 1914. A physiologist, Hodgkin received the 1963 Nobel Prize jointly with Andrew F. Huxley for their description of the mechanism of nervous activity in terms of ion movements across the axonal surface membrane. At the time of the award, he held the Foulerton Professorship of the Royal Society (1952–70) at Cambridge University. He was later appointed to the John Humphry Plummer Professorship of Biophysics (1970–81). He was knighted in 1972 and acted as master of Trinity College from 1978 to 1984. Hodgkin continues his research in a room of the Physiological Laboratory that previously had seen experiments by E. D. Adrian. Hodgkin married Marion de Kay Rous, the daughter of Peyton Rous, in 1944; they have three daughters and one son.

Hodgkin's parents were George Lloyd Hodgkin, who died when he was only four, and the former Mary Fletcher Wilson. He was educated by Gresham's School in Holt, England, and won an entrance scholarship in natural sciences to Trinity College, Cambridge University, where he matriculated in 1932 at the age of eighteen. Hodgkin received the Frank Smart Prize for Zoology and double first-class honors on his examinations and was elected to a research fellowship at Trinity.

From 1935 to 1939 he taught at Cambridge, except for a year's fellowship at the Rockefeller Institute for Medical Research in New York (1937–38). His experiments during this period supported the contention of classical membrane theory that the conduction of nerve impulses was an electrical process. While in the United States, Hodgkin visited the marine Biological Laboratory in Woods Hole, Massachusetts, and was there introduced by K. S. Cole to the giant squid axon. This preparation as originally described by J. Z. Young is still unique for nerve physiologists. The axon reached a diameter of close to one millimeter and can be dissected free from neighboring fibers over a distance of several centimeters.

The membrane theory of Julius Bernstein (1902), though based on very little in the way of experimental facts, had survived for more than thirty years. Bernstein had stated that the resting axon is surrounded by a membrane selectively permeable to potassium ions and that, in the course of activity, there is a nonselective increase of permeability to all ions in the system, thus reducing the resting potential to zero.

Hodgkin resolved to investigate this hypothesis further. During the summer of 1939 he and his former student, Andrew Huxley, began experiments at the laboratory of the Marine Biological Association in

Plymouth, England. Their work was interrupted by the outbreak of World War II. Hodgkin was first assigned to the Royal Air Force Physiological Laboratory in Farnborough and later worked on radar for the Ministry of Aircraft Production. In 1946 he returned to Cambridge, where he was appointed assistant director of research the following year, and joined forces again with Huxley.

In order to get a fair comparison between the resting potential and the amplitude of the action potential, the team directly measured the potential difference between the axoplasm and the surrounding sea water. They inserted a glass capillary tube into the axoplasm to act as an inner electrode and pushed it in an axial direction to lead off from an undamaged part. (Cole and Curtis had performed essentially the same experiment at Woods Hole in 1939).

Hodgkin and Huxley wrote a letter to *Nature* in which the "overshoot" of the membrane potential over the zero level is clearly illustrated, yet interpreted with utmost caution. The results convinced the researchers that it would be worthwhile to consider changes underlying nervous activity other than a loss of ion selectivity or "breakdown" of the membrane.

The squid season (August to November) of 1947 at Plymouth brought a quantitative test of the "sodium hypothesis." This theory tentatively stated that an excitable membrane at rest is preferentially permeable to potassium (K^+) ions (as proposed by Bernstein), but when activated undergoes a large and selective increase of permeability to sodium (Na^+) ions. The lines of evidence (Hodgkin and Katz 1949) have long become textbook knowledge. First, when external Na^+ is replaced by a nonpermeant cation (e.g., choline), the overshoot is depressed as expected for a selectively Na^+-permeable membrane. Also, the maximal rate of rise of the action potential is proportional to the extracellular concentration of sodium. Finally, excitability is lost in Na^+-deficient solutions, as Overton had shown for muscular contractibility in 1902; but his work had been largely forgotten.

By 1948 Hodgkin and Huxley were saying, "You can stimulate a nerve fiber; then the fiber does the rest of the experiment." To gain control over a surface membrane, they adapted and improved the "voltage clamping" technique developed by Cole and Marmont. Instead of observing free-running action potentials, the researchers kept the membrane voltage constant at the level of the resting potential, then stepped it to different levels, recorded the membrane current at each step for a preselected time, then stepped the voltage back to the original level. Measurements of total membrane current versus time were repeated with external solutions of different ion compositions. Hodgkin and Huxley then attempted to split the total ionic current into a sodium and a potassium component as functions of both voltage and time, on the basis of the internal and external concentrations of each ion. They further divided the component currents into conductance times driving force.

The decisive experiments were done at Plymouth in the course of the squid seasons of 1948 and 1949. They worked hard to elaborate their "ionic theory of excitation." Kenneth Cole later stated in a lecture at Cambridge, "We [Cole and Marmont] have got the voltage clamp going but you people [Hodgkin and Huxley] have asked the right questions."

The five papers that presented the Nobel Prize–winning work were published in 1952. Briefly, they stated that activity results from a voltage-dependent and transitory rise of Na^+ conductance followed (in squid axons) by a delayed rise of K^+ conductance. The experimental achievements of a few months' time appear as an impressive body of results, leaving little in the way of major gaps. Huxley in his Nobel Lecture explained: "Hodgkin and I spent a good deal of time in the early part of 1947 thinking what kind of system might give rise to an action potential." In other words, they knew exactly what to look for in their experiments of 1948 and 1949.

In the course of analyzing the current traces, they introduced mathematical language (HH equations) to describe the "on" and "off" of conductances at various voltage levels. These equations made it possible to reproduce the known behavior of the nerve admirably well, including the amplitude and time-course of the action potential and even the velocity of propagation along an axon. As Hodgkin and Huxley wrote (1952): "For the sake of illustration we shall try to provide a physical basis for these equations, but must emphasize that the interpretation given is unlikely to provide a correct picture of the membrane."

The voltage clamp experiments suggested what might happen during a single action potential. Richard Keynes and Peter Lewis then measured the inflow and outflow of radioactive isotopes with axons of the cuttlefish, a relative of the squid. Using trains of action potentials, and comparing periods of activity and periods of rest, they found a gain of 24Na and a loss of 42K, a result in close agreement with the charge displacement calculated by Hodgkin and Huxley from their voltage clamp data (in mole cm<−2> impulse<−1>).

While the squid axon work was in progress, Hodgkin adapted the Ling-Gerard micropipettes for the recording of fast voltage transient; he decreased the electrode resistance by filling the pipettes with three molar potassium chloride and used a cathode follower input stage. Together with Bill Nastuk of Columbia University, he extended the sodium hypothesis to skeletal muscle. It was Huxley, however, who was to turn his attention fully to muscle.

Hodgkin was appointed Foulerton Research Professor of the Royal Society in 1952. He continued the squid axon experiments for some years. He now understood that, as a result of one cycle of activity, an axon would have gained a minute quantity of sodium and lost a comparable quantity of potassium. In the long run, some secretion of Na^+

and reuptake of K^+ would be required. With Richard Keynes, he established that the rate at which a squid axon loses its 24Na is depressed reversibly by low temperatures or metabolic poisons. By 1960 it was further established by Hodgkin, Caldwell, Keynes, and Shaw that an injection of some of the energy-rich phosphates into a nerve fiber kept "poisoned" by cyanide will temporarily restart Na+ extrusion.

Peter Baker and Trevor Shaw, working at Plymouth in Hodgkin's absence, tried the daring experiment of squeezing the axoplasm out of a squid fiber with a roller and filling the collapsed axon with a potassium salt solution. Thus they designed the technique of internal perfusion which, in combination with voltage clamping, made the inside of the axon accessible for experimental manipulations. Perfusion experiments with solutions of different ionic compositions have shown a general agreement with predictions and have demonstrated that the membrane is a nonsymmetrical structure. Some blockers of ion movement are effective only when applied externally, others only internally.

The long summers and falls spent at Plymouth, often just waiting for squids, were not appreciated by many physiologists' families. The wives left behind at Cambridge were nicknamed "squidows." Alan Hodgkin faced not only family pressures but those of increasing administrative duties. From 1959 to 1963 he served on the Medical Research Council, and from 1966 to 1976 he served as president of the Marine Biological Association. By the sixties, he was concentrating on animals that could survive at Cambridge. With Richard Adrian, Peter Baker, Knox Chandler of Yale University, and others, he thoroughly analyzed the electrical characteristics of the single fibers of frog skeletal muscle.

Hodgkin served as president of the Royal Society from 1970 to 1975. During these years he managed to take up yet another line of research: receptor physiology or, more precisely, transduction between light absorbed by the outer segment of a retinal rod or cone and the membrane currents that lead to signaling between the receptors and the brain. This work was done in close collaboration with Denis Baylor of Stanford University.

Their work began with the finding that vertebrate rods kept in the dark pass appreciable amounts of membrane current, inward through the outer segment and outward through the inner segment. If isolated rods are sucked into a tightly-fitting pipette, it is possible to measure the extracellular current flow between the inner and outer segments. A flash of light will reduce or switch off this "dark current," thus allowing the inner segment to hyperpolarize to the potential of its own K^+ battery. Using rapid solution exchange techniques and having the outer, photosensitive, segment in contact with the bathing solution, the researchers found that the photocurrent generated by a flash is sensitive to the sodium concentration of the external medium. This result suggested that light absorption normally leads to a drop in Na^+ influx. Working with varying degrees of illumination and external changes of sodium and calcium, they established the following sequence of events. When light is partially absorbed by the pigment of an outer segment, the photoreaction increases free internal calcium that blocks the dark Na^+ current until a sodium/calcium exchange has reduced the internal calcium to a level at which the dark current will flow again.

Both Hodgkin and Huxley have repeatedly and decisively helped to solve research problems for colleagues and former associates. When a problem had reached a stage of intuitive understanding, the best thing to do would be to buy a ticket to Cambridge. The traveler would be sure to return with the right kind of questions to be asked, sometimes even with a neat set of equations in his bag.

Sir Alan Hodgkin holds the doctorate of science from Cambridge (1960) and is a fellow of the Royal Society and of the Imperial College of Science and Technology. He holds honorary membership or associate status in many foreign societies, including the National Academy of Sciences of the United States. His many other awards include the Baly Medal of the Royal College of Physicians (1955), the Royal Medal of the Royal Society (1958), the Copley Medal of the Royal Society (1965), the Order of Merit (1973), and the Helmerich Prize (1988).

SILVIO WEIDMANN

Selected Bibliography

PRIMARY SOURCES

Hodgkin, A. L. 1937. "Evidence for Electrical Transmission in Nerve. Parts 1 and 2." *Journal of Physiology* 90:183–210, 211–32.

Hodgkin, A. L. and B. Katz. 1949. "The Effects of Sodium Ions on the Electrical Activity of the Giant Axon of the Squid." *Journal of Physiology* 108:37–77.

Nastuk, W. L., and A. L. Hodgkin. 1950. "The Electrical Activity of Single Muscle Fibres." *Journal of Cellular and Comparative Physiology* 35:39–73.

Hodgkin, A. L., and A. F. Huxley. 1952. "A Quantitative Description of Membrane Current and Its Application to Conduction and Excitation in Nerve." *Journal of Physiology* 117:500–544.

Hodgkin, A. L., and R. D. Keynes. 1955. "Active Transport of Cations in Giant Axons from *Sepia* and *Loligo*." *Journal of Physiology* 128:28–60.

Baker, P. F., A. L. Hodgkin, and T. I. Shaw. 1962. "Replacement of the Axoplasm of Giant Nerve Fibres with Artificial Solutions." *Journal of Physiology* 164:330–54.

Hodgkin, A. L. 1964. *The Conduction of the Nervous Impulse*. Liverpool: Liverpool University Press.

———. 1976. "Chance and Design in Electrophysiology: An Informal Account of Certain Experiments on

Nerve Carried Out between 1934 and 1952." *Journal of Physiology* 263:1–21.

———. 1983. "Some Reminiscences of My Early Life (1914–1947)." *Annual Review of Physiology* 45:1–16.

Hodgkin, A. L., and B. J. Nunn. 1987. "The Effect of Ions on Sodium-Calcium Exchange in Salamander Rods." *Journal of Physiology* 391: 371–98.

ROBERT W. HOLLEY *1968*

The 1968 Nobel Prize in Physiology or Medicine was awarded to Robert W. Holley, Har Gobind Khorana, and Marshall W. Nirenberg "for their interpretation of the genetic code and its function in protein synthesis." Robert W. Holley was born on January 28, 1922, in Urbana, Illinois, but he grew up in California, Idaho, and Illinois, developing a love for the outdoors and an enduring interest in living things. His area of scientific specialization is the biochemistry of the nucleic acids and protein synthesis. Both his father, Charles Elmer Holley, and his mother, Viola Esther Wolfe, were teachers. Holley married Anne Lenore Dworkin, a chemist and high school mathematics teacher, on March 3, 1945. They have one son.

Holley majored in chemistry at the University of Illinois, receiving his A.B. in 1942. He did his graduate work at Cornell University, where he studied organic chemistry with Alfred T. Blonquist, and earned his Ph.D. in 1947. His graduate work was interrupted by World War II. During the war he took part in research for the United States Office of Research and Development. Holley worked with Vincent duVigneaud at Cornell University Medical College from 1944 to 1946 as a member of the team that first synthesized penicillin. In 1946–47 he held a fellowship from the National Research Council.

From 1947 to 1948 Holley was instructor and American Chemical Society Postdoctoral Fellow with Carl M. Stevens at Washington State University. He returned to Cornell University as assistant professor of organic chemistry at the Geneva Experiment Station in 1948. From 1948 to 1957 he was assistant professor, New York State Agriculture Experiment Station, and associate professor of organic chemistry. During a sabbatical year (1955 to 1956) as a Guggenheim Memorial Fellow he worked in the division of biology at the California Institute of Technology, in James Bonner's laboratory, studying protein synthesis and performing experiments to detect the acceptor of activated amino acids. He held the position of part-time associate professor of biochemistry at Cornell University from 1957 to 1964, while also serving as a research chemist for the U.S. Plant, Soil and Nutrition Laboratory, ARS, USDA. Holley rejoined the faculty of Cornell University, as full-time professor of biochemistry and molecular biology in 1964 and served as chairman of the department from 1965 to 1966. He spent 1966–67 as a National Science Foundation Senior Postdoctoral Fellow at the Salk Institute for Biological Studies and the Scripps Clinic and Research Foundation. Since 1968 he has been a resident fellow at the Salk Institute of Biological Studies, La Jolla, California.

Although trained as a chemist, Holley has always retained his basic interest in living things. After beginning his research career with the organic chemistry of natural products, he gradually turned to more biological topics, such as work on amino acids and peptides. Holley is one of the discoverers of the special type of nucleic acid now called transfer-RNA (tRNA). During his investigations of the biosynthesis of proteins, alanine transfer RNA was discovered. Holley worked on the isolation and structure of this tRNA for ten years. By the end of 1964 the nucleotide sequence had been completed. The first announcement was a modest abstract published in the March 19, 1965, issue of *Science*. Holley reported that the complete nucleotide sequence of an alanine transfer RNA, isolated from yeast, had been determined. This was the first nucleic acid for which the structure had been determined. Holley's work was also important in revealing how tRNA is involved in reading off the genetic code and transforming that information into the protein alphabet. His more recent research interest has been the factors that control cell division in mammalian cells.

In the 1970s Holley's own researches and reflections on the literature led him to the conclusion that "the factors that control growth are probably polypeptide hormones, or hormone-like materials, as well as a variety of low molecular weight nutrients." He was searching for an understanding of the ways in which complex interactions of cells with such materials led to the control of the growth of mammalian cells (Holley 1975, 487). In the 1980s he was involved in studies of specific cell growth inhibitors and had deduced the complete amino acid sequence of the BSC-1 cell growth inhibitor from the nucleotide sequence of its cDNA (Hanks et al. (1988).

Robert Holley was awarded the Nobel Prize for his development of techniques for determining the structure of nucleic acids and for his determination of the complete nucleotide sequence of alanine transfer ribonucleic acid. In the course of this research he refined the techniques that would lead to further structural determinations and progress in understanding the workings of the genetic code. Holley shared the Nobel Prize with Har Gobind Khorana of the University of Wisconsin and Marshall W. Nirenberg of the National Institutes of Health.

Although the work of these three laureates was interrelated, each was honored for work that had been carried out independently of the other two. In commenting on the work of the three laureates Maxine Singer wrote that the significance of each achievement "is enhanced by the achievement of the others. These three men together constitute a triplet of great sense" (Singer 1968).

The process of elucidating the genetic code accelerated very rapidly after Marshall Nirenberg and Heinrich Mattaei reported on their synthesis of the "protein" polyphenylalanine from polyuridylic acid. Nirenberg and Mattaei announced their demonstration of the relationship between the amino acid content of a polypeptide chain and the base composition of a polyribonucleotide at the International Biochemistry Congress in Moscow in 1961. Nirenberg also reported that transfer RNA was an obligatory intermediate in the formation of polyphenylalanine directed by polyuridylic acid. Scientists realized that by extending and refining this approach it would be possible to decipher the entire genetic code. The necessary construction of polyribinucleotides containing the four common ribonucleotides—adenylic, uridylic, cytidyltic, and guanylic acids—in specific proportions was made practical through the use of polynucleotide phosphorylase, an enzyme discovered in 1955 by Severo Ochoa and Marianne Grunberg-Manago.

In 1957 Robert Holley had described evidence for the existence of the form of cellular RNA now known as tRNAs and their possible involvement in protein synthesis. Within five years it was clear that protein synthesis involved a whole series of enzymes, each specific for one amino acid and one particular tRNA. These enzymes catalyzed the formation of a covalent linkage between the amino acid and their specific tRNAs. It seemed probable that amino acids had to be linked to their tRNAs in order to be used in protein synthesis. All the tRNAs seemed to be relatively small molecules, consisting of chains of fewer than one hundred nucleotides. They all seemed to be very similar, if not identical, at least at the ends of the chains. They also seemed to contain some unusual nucleotides. Nevertheless, given the methods available in the 1950s and 1960s, the task of purifying any one of the tRNAs and sequencing even such a relatively small polynucleotide chain was formidable. Solving all the many problems of purification and sequencing required quite novel and major technical innovations.

In 1965 Holley announced that he and his colleagues had determined the complete nucleotide sequence of a tRNA specific for the amino acid alanine. He had obtained pure alanine tRNA by the countercurrent-distribution technique. To solve the primary structure of the purified tRNA Holley devised procedures similar in concept to those introduced by Nobel laureate Fred Sanger for the determination of the sequence of amino acids in proteins. Purified tRNA was broken into pieces by different enzymes that were known to catalyze chain scission only at bonds occupied by a particular type of nucleotide residue. For example, ribonuclease T1 splits the chain at guanylic acid residues. Pancreatic ribonuclease splits the chain at both uridylic and cytidylic acid residues. Holley and his coworkers had to work out methods for separating and sequencing the small polynucleotide fragments released from tRNA by enzymatic digestion. When the fragments had been analyzed, they had to be put together in the unique linear array that constituted the original alanine tRNA. Holley noted that the nucleotide sequence for alanine tRNA was not just the first nucleotide for a nucleic acid; with appropriate modifications for DNA, the sequence also provided the first nucleotide sequence for a gene.

Having solved the complete nucleotide sequence of alanine tRNA, Holley turned to other aspects of its structure. The question of particular interest revolved around the nature of the interaction of tRNA with a messenger RNA. It seemed reasonable to suggest that the three-dimensional structure of the tRNA should have an anticodon exposed in such a way as to permit interaction with the condon in messenger RNA. The "cloverleaf" model seemed to meet these requirements. By 1968 twelve different tRNAs had been sequenced and all seemed to allow for double-stranded regions that fit the cloverleaf model. The pattern of enzyme digestion had provided some clues about the secondary structure of the tRNA: areas that were involved in double-helical configurations were presumably less exposed and more protected from digestive enzymes than other areas. Thus, Holley not only determined the primary sequence of tRNA, he also proposed several plausible models for the configuration of alanine tRNA, including the generally accepted cloverleaf model.

According to Holley, the successful solution of the structure of alanine transfer RNA "all followed quite naturally from taking a sabbatical leave." Therefore, he strongly recommended sabbatical leaves (Holley, "Alanine Transfer RNA," *Nobel Lectures*, 336).

Other honors awarded to Robert Holley include the Distinguished Service Award, U.S. Department of Agriculture (1965), the Albert Lasker Award for Basic Medical Research (1965), the U.S. Steel Foundation Award in Molecular Biology (1967), a doctor of science honorary degree from the University of Illinois, Urbana-Champaign (1970), and an American Cancer Society Research Professorship as American Cancer Society Professor of Molecular Biology (1969–87).

Holley is a member of the American Academy of Arts and Sciences, the American Association for the Advancement of Science, the American Chemical Society, the American Society of Biological Chemists, and the National Academy of Sciences.

LOIS N. MAGNER

Selected Bibliography

PRIMARY SOURCES

Holley, R. W., J. Apgar, G. A. Everett, J. T. Madison, M. Marquisee,

S. H. Merrill, J. R. Penswick, and A. Zarmir. 1965. "Structure of a Ribonucleic Acid." *Science* 147:1462–65.

Holley, R. W. 1965. "Structure of an Alanine Transfer Ribonucleic Acid." *Journal of the American Medical Association* 194:868–71.

———. 1968. "Alanine Transfer RNA." Nobel Lecture, December 12, 1968. Reprinted in *Nobel Lectures, Physiology or Medicine*, vol. 4 (1963–1970), 324–40.

———. 1972. A Unifying Hypothesis Concerning the Nature of Malignant Growth. *Proceedings of the National Academy of Science* (USA) 69:2840–41.

———. 1975. "Control of Growth of Mammalian Cells in Cell Culture." *Nature* 258:487–90.

Hanks, S. K., R. Armour, J. H. Baldwin, F. Malconado, J. Spiess, and R. W. Holley. 1988. "Amino Acid Sequence of the BSC-1 Cell Growth Inhibitor (Polyergin) Deduced from the Nucleotide Sequence of the cDNA." *Proceedings of the National Academy of Science* 85:79–82.

SECONDARY SOURCES

Holley, Robert W. 1966. "The Nucleotide Sequence of a Nucleic Acid." *Scientific American* 214:30–40.

1967. *Current Biography Yearbook* 172–74. New York: H. W. Wilson.

Grossman, L. and K. Modave, eds. 1967. *Enzymology*. Vol. 12, "Nucleic Acids," part A. New York: Academic Press.

Holley, R. W. 1968. "Experimental Approaches to the Determination of the Nucleotide Sequences of Large Oligonucleotides and Small Nucleic Acids." *Progress in Nucleic Acid Research* 8:37–47.

Singer, Maxine F. 1968. "1968 Nobel Laureate in Medicine or Physiology." *Science* 162: 433–36.

Fruton, Joseph S. 1972. *Molecules and Life. Historical Essays on the Interplay of Chemistry and Biology*. New York: Wiley-Interscience.

Smith, E. E., and D. W. Ribbons, eds. 1975. *Molecular Approaches to Immunology*. New York: Academic Press.

Corradino, R. A., ed. 1982. *Functional Regulation at the Cellular and Molecular Levels*. New York: Elsevier.

SIR FREDERICK GOWLAND HOPKINS *1929*

Sir Frederick Gowland Hopkins was born June 20, 1861, in Eastbourne, England. A biochemist, Hopkins won the Nobel Prize in 1929 for his chemical studies of nutritional substances, which conclusively established that proteinaceous and caloric foods *alone* were insufficient for normal animal growth; "accessory factors," found in certain specific foods, were essential. These factors were unknown before Hopkins's work; following his lead, several investigators isolated and characterized them as "vitamins" A through K. At the time of the award, Sir Frederick was chairman of the Biochemistry Department at Cambridge University, the position he occupied for twenty-nine years, until his retirement in 1943. He had been knighted in 1925. He was married to Jessie Anne Stevens in 1898; they had one son and two daughters. The younger daughter, Jacquetta Hawkes, is a well-known writer on history and archaeology; she is married to J. B. Priestley. Hopkins died on May 16, 1947, in Cambridge, England.

Hopkins's father, Frederick, was a London bookseller and a first cousin to Gerard Manley Hopkins, the poet. He was much interested in science but died when his son was still an infant. Hopkins was raised by his mother, Elizabeth Gowland Hopkins, in Eastbourne; as a boy, he wrote poetry and studied sea animals with a small microscope. When he was ten, they returned to London and he entered the City of London School, where he won several honors in science. His first paper, on the purple vapor produced by the bombardier beetle, was published in *The Entomologist* shortly after he left school, out of "sheer boredom."

At age seventeen, Frederick became a clerk in an insurance office, where he stayed only six months. Next he entered on a three-year indenture as assistant in a commercial analytic laboratory. This commitment must have seemed a long one in a young man's life, for he later wrote: "These years taught me something perhaps which might not have been learned elsewhere, for instance, how to obtain results in the shortest possible time." He added ruefully, "Intellectually, they were nearly sterile years."

A small legacy enabled Hopkins to enroll in a course at the Royal School of Mines. There he heard several lectures by Edward Frankland, "the only lectures on chemistry to which I ever listened." These inspired him to join a new private laboratory run by Frankland's son. He was quickly bored by the routine work, however, and struck out on his own. He was twenty-one years old.

He enrolled at the University of London to prepare for the associateship examination at the Institute of Chemistry. Hopkins's brilliant showing at these sessions led to an invitation to work with Sir Thomas Stevenson of Guy's Hospital, forensic specialist to the Home Office and an expert on poisoning. As Sir Thomas's assistant, he participated in several legal cases and was able to support himself while studying, largely on his own, for his B.Sc., which he earned in 1888.

Hopkins then applied to Guy's Hospital Medical School, where he was awarded the William Gull research studentship. He won several honors as a medical student and added to his list of publications. In 1891 *Guy's Hospital Reports* published his method for assaying the uric acid content of urine. His work on the pigments in the wings of butterflies was published in preliminary form in 1889 and presented in full to the Royal Society in 1895, by E. R. Lankester.

Hopkins graduated in medicine in 1894, at the mature age of thirty-three. He was immediately made an assistant at Guy's, where he taught physiology and toxicology for the next four years. During this period he assisted in the formation of the Clinical Research Association, which provided pathology services for practitioners. His research at Guy's concerned the crystallization of the albumins of blood serum and the halogen derivatives of proteins.

In 1898, while attending a meeting in Cambridge, he met Sir Michael Foster, professor of Physiology, who invited him to take up the lectureship assigned to the neglected field of chemical physiology (biochemistry was not then established as a separate discipline). Hopkins accepted the lectureship, which paid two hundred pounds a year. His laboratory consisted of a single small room in the Department of Physiology. He supplemented his income by supervising undergraduates and tutoring at Emmanuel College, and by doing part-time work for the Home Office.

Hopkins had been interested in nutrition since he was a medical student and at one time had hoped to investigate nutritional deficiency diseases, such as scurvy and rickets, from a clinical standpoint. He now concentrated his research efforts on dietary proteins, which were believed to be the key to understanding nutrition. After some studies on the relation of protein to uric acid output, he began work on the purification of protein components. In 1901, assisted by S. W. Cole, he isolated and identified the essential amino acid tryptophane, which is formed from dietary protein in the body. With the help of Edith Willcox, he demonstrated the critical role of the amino acids. These researchers were sufficiently impressive to the Cambridge authorities to result in the creation of a readership in biochemistry for Hopkins in 1902.

In his amino acid studies, Hopkins fed his animals synthetic diets. From his observations over several years, he concluded that a synthetic diet consisting *only* of the "basal dietary elements," that is, purified proteins or amino acids, carbohydrates, fats and salts, was, contrary to accepted wisdom, inadequate to support normal healthy growth. "Accessory food factors," as yet unknown, but found in natural diets, were also essential. Although research animals were known to survive on synthetic diets, Hopkins concluded that the diets in question had not been completely purified and some traces of the "accessory factors" remained.

After a series of experiments with mice in 1906–7, in which he fed diets with fractionally different amounts of casein and yeast, and amino acids in place of intact proteins, he announced his ideas publicly. They were met with skepticism as the caloric theory of nutrition was considered to be well established. Hopkins realized he would have to prove his case experimentally and retired to his laboratory to attempt to isolate the "accessory factors."

As Stephenson, one of Hopkins's biographers, has put it: "In his famous paper of 1912 Hopkins showed that a diet consisting of casein, extracted exhaustively with ethanol, starch, sugar, lard and inorganic salts was unable to maintain growth or support life in young rats, but became perfectly adequate when fresh milk amounting to 1–3% of the whole diet was added. The great feature of the work was the complete adequacy of the controls introduced in the selection of the animals, and the certainty, that incomplete ingestion or absorption were playing no part. As a perfect experiment of its kind it stands as a model."

Hopkins then suffered a severe illness and was not able to work for some time. When he did return to the laboratory, he reviewed the data he had collected over the years, and immediately began a study of energy consumption in rats given no milk or butter, and then fed minute increments of milk, with no change in caloric consumption or basic dietary composition. (Milk, of course, provides vitamins A, B, and D.) The results, published in the *Journal of Physiology* in 1912, established the "indispensable nature of food constituents which were then receiving no serious consideration as physiological necessities."

Even the skeptics were unable to contradict Hopkins's evidence; the era of vitamin research began immediately. McCollum and Davis in 1913 isolated the fat-soluble vitamin A, and the water-soluble vitamin B, in milk. Joseph Goldberger later demonstrated that B was not a single factor but a complex of related chemicals, two of which were related to the deficiency diseases beriberi and pellagra. Scurvy was found to result from vitamin C deficiency; rickets from a lack of D; vision defects from vitamin A deficiency. Work on vitamin mechanisms continues today.

Hopkins had been elected a fellow of Trinity College in 1910. He was now freed from all intrusions on his time unrelated to biochemistry. A group of bright young students quickly grew up in his small lab. In 1914 Hopkins and his "school" inherited the Balfour Laboratory space belonging to the Department of Physiology, which had moved to a new building.

He had begun work with Walter Morley Fletcher on the metabolism of muscular activity and rigor mortis. Fletcher and Hopkins were the first to accurately describe the production of lactic acid by the voluntary muscles, which they outlined in the Croonian Lecture before the Royal Society in 1915. Hopkins's precise analytical methods and development of a new color reaction for lactic acid were crucial to this important research.

His further research led him into the study of intracellular enzymes. In 1921 he identified a substance that appeared to be integral to rapid cellular multiplication in both plants and animals; he named this compound glutathione and later characterized it as a tripeptide of glutamic acid, glycine, and cystein. He also isolated xanthine oxidase, the enzyme catalyst for the oxidation of purines to uric acid.

In 1921 the trustee of Sir William Dunn's estate endowed a new chair in biochemistry for Hopkins, and also funded the construction of the new Sir William Dunn Institute of Biochemistry, into which the department moved in 1925. Here "Hoppy's" school finally had facilities specifically designed for their work.

Sir Frederick was a spare, quiet man, much beloved by his students. From his earliest work, he was moved by a vivid understanding of the cell as a minute, cooperatively organized factory, in which a thousand microcosmic activities were constantly in progress. He was deeply concerned with the development of biochemistry as "a separate discipline concerned with this active chemistry of the life processes, and not merely with its fuel and end-products" (Sherrington 1947, Dale 1959). His students served him well; among his many apprentices were J. B. S. Haldane and Judah Quastel, both of whom made major contributions to the field.

Hopkins was elected to the Royal Society in 1905. Among the many other honors Hopkins received for his work were the Baly Medal of the Royal College of Physicians (1915), the Royal Medal of the Royal Society (1918), the Cameron Prize from the University of Edinburgh (1922), the Copley Medal (1926), and the Order of Merit (1935).

From 1930 to 1935 Sir Frederick served as president of the Royal Society. In 1933 he presided as well over the massive British Association for the Advancement of Science. Although these responsibilities took him away from his laboratory, he was a major influence on British science in the 1930s.

Increasing blindness clouded his later years and limited his work in the laboratory, although not the affection of his students. He retired in 1943 and died four years later at age eighty-six.

WILLIAM C. GIBSON

Selected Bibliography

PRIMARY SOURCES

Hopkins, Sir Frederick Gowland. 1949. *Hopkins and Biochemistry, 1861–1947*. Cambridge: W. Heffer. Contains much of his published work.

SECONDARY SOURCES

Sherrington, Sir Charles S. 1947. "Hopkins, Sir Frederick Gowland. Obituary. *Lancet* (May 24):728–31.

Stephenson, M. Obituary Notice. *The Biochemical Journal* 42:161–169. Illus.

Dale, Sir Henry H. 1959. "Hopkins, Sir Frederick Gowland." In *Dictionary of National Biography, 1941–1950,* 406–8. London: Oxford University Press.

Baldwin, Ernest. 1966. *Gowland Hopkins.* London: VandenBerghs.

1972. "Hopkins, (Sir) Frederick Gowland." In *Dictionary of Scientific Biography,* 6:498–502. New York: Scribners.

SIR GODFREY NEWBOLD HOUNSFIELD *1979*

Hounsfield was born in Newark, Nottinghamshire, England, on August 28, 1919, the son of Thomas Hounsfield, a farmer. He was active as a radar technician and then as an electronics engineer, but became best known for the work that earned him the Nobel Prize for Physiology or Medicine in 1979, the development of computed tomography.

Hounsfield's father worked in the steel industry until failing eyesight forced him to turn to farming. A cousin had designed the Trojan car and had invented the Hounsfield tensometer, which may account for the boy's early interest in technical apparatus. Hounsfield grew up in the Nottinghamshire village of Trent. He attended the Magnus Grammar School in Newark, where he was an indifferent scholar, although he excelled in the physical sciences and was fascinated with electronics. He built his own audio recording system and for a time operated the local movie house with another teenager. He left secondary school without matriculating at a university and became a draftsman for a local builder. On his own, he studied textbooks on radio, including some intended for communications officers in the armed forces. He was twenty when World War II broke out and at once volunteered for the Royal Air Force, in which he served from 1939 to 1946. After taking a placement test for radio technicians, he was excused from the basic ("ab initio") training and assigned to a more advanced course, some of whose early graduates then became instructors as the RAF's wartime requirements for communications personnel continued to grow.

Hounsfield became such an instructor. His duties expanded as electronic navigation and radar equipment was introduced, and he also prepared for and passed the examinations for the radio communications certificate of the City and Guilds of London Institute. He was posted to the RAF's famed Cranwell Radar School, where he attracted attention by devising electrical visual aids to train maintenance technicians how to locate circuit faults. His work in the RAF earned him the Certificate of Merit in 1945, which facilitated his postwar admission to Faraday House, a four-year diploma-granting institution engaged in training mainly industry-bound electrical engineers.

Hounsfield graduated in 1951 and joined EMI Ltd, the parent company of His Master's Voice and of a worldwide network of affiliated recording companies. EMI was widening its scope by turning to the design and manufacture of products based on its wartime participation in defense electronics, and also attempting to enter the computer business. Hounsfield worked first on radar systems and then led the team that designed Britain's first all-transistor computer, the EMIDEC 1100. EMI never became a computer manufacturer, but the experience stood Hounsfield in good stead for his next project.

Starting from an interest in pattern recognition, he conceived a system in which a collimated beam of X-rays would produce a display of a cross section of the human body, to replace the conventional shadowgraph familiar since the discovery of X-rays by Konrad Röntgen in 1895. The conventional system also suffered from poor contrast, which made the differentiation of soft tissues difficult and the display of features hidden behind bones next to impossible. The latter problem had been attacked in the 1920s and 1930s by "tomography," a method in which the X-ray source and the photographic plate were moved in opposite directions during exposure, so that a particular feature would remain in focus and objects behind and in front of it would be blurred. Even then, the resulting image would not be representative of the density distribution in the objects through which the X-rays had passed, but only of an average value.

Hounsfield's great contribution was to measure the attenuation of a highly collimated beam of X-rays passing through a thin horizontal slice of a patient's head or other organ from successive directions and then to re-create a display from the resulting data by means of a computer. Although he was not a mathematician, he devised a practical method of doing it that proved to be consistent with rigorous mathematical theory. The theory had been available since 1917, buried in a paper by the Austrian mathematician Johann Radon ("Ueber die Bestimmung von Funktionen durch ihre Integralwerte längs gewisser Manningfaltigkeiten," *Berichte der sächsischen Akademie der Wissenschaften* 67 [1917]:262–77). It had been elaborated by Hounsfield's near contemporary A. M. Cormack in 1963–64 ("Representation of a Function by Its Line Integrals," *Journal of Applied Physics* 34 [1963]:2722–27 and 35 [1964]:2908–13). The method, dubbed "computed tomography," is still widely used, although the technique has been substantially changed, notably through the replacement of X-rays by tomography based on different principles, such as nuclear magnetic resonance.

The EMI machine (originally known as "computer-assisted tomography" or CAT scanner) became an extraordinary commercial success, especially after a more elaborate version was produced that could scan not only the head but the entire human body. The annual grosses in the hundreds of millions of pounds that flowed into EMI's coffers were the more remarkable since the company still had little in-house experience in computers, and even less in X-ray equipment. Much of the credit belonged to the vice chairman of EMI's electronics group, John Powell, who was a steadfast and effective champion of Hounsfield's invention. That he succeeded in persuading EMI's management and board to support the project was in part due to the company's excellent financial condition after a decade during which it dominated the popular-music market with The Beatles and other recording artists. However, as other companies, with better access to the medical community and more experience in manufacturing and marketing complex equipment, rose to the challenge, EMI's pre-eminence faded and the company ultimately abandoned manufacturing X-ray scanners altogether. In 1980, it merged with Thorn Electric Industries to become Thorn EMI Ltd.

Hounsfield's contribution was promptly recognized in Britain and elsewhere. He received the MacRobert Award for Engineering Excellence in 1972 and the Prince Philip Medal of the City and Guilds of London Institute for outstanding achievement in science, technology, and industry in 1975; he was elected Fellow of the Royal Society in 1975; he was named Companion of the Order of the British Empire in 1976; and he was knighted in 1981. Among his foreign honors were several honorary doctorates and the Exner Medal (Austria), the Lasker Award (USA), and the Deutsche Röntgen Plakette (Germany). He shared the Nobel Prize in Physiology or Medicine in 1979 with A. M. Cormack, the aforementioned physicist who had worked out the mathematical aspects of the scanning problem in 1963.

CHARLES SUSSKIND

Selected Bibliography

PRIMARY SOURCES

Hounsfield, G. N. 1968 and 1973. UK patent 1,283,915.

Hounsfield, G. N. 1973. "Computerised Transverse Axial Scanning (Tomography)." *Brit. J. Radiology* 46: 1016–22, 1023–47.

SECONDARY SOURCES

Rowbottom, Margaret, and Charles Susskind. 1981. *Electricity and Medicine: History of Their Interaction*, 253–59. San Francisco: San Francisco Press.

Susskind, Charles. 1981. "The Invention of Computed Tomography." In *History of Technology*, edited by A. R. Hall and Norman Smith, 6:39–80. London: Mansell.

1988. "Hounsfield, Sir Godfrey (Newbold)." *Who's Who* (London).

BERNARDO ALBERTO HOUSSAY

1947

A scientist and physician with special interests in physiology and pharmacology, Houssay was born April 10, 1887, in Buenos Aires, Argentina. He died there on September 21, 1971, after an illustrious career that included winning the Nobel Prize for Physiology or Medicine in 1947. The award was bestowed for his discovery of the role played by the hormone of the anterior pituitary lobe in sugar metabolism. Within Latin American academic circles, Houssay was unquestionably the most eminent scientist of his day. Largely an autodidact, he quickly rose to the top of his chosen field because of his total devotion to research and teaching. Not only did he enjoy a worldwide reputation as an endocrinologist, but, more importantly, Houssay inspired generations of his compatriots to follow him into experimental physiology. To this day his school remains highly influential in academic circles throughout Latin America.

I must also point out that Houssay's dedication to the ideals of democracy and justice prompted him to vigorously oppose fascism, Nazism, and, after the military coup of 1943, the political leadership in Argentina. For more than a decade he spoke out fearlessly against the military dictatorship and subsequent government of General Juan D. Peron, an action that cost him his academic position and forced him to continue his research in private laboratories furnished by the Sauberan Foundation of Argentina.

One of eight children—four boys and four girls—Bernardo A. Houssay was the son of Dr. Alberto Houssay, a lawyer, and Clara Laffont, both of whom had come to Argentina from France. Barely thirteen, Bernardo entered the School of Pharmacy of the University of Buenos Aires in 1901, after successfully completing his baccalaureate degree with honors at the prestigious Colegio Nacional de Buenos Aires. Before graduating at the top of his class in 1904, he sought further studies and subsequently enrolled in the university's medical school. In 1910 Houssay received his medical degree with honors. His doctoral dissertation focused on the physiological action of pituitary extracts and earned him a prize as the best thesis of that year.

In spite of his formal pharmaceutical and medical studies, Houssay remained largely a self-taught man, earning a modest living as a hospital pharmacist to provide for his continuing education. Although he lacked role models and mentors, he pursued his scientific studies with alacrity. Even before graduation from medical school, Houssay had received an appointment as assistant in the university's Department of Physiology. Then, shortly after receiving the M.D. degree in 1910, he became professor of physiology at the School of Veterinary Science of the University of Buenos Aires. Three years later Houssay was appointed chief physician at the Alvear Hospital, a municipal establishment in the city of Buenos Aires. Here, surrounded by a group of equally enthusiastic young physicians, he taught the basics of scientific medicine.

In 1915 Houssay became chief of the Laboratory of Experimental Pathology and Physiology organized at Argentina's National Public Health Laboratories, then under the direction of the Viennese bacteriologist Rudolf Krauss. Several publications from that time attest to his interests in the effects from snake, spider, and scorpion bites on blood coagulation and hemolysis, work that cemented Houssay's international reputation. At the same time, it brought the young scientist in contact with Maria A. Catan, a chemist, and in 1920 their relationship led to marriage. The couple had three sons, Alberto, Hector, and Raul, all of whom became prominent physicians. Mrs. Houssay not only dedicated her life to childrearing but helped her husband with the drafting and writing of papers.

Houssay began his academic career at the University of Buenos Aires Medical School when he was appointed professor of physiology in 1919. Shortly thereafter, the chair was expanded into an Institute of Physiology and Houssay became a full-time educator and researcher, a status gradually emulated by other colleagues in Argentina and throughout Latin America. His studies in fat metabolism and ketogenesis, the influence of the pituitary gland and sex hormones on diabetes mellitus, and thyroid and adrenal functions attracted worldwide attention and brought numerous students to his laboratory. Houssay's meticulous attention to detail and capacity for work in the laboratory became legendary. Among his early disciples were Virgilio G. Foglia, Juan T. Lewis, Venancio Deulofeu, Agustin Marenzi, Enrique Di Benedetto, and Oscar Orias.

According to Juan T. Lewis, Houssay's teaching at the Institute of Physiology started a new era in Argentine medicine. Although not a brilliant lecturer, he nevertheless stimulated others by his exemplary dedication to scientific research and exacting methods that could be applied to clinical studies. Among the principal fields of research were the role of the hypothesis on carbohydrate metabolism, which clarified the pathogenesis of human diabetes. With the help of his collaborators, Houssay discovered and identified the principal hypophyseal hormones, the work that earned him the Nobel Prize. Related work on the pancreatic secretion of insulin included the transplantation of pancreatic tissue to correct diabetic hyperglycemia.

In another long series of experiments, Houssay discovered that the hypophyseal hormones and insulin played key roles in the control of fat metabolism. Inspired by his earlier interest in the sexual functions of toads, Houssay and his colleague Galli Mainini demonstrated that a liberation of sperm in the toad occurred if the animal was injected with urine from a pregnant woman. This phenomenon was quickly exploited and became an inexpensive but accurate diagnostic test for pregnancy.

Other significant research focused on the factors regulating arterial blood pressure. Working with Eduardo Braun Menendez, Houssay explored the production of hypertension in dogs when the renal arteries were partially ligated. The results of this research revealed the presence of "renin" in kidneys, a substance acting on the blood to produce a vasopressor called angiotensin. Angiotensin, in turn, was shown to influence the adrenal glands and trigger the secretion of another hormone: aldosterone.

In addition to his busy career as a researcher and teacher, Houssay became active in the institutional developments of Argentine biomedicine. He founded the Argentine Society of Biology in 1920, and was elected member of the National Academy of Medicine in 1927, the National Academy of Letters in 1935, and the National Academy of Sciences in 1946. He also became a member of the editorial board of several scientific periodicals, including the *Revista de la Sociedad Argentina de Biologia.*

Following the military coup of 1943, Houssay and many other university professors who had signed a petition urging the military to return Argentina to a constitutional government, were dismissed from their posts. Undaunted, Houssay resisted invitations to resume his career abroad and instead founded in 1944 a privately financed Institute of Biology and Experimental Medicine in Buenos Aires with Juan T. Lewis, Virgilio G. Foglia, Oscar Orias, Eduardo Braun Menendez, and later Luis F. Leloir.

After a brief reinstatement in 1945, Houssay was again relieved of all his academic posts a year later because of his opposition to the government of General Juan Peron. He spent some time abroad, visiting European and American centers of biomedical investigation. Offered in 1949 a permanent position at the National Institutes of Health in Bethesda, Maryland, and the opportunity to assemble his entire team of researchers, Houssay wrote from the Cosmos Club in Washington to one of his students: "My life is dedicated to almost impossible goals, many of which have been unexpectedly fulfilled. I want to devote myself to the scientific development of the land in which I was born, grew up, have friends, fought and learned." Houssay returned to Argentina, working quietly at the Institute of Biology. His final vindication came in 1955, after the successful revolution that toppled Peron from power. Already sixty-eight years old, Houssay regained the directorship of his old Institute of Physiology at the University of Buenos Aires. A year later, however, he retired from this academic post.

In 1958 Houssay helped to launch the National Council for Scientific and Technical Research. This quasi public organization was charged with the task of promoting scientific research in Argentina in several areas including biomedicine. With the help of fellowships to train promising scientists abroad, the creation of new technical and scientific careers at home, and the repatriation of Argentine scientists who had left the motherland during the dictatorship of Peron, Consejo Nacional de Ciencia y Technica under Houssay flourished. Even two weeks before his death, in a conversation with the Argentine president and CONACYT officials, the future of science in Argentina was foremost on his mind.

Houssay's dictum that science had no country but a scientist did, reflected his conviction that in spite of the universality of science, knowledge was shaped by the ideals and values prevalent in those societies whose representatives engaged in research. For him the investigative enterprise was closely coupled with political freedom and a set of attitudes—competence, dedication, and self-denial—deemed necessary for its success. His scientific endeavors and political activities were thus inextricably connected. To this day, Houssay remains the symbol of Argentina's intellectual and scientific maturity, linked through his Nobel Prize and numerous foreign contacts to the world community of science.

GUENTER B. RISSE

Selected Bibliography

PRIMARY SOURCES

Houssay, Bernardo Alberto. 1942. *Escritos y Discursos*. Buenos Aires: El Ateneo.

———. 1947. "The Role of the Hypothesis in Carbohydrate Metabolism and in Diabetes." Nobel Prize Lecture, 12 December, 1947. Reprinted in *Nobel Lectures, Physiology or Medicine*, vol. 3 (1942–1962), 210–17. Amsterdam: Elsevier, 1964.

———. 1965. "Role of the Scientist in Modern Society." *Georgetown Medical Bulletin* 18:143.

SECONDARY SOURCES

Lewis, Juan T. 1963. "Bernardo Alberto Houssay." *Perspectives in Biology*, edited by C. F. Cori et al., vii–xiv. New York: Elsevier.

Foglia, Virgilio G. 1971. "Bernardo Alberto Houssay." *Acta Physiologica Latino Americana* 21:267–85.

Young, Frank, and Virgilio G. Foglia. 1974. "Bernardo Alberto Houssay, 1887–1971." *Biographical Memoirs of Fellows of the Royal Society* 20:247–70.

DAVID HUNTER HUBEL *1981*

David Hunter Hubel was born on February 27, 1926, in Windsor, Ontario, Canada. A neurophysiologist, Hubel was awarded one half of the 1981 Nobel Prize for Physiology or Medicine jointly with Torsten N. Wiesel; the other half was awarded to Roger W. Sperry. Hubel and Wiesel's work in mapping the striate cortex and describing its operation illuminated our understanding of the process of visual perception and has had important clinical impact on the early treatment of visual problems in children. The Hubel-Wiesel team also laid the foundations of the Department of Neurobiology at Harvard, where Hubel is today John Franklin Enders University Professor. At the time of the award, he held the title of George Packer Berry Professor. Hubel married Shirley Izzard in 1953; he and his wife have three sons: Carl, Eric, and Paul.

Hubel's parents, Jesse Hervey and Elsie Hunter Hubel, were Americans living in Canada, where his father worked as a chemical engineer. Despite early interests in chemistry and physics, Hubel was not determined on a career until he rather impulsively decided to enter medical school after graduation from McGill University in 1947. He became interested in neurology while attending McGill's medical school and spent two years as a resident at the Montreal Neurological Institute after completing a general internship at Montreal General Hospital.

In 1954 he was accepted for further residency training at Johns Hopkins but was soon drafted into the U.S. Army Medical Corps. From 1955 to 1958 he worked at the Walter Reed Army Institute of Research, where he used microelectrodes to study brain activity in cats over long periods.

Returning to Johns Hopkins in 1958, he began work at the Wilmer Institute with Vernon Mountcastle and Stephen Kuffler. Here he met Torsten Wiesel, a graduate of the Karolinska Institute of Stockholm, and the two began their investigations of the visual mechanism. Most of their work was done at Harvard, where the team followed Kuffler in 1959.

Previous research, by H. Keffer Hartline, Ragnar Granit, Jerome Y. Lettvin, and Kuffler himself, had described the visual process as based on the perception of change in the level of light stimulus and comparison of the boundaries of different levels of light. The initial perception by rods and cones in the eye is fed back through layer after layer of neurons. Within the cat's retina, each retinal ganglion cell is stimulated by the particular point of light stimulating the point on the outer eye that connects with that cell. The pattern of stimulation varies, however, according to the differences in the level of illumination reaching surrounding cells; a brighter light stimulus reaching the surrounding area inhibits the individual cell, and vice versa. The contrasting light and dark levels can thus form a picture for interpretation.

Studies of frogs had shown that this interpretation occurs in the optic nerve, but Kuffler's examination of the cat's retinal ganglion cells showed that they reacted to differences between light and dark but showed no ability to sort out particular shapes and movements, as did similar cells in frogs. Hubel and Wiesel theorized that the critical level of visual perception in mammals occurs within the brain, in the striate cortex, and that cortical perception is binocular, that is, based on stimuli from both eyes simultaneously (Lettvin 1981, 519).

The team implanted microelectrodes in cats and monkeys, and then exposed the animals to a variety of visual stimuli to detect the electrochemical discharge of individual nerve cells. After recording the nervous activity, they sacrificed and dissected the animals to determine the relation of anatomy and function. In other experiments they injected radioactive substances into the eyes to trace the route from the retina to the visual cortex. The path they described leads from the retinal ganglions via the optic nerve to lateral geniculate nuclei in the brain and from there to the layered neurons of the cortex itself.

Hubel and Wiesel found the cortical anatomy to be extremely complex; indeed, in their classification, they rank nerve cells as simple, complex, and hypercomplex, acting progressively to create a single visual image from the millions of small bits of information arriving from the retina. They called this process progressive convergence. Although each cell "sees" only one point in the visual field, each point is perceived by a great many cells. The various cells record information in terms of the size and shape of the stimulus, the sharpness and angle of the boundary between light and dark, or the type and direction of movement of the stimulus. Different cells have different "preferences" for the type of stimulus they will register most effectively: a straight boundary between light and dark, a shaded band, a corner, or a tongue. Moreover, although each area of the cortex receives images from both retinas, some cells respond to one eye, some to the other, some to localized parts of both images.

The cortical cells are further organized into vertical divisions of two types, named by Hubel and Wiesel ocular dominance columns and orientation columns. The orientation columns translate the information from the retina, which is essentially coded as circular points of light, into linear images. The ocular dominance columns combine the information from both eyes into the carefully textured three-dimensional picture "seen" by the mammal. The extreme complexity of the visual cortex, as described by the team, makes clear the qualitative difference between the simple binocular perception of frogs and birds with the stereoscopic vision of cats and humans (Hubel and Wiesel 1962; Lettvin 1981, 519–20).

Further experiments with kittens established that the newborn mammal has a visual cortex functionally complete but still subject to development, as the animal learns to recognize the external world. During this critical period, if the vision of one eye is impaired or obscured, the cortical cells will "learn" to disregard the faulty information received from this eye as incompatible with experience. Even if the vision is later corrected, the brain will continue to operate as if the impairment existed and the repaired eye will remain functionally blind (Hubel and Wiesel 1963, 1965).

This new understanding has changed the whole field of pediatric ophthalmology. It is now clear that an early eye problem, such as strabismus or congenital cataracts, should not be neglected until the child is older or in hopes it will improve with maturity. On the contrary, immediate intervention is necessary if normal vision is to be preserved (Lettvin 1981, 520).

After coming to Harvard as an assistant professor of neurophysiology and neuropharmacology, Hubel rose to full professor by 1965 and was named to the Berry professorship in 1968. In 1967 he followed Kuffler as chairman of the Department of Neurobiology, which the elder scientist had created three years earlier. Torsten Wiesel in turn succeeded Hubel in 1973. The close Hubel-Wiesel partnership, remembered by George Berry as "like identical twins," continued throughout these years, until Wiesel's move to Rockefeller University in 1984 (*New York Times*, October 10, 1981).

Outside of his work and his family, Hubel's major interest is music. He is a member of the National Academy of Sciences and a fellow of the American Academy of Arts and Sciences. Among the many awards he and Wiesel have jointly won have been the Jules C. Stein Research for the Prevention of Blindness Award (1971), the Lewis S. Rosenstiel Award for Basic Medical Research from Brandeis University (1972), the Jonas S. Friedenwald Memorial Award of the Association for Research in Vision and Ophthalmology (1975), the Karl S. Lashley Prize of the American Philosophical Society (1977), the Louisa Gross Horowiz Prize from Columbia (1978), and the George Ledlie Prize from Harvard (1980).

MARCIA MELDRUM

Selected Bibliography

PRIMARY SOURCES

Hubel, David H., and Torsten N. Wiesel. 1959. "Receptive Fields of Single Neurons in the Cat's Striate Cortex." *Journal of Physiology* 148:574–91.

———. 1961. "Integrative Action in the Cat's Lateral Geniculate Body." *Journal of Physiology* 155:385–98.

———. 1962. "Receptive Fields, Binocular Interaction, and Functional Architecture in the Cat's Visual Cortex." *Journal of Physiology* 160:106–54.

———. 1963. "Single-cell Responses in Striate Cortex of Kittens Deprived of Vision in One Eye." *Journal of Neurophysiology* 26:1003–17.

———. 1965. "Extent of Recovery from the Effects of Visual Deprivation in

Kittens." *Journal of Neurophysiology* 28:1060–72.

———. 1965. "Receptive Fields and Functional Architecture in Two Non Striate Visual Areas (18 and 19) of the Cat." *Journal of Neurophysiology* 28:229–89.

———. 1968. "Receptive Fields and Functional Architecture of Monkey Striate Cortex." *Journal of Physiology* 195:215–43.

Hubel, David H. 1979. "The Visual Cortex of Normal and Deprived Monkeys." *American Scientist* 67:532–43.

———. 1988. *Mind, Brain, and Vision.* New York: Scientific American Library.

SECONDARY SOURCES

Altman, Lawrence K. 1981. "Studies Advance Work on Brain, Eye Disorders." *New York Times* (October 10):50.

Anon. 1981. "Nobel Prize in Medicine: David Hunter Hubel." *New York Times* (October 10):50.

Anon. 1981. "Torsten Nils Wiesel." *New York Times* (October 10):50.

Schmeck, Harold M., Jr. 1981. "Three Scientists Share Nobel Prize for Studies of the Brain." *New York Times* (October 10):1.

Lettvin, Jerome Y. 1981. "Filling Out the Forms: An Appreciation of Hubel and Wiesel." *Science* 214 (October 30):518–20.

CHARLES BRENTON HUGGINS
1966

Charles Brenton Huggins was born on September 22, 1901, in Halifax, Nova Scotia, Canada, the son of Charles Edward and Bessie Spencer Huggins. A surgeon, medical researcher, and university professor, Huggins grew up in Halifax and received a B.A. from Acadia University in Wolfville, in western Nova Scotia, in 1920. He then moved to the United States to attend Harvard University Medical School from which he received an M.D. degree in 1924. He served as intern and resident in surgery at the University of Michigan Medical School from 1924 to 1926, and then was appointed instructor in surgery in 1926.

While at Ann Arbor, Huggins met an undergraduate student, Margaret Wellman, and the two were married on July 29, 1927. Shortly thereafter the couple moved to Chicago where Huggins had been appointed to the faculty of the newly formed University of Chicago Medical School. The Huggins have two children, Charles Edward Huggins and Emily Wellman Huggins Fine.

Almost all of Huggins's career was spent at the University of Chicago. He began in 1927 as an instructor of surgery, was promoted to assistant professor in 1929, to associate professor in 1933, and to full professor in 1936, specializing in genitourinary surgery. He accepted an appointment as professor of urological surgery and director of the Department of Urology at Johns Hopkins University in 1946, but shortly returned to Chicago. In 1951 he was named director of the Ben May Laboratory for Cancer Research at the University of Chicago and in 1962 he became the William B. Ogden Distinguished Service Professor. Though he stepped down as director of the Ben May Laboratory in 1969, he continued to carry on with his research.

Huggins received the Nobel Prize for Physiology or Medicine in 1966 for his "discoveries concerning hormonal treatment of prostate cancer," a discovery that led to a system of cancer treatment by endocrinologic methods. Emerging from his studies was the concept now basic to cancer research that some types of cancer cells differ in a crucial way from their ancestral normal cells in their response to modification of hormonal environment. Change in hormonal status can induce regression and, in some instances, cures of such cancers. This could be accomplished either by deprivation of essential hormones or through administration of large amounts of other hormones. His breakthrough marked the effective beginning of chemotherapy in cancer.

Huggins began working on diseases of the genitourinary tract through the influence of Dallas B. Pehmister, the surgical head at Chicago, and soon assumed leadership of the urological division of surgery. He began work at an exciting time because research on hormones, which had been strongly supported by the Rockefeller Foundation through the Committee for Research in Problems of Sex of the National Research Council, was leading to critical breakthroughs. One of the major centers for such research was at the University of Chicago; it was headed by Frank R. Lillie, professor of biology, who as early as 1922 had started a program in sex biology. Lillie was particularly interested in the nature and limits of hormone action and under his aegis at Chicago a vast number of studies were commissioned and published.

The Chicago group initially had concentrated on female hormones but soon also became interested in male hormones. A group of Chicago biologists and biochemists had successfully isolated the testis hormone (testosterone) in partially purified form and had begun to characterize its activities through experiments of many sorts. These experiments grew in number as the chemistry of testosterone and related androgens was rather quickly worked out.

Huggins, who had begun his career by studying the physiology of bone marrow and bone formation, had been the first to recognize the effects of physiological temperature gradients on bone marrow in living animals. From 1933 to 1953 he concentrated on the physiology and biochemistry of the male urogenital tract; much of this research was supported by the Committee for Research in the Problems of Sex. He was the first to measure reliably the many components of seminal fluid in men. In a study of coagulation of the semen, he established that the liquification of the seminal clot in man is a proteolytic phenomenon. During his research he had observed that human spermatoza for a time soon after production lived in a fluid devoid of inorganic phosphorus. After the evaculation of spermatozoa, however, there was an increase in acid soluble phosphorus in their fluid environment. This led him to a detailed study of the metabolism of phosphorus in males. When he found it difficult to obtain unmixed secretions from human males, he turned to dogs, and thereafter devised the prostatic isolation operation that allowed him to collect prostatic fluid in quantity over specified intervals for long periods of time. He found that the normal output of prostatic secretion is dependent upon testicular androgens. He also discovered that castrated dogs could maintain their prostatic function through injection of androgenic steroids but that this function could be nullified by simultaneous administration of estrogenic compounds, thus achieving the first demonstration of the competitive antagonism between the two.

The use of the dog at this juncture proved fortuitous since it is the only known animal specie which like man develops tumors of the prostate, both benign and cancerous. Since his research was focused on establishing norms, he at first had no interest in dogs with tumors and simply considered them troublesome. But as he continued experimenting he observed that both an orchiectomy and small doses of phenolic estrogen caused a shrinkage in prostatic tumors. This concept was carried over to humans where Huggins reported similar results. He developed a test for measurement of enzymes in blood serum, especially alkaline and acid phosphatases, allowing him to appraise the result of endocrine therapy for cancer of the prostate.

His first series of orchiectomies was comprised of twenty patients with prostatic cancer and with widespread metastases. Four of these men survived more than twelve years following surgery. While there were failures in the hormone therapy, on the whole the life span was extended and there was a decrease in the pain hours of those whose life spans were not noticeably extended. Recognizing that some patients did not respond to his treatment and others who initially had responded favorably to either castration or estrogen therapy had suffered a return of their cancer, he found that the adrenals, which also produce male sex hormones, were stimulated to increase their output after chemical or surgical castration. To counter this relationship Huggins in 1951 developed a surgical procedure for removing the adrenals, keeping the patients well with daily doses of cortisone and water. The adrenalectomies clearly were to be prescribed as a last resort, only after all other curative methods had been utilized. Between 1951 and 1953 the operation was performed on some eighty patients. Fifty percent of those with advanced prostate and breast cancer were helped but it did not benefit other types of cancer cases. The fact that 50 percent of his patients continued to produce the female hormone estrogen, even after the adrenals and ovaries were removed, suggested that still another body organ must be a source of secretion of these hormones.

The adrenalectomies, six of which were performed on patients in Manteno Mental Health Center (later in 1979) led to sensational charges against Huggins of practicing experimental surgery. Only two of his patients from the center had cancer of the breast or prostate; the other four had been operated on because it was hypothesized that there might be a connection between hormones and schizophrenia. This was not demonstrated by the surgery.

Huggins's greatest ability was not as a surgeon. He could see what others had not observed before, discover new connections and then act boldly on his hypotheses no matter how farfetched they seemed at the time. Usually he was successful. Once he had made the connection between hormones and cancer, he spent some time trying to find nonfeminizing substances that would suppress testosterone in males, and this led to much of modern cancer chemotherapy. He later moved into the study of breast cancer in women and began experimenting with a powerful chemical, 3 methyl choanthrene, which suppressed the production of a substance known to stimulate the secretion of female sex hormones. He also found that giving a known carcinogen, 7,12 dimethylbenz (a) anthracene (DMBA), to a special strain of rats led to the development of breast cancer. Structural similarities between chemical carcinogens, steroid hormones, and two components of the chemical deoxyribonucleic acid (DNA) were studied, leading to the finding that they had carcinogenic molecules known as "Polynuclear aromatic hydrocarbons" masquerading as hormones or hereditary material. These forced their way into body cells, changing the cells from normally functioning units to malignant tissues that grew into tumors, causing cancer in laboratory animals. Single doses of these hydrocarbons caused cancers in rats and killed them in two months, but if the rats were injected with estrogen the cancer could be destroyed.

His research into breast cancer led him to be consulted when fears were expressed that birth control pills using estrogen might cause cancer of the breasts and genitals. Never afraid to take a stand, he held that these pills would not cause significant numbers of cancers.

Though Huggins had made his breakthrough discovery in 1941, the Nobel Committee was slow to recognize his importance. Goran Liljestrand, secretary of the Nobel Committee for Medicine, in Shück's *Nobel, the Man and His Prizes* (1951), dismissed Huggins's work because among other things it had not resulted in a permanent cure. Apparently, as with many other Nobel Prizes, it took over a generation to realize the significance of his breakthroughs.

Huggins, however, had not gone unrecognized. His awards are numerous: the Gold Medal of the American Medical Association (1936 and 1940); the Award for Research from the American Urological Association (1948); the Francis Amory Award (1948); Gold Medal from the Sociéte International d'Urologie (1948); Lasker Award for Medical Research (1963); Laurea Award, American Urological Society (1969); Sheen Award, American Medical Association (1970); Sesquicentennial Commemorative Award, National Library of Medicine (1986), and numerous others. He was elected to the National Academy of Sciences in 1949 and served as chancellor of the University of Acadia from 1972 to 1979. He also had numerous awards from foreign governments.

VERN L. BULLOUGH

Selected Bibliography

PRIMARY SOURCES

Huggins, C. 1943. "Endocrine Control of Prostatic Cancer." *Science* 97: 541–44.

———. 1965. "The Business of Discovery in the Medical Sciences." *JAMA* 194 (December 13):1211–15.

———. 1967. "Endocrine Induced Regression of Cancers." *Science* 156:1050–54.

———. 1979. *Experimental Leukemia and Mammary Cancer.* Chicago: University of Chicago Press.

SECONDARY SOURCES

Shück, H. 1951. *Nobel, The Man and His Prizes.* Norman: University of Oklahoma Press.

Aberle, Sophie D., and George W. Corner. 1953. *Twenty-Five Years of Sex Research*, 171–73. Philadelphia: W. B. Saunders.

Haddow, Alexander, et al. 1982. *On Cancer and Hormones: Twenty-Seven Essays Presented to Charles Huggins on the Occasion of His Sixtieth Birthday.* Chicago: University of Chicago.

Talalay, Paul. 1965. "The Scientific Contributions of Charles Brenton Huggins," *JAMA* 192 (June 28): 1137–40.

SIR ANDREW FIELDING HUXLEY *1963*

Sir Andrew Fielding Huxley was born in London, England, on November 22, 1917. A physiologist, Huxley received the 1963 Nobel Prize jointly with Alan L. Hodgkin for their work in describing nervous activity as a function of ion movements across the axonal surface membrane. At the time of the award, Huxley was Jodrell Professor and head of the Department of Physiology at the University of London. Although now in his seventies, he continues to contribute actively in his field and is presently serving as master of Trinity College, Cambridge, where he succeeded Hodgkin in 1984. He was knighted in 1974. Huxley married Jocelyn Richenda Gammell Pease in 1947; they have one son and five daughters.

Huxley's parents were Dr. Leonard Huxley, an author and editor, and the former Rosalind Bruce. He was a King's Scholar at the Westminster School before entering Trinity College to study natural sciences. Hodgkin was his physiology tutor; after Huxley received his B.A. in 1938, the two began experiments on the giant squid axon at the Marine Biological Association Laboratory in Plymouth, England. They had only begun in the summer of 1939 when their work was interrupted by the outbreak of World War II. Huxley was assigned to operation research in Anti-Aircraft Command. In 1946 he returned to Cambridge—where he was to become assistant director of research in physiology in 1951 and director of studies at Trinity in 1952—and joined forces again with Hodgkin.

Hodgkin had been introduced to the giant squid axon by K. S.. Cole at the Marine Biological Laboratory in Woods Hole, Massachusetts, in 1938. This preparation as originally described by J. Z. Young is still unique for nerve physiologists. The axon reaches a diameter of close to one millimeter and can be dissected free from neighboring fibers over a distance of several centimeters. Hodgkin and Huxley planned to use the squid axon to test the membrane theory of Julius Bernstein (1902).

This hypothesis, though based on very little in the way of experimental facts, had survived for more than thirty years. Bernstein had stated that the resting axon is surrounded by a membrane selectively permeable to potassium (K) ions and that, in the course of activity, a nonselective increase of permeability to all ions in the system occurs, thus reducing the resting potential to zero.

In order to get a fair comparison between the resting potential and the amplitude of the action potential, the team directly measured the potential difference between the axoplasm and the surrounding sea water. They inserted a glass capillary tube into the axoplasm to act as an inner electrode and pushed it in an axial direction to lead off from an undamaged part. (Cole and Curtis had performed essentially the same experiment at Woods Hole in 1939).

Hodgkin and Huxley wrote a letter to *Nature* in which the "overshoot" of the membrane potential over the zero level is clearly illustrated, yet interpreted with utmost caution. The result convinced the researchers that it would be worthwhile to consider changes underlying nervous activity other than a loss of ion selectivity or "breakdown" of the membrane.

The squid season (August to November) of 1947 at Plymouth brought a quantitative test of the "sodium hypothesis." This theory tentatively stated that an excitable membrane at rest is preferentially permeable to potassium (K^+) ions (as proposed by Bernstein), but when activated undergoes a large and selective increase of permeability to sodium (Na^+) ions. The lines of evidence (Hodgkin and Katz 1949) have long become textbook knowledge. First, when external Na^+ is replaced by a nonpermeant cation (e.g., choline), the overshoot is depressed as expected for a selectively Na^+-permeable membrane. Also, the maximal rate of rise of the action potential is proportional to the extracellular concentration of sodium. Finally, excitability is lost in Na^+-deficient solutions, as Overton had shown for muscular contraction in 1902; but his work had been largely forgotten.

By 1948 Huxley and Hodgkin were saying, "You can stimulate a nerve fiber; then the fiber does the rest of the experiment." To gain control over a surface membrane, they adapted and improved the "voltage clamping" technique developed by Cole and Marmont. Instead of observing free-running action potentials, the researchers kept the membrane voltage constant at the level of the resting potential, then stepped it to different levels, recorded the membrane current at each step for a preselected time, then stepped the voltage back to the original level. Measurements of total membrane current versus time were repeated with external solutions of different ion compositions. Huxley and Hodgkin then attempted to split the total ionic current into a sodium and a potassium component as functions of both voltage and time, on the basis of the internal and external concentrations of each ion. They further divided the component currents into conductance times driving force.

The decisive experiments were carried out at Plymouth in the course of the squid seasons of 1948 and 1949. At this time, as they worked hard to elaborate their "ionic theory of excitation," Kenneth Cole stated in a lecture at Cambridge, "We (Cole and Marmont) have got the voltage clamp going but you people (Huxley and Hodgkin) have asked the right questions."

The five papers that presented the Nobel prize–winning work were published in 1952. Briefly, they stated that activity results from a voltage-dependent and transitory rise of Na^+ conductance followed (in squid axons) by a delayed rise of K^+ conductance. The experimental achievements of a few months' time appear as an impressive body of results, leaving little in the way of major gaps. Huxley in his Nobel Lecture explained: "Hodgkin and I spent a good deal of time in the early part of 1947 thinking what kind of system might give rise to an action potential." In other • words, they knew exactly what to look for in their experiments of 1948 and 1949.

In the course of analyzing the current traces, they introduced mathematical language (HH equations) to describe the "on" and "off" of conductances at various voltage levels. These equations made it possible to reproduce the known behavior of the nerve admirably well, including the amplitude and time-course of the action potential and even the velocity of propagation along an axon. As Huxley and Hodgkin wrote (1952): "For the sake of illustration we shall try to provide a physical basis for these equations, but must emphasize that the interpretation given is unlikely to provide a correct picture of the membrane."

The voltage clamp experiments suggested what might happen during a single action potential. Richard Keynes and Peter Lewis then measured the inflow and outflow of radioactive isotopes with axons of the cuttlefish, a relative of the squid. Using trains of action potentials, and comparing periods of activity and periods of rest, they found a gain of 24Na and loss of 42K, a result that closely agreed with the charge displacement calculated by Huxley and Hodgkin from their voltage clamp data (in mole cm<–2> impulse <–1>).

In 1947 Huxley began collaborative experiments on myelinated nerve fibers of the frog with Robert Stämpfli of Berne, Switzerland. Their work put an end to the debate over "saltatory conduction." A quantitative evaluation of current flow during propagation made it clear that the Ranvier node is the only excitable structure and that the myelin sheaths between the nodes act as electrically passive insulators.

Huxley's own explanation (1950) of his decision (1950) to shift to muscle research is based on his personal preference for optical instruments and precise measurements. It occurred to him that some important observations on muscle made in the nineteenth century were not receiving the attention they deserved. He began these studies at Cambridge and continued them at University College, London, after his appointment as Jodrell professor in 1960.

It was clear to him at the outset that an ordinary light microscope would not resolve with any confidence the changes of sarcomere pattern expected to occur during a stretch or twitch of the muscle. He constructed his own interference microscope, and, working in collaboration with Rolf Niedergerke, obtained some unexpected results. When a muscle fiber was stretched, the A bands remained constant in length, contrary to the generally held opinion at that time. A strong contraction resulted in the appearance of "contraction bands" midway between the Z lines, as if filaments of fixed length extending from each Z line collided with each other in the middle of the A bands.

Independently, and at about the same time, Hugh Huxley used the electron microscope to reveal thick filaments (myosin) and thin filaments (actin) in muscle fiber. Electron micrography showed a regular spatial relationship in the zones of overlap. A. F. Huxley and R. E. Taylor meanwhile observed that a point source of current can cause single sarcomeres to shorten in graded steps.

One of the main problems in 1948 and 1949 had been to gain control over the membrane current of a nerve axon. Thus, to gain control over the tension in an isolated muscle fiber and then to keep control during rapid changes of imposed tension was a problem made for the skills of Andrew Huxley. In London, in collaboration with Robert Simmons and Lincoln Ford, he began experiments on mechanical transients. These provided the basis for a deeper understanding of muscle contraction.

The working hypothesis Huxley has evolved is based on the thick and thin filaments, myosin and actin. He postulates sites of interaction, or cross-bridges, that have a morphological correlate. These can generate force in the direction of shortening, resulting in a sliding movement in the zone of overlap between the two types of filaments. Huxley's theory of "independent force generators" is widely accepted today in its general outline. It accounts for two experimentally demonstrated features of muscle contraction: the tetanic tension proportional to the overlap and the speed of unloaded shortening independent of overlap. As for the details of his theory, Andrew Huxley says, "The scheme is very speculative, and its value cannot be anything more than to suggest further experiments."

Huxley was named Royal Society Research Professor in the University of London in 1969, a title he held until 1983. In that year, he accepted the title of Honorary Research Fellow at University College, London, and soon after was installed in the mastership of Trinity College, Cambridge University. He served also as president of the Royal Society from 1980 to 1985.

Both Huxley and Hodgkin have repeatedly and decisively helped to solve research problems for colleagues and former associates. When a problem had reached a stage of intuitive understanding, the best thing to do would be to buy a ticket to Cambridge. The traveler would be sure to return with the right kind of questions to be asked, sometimes even with a neat set of equations in his bag.

Sir Andrew is a fellow of the Royal Society, a member of the British Biophysical Society and of the Royal Institution, and a past president of the British Association for the Advancement of Science (1976–77). He holds honorary membership or associate status in many foreign societies, including the National Academy of Sciences of the United States. Among the many other awards he has received are the Copley Medal of the Royal Society

(1973) and the Order of Merit (1983).

SILVIO WEIDMANN

Selected Bibliography

PRIMARY SOURCES

Huxley, A. F., and Stämpfli. 1949. "Evidence for Saltatory Conduction in Peripheral Myelinated Nerve Fibres." *Journal of Physiology* 108: 315–39.

Hodgkin, A. L., and A. F. Huxley. 1920. "A Quantitative Description of Membrane Current and Its Application to Conduction and Excitation in Nerve." *Journal of Physiology* 117:500–544.

Huxley, A. F. 1957. "Muscle Structure and Theories of Contraction." *Progress in Biophysics and Biophysical Chemistry* 7:255–318.

Huxley, A. F., and R. Niedergerke. 1958. "Measurement of the Striations of Isolated Muscle Fibres with the Interference Microscope." *Journal of Physiology* 144:403–25.

Huxley, A. F., and R. E. Taylor. 1958. "Local Activation of Striated Muscle Fibres." *Journal of Physiology* 144:426–41.

Huxley, A. F., and L. D. Peachey. 1961. "The Maximal Length for Contraction in Vertebrate Striated Muscle." *Journal of Physiology* 156:150–65.

Huxley, A. F., and R. M. Simmons. 1971. "Proposed Mechanism of Force Generation in Striated Muscle." *Nature* 233:533–38.

Ford, L. E., A. F. Huxley, and R. M. Simmons. "Tension Responses to Sudden Length Change in Stimulated Frog Muscle Fibres Near Slack Length." *Journal of Physiology* 269:441–515.

Huxley, Sir Andrew. 1980. *Reflections on Muscle*. The Sherrington Lectures, Series 14. Liverpool: University Press.

Huxley, Sir Andrew. 1988. *Prefatory Chapter: Muscular Contraction. Annual Review of Physiology* 50: 1–16.

FRANÇOIS JACOB *1965*

François Jacob was born June 17, 1920, in Nancy, France. A physician and cellular geneticist, he shared the 1965 Nobel Prize with André Lwoff and Jacques Monod for his contributions to the "discoveries concerning the genetic regulation of enzyme and virus synthesis." He was the only child of Jewish parents, Thérèse Franck Jacob, a nurse, and Simon Jacob, who worked in real estate. In 1947 he married the pianist Lise Bloch; his wife died in 1984. They had four children: Pierre (born 1949), Laurent and Odile (twins, born 1952) and Henri (born 1954).

Jacob was educated at the Lycée Carnot, in Paris, where he completed his baccalauréat in 1938 and began medical school. His studies were interrupted by World War II, but he obtained his M.D. from the Université de Paris in 1947. He became a research assistant at the Institut Pasteur in 1950 and simultaneously worked toward a doctorate in science, completed in 1954. In 1960 he became head of the Department of Cellular Genetics of the Institut Pasteur and since 1964, when it was founded, he has held the Chair of Cellular Genetics at the Collège de France.

Jacob began medical studies with the hope of becoming a surgeon. In his second year, two unrelated but traumatic events, the death of his mother in early June 1940 and the fall of France a few days later, prompted him to flee to England where he joined the Free French Forces of Charles de Gaulle. He served as a medical attendant and saw action in several battles in North Africa, suffering wounds in Tunisia and again in Normandy on August 8, 1944. The sequelae of these wounds caused him to abandon plans for surgery, but he did resume his medical studies after the war. He completed his M.D. in 1947 with a thesis on "tyrothricin," an antibiotic that had been isolated by René Dubos. Reluctant to practice medicine, Jacob worked for the French National Penicillin Center, but became bored and dissatisfied. He turned to research in biology and after much persistence was given an opportunity at the Institut Pasteur.

Under the direction of André Lwoff, Jacob's first project was an exploration of various aspects of a *pseudomonas* species of lysogenic bacteria. Jacob studied the various factors, such as irradiation or ultraviolet light, that "induced the prophage" and led to the appearance of virus particles in a strain of bacteria in which the virus was known to be present but dormant. This topic, together with an analysis of the "immunity" or conditions that favor silence of the virus, was the subject of his doctoral thesis, defended in May 1954.

From 1954 to 1958 Jacob collaborated with Elie Wollman, the son of a Jewish couple, both Pastorian scientists, who had disappeared during the Holocaust. Wollman and Jacob established a theory of sexuality in bacteria. Previously, it had been thought that bacteria reproduced by simple cell division without the addition of genetic material from other organisms. They were able to demonstrate that bacteria do indeed exchange genetic material between individual cells prior to division, in a process called "conjugation," during which the "male" bacterium introduces a spaghetti-like strand of chromosome into the "female" bacterium. By mechanically shaking the bacteria at various times during conjugation, something Jacob has called a "sort of *coitus interruptus*," Wollman and Jacob discovered that genes entered the cell in a specific order and that their position on the chromosome could be mapped. They gave the name "episome" to the added genetic material. Jacob observed that although different bacteria of the same species may pass their genes in a different order, the order always followed the same sequence. He concluded that the bacterial chromosome was circular (Jacob and Wollman 1961).

When Jacob came to the Institut Pasteur, Monod had already been there for five years working on enzymes and Lwoff had just discovered his ultraviolet light method for induction of the prophage in lysogenic bacteria. Jacob has described how the laboratories of these two older scientists were located at opposite ends of the same corridor and how his own, located in between the two, was the site of afternoon tea. He has used this floor-plan analogy to describe his contribution to their seemingly different work as the sudden insight, in 1958, that in their disparate situations they both had been working on manifestations of the same genetic mechanism. Jacob realized that each phenomenon, Lwoff's induction of the prophage and Monod's stimulation of enzyme production, was the result of a gene expression resulting from the removal of a repressor. This perspective led to the theoretical synthesis that began with the PA-JA-MA experiment and ended with the elegant operon theory of genetic control and messenger RNA. Essentially, this theory holds that the elaboration of an enzyme or protein is "switched on" when a repressor substance is removed from a controlling operator site, thereby triggering the transcription of the DNA code by RNA that uses the message to build the protein. Five years later he shared the Nobel Prize for this work.

In the many years since his collaboration with Monod, Jacob has published a number of other important studies in the various fields of genetics, cellular biology, virology, and oncology. It has been said that he was "profoundly disappointed" by the failure of the Pasteur team to isolate the repressor protein and identify the operator as DNA, feats accomplished by the Harvard scientists B. Müller-Hill and W. Gilbert in 1966–67 (Judson 1979, 590). Nevertheless, together with Sydney Brenner, Jacob continued to work on genetics, especially as it controls cell division. In 1963 they developed the "replicon" hypothesis to explain the control of the replication of DNA in bacteria. In a series of articles published between 1968 and 1971, Jacob, Y. Hirota, and others described the cell division of *E. coli* with special attention to membrane protein alterations and the production of DNA-less bacteria. Much of his work since 1970 has been based on mammalian cell culture technique, to which he has also made significant contributions. Cells derived from the mouse embryo and from murine teratocarcinoma (cancer) can be used as models for the exploration of fundamental problems. Jacob has applied these cell-systems to the study of differentiation, the process by which cells, whose progeny have many potential functions, specialize into those that perform only specific functions.

Jacob has written a lucid and epistemologically sensitive history of heredity, proceeding from visible structures through chromosomes to molecules (Jacob 1970). He modestly includes a discussion of his own contribution with no mention of his name. The Jessie and John Danz Lectures given in Seattle reveal his interest in philosophy of science, specifically in the theory of evolution and its limitations as science, beyond which it is used as myth (Jacob 1982). Jacob has described the process of evolution as "tinkering" ("bricolage") that "conforms to no special project." Through rearrangements of existing systems, evolution proceeds as a series of small changes that can deeply affect form, function, and behavior of the organism to produce new objects of increasing complexity (Jacob 1983).

Although Jewish by birth, Jacob is an atheist in thought and practice and has avoided political affiliations. He declined an opportunity to make his career in Israel. Monod once described him as being more "intuitive" and "visual" than himself, but Jacob has also been more reserved and private with occasional quiet forays into the realm of social responsibility (Judson 1979, 384, 402). Together with François Gros and Pierre Royer, he collaborated on a report, commissioned by French president Giscard d'Estaing, on changes in biological sciences and their implications for society. The conclusions recognized the potential impact of these changes on modes of thinking and living, and cautioned against allowing the science of biology to control the idea of humanity. The authors recommended careful attention to a prior idea of human existence, rights, and values that can bring biology into its service. Jacob is committed to international collaboration between scientists. Recently, he joined a group of investigators, including Americans and his old patron, André Lwoff, in welcoming the end of the AIDS priority dispute, which was described as a dispute between institutions rather than between individual scientists (Jacob et al. 1987). The intimate events of Jacob's personal and scientific life up to 1960 are described with candor and grace in his autobiography.

Jacob has been awarded numerous prizes and honors including the Croix de la Libération, the Prix Charles-Léopold Mayer (1962), the Légion d'Honneur, and membership in both the Royal Society (1973) and the Académie des Sciences, Paris (1977). He holds an honorary doctorate of science from the University of Chicago (1965), and other universities.

JACALYN DUFFIN

Selected Bibliography

PRIMARY SOURCES

Jacob, François, and Elie L. Wollman. 1961. *Sexuality and the Genetics of Bacteria*. New York: Academic Press.

Pardee, A. B., F. Jacob, and J. Monod. 1959. "The Genetic Control and Cytoplasmic Expression of 'Inducibility' in the Synthesis of β-galactosidase by *E. Coli.*" *Journal of Molecular Biology* 1:165–78.

Jacob, F., and J. Monod. 1961. "Genetic Regulatory Mechanisms in the Synthesis of Proteins. *Journal of Molecular Biology* 3:318–56.

———. 1961. "On the Regulation of Gene Activity." *Cold Spring Harbor Symposia on Quantitative Biology* 26:193–211.

Jacob, F., S. Brenner, and F. Cuzin. 1963. "On the Regulation of DNA Replication in Bacteria." *Cold Spring Harbor Symposia on Quantitative Biology* 28:329–48.

Jacob, François. 1965. "Genetics of the Bacterial Cell," and "Biography." Nobel Lecture, December 11, 1965. Reprinted in *Nobel Lectures in Molecular Biology, 1933–75*, 219–42, 243–44. New York: Elsevier, 1977.

Jacob, François. 1970. *The Logic of Living Systems: A History of Heredity.* Translated by Betty Spillman. London: Allen Lane, 1974. Also called *The Logic of Life* in other editions.

Jacob, François. 1979. "The Switch." In *Origins of Molecular Biology*, edited by André Lwoff and Agnes Ullman, 95–107. New York: Academic Press.

Gross, François, François Jacob, and Pierre Royer. 1979. *Sciences de la vie et societé. Rapport présenté à M. le Président de la République.* Paris: La Documentation française.

Jacob, François. 1982. *The Possible and the Actual.* The Jessie and John Danz Lectures. Seattle: University of Washington Press.

———. 1983. "Molecular Tinkering in Evolution." In *Evolution from Molecules to Man*, edited by D. S. Bendall, 131–44. Cambridge: Cambridge University Press.

———. 1987. *The Statue Within. An Autobiography.* Translated by Franklin Philip. New York: Basic Books.

SECONDARY SOURCES

Sourkes, Theodore L. 1967. *Nobel Prize Winners in Medicine and Physiology, 1901–1965*, 432–44. London: Abelard-Schuman.

Judson, Horace. 1979. *The Eighth Day of Creation.* New York: Simon and Schuster.

1981. *Biographical Encyclopedia of Scientists*, edited by John Daintith, Sarah Mitchell, and Elizabeth Tostill, 414. New York: Facts on File.

Muller-Hill, Benno. 1987. "L'enfant du paradis." *Nature* 328:389. Review of Jacob's autobiography.

NIELS KAJ JERNE *1984*

Niels Kaj Jerne is the immunologist who has contributed most to the rise of his discipline in the past two decades. His imagination has shaped our present concepts of immunity. Thousands of immunologists are still working out his premises. For his epoch-making hypotheses on the activity of the immune system he was awarded the Nobel Prize in 1984, along with Cesar Milstein and Georges Köhler, whose technological breakthroughs were made possible by Jerne's theoretical work.

Jerne was born in 1911 in London to Hans Jessen Jerne, an expert in cooling technology, and Else Marie Lindbergh, both Danes from Jutland. Jerne himself is a citizen of both Denmark and Britain. Jerne's family moved to Holland when he was three and his parents kept Danish as their mother tongue, so that Jerne grew up as a trilingual child. He still masters English, Danish and Dutch equally. Jerne went to college in Rotterdam, where he received his baccalaureate in 1928. He studied physics for two years at the University of Leiden, then moved to Copenhagen, where he married Ilse Wahlova, from Asch, Czechoslovakia, in 1935. She died in Copenhagen ten years later.

Only at the age of 27 did Jerne decide to study medicine, at the University of Copenhagen. In order to make a living, from 1943 he worked as part-time assistant at the Biological Standards Department of the Danish State Serum Institute. He remained there until 1956, even though he had taken his medical degree in 1947. Eventually, the laboratory at the institute became a gathering place for "molecular biologists" like Hans Noll and Jim Watson and the physicist-turned-biologist Max Delbrück.

The institute produced sera and vaccines and also led applied research. Jerne, along with Ole Maaloe, the head of the department, worked on the problems involved in assaying the potency of sera. The diphtheria toxin-antitoxin neutralization reaction has been called by Jerne the "classical problem of immunology" (Jerne 1951, 9). Since its description by Behring in 1890, it has remained crucial for the safe and efficient use of serotherapy. Standardized methods assumed that antidiphtheric sera of different origins were identical if they were diluted. Jerne investigated a property of sera that he called "avidity," or diphtheric toxin binding capacity, and drew the conclusion that antibodies were strikingly heterogeneous. A serum, far from being a well-defined reagent, contains a spectrum of antibodies of different avidities. Moreover, serum avidity for an antigen increases with time and on second immunization. This turned out to be the first hint of the operation of a "selective" mechanism. Jerne presented the data for his Ph.D. in 1951 at the University of Copenhagen, and became an Assistant Professor at the Danish State Institute. Jerne crossed the ocean to join Delbrück at the California Institute of Technology at Pasadena.

At Cal Tech "the air was filled with the phage particles that Delbrück had picked out as one of the weakest spots in the armour behind which Nature guards her secrets" (Jerne 1966, 301–12). The study of bacteriophages (bacteria-infecting viruses) was coming to the forefront of biology and Jerne had to apply antibodies to bacteriophages "in order to hand on the fringe" (ibid). Antibacteriophage antibodies appeared to improve the fit during the course of immunization, a phenomenon that for Jerne had "Darwinian overtones" (ibid, p. 303).

During his year at Cal Tech Jerne completed a paper called "The Natural Selection Theory of Antibody Formation" that suggested a new perspective on immunity. At that time the accepted theory for antibody formation was the so-called "instructive" theory. After Landsteiner had recognized the potentially infinite number of antigens, it seemed economical that the organism used the antigen as a template to design an antibody as it was needed. Pauling suggested that the antigen impressed a specific pattern on a master antibody, a "neutral" molecule. The theory did not fit all experimental facts, but Pauling did not pay attention when Jerne tried to explain his alternative view to him.

Jerne has always been puzzled by the existence, of the so-called natural antibodies [before any immunization], and he postulated that they display a surprising variety of specificities. He proposed a new role for the antigen: "The antigen is solely a new carrier of spontaneously circulating antibodies to a system of cells which can reproduce the antibody" (Jerne 1955, 849).

The new theory, although published in a prestigious journal with Delbrück's sponsoring, passed largely unnoticed. Jerne's paper left open the following question: How can the antigen induce antibody reproduction? Macfarlane Burnet added the word *clonal* to the *selection* theory, because it is not antibodies that are selected, but cells. These pre-committed cells are "clones" that multiply under stimulation by the antigen. As Jerne had suggested, the great variety of antibodies might be linked to the various amino-acid sequences at specific sites on antibodies, and the relevant information might be contained in the genes. Jerne thus placed his theory in the mainstream of current biological thought. This theory became official dogma in 1967 at Cold Spring Harbor, the Mecca of geneticists.

In 1956 Jerne joined the staff of the World Health Organization, where he worked on biological standardization. In 1962 he prompted an enthusiastic report on recent advances in immunology from 46 well-known experts and persuaded WHO to establish an immunology section to set up training and research centers around the world, especially in developing countries. He also served as a professor of biophysics at the University of Geneva from 1960 to 1962.

Jerne went to Pittsburgh as professor of microbiology from 1962 to

1966, and there resumed experimental work. With Alfred Nordin, Jerne worked out a practical method for detecting antibody-forming cells on agar. The method was first used to detect anti-red blood cell antibodies, but was soon extended to other antigen-antibody systems. The technique showed a hemolysis plaque around each antibody-forming cell, a clear illustration of Burnet's clone.

Jerne put an end to his trans-Atlantic sojourns in 1966 when he accepted an appointment as professor of experimental therapy at Goethe University in Frankfurt, where he directed the Paul Ehrlich Institute. Meanwhile, the Hoffmann-Laroche Company had donated a large amount of money to sponsor the founding in Basel of a non-profit institute entirely committed to the growing field of immunology. Hoffmann-Laroche approached Jerne and offered him the directorship of the institute. Jerne accepted, and remained director of the Institute of Immunology from 1971 until his retirement in 1980. There he was able to gather scientists from all over the world and to realize his ideal of scientific community life and creative exchange among peers.

In the midst of his heavy administrative work, Jerne was still able to contribute to theory. In 1971 he explained "what happened before selection" with the hypothesis that the original antibodies are directed against a set of antigens ("histocompatibility antigens") of the same species. Antibodies directed against the "self" have a function for cell to cell recognition in embryonic life; secondarily, the "anti-self" clones are eliminated. Only mutant cells survive, producing antibodies against foreign antigens. He also suggested that some organs like the thymus were specialized for breeding mutants.

The question remained of what controlled the immune system or the set of lymphocytes and their products, antibodies. Jerne started discussing immunological networks when Oudin and Kunkel's discovery of idiotypes as individual specificities of antibodies suggested to him the idea of idiotypic-antiidiotypic feedbacks. Jerne presented a brief sketch in 1973 at a colloquium in Paris (in honor of the 150th anniversary of Pasteur's birth) and published the fully elaborated version in the annals of the institute. If the concentration of antibodies with a given idiotype rises above a certain level, he wrote, the body will make an anti-idiotype antibody and an infinite network will be potentially set up: "the classic immunologist's dream" (Capra, p. 18). Thus emerges the idea of a complex self-regulating network, reactive to external stimuli but also working in the absence of an antigen whose "internal image" is built into the immune system.

During the following year, experimental data confirmed that anti-antibodies could react with the initial antigen. The network concept had profound implications on the understanding of diseases and possibly their prevention and treatment. The excitement grew among immunologists. After his retirement in 1980, Jerne was invited to the Pasteur Institute in Paris where for two years he animated a friendly circle of scholars stimulated by his predictions.

Jerne now lives in southern France with his second wife, Ursula Alexandra Kohl, born in Hanover, whom he married in Mexico in 1964 and with whom he has two sons.

Since his retirement, Jerne has been very active in international scientific cooperation and has contributed to the creation of the European Molecular Biology Organization and its laboratory at Heidelberg. In Tokyo, in 1980, he contributed to the launching of the Asian Molecular Biology Organization.

Among the many awards bestowed on Jerne are the Gairdner Foundation International Award (1970) and the Paul Ehrlich Gold Medal of the University of Frankfurt (1982). He is an honorary member of the Robert Koch Institute in Berlin (1966) and of the Royal Academy of Sciences of Denmark (1967), and a foreign member of the American Academy of Arts and Sciences (1975). He has received honorary degrees from Columbia University and the Universities of Chicago, Copenhagen, Basel and Rotterdam. He has been a member of the American Philosophical Society since 1978 and of the Royal Society since 1980.

Jerne is a provocative thinker. His ideas were greeted with incredulity, anger or amazement. He has a predilection for paradoxes: he predicted in 1969 the coming of the complete solution of immunology and went so far as to say that all the interesting issues would be settled soon, except for the grim details of the management of diseases, which would provide laborious work for doctors. This arrogant attitude, not uncommon among molecular biologists, has sometimes estranged him from his peers, and he has been called "a solitary man." But this arrogance is tempered by an exquisite sensitiveness to friendship and his openness to those beyond the scientific circle.

The Nobel Committee attributed three distinct major hypotheses to Jerne. In fact, there is a continuous thread leading from his discovery of antibody diversity to his network theory. His main concern was with the "philosophical problems of immunology" (Humphrey, p. 1). His wide reading and his background in physics (Niels Bohr's influence) oriented him in his grasp of the immunological reality as a multidimensional whole. He engaged in discussions with specialists of all disciplines, statistics and mathematics in particular. He recast the debate between instructive and selective theory into the attractive terms of the philosophical inneism/empiricism debate and welcomed the recent cognitive turn in the neurosciences.

Throughout his life, Jerne has been fascinated by the analogy between language and the immune system, an analogy that leads far back to the Kabbalist tradition and that he developed in his Nobel lecture (Jerne 1984, 1057–59). He had tried in 1960 to promote a new terminology in immunology, suggesting a coherent set of terms that would illustrate the existence of immunological families of molecules (antibodies) and the centrality of the complementarity between epitopes (antigenic sites) and paratopes (antibody sites). This terminology has indeed come into use in the past several years. His reform of scientific language included a mention of "idiotypes" or sites that "are carried by components of one individual animal" (Jerne 1960, 342), anticipating by three years the discovery of idiotypy. Recently, he has pointed to the formal analogies between the nervous and the immune systems and suggested that linguistics could help to elaborate some of the laws they have in common.

Jerne was one of the first readers of Ludvik Fleck, the Polish physician who published in 1935 on the sociology of science. Jerne himself characterized two different communities among his colleagues, which he named cis- and trans-immunologists, and analyzed their radically different *Weltanschauung* and their inability to communicate with each other.

With Jerne, the chasm between the "two cultures" is a step closer to being filled. His intellectual role in immunology may be compared with the influence of Socrates. Even if ideas are innate, their delivery requires a Socratic midwife.

ANNE MARIE MOULIN

Selected Bibliography

PRIMARY SOURCES

Jerne, Niels K. 1951. "A Study of Avidity." *Acta Pathologica Microbiologica Scandinavica* 87:9.

———. 1955. "The Natural Selection Theory of Antibody Formation." *Proceedings of the National Academy of Sciences of the U.S.A.* 41:849–56.

———. 1960. "Immunological Speculations." *Annual Review of Microbiology* 14:341–358.

———. 1963. "Plaque Formation in Agar by Single Antibody-Producing Cells." *Science* 140:405.

———. 1966. "The Natural Selection Theory of Antibody Formation: Ten Years Later." In J. Cairns, et al., eds. *Phage and the Origins of Molecular Biology*. New York: Cold Spring Harbor Laboratory.

———. 1971. "The Somatic Generation of Immune Recognition." *European Journal of Immunology* 1:1–9.

———. 1974. "Towards a Network Theory of the Immune System." *Annales de l'Institut Pasteur* 125: 373–89.

———. 1984. "The Generative Grammar of the Immune System." *Science* 226:1057–59.

SECONDARY SOURCES

Bibel, O. J. 1988. *Milestones in Immunology: A Historical Explanation*. Madison: Science Tech.

Capra, F. 1984. *The Antibody Enigma*. New York: Plenum.

Humphrey, J. 1982. "To Niels Jerne on the Occasion of His Seventieth Birthday." *European Journal of Immunology* 12:1.

Moulin, A. M. Forthcoming. "The Immune System: A Key Concept for the History of Immunology." *History and Philosophy of the Life Sciences*. Firenze.

Silverstein, A. M. 1988. *A History of Immunology*. New York: Academic Press.

Steinberg, C. M., and I. Lefkovits, eds. 1981. *The Immune System: A Festschrift in Honor of Niels Kaj Jerne on the Occasion of His Seventieth Birthday*. Basel: Karger.

1987. "Niels K. Jerne." In *Nobel Prize Winners. An H. W. Wilson Biographical Dictionary*, 509–11. New York: Wilson.

SIR BERNARD KATZ *1970*

Sir Bernard Katz was born Bernhard Katz on March 26, 1911, in Leipzig, Germany. He was the only child of Max Katz, a Russian Jewish fur merchant, and Eugenie Rabinowitz Katz. In 1935 he emigrated to England, where he began physiological and biophysical research at University College, London. With the exception of an early sojourn in Australia, his entire career was spent in the university's Biophysics Department. His research has focused on the way in which chemical transmitter substances are stored and released, and on the mechanisms of their functions at neural synapses, primarily at the terminals where nerves activate muscles (the neuromuscular junction). Both for his specific discoveries and for the general principles of the nervous system which they illuminated, he shared the Nobel Prize in 1970 with Ulf von Euler and Julius Axelrod.

Katz's early education at a humanistic preparatory school, the Albert Gymnasium in Leipzig, was largely classical, centering on Greek and Latin. He graduated in 1929 and enrolled as a medical student at the University of Leipzig, where he soon became interested in experimental physiology. He won the Garten Prize in 1933, and in 1934 wrote an M.D. dissertation that was published in a leading journal. Despite these achievements, Hitler's seizure of power, and the rising climate of anti-Semitism, made it clear to Katz that he had no future in Germany. After receiving his degree, he emigrated to London with the help of Chaim Weizmann.

He received a small scholarship to work in the laboratory of Archibald V. Hill, the Nobel laureate, at University College. There he was initiated into biophysics research on electrical stimulation of nerves and on neuromuscular transmission, and became the colleague of two brilliant generations of British physiologists, Henry Dale, Wilhelm Feldberg, John Eccles, Alan Hodgkin, and his valued mentor Hill. Katz earned his Ph.D. in 1938 and won a Carnegie Research Fellowship for further study of neuromuscular transmission.

Just before the outbreak of war in 1939, he accepted an invitation to join Eccles at the Kanematsu Memorial Institute of Pathology in Sydney, Australia. Here he found a small research group, including Stephen Kuffler, another émigré. Katz was able to continue his work after the war started but in 1942 enlisted in the Royal Australian Air Force. For four years he put his knowledge of advanced electronics to work as a radar officer. Demobilized in 1945, he married Marguerite Penly; they now have two sons, David and Jonathan.

In early 1946, at Hills' invitation, he came back to the University College as assistant director of research in biophysics. Soon thereafter, he helped Hodgkin and Alan Huxley, now at Cambridge, in their investigations (1947–49) of the ionic basis of the action potential (electrical nerve "impulse") in the giant squid axon. Hodgkin and Huxley showed that the "impulse" is caused first by sodium ions (Na^+) flowing into the nerve, and then by potassium ions (K^+) flowing out—all within a few milliseconds. The sodium theory and its mathematical formulation, as developed by Hodgkin and Huxley in the 1950s, won them the Nobel Prize in 1963.

Katz now became a British citizen. In 1950, he was appointed to a readership in physiology, and in 1952, promoted to professor and chairman of the newly established Department of Biophysics. Throughout the next three decades, the small department became an international center for neurophysiological research, attracting visiting investigators and graduate students. Many of Katz's own studies during this long and productive period were carried out with a series of gifted collaborators, including Paul Fatt (1949–52), Jose del Castillo (1952–57), and Ricardo Miledi (1959–72).

His colleagues and students speak warmly of this modest, pleasant man. As one said at the time of the Nobel award, "He really cares about his work, that it's done correctly. And he always mentions the work of colleagues, and we appreciate that very much." He was lecturing at the University of California when the Nobel announcement came; that morning, he left the press conference early, so as not to keep an undergraduate waiting for a scheduled appointment.

Katz's life work addressed the century-old problem of how messages in single nerve fibers (axons) are carried over the gap, or synapse, that separates the neural terminal from another nerve, or from an effector organ such as a muscle. This synaptic transmission was long believed to be electrical, but, in the 1920s and 1930s, Otto Loewi, Dale, and Feldberg had shown that some nerve-to-nerve synapses, as well as the neuromuscular junction, act by chemical transmission. As the nerve impulse arrives at the terminus, it releases acetylcholine (ACh), which diffuses across the synaptic break and triggers an electrical response in the target cells. When Loewi and Dale were awarded the Nobel in 1936 for these discoveries, the facts seemed well established, but the actual mechanisms remained obscure.

One of the skeptics was John

Eccles, who continued to defend electrical transmission. The research in Sydney had focused on stimulating the motor nerves of cats, and then, using external electrodes, recording the synaptic potentials (responses) on the muscle side. Katz and Kuffer had found that the localized neuromuscular junction in the frog, the motor end-plate, was a better preparation for such studies. Before the group was broken up by the war, Eccles, Katz, and Kuffler had shown that the end-plate potential was a rapid, localized depolarization on the postsynaptic side, that spread passively as allowed by the muscle's electrical properties, and then initiated the propagated muscle response (action potential) that caused contraction. These end-plate potentials (EPPs) could accumulate both temporally and spatially, and were sensitive to blocking or enhancement by drugs.

When Katz and Paul Fatt returned to the problem of the end-plate potential in London in late 1949, they had a new analytic tool. Improving on a technique invented in the United States, Hodgkin had developed minute, electrolyte-filled glass pipettes, whose tips were only 2/100,000 of an inch (0.5 microns) in diameter, and which could be used to record from the *insides* of cells (intracellularly). Fatt learned to make these microelectrodes, and he and Katz could then implant them in the motor end-plate and record potentials directly, and with a high degree of localization. They demonstrated that the end-plate potential had a magnitude of about 20–30 millivolts (mVs or thousandths of a volt), that it arises when the postsynaptic membrane becomes permeable to ions, and that it initiates the muscle spike. It was an elegant, exemplary series of experiments that applied the new methods of electrical/ionic analysis to acetylcholine-mediated synaptic transmission.

But the intracellular technique also provided a surprise. In the spring of 1950, as Katz and Fatt were making routine observations between experiments, they noticed that their oscilloscope showed small, irregular fluctuations of about 0.5 mV. Upon analysis, these turned out to have exactly the same shape as the EPP, and they were dubbed "miniature end-plate potentials" (minEPPs). They were too big to be caused by single moelcules of acetylcholine; they had to be the result of groups of ACh molecules hitting the end-plate. The minEPPs occurred randomly, with an average frequency of about one per second. They were affected by drugs in the same way as the EPP. Also, they only occurred in the presence of calcium.

Katz and Fatt realized that they had discovered a series of baseline nerve potentials, triggered by spontaneous small "bursts" of ACh. They named the individual packets of ACh molecules "quanta." (Katz later estimated that each quantum contained about 104 molecules.) Further, they suggested, the normal EPP was the result of a neural impulse depolarizing the presynaptic terminal and causing the discharge of a large number of quanta all at once. These conclusions were published in 1950.

Jose del Castillo then joined the team in a new series of experiments to confirm these ideas. By stimulating the neural fibers while in a low calcium and high magnesium solution, they were able to reduce and "spread out" the EPP in such a way as to identify the separate bursts of quanta. While their findings supported the hypothesis, they also showed unexpected fluctuations in the number of quanta discharged with each neural stimulation.

Katz and del Castillo developed the "quantum hypothesis" of neural transmission, which proposes that each motor nerve contains a large number of quanta, for each of which there is a finite probability that it will be released by an action potential. Stated in these terms, the hypothesis was provable by a series of experiments, combined with statistical analysis, which showed by 1954 that quanta behavior did indeed obey the rules of probability theory.

The following year the first primitive electron micrographs of the neuromuscular junction showed that the neural terminal contained small vesicles. Katz and del Castillo suggested in 1956 that these vesicles might represent the packaged quanta of ACh, which were released into the synaptic gap when the vesicle fused with the presynaptic membrane and discharged its contents (exocytosis). The rapidly developing story was summarized by Katz in the Herter Lectures at Johns Hopkins in 1958, and in the Croonian Lecture before the Royal Society in 1961.

Over the next decade Katz and Ricardo Miledi took on the task of consolidating, expanding, and detailing the picture that had been outlined in the 1950s. With the aid of electron microscopists, they clarified the nature of the storage vesicles in the nerve terminals. They extended the pharmacological studies of the release and effects of ACh quanta. The distribution of ACh-reactive sites on the muscle was mapped, showing the concentration at the motor end-plate. The team also demonstrated that depolarization of the nerve resulted in the flow of calcium ions into the nerve, which was essential to the release of multiple quanta. The long recognized, but poorly understood, synaptic delay now appears to be a function of the brief pause between depolarization and the release of quanta triggered by the entry of the calcium ions.

Finally, most convincing to skeptics who were loath to generalize from the frog neuromuscular junction, Katz and Miledi showed that the model also applied for nerve/nerve synapses, in spinal neurons in vertebrates, and in ganglia in squid. These findings were replicated by other investigators at a variety of synapses in several different species. ACh was found to be present in high concentrations on neural surfaces and to be released in intracellular impulse transmission in the parasympathetic nervous system, and in transmissions at neural junctions with smooth muscle, skeletal muscle, and exocrine glands.

The various studies served to confirm the quantum hypothesis and to establish a general model of neural chemical transmission: arrival of a nerve action potential, depolarization of the neural terminal, influx of calcium, exocytosis of vesicles containing transmitter quanta, diffusion of the quanta across the synapse, interaction with receptors that open channels within the target, flow of sodium and potassium ions through these channels to produce the synaptic potential, leading to a new spike on the other side of the synapse.

Bernard Katz was elected a fellow of the Royal Society in 1952 and served as its biological secretary for several years in the 1960s and 1970s. He was knighted in 1969. Among the many other honors he had received for his work are the Feldberg Foundation Award (1965), the Baly Medal from the Royal College of Physicians (1967), and the Copley Medal from the Royal Society (1967). He retired from University College in 1978, but remains active lecturing and writing.

In addition to the more than one hundred research papers that Katz has written with his collaborators, he has also been successful in integrating his group's discoveries into the larger field of neurophysiology and in bringing the whole before a wider public. He has written several excellent overviews for *Scientific American*, as well as his widely praised introduction to the field, *Nerve, Muscle, and Synapse* (1966).

The techniques and approaches pioneered by Katz and his colleagues have proven central to neurophysiology in the second half of the twentieth century. The model of chemical transmission they developed is not universal but it is widely applicable. Where new mechanisms have been discovered through research, it has often been through the use of the methods of intracellular recording, drug applications, and statistical analysis that were elaborated by Bernard Katz.

ROBERT C. FRANK, JR.

Selected Bibliography

PRIMARY SOURCES

Katz, Bernard. 1939. *Electric Excitation of the Nerve: A Review*. London: Oxford University Press.

Fatt, Paul, and Bernard, Katz. 1951. "An Analysis of the Endplate Potential Recorded with an Intracellular Electrode." *Journal of Physiology* 115:320–370.

———. 1952. "Spontaneous Threshold Activity at Motor Nerve Endings." *Journal of Physiology* 117:109–28.

Del Castillo, Jose, and Bernard, Katz. 1954. "Quantal Components of the Endplate Potential." *Journal of Physiology* 124:560–73.

———. 1954. "Changes in Endplate Activity Produced by Presynaptic Polarization." *Journal of Physiology* 124:586–604.

Katz, Bernard. 1958. "Microphysiology of the Neuromuscular Junction." *Bulletin of the Johns Hopkins Hospital* 102:275–312.

———. 1966. *Nerve, Muscle, and Synapse*. New York: McGraw-Hill.

———. 1969. *The Release of Neural Transmitter Substance*. Springfield, Illinois: Thomas.

———. 1985. "Reminiscences of a Physiologist, Fifty Years After." Bayliss-Starling Memorial Lecture. *Journal of Physiology* 370 (1986): 1–12.

SECONDARY SOURCES

1970. "The Three Recipients of the Nobel Prize: Sir Bernard Katz." *New York Times* (October 16):27.

Martin, A. R. 1970. "Nobel Prize: Three Share 1970 Award for Medical Research. 2. Katz." *Science* 170 (October 16):423–24.

Schmeck, Harold M., Jr. 1970. "Award Honors Research in Brain and Nerve Cells." *New York Times* (October 16): 27.

EDWARD CALVIN KENDALL

1950

Edward C. Kendall was born on March 8, 1886, in South Norwalk, Connecticut, the third child of Eva Frances Abbott and George Stanley Kendall, a dentist. Married to Rebecca Kennedy on December 30, 1915, he fathered four children: Hugh, Roy, Norman, and Elizabeth. Kendall's research in biochemistry focused on endocrinology. He received the 1950 Nobel Prize for Physiology or Medicine for "discoveries relating to the hormones of the adrenal cortex, their structure, and biological effects." He died on May 4, 1972, in Princeton, New Jersey.

Kendall developed his strong interest in chemistry during high school. Matriculating at Columbia University in 1904, he remained there until 1910, receiving a B.S. (1908), M.S. (1909), and Ph.D. (1910) in chemistry. His lifelong interest in biochemistry was stimulated by the tutelage of H. C. Sherman and culminated in a doctoral dissertation on pancreatic amylase.

After graduation he moved to Detroit, Michigan, where he worked as a research chemist at the pharmaceutical firm Parke, Davis, and Company. Fueled by current concerns about "feeblemindedness," endocrinology was then developing into an important field. Thyroid disease, with its well-established link to cretinism, was an especially important area of research. (Theodor Kocher, for example, was awarded the 1909 Nobel Prize for his work on the thyroid.) Kendall was assigned to isolate the active agent of the thyroid gland. Because chemists at early twentieth-century pharmaceutical houses typically focused on routine analyses needed to ensure product potency and purity, Kendall was the only Ph.D. in his lab. Disappointed by this absence of a research context, and resentful of his low status—he was required to punch a time clock—Kendall quit Parke, Davis after four months.

Returning to New York in 1911, he soon found a position at St.

Luke's Hospital. Here, across the street from his alma mater, he initially found a more congenial environment. Working during an era when basic science was increasingly perceived as fundamental to medicine, Kendall was convinced that his research on the thyroid would yield clinically useful results, and his early work progressed rapidly. Unfortunately, many of Kendall's clinical colleagues were skeptical of laboratory science as the new paradigm for medicine. Therapeutic thyroid preparations had been available since the 1890s and Kendall's successful isolation of a highly potent fraction of thyroid extract in 1913 seemed to some merely a minor advance. The hospital administration added to Kendall's dissatisfaction when it requested he perform routine chemical analysis of patient foodstuffs. When their salary offer for 1914 contained no raise, Kendall decided to leave.

On February 1, 1914, he joined the Mayo Clinic as the head—and sole member—of its newly opened section of biochemistry. The strong support of the Mayo brothers and Louis B. Wilson, director of the clinic's laboratories, ensured that Kendall avoided mundane clinical tasks and focused on research. Kendall rewarded their confidence in him by isolating crystalline thyroxine in December 1914. This demonstration of how biochemistry could inform clinical medicine was considered of sufficient importance and quality that he nearly received the Nobel Prize for his accomplishment (Zuckerman, Harriet, *Scientific Elite: Nobel Laureates in the United States* [New York: The Free Press, 1977], 298).

This early success ensured the acceptance of Kendall and his research-oriented section of biochemistry within the Mayo Clinic community. Kendall received a more secure appointment—eventually being promoted to professor of physiologic chemistry in 1921—a raise, and began to hire additional faculty. More importantly, documenting the clinical potency of crystalline thyroxine had created ties to clinicians and physiologists, establishing an interdisciplinary model that would prove critical to Kendall's future work.

Beginning in 1915 Kendall and his colleagues turned their attention toward defining the chemical structure of thyroxine. Unfortunately, despite years of intensive effort, this goal eluded them. Kendall was bitterly disappointed when in 1925 C. R. Harrington of University College, London, announced the proper formula and described the steps required to synthesize thyroxine.

The next several years were spent working on the biochemistry of metabolism in an effort to understand how thyroxin influenced the basal metabolic rate. Kendall focused on glutathione, and in 1929 succeeded in defining its chemical structure. Although this was an important result for biochemists, his Mayo colleagues—like the clinicians at St. Luke's a decade earlier—began increasingly to question the clinical relevancy of the section of biochemistry. As the Great Depression deepened, Kendall was again faced with selecting a research trajectory that would seem attractive to physicians.

Research into the hormones of the adrenal cortex fit this trajectory. In January 1930 published reports demonstrated that adrenal extracts could treat adrenal insufficiency. Isolating the active substance from crude extracts was of obvious clinical importance and resembled the problem Kendall had previously conquered in his thyroid work. Furthermore, Kendall's laboratory had some familiarity with adrenal glands because Albert von Szent-Györgyi, attracted by the accessibility of bovine adrenal glands provided by the proximity of midwestern packing houses, had spent much of 1929 working in the section of biochemistry.

Kendall's early efforts in adrenal research benefitted from the interdisciplinary context he had helped to create. The Mayo Clinic maintained an Institute of Experimental Medicine that allowed Kendall's group to develop a colony of adrenalectomized dogs. A cooperative venture between surgeons, physiologists, and biochemists, the colony was central to Kendall's investigations. The response of these dogs to experimental preparations served as a bioassay, allowing Kendall to constantly test the potency of the compounds he was isolating.

Work during the early 1930s was hindered by the assumption that there was a single adrenal hormone, dubbed "cortin." It was not until the mid-1930s that it became clear that the adrenal cortex contained multiple active compounds. A worldwide competition to define these substances ensued. One key step was the conclusive demonstration in 1934 that the important compounds were steroid derivatives. This provided an edge to those groups skilled in steroid chemistry, and in 1937 Tadeus Reichstein's group of university-based organic chemists published a series of papers that characterized several critical compounds.

Recognizing the superior ability of Reichstein's group in organic chemistry, Kendall nearly stopped working on the problem at this juncture. He elected to continue primarily because he believed his group had three key resources Reichstein lacked: 1) easy access to raw materials, 2) a clinical context, and 3) the dog colony. Kendall was further encouraged when in the late 1930s it was revealed that although Reichstein's group had isolated one important hormone—desoxycorticosterone—this hormone influenced only the body's mineral metabolism. Because adrenal hormones were known to also influence carbohydrate metabolism, it was clear that some important hormones remained unidentified.

The war years spurred further research. Rumors that the Nazis were using adrenal hormones to fortify Luftwaffe aviators caused the National Research Council to assign adrenal research top priority in 1941, a rating matched only by penicillin and antimalarial agents. Despite a massive research effort, the initial results were disappointing. Clinical research suggested that adrenal hormones would not improve the fighting capacity of soldiers. Reichstein's 1943 synthesis of another important compound, called compound A, embarrassed and discouraged the American researchers. By 1944 only the groups at Merck and Company, a pharmaceutical concern, and the Mayo Clinic continued to work on adrenal hormones.

The persistence of the Mayo and Merck researchers was rewarded by the successful synthesis of cortisone in 1948. Kendall's delight at the culmination of nearly twenty years of research was soon tempered by an initially cool response from clinicians. Because the wartime studies had not suggested alternative uses, cortisone seemed suitable only for the treatment of adrenal insufficiency, a relatively uncommon condition.

The final key to the recognition of cortisone's enormous therapeutic potential awaited Kendall's interaction with Phillip Hench. Hench, an arthritis expert at the Mayo Clinic, had long been searching for a reason why patients with rheumatoid arthritis improved in two disparate conditions, jaundice and pregnancy. As early as 1941 the two men had agreed that perhaps cortisone was related to these improvements and decided to test its therapeutic efficacy. Disappointed by the lukewarm response to cortisone in 1948–49, Kendall was anxious to pursue any potential therapeutic benefit of cortisone. Kendall and Hench decided to try cortisone on a woman severely incapacitated by rheumatoid arthritis. To their amazement, the response was dramatic. Further trials confirmed cortisone's efficacy in rheumatoid arthritis and Kendall and Hench prepared to announce their discovery.

Word about a possible arthritis cure spread rapidly, and when Kendall and Hench presented their findings at the national meeting of the Association of American Physicians enormous publicity ensued. As the new "miracle" drug, cortisone was touted for nearly every ailment. Enormous demand left Merck and Company incapable of producing adequate amounts of cortisone. Following the wartime example of penicillin, Merck requested the National Academy of Science to convene a committee to oversee the distribution of cortisone. Although the problem of shortages was relatively short-lived, delineating the proper role of cortisone in medical care proved more difficult. Several years passed before some of cortisone's significant side effects were determined. Many initial claims of cortisone's utility ultimately proved unfounded. Yet despite these early difficulties, the ability of cortisone and its related compounds, the corticosteroids, to suppress inflammation has provided physicians and scientists a fundamental tool for medical practice and research.

After receiving the Nobel Prize in 1950, Kendall was forced to retire from the Mayo Clinic in 1951 because he had reached the mandatory retirement age. He then moved to Princeton University where he was appointed visiting professor of chemistry. There he continued his collaboration with Merck scientists and studied nonsteroid components of adrenal extracts until his death in 1972.

Kendall's contributions were key demonstrations of the clinical relevance of biochemistry. During his lifetime his successes greatly strengthened the argument that support of basic research is fundamental to the advancement of medical science and helped secure the position of biochemistry within academic medicine.

STEVEN C. MARTIN

Selected Bibliography

PRIMARY SOURCES

Kendall, Edward C. 1915. "The Isolation in Crystalline Form of the Compound Containing Iodin which Occurs in the Thyroid: Its Chemical Nature and Physiological Activity." *Transactions of the Association of American Physicians* 30:420–49.

———. 1936. "The Identification of a Substance which Possesses the Qualitative Action of Cortin." *Journal of Biological Chemistry* 116:267–76.

Kendall, Edward C., H. L. Mason, and C. S. Myers. 1949. "The Effect of Hormone of the Adrenal Cortex (17-hydroxy 11-dehydrocorticosterone: Compound E) and of Pituitary Adreno-corticotropin Hormone on Rheumatoid Arthritis: Preliminary Report." *Proceedings of Staff Meetings of the Mayo Clinic* 24:181–97.

Kendall, Edward C. 1950. "The Development of Cortisone as a Therapeutic Agent." Nobel Lecture, 1950. In *Nobel Lectures, Physiology or Medicine*, vol. 3 (1942–1962). Amsterdam: Elsevier, 1964.

———. 1971. *Cortisone*. New York: Scribner.

SECONDARY SOURCES

Taylor, H. 1972. "Edward C. Kendall, 1886–1972." In *Yearbook, American Philosophical Society*, 216–20.

Ingle, D. 1975. "Edward C. Kendall." *Biographical Memoirs. National Academy of Science* 47:249–92. Includes bibliography.

Kohler, Robert E. 1978. "Kendall, Edward Calvin." In *Dictionary of Scientific Biography* (*Supplement 1*), edited by Charles Gillespie, New York: Scribner.

Swazey, Judith P., and Karen Reeds. 1978. "Disease and the Ductless Glands." In *Today's Medicine, Tomorrow's Science: Essays on Paths of Discovery in the Biomedical Sciences*, Chapter 4. Washington, D.C.: U.S. Department of Health, Education, and Welfare.

HAR GOBIND KHORANA *1968*

Har Gobind Khorana was born in Raipur, in the Punjab region of India, now part of West Pakistan. His birthdate was recorded as January 9, 1922. Khorana is an organic chemist who has specialized in proteins and nucleic acids. The 1968 Nobel Prize in Physiology or Medicine was awarded to Har Gobind Khorana, Robert W. Holley, and Marshall W. Nirenberg "for their interpretation of the genetic code and its function in protein synthesis."

Khorana's parents were Shri Ganput Rai Khorana and Shrimat Krishna Devi Khorana. His father was a village agricultural taxation clerk in the British colonial government. His parents were poor but dedicated to education. They were practically the only literate family in their small village. Khorana recalled receiving his first four years of schooling under a tree where the local teacher established his "classroom." Khorana married Esther Elizabeth Sibler in 1952. He credits his wife with bringing a sense of purpose into his life at a time when he felt "out of place everywhere and at home nowhere" (Khorana 1968, 371). They have three children.

Khorana received the B.Sc. with honors in 1943 and the M.Sc. with honors in 1945 from Punjab University, in Lahore, India, where he was much influenced by Professor Mahan Singh. A Government of India Fellowship enabled him to study at Liverpool University, England. Working under the supervision of Roger J. S. Beer, he earned his Ph.D. in 1948. From 1948 to 1949 he was a postdoctoral fellow at the Federal Institute of Technology, Zurich, working with Vladimir Prelog. From 1950 to 1952 he was a Nuffield Fellow at Cambridge University, working with (Lord) Alexander Todd, a future Nobel laureate, and G. W. Kenner. At Cambridge he developed his interest in proteins and nucleic acids. At the invitation of Gordon M. Shrum, Khorana accepted the position of researcher in the organic chemistry section of the British Columbia Research Council and the University of British Columbia, Canada. During this period (1952–60) Khorana established a group of researchers studying biologically interesting phosphate eaters and nucleic acids. It was here in 1959 that Khorana first received international recognition for the synthesis of coenzyme A, work carried out in collaboration with John G. Moffatt.

Khorana and four of his associates moved to the University of Wisconsin-Madison in 1960 where he became professor and co-director at the Institute for Enzyme Research. From 1962 to 1970 he was held an appointment as professor in the Department of Biochemistry, at the University of Wisconsin. In 1964 he was a visiting professor at Stanford University. In 1966 he was visiting professor at Harvard Medical School. Since 1970 he has been Alfred P. Sloan Professor, Departments of Biology and Chemistry, at MIT. From 1974 to 1980 he was also Andrew D. White Professor-at-large at Cornell University. Khorana is the author or coauthor of over five hundred scientific publications.

Although the work of the three 1968 Nobel laureates was interrelated, each man was honored for work carried out independently. Nevertheless, as Maxine Singer wrote, the significance of each achievement "is enhanced by the achievement of the others. These three men together constitute a triplet of great sense" (Singer 1968, 433). While Nirenberg provided an ingenious method that initiated the highly creative period in which the genetic code was deciphered, it was Khorana who conducted much of the final, technically sophisticated work. Khorana replicated each of the sixty-four possible genetic signals, or triplets, by synthesizing polynucleotides of known composition. Thus, Khorana confirmed and extended Nirenberg's findings. He demonstrated the exact order of nucleotides in each triplet and proved that the code consists of three-letter, nonoverlapping words, read in a determined linear fashion. The code was also found to be redundant, that is, certain amino acids had more than one triplet, and certain triplets were found to be "punctuation marks" for beginning and ending polypeptide chain synthesis. Khorana systematically devised the methods that led to the synthesis of large, well-defined nucleic acids.

Khorana's announcement on June 2, 1970, of the synthesis of the first wholly artificial gene was hailed in the scientific community and the popular press as one of the greatest scientific landmarks of molecular biology and the possible prelude to therapeutic or dangerous manipulations of the genetic material. The DNA molecule that Khorana synthesized was the gene that coded for alanine transfer RNA in yeast because the RNA sequence was already known through the work of Robert Holley.

Prior to 1960 techniques for studying the structure of the nucleic acids were still extremely limited. Khorana developed the synthetic approach to elucidating the structure of the nucleic acids. His laboratory developed techniques for the chemical synthesis of both the RNA and DNA form of the polynucleotides.

Synthetic and enzymatic methods were ingeniously combined as a means of circumventing the formidable problems posed by purely chemical synthesis of polyribonucleotides. For example, RNA-polymerase and synthetic polydeoxyribonucleotides of known sequence could be used to direct the synthesis of long, complementary polyribonucleotides. Many such polymers were tested and the results were extended with polymers containing repeating tetranucleotide sequences. This generated a repeating array of four triplets. The resulting polypeptides contained a repeated tetraamino acid sequence. Khorana's work provided the unequivocal evidence for established codon assignments and led to the definition of some codons that had not previously been determined. Of particular interest, some triplets were shown to serve as punctuation marks for initiating and terminating polypeptide chain synthesis. Khorana's work provided a direct demonstration that three nucleotides specify an amino acid, specified the direction in which messenger RNA is read, proved that codewords could not overlap, and showed that, through an RNA intermediary, the sequence of nucleotides in DNA specified the sequence of amino acids in a protein.

Summarizing the remarkable progress that had been made in polynucleotide synthesis and understanding the genetic code by 1968, Khorana remarked that the problem of the genetic code could be regarded as essentially solved, at least for *Escherichia coli*. Thus the essential question was what the direction of further work in the field of polynucleotide synthesis should be. Khorana suggested that problems for the immediate future included: the punctuation marks on DNA, recognition of DNA by repressors, DNA modifying enzymes, transcription enzymes such as RNA polymerase, and the puzzle of viral RNAs. More fundamental and obscure problems included the precise mechanism of genetic recombinations, DNA replication, and the control of DNA replication (Khorana 1968a, 79). His own untiring dedication to research contributed much to the solution of many of these problems.

Khorana's most recent research, for which he was awarded the Paul Kayser International Award of Merit in Retina Research in 1988, concerns the chemistry and molecular biology of rhodopsin, the light-transducing pigment of the retina, and bacteriorhodopsin, a light-sensitive protein found in a bacterium. Using the tools of molecular biology that he did so much to forge, Khorana has synthesized the gene for bovine rhodopsin and studied the mechanisms of action and expression.

In a rare press interview, the modest and often shy scientist told a reporter "I do have a basic faith that survival of our civilization is not even going to be possible without proper use of science" (*Current Biography Yearbook*, p. 222).

Other honors awarded to Har Gobind Khorana include the Merck Award, Chemical Institute of Canada (1958), elected to the National Academy of Sciences (1966), the American Chemical Society Award for Creative Work in Synthetic Organic Chemistry (1968), the Lasker Foundation Award for Basic Medical Research (1968), the American Academy of Achievement Award, Philadelphia, Pennsylvania (1971), the Padma Vibhushan Presidential Award, India (1972), the J. C. Bose Medal, Bose Institute, Calcutta, India (1972), the Willard Gibbs Medal of the Chicago Section of the American Chemical Society (1974), and the National Medal of Science (1987).

Dr. Khorana holds honorary degrees from Simon Fraser University, Vancouver, Canada (1969), the University of Liverpool, England (1971), the University of Punjab, India (1971), the University of Delhi, India (1974), Calcutta University, India (1974), Vikram University, India (1974), the University of Chicago (1976), the University of

British Columbia, Vancouver, Canada (1977), and New England College, Henniker, New Hampshire (1984).

He has been elected to membership in the National Academy of Sciences (1966, the American Association for the Advancement of Science (1966), the American Academy of Arts and Sciences (1967), Deutsche Akademie der Naturforscher, Leopoldina, Germany (1968), the Indian Academy of Science (1976), the Pontifical Academy of Sciences, Rome (1978), the Royal Society, London, England (1978), the Royal Society of Edinburgh (1982), and the Order of San Carlos, Colombia, South America (1986).

LOIS N. MAGNER

Selected Bibliography

PRIMARY SOURCES

Khorana, H. G. 1961. *Some Recent Developments in the Chemistry of Phosphate Eaters of Biological Interest.* New York: John Wiley.

Smith, M., and H. G. Khorana. 1963. "Preparation of Nucleotides and Derivatives." *Methods of Enzymology* 6:645–70. New York: Academic Press.

Ghosh, H. P., D. Soll, and H. G. Khorana. 1967. "Studies on Polynucleotides. 67. Initiation of Protein Synthesis in Vitro as Studies by Using Ribopolynucleotides with Repeating Nucleotide Sequences as Messengers." *Journal of Molecular Biology* 25:275–98.

Khorana, H. G., 1968a. "Polynucleotide Synthesis and the Genetic Code." *Harvey Lectures*, series 62, 79–105. New York: Academic Press.

Khorana, H. Gobind. 1968b. "Nucleic Acid Synthesis in the Study of the Genetic Code." Nobel Lecture, December 12, 1968. Reprinted in *Nobel Lectures, Physiology or Medicine*, Vol. 4 (1963–1970), 341–71. Amsterdam: Elsevier, 1972.

Khorana, H. G. 1988. "The Kayser Lecture. Studies on Bacteriorhodopsin and Rhodopsin." *Proceedings of the Retina Research Foundation Symposium.* 1:63–89.

SECONDARY SOURCES

Chargaff, E. 1955. *The Nucleic Acids*, Vol. 1. New York: Academic Press.

Singer, Maxine F. 1968. "News and Comment. 1968 Nobel Laureate in Medicine or Physiology." *Science* 162:433–36.

1970. *Current Biography Yearbook*, 222–24. New York: H. W. Wilson.

Fruton, Joseph S. 1972. *Molecules and Life. Historical Essays on the Interplay of Chemistry and Biology.* New York: Wiley-Interscience.

Kornberg, A., B. L. Horecker, L. Cornudella, L. and J. Oro, eds. 1976. *Reflections on Biochemistry. In Honour of Severo Ochoa.* Oxford: Pergamon Press.

HEINRICH HERMANN ROBERT KOCH *1905*

Heinrich Hermann Robert Koch was born on December 11, 1843, in Clausthal, Germany. Praised by contemporaries as one of the most notable medical scientists of his time, Robert Koch provided the methods and basic discoveries for the newly evolving science of bacteriology. He received the 1905 Nobel Prize for Physiology or Medicine for his pioneering work on tuberculosis, including the discovery and isolation of the etiological agent of the disease, the tubercle bacillus, in 1882. He died in Baden-Baden, Germany, on May 27, 1910, of a heart ailment.

Koch's father, Hermann, was a prominent mining official and his mother, Mathilde Biewend, was the daughter of an iron-mine inspector. Both were natives of Clausthal, an old mining town in the Oberharz region. Robert grew up in a large household—he had eight brothers and two sisters—and was encouraged to be self-reliant. He spent a great deal of time outdoors, collecting plants, stones, and insects. Having taught himself reading and writing, he entered a local school in 1848, transferring to the Gymnasium three years later. In 1862 Koch enrolled at the University of Goettingen to study natural sciences, but transferred to medicine a year later.

In the course of his medical studies, Koch came into close contact with Jacob Henle, a prominent anatomist who had postulated the existence of living agents as responsible for contagious diseases. During his medical studies he won a prize writing a paper on the distribution of nerve ganglia in the uterus. Moreover, Koch conducted some chemical experiments concerning the metabolism of succinic acid in humans, the subject of his doctoral dissertation. After graduation in 1866, he visited Berlin to attend clinical rounds at the famous Charité Hospital as well as lectures in pathological anatomy given by Rudolf Virchow, Germany's most celebrated physician.

Koch's initial years in practice took him to Hamburg, Hannover, Braetz, Niemegk, and Rakwitz. In 1867 he married Emmy Fraatz, a daughter of the superintendent of Clausthal. After serving briefly in the Franco-Russian War of 1871, he was appointed district medical officer at Wollstein (now Wdsztyn, Poland) in 1872. This position, in an idyllic countryside, provided Koch with enough time to pursue his scientific interests, especially the study of algae and parasites.

Armed with a microscope, incubator, mice, and a camera, Koch focused his attention on anthrax, an enzootic disease affecting the flocks of sheep in his district. Not only was he able to detect the rodlike microorganisms believed to cause the illness, but he cultured them and accurately described their life cycle, including the puzzling spore formation. Looking for a publisher of these observations, he arranged a visit to Breslau (now Wroclaw, Poland) in 1876 and successfully demonstrated his methods and preparations to Ferdinand Cohn, the famous botanist. His anthrax findings as well as methods for dry fixing and staining bacteria were immediately published in Cohn's *Beitraege zur Biologie der Pflanzen*.

Koch's growing scientific reputation was further enhanced through the 1877 publication of a monograph on the bacteriology of infected wounds. His experiments clearly showed that the contagion was due to specific microorganisms, a conclusion gratefully acknowledged by leading surgeons of the day such as Joseph Lister and Theodor Billroth. In spite of such findings, Koch failed to gain an academic position. Finally, in 1880, Julius Cohnheim, a pathologist at the University of Breslau, was able to persuade the German government to provide Koch with an advisory job—Regierungsrat—in the Imperial Health Department at Berlin.

The next two years proved extraordinarily fruitful. Koch and his assistants Friedrich Loeffler and Georg Gaffky immediately went to work on gathering further information about the nature and actions of pathogenic bacteria. The aim of the health department was to establish methods designed to avoid contamination and design proper disinfection processes. Among Koch's findings useful in surgery was the sterilizing capacity of steam and the disinfectant properties of mercuric chloride. His pure culture methods received worldwide recognition during the 1881 International Medical Congress in London, where he met Lister and Louis Pasteur.

Identification of the tubercle bacillus by Koch in 1882 constituted a milestone in the development of bacteriology. His findings, first presented to the Berlin Physiological Society on March 24 of that year, were quickly verified around the globe and soon employed in the diagnosis of this highly prevalent disease. However, investigators and physicians often had difficulties in achieving the pure cultures required by Koch's postulates.

Another major scourge, cholera, also yielded its secrets. Heading a German government commission, Koch went to Egypt in 1883 to investigate an epidemic of the disease in Alexandria. His discovery and isolation of a comma-shaped bacillus in the small intestine of victims was confirmed during a subsequent outbreak in India and led to measures designed to protect the contamination of drinking water sources. Koch was awarded the German Order of the Crown by the kaiser and greatly commended by the international medical community. In 1885 he was selected to occupy a new academic chair in hygiene at the University of Berlin.

Despite oppressive teaching and administrative duties, Koch returned to his experimental studies to seek a specific remedy for the disease whose cause he had already discovered: tuberculosis. Invited in 1890 to address the Tenth International Medical Congress, then meeting in Berlin, on bacteriological research, he ended his talk by announcing that after testing many chemicals he had "at last hit upon a substance which has the power of preventing the growth of tubercle bacilli." Despite the tentative nature of Koch's statement and his failure to disclose the precise nature of the remedy, the discovery was widely hailed and he received numerous honors, including a pledge from the German government to erect a new institute solely devoted to bacteriological research. Patients by the thousands flocked to Berlin determined to obtain the miracle drug.

Within less than a year, reports from various European medical centers began to cast doubt on the efficacy of tuberculin, the apparent cure composed of a glycerin extract of killed tubercle bacilli. Physicans gradually began to recognize the diagnostic properties of the tuberculin lymph but rejected Koch's therapeutic claims. Although the German government in 1891 finally appointed Koch director of the newly created Institute of Infectious Diseases in Berlin, his scientific reputation suffered irreparable harm. His subsequent career was devoted to administrative tasks and extensive foreign travel in connection with efforts to control a host of tropical diseases.

When cholera reached Hamburg in 1892, Koch became involved in the fight to convince city authorities about the importance of uncontaminated water supplies and the isolation of ambulant cases. A rinderpest outbreak in South Africa (1896), bubonic plague in India (1897), Texas cattle fever and malaria in East Africa (1898)—all came to his attention. In 1901 the Kaiser Wilhelm Military Academy in Berlin elected him to membership at the rank of major general in tribute to his many contributions to military hygiene.

In matters regarding tuberculosis, however, Koch remained adamant about the immunity of humans to bovine tubercle bacilli. His presentations at the first International Congress on Tuberculosis in London (1901) and the sixth Congress in Washington (1906) generated a fair amount of disagreement and opposition from prominent personalities such as Joseph Lister and Hermann Biggs. Indeed, Koch's ideas were in sharp contrast with findings documented by many scientists concerning the dangers from infected cow's milk.

Koch spent his last years traveling extensively around the world. Officially retired at age sixty from government service, he continued to stay in touch with his disciples and took interest in worldwide campaigns to eradicate disease. In 1903 he went to Southern Rhodesia to study another cattle disease: Rhodesian redwater. Three years were spent in equatorial Africa researching relapsing fever in Uganda, the Belgian Congo, and Tanganyika. Visits to the United States and Japan followed. Wherever Koch went, he received honors and awards. Toward the end of his life, he was still busy supervising the production and clinical trials of tuberculin.

Paul Ehrlich, one of Koch's collaborators and himself a Nobel Prize winner, placed him among the "few princes of medical science" who established the bases of modern medicine. A whole generation of colleagues and disciples applied Koch's exacting methods designed to identify and culture the most important microorganisms implicated in human disease. Compulsion, tenacity, and an endless capacity for work were traits that Koch instilled in those who labored with him. Outside his close circle of associates, he was perceived as authoritarian and arrogant, reluctant to change his views, and prone to borrow ideas from other scientists without acknowledging their source.

His efforts to place bacteriology upon a sound footing were only the prelude to a much more ambitious undertaking: the prevention and treatment of infectious diseases. His own failed endeavor to find a cure for tuberculosis was the most prominent example. Support for the production of diphtheria antitoxin, purified quinine, and Ehrlich's chemotherapeutic compounds were other examples of Koch's research program. Moreover, in the field of public health, his knowledge of the etiological agents of infection—notably tropical diseases—helped nations to draft pertinent health legislation and stimulate governmental action. Thus, Robert Koch's career reflects the ideals of a gifted investigator who not only advanced science but successfully shaped public policies based on his discoveries.

GUENTER B. RISSE

Selected Bibliography

PRIMARY SOURCES

Koch, Robert. 1932. "The Aetiology of Tuberculosis." *American Review of Tuberculosis* 25:285–323.

———. 1987. *Essays of Robert Koch.* Translated by K. Codell Carter. Westport, Connecticut: Greenwood Press.

SECONDARY SOURCES

King, Lester S. 1952. "Dr. Koch's Postulates." *Journal of the History of Medicine and Allied Sciences* 7:350–361.

Dolman, Claude E. 1973. "Robert Koch." In *Dictionary of Scientific Biography*, 7:420–35.

Penn, M., and M. Dworkin. 1976. "Robert Koch and Two Visions of Microbiology." *Bacteriological Reviews* 40:276–83.

Maulitz, Russell M. 1983. "Robert Koch in the United States of America." *NTM Zeitschrift fur Geschichte der Naturwissenschaften, Technik, und Medizin* (Leipzig) 20:75–84.

Rosenkrantz, Barbara Gutmann. 1986. "Koch's Bacillus: Was There a Technological Fix?" In *The Prism of Science*, edited by E. Ullmann-Margalit, 147–50. Dordrecht, Holland: Reidel Publishing.

Brock, Thomas D. 1988. *Robert Koch. A Life in Medicine and Bacteriology.* Madison, Wisconsin: Science Tech. Publishers.

EMIL THEODOR KOCHER *1909*

In 1909 Emil Theodor Kocher became the first surgeon to receive the Nobel Prize in Physiology or Medicine. Born in Berne, Switzerland, on August 23, 1841, he obtained his undergraduate education there and completed medical studies at the University of Berne in 1865. He ranked at the top of his class, with special citations in classical languages and art. Having committed himself at an early age to a career in academic surgery, he carefully planned a tour of the major surgical clinics in Europe. He first visited the most outstanding clinic in the world of that day, the Charité Hospital in Berlin, where the highly respected Bernhard von Langenbeck was professor of surgery at the University of Berlin. Langenbeck was considered the master surgeon in Europe, having personally devised over thirty original operations and developed a surgical training program that was the source of a number of the leading academic professors on the Continent. Kocher then went to England, where he observed Sir James Paget and Spencer Wells, both noted surgeons of the time, and next visited Paris, where he spent time with Louis Pasteur, the outstanding scientist in the world of that era.

The following year Kocher returned to Berne and applied for the position of assistant in the surgical clinic. Following his appointment, he rapidly became recognized as an outstanding clinical surgeon and a remarkable teacher. In 1872 Albert Lücke, professor of surgery in Berne, who had been trained in Germany and had established a school in Berne with a strong Germanic background, reached the age of retirement. After much deliberation the university selected Professor König, then an associate of Langenbeck in Berlin, as his replacement. However, the faculty in the Surgery Department held the strong view that Kocher should be appointed. Together with the medical students, they advanced the point that a Swiss successor should be chosen if a capable one were available. They were confident that Kocher was fully qualified. Moreover, the surgical giant, Theodor Billroth, wrote a letter about Kocher saying: "He writes clearly as well as thinks clearly and that is why he would make a scientific type of teacher" (quoted in Bonjour 1950). With the tide running strong for Kocher, the board of regents overruled the original choice and appointed Kocher to this prestigious surgery chair at the astonishing age of thirty-one. Quite rapidly he attracted worldwide attention to the Berne Clinic by devising new surgical procedures that were characterized by attention to detail, and by conducting operations that were flawlessly performed and that yielded excellent results. Kocher held the chair as professor of surgery in Berne from 1871 until 1916, a total of forty-five years, a remarkable record.

Kocher's most notable contributions were in the field of thyroid surgery, where he soon became the unquestioned leader. Switzerland has long been known for its high incidence of goiter, primarily due to iodine deficiency especially in the mountainous regions. His first thyroidectomy was performed in 1872, the year following his appointment as professor of surgery at Berne. Within a short time he had done a large number of thyroidectomies for goiter with remarkable results. It is interesting that the operative mortality was originally 13 percent, but by 1898 Kocher reported a series of six hundred patients with only a single death. His near perfect results were achieved by careful attention to control of blood loss and protection of the parathyroid glands. He also emphasized avoidance of injury to the recurrent laryngeal nerves, which could lead to changes in the voice and, in its most severe form, to tracheal obstruction, especially if both recurrent nerves were injured. At the end of his career Kocher had performed more than five thousand thyroidectomies for goiter with an amazingly low mortality of only 1 percent.

In addition to his contributions as a clinical surgeon, Kocher was also a distinguished physiologist. Quite early in his work on the thyroid he recognized that following thyroidectomy one-third of his patients developed signs and symptoms of what was later to be recognized as thyroid insufficiency. He stated quite poignantly, "the generalized use of surgery for goiter has to do with the physiological importance of the thyroid gland. Unfortunately, the physiologists know almost nothing about it, and this has probably been the main reason why surgeons have simply assumed that the thyroid gland has no function whatever. As soon as it has been learned that from the standpoint of technique total extirpation could be carried out successfully there was no longer reason to hesitate to remove the entire organ when both lobes are diseased" (Kocher 1883). Nevertheless, Kocher was quick to recognize that problems could arise in patients upon whom he had operated and said in a postoperative follow-up:

> Of the 18 patients with total excision who presented themselves for examination, only two show a state of health as good as or better than before the operation.
>
> The remaining 16 patients with total excision of the diseased thyroid gland all show more or less severe disturbances in their general condition, the analysis of which has been drawn from precise records in each individual case. The time elapsed since the operation ranges from 3½ months to 9 years and 2 months, and the severity of the symptoms is far graver in the oldest cases. They [symptoms] are obviously progressive. All younger patients who were operated upon more than two years ago show these manifestations to a pronounced degree. . . . As a rule, soon after discharge from the hospital, but in occasional cases not before the lapse of 4 or 5 months, the patients begin to complain of fatigue, and especially of weakness and heaviness in the extremities. . . . The mental alertness decreases. This is particularly striking in children of school age, inasmuch as they drop in

> class standing, and that the teachers note a progressive diminution of their intellectual capabilities. . . . In the majority of the cases, the swelling is a permanent puffiness of the face. Second only to the clumsiness, it is this which creates the impression among more distant acquaintances that the patient has become an idiot. . . . If we are to give a name to this picture, we cannot fail to recognize its relation to idiocy and cretinism: the stunted growth, the large head, the swollen nose, thick lips, heavy body, the clumsiness of thought and speech, in the presence of a well-developed musculature undoubtedly point to a related evil. It is interesting that the individuals are not really stupid, which has often been emphasized by their families; they are fully conscious of the retardation of their mental capabilities and especially of the slowness of their comprehension, deliberation, and particularly, of their speech. (Kocher 1883)

With this description Kocher had defined postoperative thyroid hormone insufficiency or hypothyroidism.

As Kocher's fame spread, the leading surgeons throughout the world visited his clinic, including the noted William S. Halsted of Johns Hopkins Hospital in Baltimore. They became close friends and collaborators, and Halsted later became the most outstanding surgeon in the United States.

Kocher also deserves credit for many surgical innovations. He devised a special clamp, which is still used and bears his name, and described several incisions, which bear his name and continue to be used, notably the Kocher collar incision for thyroidectomy, a Kocher right subcostal incision for cholecystectomy, and surgical reflection of the duodenum, the Kocher maneuver. Moreover, he carefully observed that hypothyroidism could be traced to deficiency of the gland, whether congenital or due to an operation, but could also be the result of a goiter in which the gland does not produce sufficient thyroid hormone as occurs with iodine insufficiency. These observations led directly to the fundamental discoveries of Murray, Gley, and Vassale, who administered thyroid extract in various forms to overcome this deficiency and showed that it was effective. Ultimately, the essential constituent, the thyroid hormone *thyroxine*, was isolated by Kendall in 1914. Following this, Marine showed that small amounts of iodine in the diet was effective in the prevention of goiter. These observations led to the creation of *iodized* salt which is widely used today. Harrington and Barger later synthesized thyroxine which made it available pharmaceutically in pure form, replacing the crude extract obtained from animal thyroid glands.

In his own description of work for which he received the Nobel Prize in 1909, Kocher said,

> We ourselves have communicated a continuous series of 300 and more goiter operations without a fatality. Important though this result has been for suffering humanity, yet it has been far exceeded by the understanding which has grown, anew on practical and clinical soil, concerning the vital *physiological* function

> of the thyroid. . . . Early in 1883, at the Congress of the Deutsche Gesellschaft fur Chirurgie we announced that some 30 of our first 100 patients operated on for goiter, whom we were able to follow up and reinvestigate, presented a syndrome which can be precisely characterized, and which we designated simply with the name *cachexia strumipriva* [literally, a bad condition due to removal of a struma or goiter]. This appeared in a well-marked form only in those patients from whom we had removed the whole thyroid, and on the other hand only with temporary manifestations in those in whom the whole goitrous structure was supposed to have been removed, but where in fact a portion had remained, which continued to grow. (Kocher 1909)

Kocher commented further, "The impulse was provided for the impressive investigations by the Committee of the Clinical Society, which came to the conclusion that myxoedema and sporadic cretinism, and probably cachexia strumipriva too, were identical, and that there were close relationships with endemic cretinism."

Kocher's famous textbook of surgery, first published in 1892, entitled *Text-Book of Operative Surgery*, became a classic and was used worldwide. The German pioneer thoracic surgeon, Ferdinand Sauerbruch, said of Kocher, "The center of Kocher's personality is his merciless strength directed against himself. By hard work he developed all the possibilities in himself" (quoted in McGreevy and Miller 1969; Bonjour 1950). Kocher took few vacations with those he did take usually associated with national meetings or to prepare papers for publication (Bonjour, 1950).

On his forty-third birthday, Kocher stated:

> Twenty-four years ago I started my medical studies. For the past twelve years I have been a professor. Today, I move into a new hospital. At this point a new episode in my activity begins which puts considerable demand on me. I enter this period with much richer experience but also with an older body and matured spirit. Instead of the hopes of my colleagues and the citizens, which supported me in the beginning, they now expect of me. Instead of the popularity of a young and striving spirit I am now surrounded by half-critical, half-hopeful observations of my actions. Instead of support I feel demands. I must be prepared for this in this new position. I can expect support and pleasure only from my family and circle of friends. From others, I must count on help, demands and giving. (quoted in Bonjour 1950).

A summary statement concerning Kocher's selection for the Nobel Prize should be emphasized, particularly for today's young investigators. The Nobel Committee cited Kocher "for his work on the physiology, pathology, and surgery of the thyroid gland." He was the first surgeon to receive this most distinctive of all scientific honors. At the time of his death an obituary written by Sir Berkeley Moynihan, the distinguished British surgeon, concluded: "the world loses its greatest surgeon" (Obituary 1917).

H. KIM LYERLY
DAVID C. SABISTON

Selected Bibliography

PRIMARY SOURCES

Kocher, T. 1883. "Postoperative Results of Extirpation of the Thyroid." *Archiv klinische Chirurgie* 29:254–337. Reprinted in *Great Ideas on the History of Surgery*, translated by L. M. Zimmerman and I. Veith. Baltimore: William & Wilkins.

———. 1909. "Concerning Pathological Manifestations in Low-grade Thyroid Diseases." Nobel Lecture. Reprinted in *Nobel Lectures in Physiology or Medicine*. Vol. 1, 1901–1921. Amsterdam: Elsevier (1967): 330–383.

SECONDARY SOURCES

1917. "Professor Theodor Kocher." Obituary. *British Medical Journal* 2:168–69.

Bonjour, E. 1950. *Theodor Kocher*. Bern: Paul Haupt.

McGreevey, Patrick S., and Fletcher A. Miller. 1969. "Biography of Theodor Kocher." *Surgery* 65 (June): 990–999.

GEORGES KÖHLER *1984*

Georges Köhler shared a Nobel Prize in 1984 with the immunologists Niels K. Jerne and Cesar Milstein for his joint discovery (with Milstein) of a new immunological technique for antibody production (hybridomas) which rapidly showed itself most fruitful in many fields of biology and medicine.

Georges Köhler was born in Munich in 1946. His father, Karl Köhler, was a German of Czech origin and his mother Raymonde Laporte, was French. He grew up in Kehl, on the German side of the Rhine border. Köhler entered the University of Freiburg in 1969 and obtained a diploma in biology in 1971 with work on DNA repair in *Escherichia coli*, the favorite subject of molecular biologists.

He chose immunology as his field of interest and asked Fritz Melchers, from the Institute of Immunology in Basel, to supervise his work. After starting immunological study of the galactosidase enzyme he became aware of the enormous variety of antibodies that an animal can produce against a single antigen. His interest was aroused by the genetic mechanisms responsible for this diversity. He wanted to study how mutations acting on a single cell and its progeny can determine this variety. For this purpose, he needed a pure line of cells producing identical antibodies, but this pure line did not exist.

Antibodies (or immunoglobulins) are the main component of the immune system that maintains the integrity of the organism. They are composed of two pairs of heavy and light chains, each itself composed of one "variable" and one "constant" part that are controlled by different sets of genes. Antibodies had been a significant tool in diagnosis and research long before Köhler became interested in them. But the main source of antibodies was serum derived from immunized animals; this serum contained antibodies directed against many different antigens and therefore defied standardization.

The turning point of Köhler's career resulted from his meeting Cesar Milstein when the latter visited the Basel Institute in 1973 for a seminar. Milstein invited Köhler to come and work with him in Cambridge, England, for the following year on the problem of mutations in antibody genes.

In 1962 Potter had developed a method for obtaining myelomas (antibody-producing tumors) by injecting mineral oil into mice and had then distributed these myeloma lines (an invaluable source of material for the study of antibodies) among researchers. Milstein and Cotton subsequently obtained hybrids by fusing mouse and rat myeloma cells for the purpose of investigating the genetic mechanism of antibody diversity and the complex interaction (scrambling) of the different genes involved. This study in itself proved disappointing; each chain in the antibody produced exhibited constant and variable regions belonging to the same species; only light chains and heavy chains could belong to two different species. But the hybrids refuted the dogma of "allelic exclusion" by secreting both types of parental antibodies. Building from this demonstration that the genetic information from both parents could be codominantly expressed, Köhler had the idea to fuse myeloma cells and normal antibody-producing lymphocytes. By immortalizing lymphocytes, he would construct an ideal line for the immunogenetical study of antibodies.

Köhler obtained a long-term fellowship from the European Organization of Molecular Biology (EMBO) to work at the Medical Research Council at Cambridge and began his research in spring 1974. He did not invent a totally new technique, but he did bring to maturity a method for producing antibodies of a predefined specificity in unlimited quantity. The method consisted of the fusion of cancer cells ("immortal" cells) with plasma cells to produce antibodies of a desired specificity. These hybrid cells from animals immunized against a target antigen or hybridomas could be established as a continuous line secreting one particular type of antibodies. These antibodies were named monoclonal antibodies to point out their homogeneity, they were produced by a single clone and its progeny.

Köhler began by selecting a myeloma line that had specificity for a known antigen and tried to cultivate it. At first he was not able to grow it. He then decided to attempt a hybridization similar to P_3, a myeloma line developed by Cotton (since in Australia) and Milstein. This line was ideal because the sequence of the protein was well known, but Köhler failed to identify its antigen-binding activity. He developed a mutant of P_3 that was appropriate for Littlefield's selective medium in which only hybrids can grow. The idea of hybridizing myeloma cells with preimmunized lymphocytes came to him forcefully at the start of fall 1974, one evening when, in his own words, he was at home between wakefulness and sleep, in the state most propitious for free idea association.

Milstein suggested that he first discover which antigen reacted with the myeloma line, but Köhler stuck firmly to his idea of developing hybrids that would produce antibodies of his choice. The idea was interesting, and some other immunologists had pursed similar attempts, but without success. Köhler had to face some well-known problems: lymphocytes were bad fusers and the screening of the hybrids would be tedious and might consume all the time allotted for Köhler's postdoctoral work. It was a gamble; but Köhler accepted the challenge and Milstein gave him active support and guidance.

For his first attempt, Köhler chose sheep red blood cells as the immunogen, an antigen long familiar to immunologists. Bordet had expanded immunology by choosing such a nonbacterial antigen with which he was able to achieve classical immunization and antibody production. Such antibodies could be easily detected by an assay devised by N. K. Jerne and A. Nordin in 1963. Around Christmas 1974, Köhler could see with delight that hybrids had formed. After a few weeks he observed that some hybrids were actually reacting with red blood cells. The first genuine productive hybridomas had been produced. The next step was to test the technique for other kinds of antigens.

After initial success, the experiments went badly, In the meantime Köhler had returned to Basel and was pursuing his own research independently. He tried various modifications in his cultures. The most interesting was the use of another fusing agent, the synthetic chemical propylene-glycol. Finally, he traced his problems to a toxic batch of one reagent, and the matter was settled.

Köhler was later responsible for an important improvement of his technique of producing monoclonal antibodies; he created "silent" myeloma lines that do not secrete any antibody of their own and facilitate the selection of the appropriate clones. But he refused to become a mere "monoclonal antibody maker" and maintained his initial interest in the genetics of the immune response. He studied the heavy and light components of immunoglobuline and from his study of mutants losing their capacity of synthesizing one chain he made suggestions regarding the regulation of the production of the different chains.

Köhler received the Gairdner Foundation Award as a joint prize with Milstein. Initially, he did not receive as many awards as Milstein, who benefitted from his seniority in the field. Köhler was awarded the Nobel Prize in Physiology or Medicine with Milstein and Jerne in 1984, at age thirty-eight. In his Nobel Lecture, he surveyed monoclonal antibodies and pointed out their advantages over the conventional sera. The monoclonal antibodies permit exploration of the whole repertoire of antigenic specificities. Culturing techniques enable production of unlimited quantities of pure, highly precise strains of monoclonals; these will replace the conventional sera in many medical areas for the diagnosis and possibly for the treatment of many diseases. Hybridomas secrete high levels of antibodies and are easily manipulated. They can be diversified by several methods, including selecting mutants, adding segments of chains through genetic engineering, etc. Köhler was sensitive to the impressive possibilities for "spin-off" of the new technology in many areas; the most important for him was that the original hybridomas could become "the starting-point of man-made secondary antibodies, each manufactured to satisfy a special requirement" (Köhler 1986, 1286).

He remained in Basel until 1985, when he became director of the Max Planck Institute for Immunobiology in Freiburg, Germany. While maintaining his profound interest in immunogenetics, he turned to novel lines of research with his collaborators. He investigated the impact of synthetical estrogens on various tissue receptors, notably in bone, and evaluated a whole range of molecules that could be active as drugs in rheumatoid diseases. At the same time, he is still pursuing his lifelong interest in the genetic origin of antibody diversity.

Köhler was awarded the Nobel Prize at the age of 38, a somewhat unusual case in scientific history. He was not disturbed in his subsequent work and behavior by this early crowning of his career and pursued steadily his own line of interest with his new team in Germany. He has been described by his colleagues as a congenially modest and honest researcher who welcomed his award with total happiness and a touch of humor without losing his psychological balance.

Köhler and his wife Claudia have three children. He is a devoted father and he deliberately chose the quiet life of a small village in the Basel suburb for his family.

Köhler is a member of the European Organization of Molecular Biology (EMBO).

ANNE MARIE MOULIN

Selected Bibliography

PRIMARY SOURCES

Köhler G. and C. Milstein. 1975. "Continuous Cultures of Fused Cells Secreting Antibody of Predefined Specificity." *Nature* 256:495–497.

———. 1986. "Derivation and Diversification of Monoclonal Antibodies." *Science* 233:1281–1286.

SECONDARY SOURCES

Sinkovics, J. G. 1981. "Early History of Specific Antibody-Producing Lymphocyte Hybridomas." *Cancer Research* 41:1246–1247.

Wade, N. 1982. "Hybridomas: the Making of a Revolution." *Science* 215:1073–1075.

———. 1984. "The 1984 Nobel Prize in Medicine." *Science* 226:1025–1028.

Nicholas, R. 1986. *Hybridoma Technology: an Annotated Listing of Key Papers 1975–1985* New York: Mansell.

Bibel, D. J. 1988. *Milestones in immunology. A Historical Explanation.* Madison: Science Tech Publishers.

Mackenzie, M., Cambrosio, A. and P. Keating. Forthcoming. "Scientific Information and Intellectual Property: the Case of the Hybridoma/Monoclonal Antibody Technique." *Social Studies of Science* (forthcoming).

ARTHUR KORNBERG *1959*

Arthur Kornberg was born on March 3, 1918, in Brooklyn, New York. His area of scientific specialization is the biochemistry of nucleic acids. The 1959 Nobel Prize in Physiology or Medicine was awarded to Arthur Kornberg and Severo Ochoa "for their discovery of the mechanisms in the biological synthesis of ribonucleic acid and deoxyribonucleic acid." Kornberg and Ochoa helped to elucidate the enzymatic machinery that makes DNA and RNA. On November 21, 1943, Arthur Kornberg married Sylvy R. Levy, later a research associate in biochemistry. The Kornbergs have three children.

Kornberg's parents, Joseph Kornberg and Lena Katz Kornberg, emigrated to the United States from Austrian Galicia. His father worked in the sweatshops of the Lower East Side of New York as a sewing machine operator. Later the Kornbergs opened a small hardware store in Brooklyn. Kornberg received a B.S. degree from the College of the City of New York in 1937 and an M.D. degree from the University of Rochester in 1941. From 1941 to 1942 he was an intern at Strong Memorial Hospital in Rochester. In 1942 he served briefly as a lieutenant in the United States Coast Guard. From 1942 to 1953 he was a commissioned officer in the United States Public Health Service, assigned to the National Institutes of Health in Bethesda, Maryland. He spent the years 1942 to 1945 in the nutrition section performing research on rat nutrition. In 1946 Kornberg studied enzymology with Severo Ochoa in New York and in 1947 with Carl and Gerty Cori in St. Louis. These experiences transformed him from a "vitamin hunter" to an "enzyme hunter." After working with the Coris, Kornberg organized an enzyme section at the NIH for research on coenzyme biosynthesis. From 1947 to 1953 he was chief of the new enzyme and metabolism section of the National Institute of Arthritis and Metabolic Diseases, NIH.

In 1953 Kornberg became professor and head of the Department of Microbiology at Washington University, in St. Louis, where he remained until 1959. During this period he elucidated the pathways of nucleotide biosynthesis and began his studies of nucleic acid biosynthesis and replication. Since 1959 he has been professor of biochemistry at Stanford University, where he also served as chairman of the department from 1959–69.

Kornberg's research has helped to elucidate the enzymatic machinery responsible for the biological synthesis of deoxyribonucleic acid. He notes that people were sometimes surprised at his lack of formal training in science and the fact that he had begun his career as a practicing physician, serving as a hospital intern before his appointment as a ship's doctor for a crew of five hundred during his wartime stint in the Coast Guard. However, by the time he went to sea he had already published a paper, "Latent Liver Disease in Persons Recovering from Catarrhal Jaundice and in Otherwise Normal Medical Students, As Revealed by the Bilirubin Excretion Test," in the May 1942 issue of the *Journal of Clinical Investigation.* This paper grew out of observations of his own mild jaundice and a strong desire to avoid gall bladder surgery. Although his original career goal was to practice clinical medicine, when he obtained a position at the National Institute of Health he became an eager member of the tribe of vitamin hunters and an enthusiastic biochemist. Biochemistry, a field that had seemed so barren to him during his medical studies, had been transformed into a dynamic inquiry into macromolecules and complex metabolic pathways.

Although Kornberg claims that he had "never known a dull enzyme," he would have to admit that some enzymes are more exciting than others. Certainly the decades spent with DNA polymerase must have been the most rewarding (Kornberg 1976, 243). Kornberg also studied the mechanisms of formation of important coenzymes, the enzymatic reactions in the Krebs cycle, and phospholipid biosynthesis. He discovered the enzyme DNA polymerase, which catalyzes formation of short DNA molecules.

By the late 1950s, about one hundred years after Friedrich Miescher discovered the nucleic acids, it was known that DNA served as the carrier of hereditary information in most living things. DNA was believed to be the carrier of the master pattern in the cell nucleus that allowed each cell to reproduce itself in its own image. It was also thought to play some role in the production of RNA, which seemed to be essential in the production of protein, the basic material for all living tissue. Moreover, in some viruses, such as the poliomyelitis virus and the tobacco mosaic virus, RNA also seemed to serve as the hereditary material. However, because of the complexity of living cells, and the technical problems posed by macromolecules, it was very difficult to find ways of studying DNA and RNA in isolation. When Kornberg discovered an enzyme that produced DNA from its much smaller constituents, a new field of investigation was opened up to biochemists. Severo Ochoa found an enzyme that played a similar role for investigations of RNA.

In 1956 Kornberg succeeded in demonstrating the existence of DNA polymerase in the common intestinal bacterium *Eschericia coli.* The enzyme produced DNA when provided with precursors, magnesium salts, and an appropriate primer to start the reaction. Research on nucleic acid synthesis, conducted independently by Kornberg and Ochoa, made it possible to use purified enzymes for the in vitro synthesis of polynucleotides that appeared to be virtually identical with DNA and RNA both physically and chemically.

It may surprise younger scientists to note that when Arthur Kornberg gave his Nobel Lecture in 1959, the evidence that DNA was the genetic material was considered substantial but not yet unequivocal. Kornberg's investigations of purified DNA polymerase demonstrated how the isolated enzyme catalyzed the synthesis of this nucleic acid in response to directions from preexisting DNA. These studies had effectively eliminated the last remnants of "vitalism" from discussions of the synthesis of DNA. Assuming that DNA was the genetic material, Kornberg compared DNA to a tape recording carrying a message in which there were specific instructions for tasks to be done. This recording could also be used to make exact copies so that the information could be used repeatedly and independently. Scientists had asked whether the two functions of DNA, the expression of the code (protein synthesis) and the replication of the code (preservation of the genome) were closely integrated or separable. Research had made it possible by 1959 to at least partially understand the mechanism of DNA at the enzymatic level, but much about the mechanism by which DNA directed protein synthesis was still a mystery.

Concerning the structure of DNA, it was well known that the purine content was always equal to the pyrimidine content. The double-helical model of James Watson and Francis Crick had provided an explanation for this relationship. Unlike Watson, Kornberg had a profound respect for the necessity of understanding the basic chemistry and the biosynthesis of the system's simple nucleotides and coenzymes as prerequisites to elucidating the biosynthesis of DNA itself. Crude extracts of bacteria were understandably better at destroying DNA than carrying out the biosynthetic reaction Kornberg and his coworkers were seeking. However, using labeled substrates of high specific radioactivity, they succeeded in detecting a minute amount of synthesis. According to Kornberg, "Through this tiny crack we tried to drive a wedge, and the hammer was enzyme purification" (Kornberg 1959, 1503). The enzymatic approach provided the key insights into the problem of DNA replication and the properties of the DNA-synthesizing enzyme purified from *Escherichia coli*. This enzyme catalyzed the synthesis of a new DNA chain in response to directions from a DNA template. The instructions were dictated by the hydrogen-bonding relationship of adenine to thymine and guanine to cytosine, as predicted by the Watson-Crick model of the DNA double helix. Just how much could be accomplished by refining this system was made evident when Kornberg, Mehran Goulian, and Robert L. Sinsheimer announced at a news conference on December 14, 1967, that they had succeeded in synthesizing biologically active DNA in vitro. A full report was published in the December 1967 issue of the *Proceedings of the National Academy of Sciences*. The popular press portrayed this remarkable achievement as a giant step towards creating life in a test tube.

According to Kornberg, by the 1980s progress in understanding DNA replication had reached a new peak because of "two major influences on biochemistry in the past decade: genetic engineering and the pronounced drift to cellular biology. Genetic engineering and related technologies have made it possible to obtain scarce enzymes in generous quantities, to create DNA templates with sizes and sequences needed for exploring DNA structure and enzyme function, and to tailor plasmids and viruses for probing cellular functions (Kornberg 1984, 122). Taking full advantage of these technological and conceptual advances, Kornberg continues to explore the basic science of DNA replication. His current research interest focuses on the multienzyme pathways of DNA replication as a means of understanding the mechanics and control of DNA replication and metabolism. He has been reported to have said that "If asked to name varieties of mental torture, most scientists would place writing at the top of the list" (Byrne 1988, 420). However, he has been a prolific writer of scientific articles, reviews, and books, and is working on an autobiography entitled *Never a Dull Enzyme*.

Other honors awarded to Arthur Kornberg include the Paul-Lewis Laboratory Award, American Chemical Society (1951), the Silver Medal, Federal Security Agency (1952), the Lucy Wortham James Award, James Ewing Society (1968), the Max Berg Award (1968), the Science Achievement Award, American Medical Association (1968), the Borden Award, American Association of Medical Colleges (1968), the Albert Gallatin Medal, New York University (1970), and the National Medal of Science, United States (1979).

Kornberg is a member of the National Academy of Sciences and the American Philosophical Society, and a foreign member of the Royal Society (London). He serves on the Board of Governors of the Weizman Institute and is scientific advisor to the DNAX Research Institute of Molecular and Cellular Biology.

LOIS N. MAGNER

Selected Bibliography

PRIMARY SOURCES

Kornberg, Arthur. 1959. "Biologic Synthesis of Deoxyribonucleic Acid." Nobel Lecture, December 11, 1959. Reprinted in *Science* 131:1503–8.

———. 1962. *Enzymatic Synthesis of DNA.* New York: Wiley.

Kornberg, A., B. L. Horecker, L. Cornudella, and J. Oro, eds. 1976. *Reflections on Biochemistry In Honour of Severo Ochoa.* Oxford: Pergamon Press.

Kornberg, Arthur. 1976. "For the Love of Enzymes." In *Reflections on Biochemistry*, edited by A. Kornberg, B. L. Horecker, L. Cornudella, and J. Oro, 243–51. Oxford: Pergamon Press.

———. 1980. *DNA Replication.* New York: W. H. Freeman.

———. 1982. *Supplement to DNA Replication.* San Francisco: W. H. Freeman.

———. 1984. "DNA Replication." *Trends in Biochemical Sciences* 9:122–24.

———. 1987. "Enzyme Systems Initiating Replication at the Origin of the *Escherichia Coli* Chromosome." *Journal of Cell Science Supplement* 7:1–13.

———. 1988. "Minireview: DNA Replication." *The Journal of Biological Chemistry* 263:1–4.

SECONDARY SOURCES

McElroy, W. D., and B. Glass, eds. 1957. *The Chemical Basis of Heredity.* Baltimore: Johns Hopkins Press.

Anon. 1959. "Ochoa and Kornberg Win Nobel Prize." *Science* 130:1099–1100.

1968. *Current Biography Yearbook*, 210–12. New York: H. W. Wilson.

Fruton, Joseph S. 1972. *Molecules and Life. Historical Essays on the Interplay of Chemistry and Biology.* New York: Wiley-Interscience.

McMacken, R., and T. J. Kelly. 1987. *Replication and Recombination: UCLA Symposia on Molecular and Cellular Biology, New Series.* Vol. 47. New York: Alan R. Liss.

Byrne, Gregory. 1988. "Random Samples." *Science* 241:420.

ALBRECHT KOSSEL *1910*

Karl Martin Leonhard Albrecht Kossel was born September 16, 1853, in Rostock, Germany. A biochemist and physiologist, Kossel received the Nobel Prize in 1910, for his work in isolating and identifying the chemical components of the cellular nucleus, which led to our modern understanding of the transmission of genetic information. At the time of the award, he was professor of physiology at the University of

Heidelberg, a position he held from 1901 until 1925. He married Luise Holtzmann in 1886; the couple had two children, a daughter and a son, Walther, who made major contributions to the field of theoretical physics. Kossel died July 5, 1927, in Heidelberg, Germany.

Kossel was the only son of Albrecht Kossel, a merchant and Prussian consul, and Clara Jeppe Kossel. His boyhood interest was botany, but his father wanted him to study medicine. Young Albrecht enrolled at the University of Strasbourg so that he could satisfy his father but also attend the lectures of the mycologist Anton de Bary. While at Strasbourg, however, he studied with Felix Hoppe-Seyler, whose influence led him into biochemistry. He worked as Hoppe-Seyler's assistant from 1877 to 1883, after passing the state medical examination in Rostock. He received his medical degree in 1878 and submitted a thesis (Habilitationsschrift) for his Ph.D. in 1881. His early research concerned salt diffusion and the digestion of fibrin.

Emil du Bois Reymond brought Kossel to Berlin as director of the chemical division of the Physiological Institute; he became an assistant professor in physiology at the University of Berlin in 1887. In 1895 he was appointed to the chair in physiology at the University of Marburg, where he remained until called to Heidelberg to replace Wilhelm Kuhne. Throughout most of his career, Kossel was classified as a physiologist, since biological chemistry did not have the status of an independent discipline; but it was his precision in organic chemical analysis that exemplified his work and made his major discoveries possible. (Olby 1973, 466; "G. B." 1927)

Hoppe-Seyler and his student, Friedrich Miescher, had already isolated "nuclein" from the cell nucleus in the 1860s. Kossel began his investigations of yeast cell nuclei while he was with Hoppe-Seyler in 1879. He separated the substance into two parts: protein and nucleic acid, which was made up of a carbohydrate, phosphoric acid, and nitrogen compounds. He further isolated and identified the nitrogenous components: two purines—adenine and guanine—and three pyrimidines—thymine, cytosine, and uracil (uracil is actually the substance in RNA which takes the place of thymine in DNA). (A purine's atoms are arranged in two rings and a pyrimidine's in a single ring.) Thymine was first discovered by Kossel. He and his students also identified as such the secondary breakdown products of nucleic acid, which included the substances xanthine and hypoxanthine. As they established in their analyses of a variety of animal and plant substances, this nuclear structure is basic for all organic cells.

Kossel foresaw the importance of his work but was limited by the knowledge and methodology of the time in pursuing its implications. He suggested correctly that the function of nuclein was linked to new cell formation and that the nuclein molecule could be subdivided into twelve units. But it was left to others to establish the truth and significance of his ideas (Olby 1973, 466–67).

He did succeed in establishing the distinction between true nuclein and the similar substances identified in egg yolks and milk caseins, which he identified as unnucleated breakdown products of true nucleic acids. He also identified the carbohydrate in yeast nucleic acid as a pentose and postulated the existence of a hexose sugar in another acid preparation (2-deoxyribose).

In 1884 Kossel began to investigate more fully the proteins in nuclein. He was able to isolate histone from the blood cells of geese and break this substance down into the amino acids leucine and tyrosine. Histone is similar to a substance Miescher had called protamine, which is a basic component of fish sperm cells. Kossel applied his careful analytic methods to protamine and obtained arginine, lysine, and histidine. He was then able to develop the classical method of separating these hexone bases by means of phosphotungstates and silver compounds. With his English student, H. D. Dakin, he used the ferment arginase to hydrolyze arginine into urea and ornithine. Later he also identified and isolated arginine from herring roe.

Kossel's deep interest in amino acids led to his construction of a complex theory of reproduction based on their synthesis and breakdown. He attempted to justify this empirically in quantitative analyses of salmon embryos. Kossel also believed that the key to biological specificity lay in the amazing diversity of the proteins, the polypeptides (Olby 1973, 466–67).

He was correct in his assertion that the amino acids and the nuclear components he had isolated were basic biological "building blocks." The genetic key, of course, was not in the proteins but in the nucleic acids, today classified as deoxyribonucleic or ribonucleic, depending on the structure of the carbohydrate (a pentose). RNA and DNA are the basis of our understanding of genetics, growth, and normal metabolism and are increasingly recognized as important in disease pathology. All these findings followed from Kossel's work.

Kossel was a modest, reserved, and highly conscientious man who participated actively in the international scientific community, particularly as a proponent of the definition of biochemistry as an independent field, and of the cooperation of physiologists and biochemists in separate attacks on similar problems. As he said in his Nobel Lecture, "We have arrived at problems the solution of which can only be obtained by various methods of research working together. The representatives of morphological sciences see under the microscope a structure deposited in the cell [the nucleus] and study the dependence of its form on the conditions of the elementary organism. The biochemist tries to define the composition of the structure, its position in the chemical components of the cell, but this task demands theories of structural chemistry and the aid of synthetic methods" (Kossel 1910, 405).

Kossel was instrumental in establishing separate chairs of biochemistry in several German universities. He was the editor of *Hoppe-Seyler's*

Zeitschrift für physiologische Chemie for over thirty years and in 1907 chaired the seventh International Congress in Physiology in Heidelberg. After his retirement from the university in 1925, he was made director of the new Heidelberg Institute for Protein Investigation, which had grown out of his work, and served in this capacity until his death of a heart attack two years later.

MARCIA MELDRUM

Selected Bibliography

PRIMARY SOURCES

Kossel, Albrecht. 1883–84. "Über einen peptonartigen Bestandtheil des Zellkerns." *Zeitschrift für physiologische Chemie* 8:511–515.

———. 1893. "Über die Nucleinsaure." *Archiv für Anatomie und Physiologie*, 157–64.

Kossel, Albrecht, and H. Steudel. 1902–03. "Über einen basichen Bestandtheil tierischen Zellen." *Hoppe-Seyler's Zeitschrift für physiologische Chemie* 37:177–89.

Kossel Albrecht. 1910. "The Chemical Composition of the Cell Nucleus." Nobel Lecture, December 12, 1910. Reprinted in *Nobel Lectures in Physiology or Medicine*, vol. 1 (1901–1921), 394–405. Amsterdam: Elsevier, 1967.

———. 1911–12. "The Chemical Composition of the Cell." *Harvey Lectures*, ser. 7 New York: Academic Press. 33–51.

———. 1912. "Lectures on the Herter Foundation." *Johns Hopkins Hospital Bulletin* 23:65–76.

———. 1928. *The Protamines and Histones*. London: Longmans, Green.

SECONDARY SOURCES

"G. B." 1927. "Obituary: Prof. Albrecht Kossel." *Nature* 120 (August 13): 233.

Edlbacher, S. 1928. "Albrecht Kossel zum Gedächtnis." *Hoppe-Seyler's Zeitschrift für physiologische Chemie* 177:1–14.

Felix, Kurt. 1961. "Albrecht Kossel: Life and Work." In *Great Chemists*, edited by Eduard Farber, 1033–37. London: Interscience Publishers, 1961.

Olby, Robert. 1973. "Kossel, Karl Martin Leonhard Albrecht." In *Dictionary of Scientific Biography*, 7:466–68. New York: Scribners.

SIR HANS ADOLF KREBS 1953

Hans Krebs was born on August 25, 1900, in Hildesheim, Hanover, the second of three children of Georg Krebs, a successful ear, nose, and throat specialist, and Alma Davidson Krebs. As a boy he enjoyed a wide variety of activities, including hiking, cycling, bookbinding, and encyclopedic reading. In Mittelschule and the classical Gymnasium Hans did well on all his subjects but was not outstanding in any single area. At age fifteen he decided to follow his father's footsteps into medicine and then to join his thriving practice.

Drafted into the army in September 1918, Krebs was discharged two months later when World War I ended. In December he entered the University of Göttingen. After two semesters he moved to the University of Freiburg to complete his preclinical studies. Several of the professors he had in Freiburg, including Franz Knoop, a pioneer in the investigation of intermediary metabolism, described their own discoveries in their lectures, arousing in Krebs a desire to participate in research himself. During the summer semester of 1920 he carried out, under the direction of Wilhelm von Möllendorff, an experimental project in which he stained striated muscle tissue with various dyes in order to ascertain the relation between their staining properties and their physical or chemical ones.

After his first clinical semester Krebs moved again, to the University of Munich, in order to follow the lectures of several distinguished clinicians on the Munich faculty. His conviction grew that he would enter academic medicine so that he could combine clinical work with medical research. Obtaining his M.D. in 1925, he served a required year of hospital service in Berlin. He found the time there also to carry out experiments on the reaction of gold sol suspensions with cerebral spinal fluid, a reaction then in use as a diagnostic test for syphilis. In collaboration with the head of his section, he investigated the penetration into the cerebrospinal fluid of dyes injected into the bloodstream of dogs. These investigations, largely conceived on his own, resulted in several published papers.

Aware since his work with Möllendorff that he needed to know more chemistry in order to pursue medical research, he enrolled in 1925 in a special chemistry course in Berlin for medical students with such aims. Through chance contacts made by a friend, he had the opportunity to become, at the beginning of 1926, a paid research assistant in the laboratory of the outstanding biochemist Otto Warburg, at the Kaiser Wilhelm Institut für Biologie at Dahlem. Here Krebs learned the methods of manometry and tissue slices that Warburg employed to study cellular respiration and glycolysis. Krebs remained in Warburg's laboratory until March 1930. He came to admire and to emulate Warburg's disciplined approach to scientific research, his capacity to concentrate on problems of central importance, and his insistence on writing succinct, lucid scientific papers.

Not expecting that a career in biochemistry alone was practicable, Krebs took a position at a municipal hospital near Hamburg, where he had heavy clinical duties but also an opportunity to pursue some research on his own. A year later he moved to the laboratory of Siegfried Thannhauser at the University of Freiburg. Although he had clinical responsibilities here also, he had sufficient support to undertake a major research problem. He decided to apply the manometric tissue slice methods he had learned from Warburg to one of the long-standing unsolved problems of metabolism, the synthesis of urea. Late in November 1931, he and his assistant, Kurt Henseleit, discovered that the amino acid ornithine, in the presence of ammonia, increased strikingly the output of urea from liver tissue slices. During the following weeks he established that ornithine acts catalytically. By April 1932 he had formulated the theory that a cyclic process involving ornithine, citrulline, and arginine produces urea from amino nitrogen, carbon dioxide, and ammonia. The discovery attracted widespread attention and quickly established Krebs as a major investigator in metabolic biochemistry.

During the following year Krebs pursued related problems, including the deamination of amino acids, and began to attract students, forming a small research group. His progress was rudely interrupted in April 1933 when the recently installed Nazi regime passed a law for the reform of the civil service that caused him to be dismissed from his post. In June he resumed his career in England in the Biochemistry Department of Frederick Gowland Hopkins at Cambridge University, supported by a Rockefeller grant. Adapting readily to English life and culture and finding the atmosphere of the Cambridge laboratory inspiring, Krebs flourished there, began again to attract younger collaborators, and made several further discoveries. He showed that glutamine is synthesized from glutamic acid in kidney and other tissues, and that hypoxanthine is an intermediate in the formation of uric acid in birds.

In October 1935 Krebs accepted a position in the Department of Pharmacology at Sheffield University, where he had ample space to pursue his own work and to begin to build a research team. A year later he took up one of the central problems of the time, the oxidative metabolism of carbohydrates. For a time he attempted to extend the pattern of paired oxido-reduction reactions characteristic of the recently established Embden-Meyerhof glycolytic pathway to the later stages of carbohydrate breakdown. By the spring of 1937 this direction was turning out to be less promising than he had hoped. In April a paper published by Carl Martius and Franz Knoop stimulated Krebs to a fresh attack on the problem. Citric acid had long been known to stimulate tissue respiration; but because it was difficult to envision how that substance might be broken down, it had largely been left out of previous hypotheses concerning oxidative decomposition, which were oriented mainly around the dicarboxylic acids: succinic, malic, fumaric, and oxaloactetic acid. Martius and Knoop showed that citric acid is oxidatively degraded, in several steps, to form α-ketoglutaric acid. Krebs perceived at once that the decomposition of citric acid could be connected through α-ketoglutaric acid to the dicarboxylic acids, and that oxaloacetic acid could react with a "triose" to reform citric acid, producing a closed cycle of reactions. In formulating this theory Krebs was also strongly influenced by the recent discovery by Albert von Szent-Györgyi that fumaric acid catalytically increases the respiration of minced pigeon breast muscle.

With the assistance of his first graduate student, William Arthur Johnson, Krebs was able to gather within six weeks sufficient experimental evidence for his theory—including the demonstration in pigeon breast muscle that citric acid is synthesized anaerobically from oxaloacetic acid—to publish a paper proposing the "citric acid cycle." Although Krebs himself initially viewed the cycle as involved primarily in carbohydrate metabolism, eventually it became clear that it is the common final pathway for the oxidative conversion of all major classes of foodstuffs to carbon dioxide and water, and that it is also connected with numerous synthetic pathways.

In 1938 Krebs married Margaret Fieldhouse, the daughter of a Yorkshire family and teacher of domestic science in a nearby convent school. They had three children: Paul, Helen, and John.

During World War II Krebs took part in research directed toward special diets that might be employed to supplement scarce supplies of ordinary food. Near the end of the war the Medical Research Council established a "Unit for Research in Cell Metabolism" under his direction at Sheffield. During the postwar decades Krebs, and the increasing numbers of students who came to learn the methods pursued in the unit, extended his prewar discoveries, especially to the metabolism of microorganisms. In the early 1950s Krebs became particularly interested in the question of how some microorganisms can synthesize all of their required organic molecules from acetic acid as the sole organic nutrient. Although acetic acid could enter the citric acid cycle, that cycle could not provide a synthesis of carbohydrates. He suggested this problem to a former student, Hans Kornberg, who discovered in his laboratory a modification of the citric acid cycle, which they named the glyoxylate cycle.

In 1953 the Nobel Prize in Physiology or Medicine was awarded jointly to Hans Krebs, for the discovery of the citric acid cycle, and to Fritz Lipmann, for the discovery of acetyl-coenzyme A which elucidated the detailed mechanism of the critical synthetic step in the cycle. Among the many other awards Krebs received for his work were the Lasker Award (1954); the Royal Medal of the Royal Society (1954);

the Gold Medal from the Netherlands Society for Physics, Medical Science and Surgery (1958); and the Copley Medal (1961). He was knighted in 1958.

Soon after winning the Nobel, Krebs accepted the chair of biochemistry at Oxford and brought with him the research team of the metabolic research unit. At Oxford, Krebs became particularly interested in the regulation of metabolic pathways, examining the factors that determine the directions in which particular pathways proceed. He drew attention especially to the importance for the control of the ratios of reduced and oxidized forms of the coenzyme components of such catalysts as the pyridine nucleotides, and of the ratios of ATP and ADP and inorganic phosphate. In 1963, he explained the regulation of gluconeogenesis, identifying the pace maker reactions involved in a feedback mechanism.

After reaching the mandatory retirement age at Oxford in 1967 Krebs was able to continue his work with his own metabolic research unit in a laboratory at the Radcliffe Hospital. He continued actively to direct the work of this unit for fourteen years.

In 1979 Jack Baldwin, an organic chemist at Oxford, offered Krebs an explanation, based on the mechanisms of organic reactions, for the fact that acetic acid cannot be oxidized metabolically without undergoing a synthetic reaction. Building on this suggestion, Krebs developed the viewpoint that cyclic processes provide the most efficient possible means for utilizing the energy of foodstuffs within the constraints under which the metabolic accumulation and release of energy occur. This led him to publish a paper in April 1980 offering an evolutionary explanation for the occurrence of the citric acid cycle.

Krebs pursued his scientific activity with undiminished energy until September 1981. Then, after a short illness, he died on November 22, in his eighty-first year.

Hans Krebs combined the discipline to carry on a steady investigative pace with the imagination to connect his results with contemporary developments so as to produce broadly unifying theories. He was most innovative in his prewar work, but his later investigations significantly broadened the scope of his earlier discoveries and insights. For some of those who worked with him he was a hard taskmaster, who expected quality work as a matter of course. He was also, however, gentle and considerate. He laughed easily at the commonplace events of daily laboratory life but did not allow them to divert him from his central purposes. His integrity and his genuine modesty inspired in many who worked with him a lifelong loyalty. He was recognized in his own time as one of the most important architects of the field of intermediary metabolism.

FREDERIC L. HOLMES

Selected Bibliography

PRIMARY SOURCES

Krebs, H. A., and L. V. Eggleston. 1944. "Metabolism of Acetoacetic Acid in

Animal Tissues." *Nature* 154 (August 12):209–210.

Krebs, H. A., *et al.*, "Urea Synthesis in Mammalian Liver." *Nature* (June 14):808–809.

Krebs, H. A. 1950. "Tricarboxylic Acid Cycle." *Harvey Lectures* ser. 44: 165–199. New York: Academic Press.

———. 1968. *The Metabolic Roles of Citrate.* London: Academic Press.

———. 1970. *Essays in Cell Metabolism.* New York: Wiley.

Krebs, H. A., and Anne Martin. 1981. *Reminiscences and Reflections.* Oxford: Clarendon Press. This volume also contains a complete bibliography on pages 269–289.

An extensive collection of Krebs' laboratory notebooks, correspondence, and other personal papers, is deposited in the Sheffield University Archives, with an unpublished catalog compiled by Jeannine Alton and Peter Harper.

SECONDARY SOURCES

Benner, Steven. 1976. "The Tricarboxylic Acid Cycle." *Yale Scientific* 50:4–10, 34–35.

Holmes, Frederic L. 1980. "Hans Krebs and the Discovery of the Ornithine Cycle." *Federation Proceedings* 39: 216–225.

Kornberg, Sir Hans, and P. H. Williamson. 1984. "Hans Adolf Krebs, 25 August 1900–22 November 1981." *Biographical Memoirs of Fellows of the Royal Society* 30:351–389.

SCHACK AUGUSTUS STEENBERG KROGH *1920*

Schack Augustus Steenberg Krogh was born on November 15, 1874, in Grenas, Denmark. A physiologist and zoologist, Krogh received the Nobel Prize in 1920 for his work on the regulation of circulation in the capillaries, a discovery of considerable importance for our understanding of the total body metabolism. He spent his entire career at the University of Copenhagen, holding the position of professor of animal physiology from 1916 until his retirement in 1945. Krogh married Dr. Marie Jørgenson in 1905; she collaborated with him in many of his investigations. The Kroghs had one son, Erik, and three daughters, Bodie, Ellen, and Agnes. Krogh died September 13, 1949, in Copenhagen.

Krogh's father, Viggo Krogh, was a brewer; his mother, Marie Drechman Krogh, taught the boy to read and write at the age of five. He was educated at local schools but spent much of his free time observing birds and animals and attempting chemistry and physics experiments. He considered careers in medicine or the navy; but a family friend, William Sorenson, rekindled his interest in zoology and specifically in animal physiology. Krogh completed his master's degree in zoology at the University of Copenhagen in 1899 and became an assistant in the laboratory of Christian Bohr, who had been his professor.

Krogh's great talents lay in his quantitative precision and his skill at designing and improving apparatus for his experiments. He applied these talents to the study of physical problems in biology, which he found more interesting and suggestive than biochemical experiments (Snorrason 1973, 501).

Krogh's early work dealt with respiration and gaseous exchanges in metabolism. His Ph.D. thesis in 1903 discussed the cutaneous and pulmonary respiration of the frog. In 1904 he published with Bohr and K. A. Hasselbach a paper that established that oxygen metabolism in the blood is dependent upon carbon dioxide pressure.

In 1906 he received the Seegen Prize from the Vienna Academy of Sciences, for a paper on the pulmonary exchange of nitrogen, which brought him considerable renown. For this study, Krogh had to construct a very small apparatus that could be completely immersed in water to ensure accurate temperature control. He was then able to demonstrate that nitrogen plays no role in respiratory exchange (Snorrason 1973, 501–2; Rehberg 1951, 86).

He continued his experiments on oxygen and carbon dioxide exchange, now working with Marie Krogh, and in 1910 published definitive results that challenged the theories of Bohr and others: exchange was based on "diffusion and diffusion alone," rather than on any secretory or other integral regulatory process. Again, this research had been impossible until Krogh designed and built the instruments for microanalysis of gases and gaseous pressure (Krogh 1908; Krogh and Krogh 1910).

He had been appointed associate professor at the university in 1908 but had to wait two years for his own laboratory. Even after he received a small, simply equipped facility, he worked often in a lab at his home. From 1910 to 1920 he conducted studies of respiration and muscle work with Johannes Lindhard, perhaps among the first investigations in sports medicine; completed with his wife an analysis of arctic metabolism, based on earlier trips to Greenland; and began his pioneering work on capillary action.

In his researches with Lindhard he had begun to consider questions of circulation, volume, and oxygen supply to the tissues. Conventional wisdom held that blood flowed continuously through all the capillaries, as it did through the arteries and veins. Krogh theorized that it would be more efficient and economical if some capillaries closed while a muscle or organ was at rest. His observations of animals while exercising or under stress showed that blood flow increased to the body system involved. Increased blood flow would be of little value without increased oxygen supply, but Krogh's quantitative analysis found that only a part of the additional oxygen was provided by respiration. Where then did the extra oxygen come from? He perceived that the answer might provide additional support for his closed capillary hypothesis.

Careful study of living animals showed that many invisible capillaries suddenly dilated and became visible when a muscle was stimulated. Krogh then began intensive microscopic studies. Previous capillary studies had not been precise enough, he believed, in controlling the animal's actions. Krogh injected an isotonic ink into the arteries of frogs, then immediately stopped the animal's heart and dissected the muscles and organs. He found that capillaries in resting organs were small and partially closed, while those in muscles stimulated just before death were black with ink-filled capillaries. He thus determined that capillaries are open during work and partially closed during rest, demonstrating the critical role of capillary control in body metabolism and oxygen consumption.

His initial results were published in 1918. His major work, *The Anatomy and Physiology of Capillaries*, which discussed further research on the role of the nervous system and of hormones in capillary control, was not published until 1922, however, after the Nobel Prize. This beautifully written book has become a classic in the field (Snorrason 1973, 502–3; Rehberg 1951, 90–91).

Krogh's work owed a debt to his wife, a physician, who perceived the importance of his discovery to clinical medicine. The new understanding of capillary control aided medical treatment of blood pressure, shock, inflammation, allergies, and some hemorrhagic and cardiac disease. Further research demonstrated that many pathologic symptoms are a result of changes in the ability of the capillaries to open and close at need.

In 1924 the Rockefeller Foundation offered funding for the modern laboratory Krogh had so long needed. The Rockefeller Institute in Copenhagen, which opened in 1928, was designed by Krogh himself and contained space for six laboratories.

He continued his muscle work research in the 1920s, developing new methods for determination of the total osmotic tension of blood. He devoted the rest of his life to zoophysiological research, studying insect respiration, the metabolism of aquatic animals, and the flight of birds and insects. During World War II, he had to escape to Sweden to avoid capture by the Germans; there he took the opportunity to carry out plant physiology studies.

Krogh also contributed more directly to the public welfare of his native land. His wife had become diabetic and, in 1922, he visited the United States to study insulin. Through his efforts, factories were established in Denmark to manufacture insulin. He also worked on the physiological aspects of heating houses for the Academy for the Technical Sciences, designing a microclimatograph for field measurements of temperature and humidity. Although he retired from active teaching in 1934, he remained a resource for other teachers and had a lasting influence on high school science through his textbook, *Laerebog i Menneskets Fysiologi* (first published in 1908).

Throughout his life, Krogh worked in his laboratory from early morning to late evening, barely stopping to allow it to be cleaned. He nevertheless found time to read history, archaeology, and British and American literature, and was particularly fond of Kipling. He liked to spend his summer vacations boating and observing aquatic life.

Krogh was elected to the Royal Danish Society of Sciences but resigned because he found its philosophy too conservative. He was always rather disdainful of honors, although he was pleased to accept lectureships and honorary degrees. Among the awards he did accept was the Baly Medal from the Royal College of Physicians in 1945 (Snorrason 1973, 503–4; Rehberg 1951, 100–102).

MARCIA MELDRUM

Selected Bibliography

PRIMARY SOURCES

Krogh, August. 1908. "On the Microanalysis of Gases." *Skandinavisches Archiv für Physiologie* 20:279.

Krogh, August, and Marie Krogh. 1910. "On the Mechanism of Gas Exchange in the Lungs." *Skandinavisches Archiv für Physiologie* 23:248.

Krogh, August. 1916. *The Respiratory Exchange of Animals and Man.* London: Longmans Green.

———. 1922. *The Anatomy and Physiology of Capillaries.* New Haven: Yale University Press.

———. 1929. "The Progress of Physiology." *Science* 70:203.

———. 1941. *The Comparative Physiology of Respiratory Mechanisms.* Philadelphia: University of Pennsylvania Press.

SECONDARY SOURCES

Hagedorn, H. C., "August Krogh". *Meddeleiser fra Akademiet for de Tekniske Videnskaber* 1 (1949):33–38. With bibliography of Krogh's work pp. 39–50.

Liljestrand, G. 1950. "August Krogh." *Acta Physiologica Scandinavica* 20:109–20.

Rehberg, H. Brandt. 1951. "August Krogh, November 15, 1874–September 13, 1949." *Yale Journal of Biology and Medicine* 24:83–102.

Snorrason, E. 1973. "Krogh, Schack August Steenberg". In *Dictionary of Scientific Biography*, 7:501–4. New York: Scribners.

KARL LANDSTEINER *1930*

Karl Landsteiner was born on June 14, 1868, in Vienna, Austria. A bacteriologist and serologist, Landsteiner received the Nobel Prize in 1930 for his discovery of the human blood groups, which made possible lifesaving blood transfusions and modern surgical procedures, and laid the groundwork as well for a multitude of diagnostic and forensic serological tests. He also described the Rhesus (Rh) factor and made major contributions to the understanding and treatment of poliomyelitis and syphilis, among other diseases. Landsteiner has been called the father of immunology for his many pioneering investigations. Although much of his work was done in Vienna, at the time of the award he was a member of the research staff at the Rockefeller Institute for Medical Research, a position he held until his death. He married Helene Wlasto in 1916; they had one son, Ernst Karl. Karl Landsteiner died June 26, 1943, in New York City.

Landsteiner was the son of Leopold Landsteiner, a journalist and newspaper publisher. The elder Landsteiner died when Karl was six and he was raised by his mother, Fanny Hess Landsteiner, to whom he remained devoted throughout his life. He received his medical degree from the University of Vienna in 1891, followed by a short period of clinical training at the Second Medical University Clinic. Interested in developing his knowledge of chemistry, he left Vienna to work with Emil Fischer in Wurzburg, Eugen Bamberger in Munich, and Arthur Hantzsch in Zurich. These studies occupied him for two years.

He returned to Vienna in 1894 and resumed his clinical apprenticeship with Eduard Albert at the First Surgical University Clinic. In 1896 he accepted an appointment as assistant to Max von Gruber in the new Department of Hygiene at the University of Vienna. There he became interested in the new science of immunology. Recent work by Emil von Behring had established that the body produces its own antigens to fight disease when vaccinated or infected, the first scientific demonstration of "the healing power of nature" (Speiser 1973, 622–23).

In order to gain more experience in physiological pathology, Landsteiner joined the university's Pathological-Anatomical Clinic in 1897, under the tutelage of Anton Weichselbaum, who had isolated the bacteria that causes meningitis. He conducted 3,639 autopsies during his years at the clinic, which contributed materially to his understanding of human physiology as well as anatomy. Weichselbaum encouraged him to pursue his interest in antibodies and he began his work with blood serum.

Jules Bordet had observed the agglutination, or clumping, and dissolution, or hemolysis, of animal red blood cells when they were injected into a foreign host, such as an animal of a different species. In 1900 Paul Ehrlich noted the same phenomenon occurring with a host of the same species (isoagglutination). In that same year Landsteiner published a paper in which he asserted in a footnote that human isoagglutination was the result of physiological differences in human blood types. He performed extensive blood testing and the following year, in his pioneering article, "Über Agglutinationserscheinungen normalen menschliches Blutes," differentiated three blood types—A, B, and C (later O)—in terms of the reaction of sera with red cells. The serum from type A included antibodies against B and therefore clumped cells from type B but not from O or A; the inverse was true of type B sera: type O sera contained both anti-A and anti-B antibodies and agglutinated both other types. Landsteiner's rule therefore states that serum contains only antibodies that will not attack its own type or blood group.

In 1902 Landsteiner's associates, A. Decastello and A. Sturli, on the basis of further tests, described a fourth group, AB. AB was agglutinated by anti-A and anti-B sera, but its own sera contained no antibodies and did not clump the cells of other groups. On the basis of Landsteiner's characterization, safe blood transfusion now became feasible. Surgeons were now able to perform operations on the heart and lungs, involving extensive blood loss; complete blood exchanges on newborns were also now possible. His work led also to a greater understanding of shock, jaundice, and other clinical problems. His observations indicated that blood type is hereditary; this fact proved useful in cases of disputed paternity.

Landsteiner was convinced that further research on antibodies would lead to even more individual differences in human blood, making it possible to take a "serological fingerprint." In this conviction, he has been proven very nearly correct (Speiser 1973, 623).

Landsteiner worked for Weichselbaum until 1908 and made many experiments that furthered knowledge of immunology and were applicable to clinical medicine. In 1904 he investigated paroxysmal cold hemoglobinurira, working with Julius Donath. In this disease, hemoglobin is spilled in the urine after a patient has been exposed to cold, a phenomenon that Ehrlich attributed to vascular pathology. Landsteiner demonstrated in vitro that the disease was caused by an antigen that attacked the blood cells in the body but combined with them at low temperatures. The result of this research was the Donath-Landsteiner diagnostic test.

In 1905–06 Landsteiner worked with Ernest Finger of the Vienna Dermatological Clinic and several other associates on the characterization of *Spirochaeta pallida*, the agent that causes syphilis. They were able to describe the mechanism that results in the Wassermann reaction and, in 1907, Landsteiner isolated the antigen used in this test from a bovine heart preparation. The discovery of this readily available source made the Wassermann feasible for clinical use (Speiser 1973, 624).

In 1908 Landsteiner was appointed prosector of the Royal Imperial Wilhelminen Hospital and, in 1909, promoted to staff pathologist, with the rank—but not the salary—of professor. For most of the next decade his research dealt with poliomyelitis. He succeeded in transmitting the disease to rhesus monkeys, using a preparation of brain and spinal cord tissue from a human victim. But he was unable to find a bacterial agent and therefore hypothesized that the disease was caused by one of the "invisible" viruses, a class of microbes much smaller and harder to isolate than the now well-known bacteria. Before World War I, he cooperated with the Pasteur Institute in creating a serum diagnostic test and a way of collecting the virus for further study.

The war disrupted life in Vienna and, at its end, Landsteiner and his family emigrated to the Hague, where he worked at the R. K. Ziekenhuis for three years. While there, he isolated the antigenic components, haptens, which he had earlier identified in vivo. He experimented also with hemoglobins specific to different animals. The Netherlands proved little better than Austria, however, so in 1922 he accepted an offer to join the Rockefeller Institute for Medical Research in New York. He became an American citizen in 1929 and was elected president of the American Association of Immunologists the same year.

At Rockefeller, he was able to continue his characterization of human blood and isolation of individualizing factors. Among other contributions, he identified the irregular agglutinins alpha-1 and alpha-2 with Philip Levine in 1926, and contributed to the discovery of the Hunter-Henshaw factor specific to blacks in 1934.

His most famous contribution of this period came in 1940, when he, Alexander Wiener, and Philip Levine found and described the Rhesus (Rh) factor, which was of crucial importance to blood transfusions and also, of course, in the etiology of the jaundice now known as Rh disease in newborn children (Speiser 1973, 624).

Landsteiner was a quiet, reserved, man, who set rigorous standards for his work and remained dedicated to research throughout his life. Among the many other awards he received for his work were the Hans Aronson Prize (1926); the Paul Ehrlich Gold Medal (1930); the Dutch Red Cross Medal (1933) and the Cameron Prize from the University of Edinburgh (1938). He was a member of the National Academy of Sciences, the Royal Society of London, the New York Academy of Medicine, and at least ten other major scientific societies. He died after suffering a heart attack in his laboratory in 1943.

MARCIA MELDRUM

Selected Bibliography

PRIMARY SOURCES

Landsteiner, Karl. 1930. "On Individual Differences in Human Blood."

Nobel Lecture, December 11, 1930. Reprinted in *Nobel Lectures in Physiology or Medicine*. Vol. 2: 1922–1941:234–245. Amsterdam: Elsevier, 1965.

———. 1982. *The Specificity of Serological Reactions*. New York: Dover. This edition contains a new bibliography.

SECONDARY SOURCES

Rous, Peyton E. 1947. "Karl Landsteiner." *Obituary Notices of Fellows of the Royal Society of London*, 5:295–324. London: Royal Society.

Speiser, Paul. 1961. *Karl Landsteiner*. Vienna: Hallenek Brothers.

———. 1973. "Landsteiner, Karl." In *Dictionary of Scientific Biography*, 7:622–25. New York: Scribner's.

CHARLES LOUIS ALPHONSE LAVERAN *1907*

Charles Louis Alphonse Laveran was born on June 18, 1845, in Paris, France. A military physician and parasitologist, he won the Nobel Prize in Physiology or Medicine in 1907 for his work as initiator and pioneer of the pathology of protozoa. A significant part of this work was his discovery of parasites as the cause of malaria. He died May 18, 1922, in Paris.

Laveran was the second child and only son of Louis-Theódore Laveran, a career military physician, who had positions in Paris, Metz, and Algeria before becoming a professor and then director at Val-de-Grâce, the center for training in military medicine in Paris. His mother (née Marie-Louise Anselme Guénard de la Tour) came from a distinguished military family.

Alphonse Laveran devoted himself to his work and research throughout his life. Duty and discipline were watchwords in his career. He was severe in manner, rarely smiled, and was reserved in speech. However, he could be most encouraging to collaborators and students who showed genuine scientific curiosity and who were willing to work as hard as he was, and among friends he could become more relaxed and sociable. He did not marry until age forty. In 1885, at his mother's urging, he wed a younger woman of twenty-seven, Sophie-Marie Pidancet, who dedicated herself to the furtherance of his work. The couple had no children.

In his childhood, Alphonse Laveran spent five years in Algeria as the family followed Louis Laveran in his postings. His secondary schooling was obtained first at the Collège Sainte-Barbe and then at the Lycée Louis-le-Grand in Paris. He decided to follow in his father's footsteps, and entered the military medical school in Strasbourg in 1863. In 1867 he submitted his doctoral thesis on the regeneration of nerves. He then embarked on his army medical career. After a short period at Val-de-Grâce, he was made *aide-major* at the Saint-Martin military hospital in Paris. His self-discipline and his precise and methodical character were already apparent in these early positions.

His military medical training was soon put to the test in the Franco-Prussian war of 1870 when he was assigned as part of the medical support group for the eastern army. Battle and field hospital experience taught him the realities of disease in wartime among the troops. After another short period in the Saint-Martin hospital during the Commune, he was attached in 1873 to the Tenth Hussars Regiment at Pontivy. Then in the following year, after a competitive examination, he obtained the position of *professor agrégé*, formerly held by his father, at Val-de-Grâce. Laveran taught epidemiology for four years at the school; his first book, *Traité des maladies et épidémies des armées* (1875), grew out of his teaching. At the same time, he directed a "fever" ward at the Val-de-Grâce hospital and demonstrated his remarkable clinical diagnostic abilities. During this period he also improved the knowledge of histology he had gained in Strasbourg by studying the subject at Charles Ranvier's laboratory at the Collège de France. This training was to prove valuable in his malaria research.

In 1878 he was sent to Algeria, one of the major French colonies, to direct the medical service first at Bône, then Biskra, and finally Constantine. This posting was his initiation into the world of tropical diseases and his first confrontation with the virulent forms of malaria that caused high mortality. In order to find more reliable means of diagnosis for malaria, Laveran set up a modest laboratory and began to study changes in the blood of malaria patients with a microscope of limited power. The pigmented particles seen by Laveran in such blood had been noticed before but their significance was still under debate. In addition to pigmented particles, Laveran also found other bodies that varied in shape and were capable of movement. He identified these changing forms as different phases of parasitical activity and the pigmented particles as the result of their effect on red corpuscles. From 1879 on he believed that parasites were the cause of malaria. According to his own account, confirmation of his ideas was obtained from the blood of a patient in the Constantine hospital on November 6, 1880, when he saw clearly the parasite with its four moving filaments. On a visit to Rome in 1882 and during the rest of his tour of duty in Algeria until 1883 he established by repeated testing the parasites' constant presence in the blood of malaria sufferers at the onset of fever and in patients who had not been treated with quinine.

Laveran's discovery was first announced to the Academy of Medicine in Paris on November 23, 1880. Further accounts were given in a paper for the Société Médicale des hôpitaux in late 1880 and in a presentation by Laveran to the Academy of Sciences in 1881. In 1881 he published a short book, *Nature parasitaire des accidents de l'impaludisme: description d'un nouveau parasite trouvé dans le sang des malades atteints de fièvre palustre*, answering early skepticism about his claims. The summary of all his Algerian research was presented in his authoritative work *Traité des fièvres palustres* (1884) which appeared after his return to Paris to take up a professorship of military hygiene at Val-de-Grâce.

For several reasons, Laveran's work was not immediately accepted by other scientists seeking the cause of malaria. First, he used fresh blood in his research and not stained preparations. This choice aided his recognition of the living nature of the organism he saw but made identification and corroboration of the several forms of the parasite difficult. Other researchers took issue with his microscopical findings. Moreover, in the early years of the germ theory, bacteria—not protozoa—were being actually pursued as the agents of disease. In 1879 a bacterial cause for malaria had been announced by Edwin Klebs and Corrado Tommasi-Crudeli and in the early eighties research was being undertaken to establish their findings. It took until the late 1880s and the development of better microtechniques before the bacteriologists became persuaded of Laveran's claims for protozoa. In 1884 Laveran himself persuaded Pasteur and Emile Roux of the correctness of his views when a rare case of malignant malaria in a soldier in Paris gave him the opportunity for a personal demonstration of the parasite.

Laveran was not the leader in the search to answer the many questions raised by his discovery as to where the parasite existed outside man and how the disease was transmitted. His return from Algeria meant he no longer had ready access to malarial patients, although he did try to continue his work by investigating avian parasites similar to those of malaria. He suggested in 1884 that the vector of malaria was the mosquito, but it was the work of Patrick Manson, Giovanni Grassi, and Ronald Ross that elucidated the life cycle of the parasite and the transmission of the disease by the *Anopheles* mosquito.

By early 1890 Laveran's work brought him recognition from the leading scientific and medical societies of Paris as well as more broadly in the international scientific community, but the army military medical service did not acknowledge his contributions in the way that he hoped. When his professorship at Val-de-Grâce ended in 1894, he was only offered temporary administrative posts at Lille and Nantes instead of the laboratory and hospital facilities he desired to pursue his research. Deeply dissatisfied, and showing the fierce independence that characterized his personality, he resigned from the military medical service on December 15, 1896, much to the consternation of his friends and colleagues.

His research career was by no means over. The Pasteur Institute in Paris offered him laboratory space and independence, naming him honorary chief of research. The institute soon became in a sense his new home and his fellow investigators his family. Laveran in company with other scientists began a broad investigation of other infectious diseases of man and animals that had been discovered to be caused by parasites; this research continued until the end of his life. Laveran elucidated the life cycles and disease activities of many trypanosomes as well as therapeutic and prophylactic measures against the diseases they caused; he contributed particularly to the understanding of the transmission of sleeping sickness. He also studied the parasites of leishmania found in India, Africa, and America. It was for his work in elaborating protozoology following his malaria investigations that he was awarded the Nobel Prize in 1907. In addition to numerous papers, he published two books on this later research, *Trypanosomes et trypanosomiases* (1904 and 1912), in conjunction with Félix Mesnil, and *Leishmanioses: Kala-Azar: Bouton d'Orient; Leishmaniose américaine* (1917).

Laveran donated half the money from his Nobel Prize to the setting up of a fully equipped laboratory for research in tropical medicine at the Pasteur Institute. He also founded the Société de pathologie exotique in 1908, of which he was president for twelve years, and established its journal for reporting of research results in the field. The laboratory and the society became centers for the development of French research into tropical medicine in the decade up to 1920 with Laveran as the leader.

In World War I Laveran was active as a member of a commission on hygiene and prophylaxis for soldiers. He also organized preventive measures against malaria in locales where French troops would encounter the disease. French government recognition of Laveran came in 1912 when he was made Commander of the Legion of Honor; his medical colleagues appointed him honorary director of the Pasteur Institute in 1915 on his seventieth birthday and president of the Academy of Medicine in 1920. Laveran continued his research work until a short illness led to his death in May 1922.

CAROLINE HANNAWAY

Selected Bibliography

PRIMARY SOURCES

Laveran's early short announcements of his discovery are to be found in:

Laveran, Alphonse. 1880. "Sur un nouveau parasite trouvé dans le sang de plusieurs malades atteints de fièvre palustre." *Bulletin de l'Académie de médecine* 2d series, 9:1268.

———. 1881. "Deuxième note. . ." *ibid.*:1346.

———. 1881. "Description d'un nouveau parasite découvert dans le sang des malades atteints d'impaludisme." *Comptes rendus hebdoma*

daires des séances de l'Académie des Sciences 93:627–34.
———. 1875. *Traité des maladies et épidémies des armées.* Paris: G. Masson.
———. 1879. *Nouveaux éléments de pathologie et de clinique médicales,* 2 vols. Paris: J. B. Baillière.
———. 1881. *Nature parasitaire des accidents de l'impaludisme.* Paris: G. Masson.
———. 1884. *Traité des fièvres palustres.* Paris: G. Masson.
———. 1896. *Traité d'hygiène militaire.* Paris: G. Masson.
———. 1898. *Traité du paludisme.* Paris: G. Masson.
Laveran, Alphonse, and Félix Mesnil. 1904 and 1912. *Trypanosomes et trypanosomiases.* Paris: G. Masson.
Laveran, Alponse. 1907. "Protozoa as Causes of Diseases" in *Nobel Lectures, Physiology or Medicine, 1901–1921.* Amsterdam: Elsevier, 1967. Pp. 257–74.
———. 1917. *Leishmanioses: Kala-Azar; Bouton d'Orient; Leishmaniose américaine.* Paris: G. Masson.

SECONDARY SOURCES

A bibliography of Laveran's numerous scientific papers (with some inaccuracies) is to be found in:
Phisalix, Marie. 1923. *Alphonse Laveran: sa vie, son oeuvre.* Paris: Masson. Pp. 233–62.
Roux, Emile. 1915. "Jubilé de M. le Professeur A. Laveran." *Annales de l'Institut Pasteur* 29:405–14.
Roux, Emile. 1922. "Alphonse Laveran (1845–1922)." *ibid.* 36:459–61.
Calmette, A. 1922. "Nécrologie: Le Professeur A. Laveran." *Bulletin de la Société de Pathologie exotique* 15:373–78.
Manson-Bahr, Philip. 1963. "The Story of Malaria: The Drama and the Actors." *International Review of Tropical Medicine* 2:329–91.
Percebois, G. 1980. "Laveran et le pays messin." *Journal de médecine de Strasbourg* 11:311–16.
Smith, Dale C., and Lorraine B. Sanford. 1985. "Laveran's Germ: The Reception and Use of Medical Discovery." *American Journal of Tropical Medicine and Hygiene* 34:2–20.

JOSHUA LEDERBERG *1958*

Joshua Lederberg was born on May 23, 1925, in Montclair, New Jersey. A microbiologist and geneticist, Lederberg shared the Nobel Prize in 1958 with George Wells Beadle and Edward Lawrie Tatum for his discoveries regarding the sexual reproduction and genetic recombination of bacteria, which established the groundwork for much later work in genetic engineering. Lederberg, only thirty-three at the time of the award, was then professor and chairman of the Department of Medical Genetics at the University of Wisconsin, a department which had been newly established under his leadership. He was shortly after appointed chairman of the Department of Genetics at Stanford University. In 1946 Lederberg married Esther Miriam Zimmer, a student of Beadle and Tatum and a geneticist in her own right. The marriage ended in divorce in 1968. He married Dr. Marguerite Stein Kirsch, a clinical psychiatrist, later that year, and adopted her son, David; they also have a daughter, Ann.

Lederberg was raised in New York City by his parents, Zwi Hirsch and Esther Goldenbaum Lederberg. He entered Columbia University at the age of sixteen in 1941, planning to study chemistry as preparation for a medical career in cancer or neurological research. Francis J. Ryan, a Columbia professor who had taken a fellowship with Beadle and Tatum at Stanford, aroused his interest in microbial genetics, then still a no-man's land between classical genetics and medical microbiology. After receiving his B.A. in zoology in 1944, Lederberg began his medical studies at Columbia, but continued working with Ryan to learn research methods in genetics. Until 1945 he was also serving in the U.S. Navy Hospital Corps.

In that same year, D. T. Avery, and C. M. MacLeod, and M. J. MacCarty published their findings that DNA in a culture medium was responsible for apparent genetic transformations in the pneumococcus bacteria. Lederberg had been working with *Neurospora* and was inspired to investigate the genetic recombination of bacteria. During the summer of 1945 Ryan learned that Tatum was leaving Stanford to set up a new program in microbiology at Yale, and that he was working with genetic studies of *Escherichia coli.* He suggested to Lederberg that he apply to work with Tatum, since they were thinking along the same lines. Tatum agreed to accept the young student, and Lederberg obtained a Jane Coffin Childs Research Fellowship, allowing him to transfer to Yale as a Ph.D. candidate in 1946.

For many years bacteria had been "considered biologically exceptional organisms, with no genes, nuclei, or sex." This idea began to change when Andre Lwoff identified in 1938 what appeared to be an evolutionary loss, through mutation and natural selection, of the ability to synthesize essential nutrients in certain microorganisms. Beadle and Tatum in 1941 had then produced nutritionally deficient mutations of *Neurospora*; this was the project on which Francis Ryan had worked as a fellow. This study, and the findings on DNA, pointed to the next step: to demonstrate sexual recombination and inheritance of characteristics, analogous to the Mendelian model, in bacteria. This was the challenge undertaken by Tatum and Lederberg.

They selected auxotrophic (nutritionally deficient) mutations in *E. coli* strain K-12 as their subject. The mutations were easy to identify and differentiate because each had very specific nutritional requirements. By growing and culturing two separate mutations of the K-12 strain separately and together, and observing the mutations in the colonies generated, Tatum and Lederberg identified a prototrophic (nutritionally independent) mutation that could be "satisfactorily explained only as resulting from a sexual mating process, followed by reassortment or segregation of genetic material" (Lederberg and Tatum 1954).

These results were announced at the Cold Spring Harbor Symposium on Microbial Genetics in July 1946, and published three months later in *Nature.* A number of other geneticists replicated and extended their conclusions, eventually identifying four methods of genetic transformation in bacteria: 1) absorption from a culture medium, as in the pneumococcus experiments; 2) genetic recombination (*E. coli,* as it happens, is one of the few bacteria where this occurs); 3) introduction by an infecting phage (bacterial virus), a process first confirmed by Joshua and Esther Lederberg in *Salmonella* in 1953; and 4) chemical change, or mutation, of the bacteria's own DNA. This understanding of bacterial DNA transformation led to a variety of discoveries in genetics, virology, and microbiology, and eventually to breakthroughs in genetic engineering (Lederberg and Tatum 1946; Lederberg 1986).

Lederberg received his Ph.D. from Yale in 1948. The previous year he had accepted a position as assistant professor of genetics at the University of Wisconsin, where he continued his investigations in collaboration with his wife, Esther. Lederberg's interests were never narrowly defined, however. At Wisconsin, he became interested in computer science and participated in research on artificial intelligence. He was promoted to associate professor in 1950 and to full professor in 1954. In 1957 he travelled to Melbourne University in Australia, where he worked on the culture of monoclonal antibodies. On his return, he organized the new Department of Medical Genetics and served as its first chairman.

In 1959 he was recruited to organize a Department of Genetics at Stanford University. He served again as the inaugural chairman, also as professor of biology and of computer science. In 1962 he became director of the Kennedy Laboratories for Molecular Medicine.

Lederberg has also been an overachiever in public service. He was a significant advisor to the Arms Control and Disarmament Agency during the negotiation of the biological weapons disarmament treaty. He advises the U.S. Defense Science Board and played an active role in scientific aspects of the Mariner and Viking missions to Mars. These are only the highlights of a long career of service on government boards and as a consultant for industrial applications of biologic and genetic technology. In his writing he has actively promoted open communications on scientific issues between science, government, and the lay public. In 1978 his scientific, administrative, and public service contributions were recognized when he was named president of Rockefeller University, one of the most prestigious and influential positions in American science.

Lederberg was elected to the National Academy of Sciences in 1957. His many awards include the Eli Lilly Award (1953), the Pasteur Award of the Society of Illinois Bacteriologists (1956), and the Procter Prize (1982). He holds honorary degrees from Turin, Tufts, Yale, Wisconsin, Columbia, Yeshiva, Mt. Sinai, Rutgers, New York, and Pennsylvania universities and from the Jewish Theological Seminary.

JAMES J. POUPARD

Selected Bibliography

PRIMARY SOURCES

Lederberg, Joshua, and Edward L. Tatum. 1946. "Gene Recombination in *E. coli.*" *Nature* 158 (October 19):558.

Lederberg, Joshua, and Edward Lawrie Tatum. 1954. "Sex in Bacteria: Genetic Studies 1945–1952." *Science* 118:169–75.

Lederberg, Joshua. 1957. "Viruses, Genes, and Cells." *Bacteriological Reviews* 21:133–39.

———. 1986. "Forty Years of Genetic Recombination in Bacteria." *Nature* 324 (December 18):627–28.

———. 1987. "Genetic Recombination in Bacteria: A Discovery Account." *American Review of Genetics* 21:23–46.

SECONDARY SOURCES

1959. "Lederberg, Joshua." In *Current Biography Yearbook*, 251–52. New York: H. W. Wilson.

1981. "Lederberg, Joshua." In *Biographical Encyclopedia of Scientists*, 479–81. New York: Facts on File.

RITA LEVI-MONTALCINI *1986*

The 1986 Nobel Prize in Physiology or Medicine was awarded jointly to Rita Levi-Montalcini and Stanley Cohen for their discovery of cell growth factors. Levi-Montalcini was only the fourth woman to receive the Nobel Prize in Physiology or Medicine. Levi-Montalcini has never married. In her autobiography she explained why: "My experience in childhood and adolescence of the subordinate role played by the female in a society run entirely by men had convinced me that I was not cut out to be a wife. Babies did not attract me, and I was altogether without the maternal sense so highly developed in small and adolescent girls" (Levi-Montalcini 1988, 35). She now lives with her twin sister, Paola, in Rome.

Rita Levi-Montalcini was born on April 22, 1909, in Turin, Italy. Her area of scientific specialization is experimental neurology. Her parents were Adamo Levi, an engineer, and Adele Montalcini. Levi-Montalcini graduated from the University of Turin, Italy, in 1936. She left Italy for Brussels in 1939 when Jews were barred from academic and professional careers, but she returned to Italy shortly before Belgium was invaded by Germany. She set up a laboratory in her bedroom and began studying the effect of peripheral tissues on the development of nerve centers in collaboration with her mentor, Giuseppe Levi. Levi-Montalcini received her M.D. from the University of Turin in 1940. Two other Nobel laureates, Salvador E. Luria and Renato Dulbecco, were also medical students in Turin with Levi-Montalcini. Driven from Turin by the heavy bombing in July 1942, she built another laboratory in a small farmhouse despite the deplorable wartime conditions. When Italy was occupied by the Nazis, she and her family fled to Florence and lived a precarious underground existence for the rest of the war. She endangered her own health during the epidemics that flourished in the aftermath of the war by serving as a volunteer physician.

A paper she had written with Giuseppe Levi came to the attention of Viktor Hamburger, chairman of the Zoology Department at Washington University in St. Louis. In 1946 he invited Levi-Montalcini to join his laboratory. From 1947 to 1951 she was a research associate in zoology at Washington University. She was promoted to associate professor in 1951 and to full professor in 1958. In 1981 she moved to the Institute for Cell Biology, National Council of Scientific Research, in Rome.

Rita Levi-Montalcini won the Nobel Prize in recognition of her research in experimental neurology, her discovery of the effect of a nerve growth factor—isolated from the mouse salivary gland—on the sympathetic nervous system, the effect of an antiserum on the nerve growth factor, and the study of other specific growth factors. In popular press announcements of the Nobel Prizes for 1986 Rita Levi-Montalcini's life was compared to vintage Hollywood drama and her research was said to hold out promises of therapeutic advances in problems from burns to cancer (Levine 1986, 67).

Levi-Montalcini has focused almost exclusively on one issue throughout the course of her forty years in research. Although she has always maintained her own focus on the intriguing question of how nerve cells grow, her work has led to new insights into research on cancer, tissue regeneration, and neurological diseases.

In 1934 Viktor Hamburger substituted the chick embryo for the amphibian larva as the "object of choice for the analysis of the effects of limb bud extirpation on spinal motor neurons and sensory nerve cells innervating the limbs" because the chick embryo had many advantages over the amphibian larva in neurological investigations. Hamburger's studies of the effects of limb bud extirpation provided some suggestive evidence for a novel form of control mechanism by which peripheral tissues affected developing nerve centers. In 1947 Hamburger asked Levi-Montalcini to collaborate on an investigation of this problem. Within two years Levi-Montalcini and Hamburger had confirmed the hypothesis she and Giuseppe Levi had previously set forth. However, it was also clear that the techniques available were not powerful enough for an in-depth exploration of the tremendously complex neurogenetic process. At this point she was tempted to abandon experimental neurology and move on to the apparently greener pastures of the phage field, but successfully resisted the temptation "thanks to unpredictable and fortunate events that occurred at the same time and opened a new era in developmental neurobiology" (Levi-Montalcini 1987, 1155).

In 1948 Hamburger's former student, Elmer Bueker, published a report of his ingenious experiments in which fragments of mouse sarcoma 180 had been grafted into the body wall of three-day chick embryos. Histological analyses of embryos fixed three to five days later revealed that sensory nerve fibers from adjacent dorsal root ganglia had entered into the neoplastic tissue, but no motor nerve fibers had gained access to the tumor. These observations suggested that the mouse sarcoma offered favorable conditions for the growth of sensory fibers. When Levi-Montalcini and Hamburger reinvestigated this phenomenon they discovered additional effects that the mouse tumor graft had elicited. These findings could not be accounted for by an existing hypotheses of embryonic development. Transplants of normal embryonic tissues did not call forth the same responses. Sympathetic fibers as well as sensory fibers entered the neoplastic tissues and built up a remarkable network. Although nerve fibers did not establish synaptic connections with tumor cells, they appeared to branch at random between them. Moreover, the sensory and sympathetic ganglia that had innervated the tumor progressively increased in volume, often, in the case of sympathetic ganglia, reaching a size about six times larger than that of some control ganglia.

Another remarkable finding was that in embryos bearing transplants of mouse sarcoma 180 or sarcoma 37, viscera that were normally devoid of innervation were infiltrated by sympathetic nerve fibers at early embryonic stages. Thick sympathetic fiber bundles were even found inside the veins of the host embryos. Even sympathetic chain ganglia that were not in contact with the tumor transplant enlarged. These remarkable findings seemed consistent with the hypothesis that the neoplastic cells released a soluble, diffusible agent that altered the differentiation and growth patterns of target cells. This hypothesis was confirmed by experiments in which the mouse sarcoma was transplanted onto the chorioallantoic membrane of four- to six-day chick embryos so that direct contact between embryonic and neoplastic tissues was precluded, but connections existed through the circulatory system. The same anomalous effects were elicited by the tumor transplants under these conditions. Dried pellets or extracts of the tumors did not have the same effects.

Because the University of Washington did not have the tissue culture facilities that Levi-Montalcini needed to pursue the nerve growth stimulating factor, she took her experimental materials to Carlos Chagas's laboratory at the University of Brazil in Rio de Janeiro, where Bertha Meyer had built a well-equipped tissue culture unit. The development of tissue culture bioassay procedures provided "a practical and invaluable tool for uncovering the identity of this factor and paved the way for the study of its mechanism of action." However, the picture became somewhat confused by the observation that normal mouse tissues could induce a similar, but weaker effect than the mouse sarcomas. Further research revealed that nerve growth factor was present in both normal and tumor tissues.

For two years Levi-Montalcini and her coworkers attempted to determine the chemical nature of the nerve growth factor (NGF) released by the mouse sarcomas. Stanley Cohen isolated a nucleoprotein fraction from the mouse tumors that contained the nerve growth–promoting activity. Serendipitously, Cohen attempted to use snake venom to determine whether nucleic acids or proteins were responsible for the nerve growth–promoting activity. (Snake venom contains enzymes that degrade nucleic acids.) The startling result was that the addition of minute amounts of venom to the active fraction caused a remarkable increase in activity. The venom itself proved to be a very potent source of NGF. Cohen isolated a nondialyzable heat-labile protein with a molecular weight of about 20,000 having nerve growth–promoting activity. Mouse submandibular salivary gland extract proved to be an even better source of NGF. These glands are homologous with the snake venom glands. The salivary gland factor was a protein with a molecular weight of about 44,000. Because salivary gland factor could be produced in larger quantities and was only moderately toxic, its biological activity could be studied in neonatal, young, and adult mammals.

Levi-Montalcini recalled that "NGF did not at first find enthusiastic reception by the scientific community. . . . The finding that a protein molecule from such diverse and unrelated sources as mouse sarcomas, snake venom, and mouse salivary glands elicited such a potent and disrupting action on normal neurogenetic processes did not fit into any conceptual preexisting schemes, nor did it seem to bear any relation to normal control mechanisms at work during ontogenesis." Proving that this bizarre factor played an essential role in the normal life of its target cells provided an even greater challenge for Levi-Montalcini and Cohen. These demonstrations were carried out in vitro and in vivo with specific antisera to salivary NGF. When neonatal rodents received daily injections of this antiserum, the result was a nearly total disappearance of sympathetic para- and prevertebral chain ganglia. This effect was dubbed "immunosympathectomy." It was shown to be the result of the inactivation of a NGF-like protein needed for the differentiation and survival of sympathetic nerve cells.

The effects of NGF have proved to be wide and diversified, but cells are most responsive during their early period of differentiation. In more recent experiments, the effect of NGF on neurons of the central nervous system and cells originating from the hematopoietic system have been emphasized. The sequencing of mouse submandibular gland NGF in 1971 led to the identification of NGF complementary DNA and the cloning of mouse, human, bovine, and chicken genes. These genes exhibit a high degree of homology, but much remains to be studied about the nature of NGF and its gene.

With the catalog of "growth factors" continuing to increase, Levi-Montalcini suggests that the most obvious targets of future research are the search for other NGF target cells and the search for other NGF-like molecules and their genetic regulation.

Levi-Montalcini is a member of the National Academy of Science, Society for Developmental Biology, the American Association of Anatomists, and the Tissue Culture Association. Weeks before the announcement of the 1986 Nobel Prize, Rita Levi-Montalcini and Stanley Cohen were awarded the Lasker Prize in basic science.

LOIS N. MAGNER

Selected Bibliography

PRIMARY SOURCES

Cohen, S., R. Levi-Montalcini, and V. Hamburger. 1954. "A Nerve Growth Stimulating Factor Isolated from Sarcomas 37 and 180." *Proceedings of the National Academy of Sciences* 40:1014–18.

Cohen, Stanley, and Rita Levi-Montalcini. 1956. "A Nerve Growth Stimulating Factor Isolated from Snake Venom." *Proceedings of the National Academy of Sciences* 42:571–74.

Levi-Montalcini, R. 1964. "The Nerve Growth Factor." *Annals of the New York Academy of Sciences* 113: 149–68.

———. ed. 1980. *Nerve Cells, Transmitters and Behavior*. Proceedings of a Study Week at the Pontifical Academy of Sciences. October 9–14, 1978. Amsterdam: Elsevier.

Levi-Montalcini, Rita, Piertro Calissano, Eric R. Kandel, and Adriana Maggi, eds. 1986. *Molecular Aspects of Neurobiology*. New York: Springer-Verlag.

Levi-Montalcini. 1987. "The Nerve Growth Factor Thirty-five Years Later." *Science* 237:1154–62.

Levi-Montalcini, Rita. 1988. *In Praise of Imperfection: My Life and Work*. New York: Sloan Foundation Sciences Series/Basic Books.

SECONDARY SOURCES

Worden, F. G., J. P. Swayzey, G. Adelman, eds. 1975. *The Neurosciences: Paths of Discovery*. Cambridge: MIT Press.

Server, A. C., and E. M. Shooter. 1977. "Nerve Growth Factor." In *Advances* in *Protein Chemistry*, vol. 31, edited by C. B. Anfisen, J. T. Edsal and F. M. Richards, 339–409. New York: Academic Press.

Li, C. H., ed. 1984. *Hormonal Proteins and Peptides*, vol. 12. New York: Academic Press.

Levine, Joe. 1986. "Lives of Spirit and Dedication." *Time* (October 27):66–68.

Newmark, Peter. 1986. "Nobel Prizes. Growth Factors Bring Rewards." *Nature* 323:572.

Gilman, Alfred G., Erwin Heher, Tomas Hikfelt, Joseph B. Martin, and Viktor Hamburger. 1988. *Fidia Research Foundation Neuroscience Award Lectures*, vol. 2 (1986–87). New York: Raven.

FRITZ ALBERT LIPMANN *1953*

Fritz Albert Lipmann was born on June 12, 1899, in Konigsberg, Germany. A biochemist, Lipmann received the Nobel Prize in 1953 for his discovery of CoA, the coenzyme that activates acetylation reactions in the cell, thus assisting to release stored energy to power a variety of cellular functions. His work complemented and extended that of his colaureate, Sir Hans Krebs, who had described the process by which food is converted to cellular energy. At the time of the award, Lipmann was professor of biological chemistry and head of the Biochemical Research Laboratory at Harvard; he subsequently joined the faculty of Rockefeller University. Lipmann met and married his American wife, Elfreda Hall, in Berlin in 1931; he himself became an American citizen in 1944. The Lipmanns had one son, Stephen Hall. Fritz Lipmann died July 24, 1986, in Poughkeepsie, New York.

Lipmann's parents, Leopold and Gertrude Lachmanski Lipmann, were German Jews; his father was a lawyer. He began to study medicine at the University of Konigsberg in 1917, where he was deeply impressed by "a dramatic chemistry course" given by a Professor Klinger. Lipmann interrupted his education briefly for army service in the closing days of World War I, returned to medical school in Munich, and finally received his degree from the University of Berlin in 1922. He then began his "Wanderjahre," to work with and learn from Germany's leading biochemists, which were to last ten years.

Lipmann first accepted a fellowship to study pharmacology with Ernst Lacquer in Amsterdam; he then returned to Konigsberg to work under Hans Meerwein, and later joined Otto Meyerhof's laboratory at the Kaiser Wilhelm Institute for Biology in Berlin-Dahlem. Here he studied the failure of lactic acid in muscle to oxidize in the presence of flouride. The University of Berlin awarded him a Ph.D. in chemistry in 1927.

In 1929 he followed Meyerhof to the Kaiser Wilhelm Institute for Medical Research in Heidelberg, where he met Hans Krebs. In 1931 Albert Fischer recruited him back to the Kaiser Wilhelm in Berlin as his assistant in tissue culture. During a year in New York as a Rockefeller Fellow (1931–32), where he worked with P. A. Levene on phosphorylation reactions, Lipmann identified the presence of serine phosphate in phosphoproteins. He was then invited to work with Fischer in his new job at the Biological Institute of the Carlsberg Foundation in Copenhagen in 1932.

He had been concentrating for some time on the processes of intermediary metabolism in the cell. Although biologists had understood for years that food chemicals were metabolized in the cell to produce energy, the actual mechanisms were unknown. Two processes of glucose metabolism had been identified, both beginning with its conversion to pyruvic acid. If oxygen is present, the molecule is then further broken into carbon dioxide and water. This process, respiration, releases all the available energy supplied by the glucose. If no oxygen is present, a fermentation reaction occurs, in which the pyruvate is metabolized into lactic acid or another organic acid. This reaction appears to be only a partial utilization of the available energy. Fermentation will not occur while oxygen is present; this is known as the "Pasteur effect."

In Fischer's laboratory, Lipmann studied the oxidation of pyruvate in the bacteria *Lactobacillus delbrueckii*. With surprise, he observed that the oxidation reaction was completely dependent on the presence of phosphate. After some experimenting, he confirmed that an intermediate step in the oxidation was the formation of acetyl phosphate. He did not immediately understand the significance of this finding (Lipmann 1939; 1953, 413–16).

Lipmann had at one point considered returning to Germany, but the growing Nazi hostility towards Jews impelled him to remain in Copenhagen. The outbreak of World War II and the threat of German occupation of Denmark forced Lipmann and his wife to emigrate to the United States. Like many European scientists of the time, he arrived in New York with little money and no official status, dependent on the goodwill and support of the American scientific community. Lipmann was able to obtain a position as research associate in the Department of Biochemistry at Cornell Medical College. In 1941 he was appointed to a similar position at Harvard Medical School, with concurrent responsibilities at Massachusetts General Hospital. He also advised the Office of Scientific Research and Development during the war (*New York Times* October 23, 1953).

He continued his work with the interesting and puzzling acetyl phosphate. Phosphorylation was known to occur in fermentation reactions; yet he had definitely, by 1941, confirmed its essential role in respiratory reactions as well. Lipmann hypothesized that the phosphate bond was the cell's "dynamo"; that it was able to store and then release great quantities of energy as required for a variety of metabolic reactions (Lipmann 1941).

For some years he and his colleagues, including Nathan Kaplan, David Novelli, and Constance Tuttle, experimented with acetyl phosphate as the agent for acetyl transfer, that is, as the catalyst for the various acetylation reactions that power cellular metabolism. They were not markedly successful until they noted the involvement of a heat-stable "cofactor," which appeared to be always present in fresh tissues but disappeared after aging. It appeared to participate in acetylation of choline and sulfanomide and in the synthesis of acetoacetate; and it could not be replaced by any other substance.

In 1945 the team isolated this factor, which they named "CoA," the coenzyme of acetylation. They now hypothesized that "in animal tissue, the energy transmission from phosphate to acetyl occurs through a continuous enzyme bound reaction chain." Subsequently, with the assistance of Beverley Guirard, they analyzed their discovery, described its action and structure, and finally synthesized CoA in the laboratory.

CoA consists of pantothenic acid, one of the B complex vitamins, sulfur, and several proteins, bound by phosphate links. It is present in all living cells, where it acts to combine with all acetyl groups entering the cell, from whatever source, to create molecules that can be temporarily "stored" in energy-rich phosphate bonds, then converted as required into "working" energy in any one of the many metabolic processes. Thus the cell is able to conserve and utilize all its energy effectively. CoA is essential to citric acid synthesis, the first step in the Krebs cycle, also to the oxidation of fatty acids, amino acids, and steroids, as well as pyruvate (Lipmann and Novelli 1950; Lipmann 1953, 420–24, 433–35).

Lipmann was promoted to associate professor in 1945 and to full professor in 1949. His primary interest remained intermediary metabolism, which led him into work on the energy regulation functions of the thyroid hormones, vitamin B-complex, the biological transfer of the sulfate group, embryo cell metabolism, and peptide and protein synthesis. He also became interested in the generation and structure of cancer cells. As he commented when he won the Nobel Prize, "[in basic research] You have to follow your nose; you don't map it out. You try one experiment, then another and bring some sense into it" (*New York Times* October 23, 1953).

Away from the laboratory, his principal recreation was listening to music. His appointment as professor of biochemistry at Rockefeller University in 1957 allowed him to devote more time to research projects. He retired to an emeritus position in 1970 and moved to a country home in Rhinebeck, New York, but maintained his laboratory at the university until shortly before his death at age eighty-seven.

Lipmann was a member of the National Academy of Sciences, the American Society of Biological Chemists, the New York Academy of Science, the American Philosophical Society, the Danish Royal Academy of Sciences, and a foreign member of the Royal Society of London. Among the many other awards he received for his work were the Carl Neuberg Medal of the American Society of European Chemists (1948), the Mead-Johnson Award from the American Academy of Pediatrics (1948), and the National Medal of Science (1966).

MARCIA MELDRUM

Selected Bibliography

PRIMARY SOURCES

Lipmann, Fritz A. 1936. "Fermentation of Phosphogluconic Acid." *Nature* (October 3):588–89.

———. 1937. "Colored Intermediate on Reduction of Vitamin B1." *Nature* (November 13):849.

———. 1939. "Coupling Between Pyruvic Acid Dehydrogenation and Adenylic Acid Phosphorylation." *Nature* (February 18):281.

———. 1941. "Metabolic Generation and Utilization of Phosphate Bond Energy." *Advances in Enzymology* 1:99–162.

Lippmann, Fritz A., and Nathan O. Kaplan. 1949. "Intermediary Metabolism of Phosphorus Compounds." *Annual Review of Biochemistry* 118:267–298.

Lipmann, Fritz A., and G. David Novelli. 1950. "Catalytic Function of Coenzyme A in Citric Synthesis." *Journal of Biological Chemistry* 182 (January):213–28.

Lipmann, Fritz A. 1950. "Biosynthetic Mechanisms." *Harvey Lectures*, Series 44, 99–123. New York: Academic Press.

———. 1953. "Development of the Acetylation Problem: A Personal Account." Nobel Lecture, December 11, 1953. Reprinted in *Nobel Lectures in Physiology or Medicine*, vol. 3 (1942–1962), 413–28. Amsterdam: Elsevier, 1964.

———. 1971. *Wanderings of a Biochemist*. New York: Wiley.

SECONDARY SOURCES

1953. "Dr. Lipmann Cites Experiments." *New York Times* (October 23):21.

1954. "Lipmann, Fritz (Albert)". In *Current Biography Yearbook*, 413–14. New York: H. W. Wilson.

OTTO LOEWI *1936*

Otto Loewi was born in Frankfurt-am-Main in 1873, the son of Jacob Loewi, a wine-merchant, and his wife Anna (née Willstaedter). While early in life inclined toward the humanities, he studied medicine at Strasbourg and Munich Universities and graduated in 1896. He was already embarked on his career in pharmacology when he met Guida Goldschmiedt, whom he married in 1908; they had four children. In 1909 he was appointed to the chair in pharmacology at the University of Graz in Austria, where, among other projects, he was particularly concerned with drug effects on the heart. His work demonstrated that the application of external drugs could mimic normal functioning, especially the effects of the nervous system. This was directly related to the experimental advances being made by Henry Dale in England. The two men shared the 1936 Nobel Prize in Physiology or Medicine for their work on elucidating the chemical basis of the transmission of the neural impulse. Loewi died in New York in 1961.

Loewi's early education emphasized the classics and fine arts; as a young man he wished to study art history. Persuaded by his parents, he finally agreed to study medicine instead. Before graduation he had his first experience with research, working on a pharmacological project—the effects of drugs on the isolated heart of the frog—suggested to him by Professor Oswald Schmiedeberg. But clinical work also appealed to him; although stimulated by his period in the laboratory and by those with whom he had come into contact, he accepted a medical position in the City Hospital of Frankfurt. The nature of this work, in a tuberculosis ward, soon dispirited Loewi and he sought a return to research, applying for and obtaining a position with the eminent pharmacologist H. H. Meyer in Marburg.

Loewi remained with Meyer for twelve years, working mainly on metabolic problems, including a study of the induction and amelioration of experimental diabetes. By 1902 he had acquired a broad experience in nutritional research, principally using biochemical techniques. He decided to visit England to learn more about physiological methods and equipment; he met with Sir Frederick Gowland Hopkins in Cambridge, Ernest Starling and Henry Dale in London and T. R. Elliott, then beginning his work on autonomic nerves and their chemical stimulation.

Returning to Marburg, Loewi commenced an important study of kidney function and the effects of diuretics, and he also began an analysis of chemical effects on the autonomic nervous system. As Dale was to do later, Loewi and Meyer examined norepinephrine (noradrenaline) and remarked on its similarity to epinephrine (adrenaline). But, also like Dale, they knew the chemical only as a synthetic product of the pharmaceutical factory and therefore did not investigate it further.

In 1909 Loewi accepted the chair of pharmacology at Graz, where he continued his research on a wide range of topics: carbohydrate metabolism and experimental diabetes, the nutritional requirements of different organs, and cardiovascular pharmacology and the physiological control mechanisms of heart function. After the discovery of insulin in 1922 by F. G. Banting and C. H. Best, he produced a series of papers on its mode of action, mostly in collaboration with H. Hausler. By this stage in his career he had made important contributions to biochemical pharmacology across a broad front of investigations, and had particularly examined the physiology and pharmacology of the frog's heart and its neural stimulation. But none of this work was directly concerned with chemical neurotransmission, for which he received the Nobel Prize. He was, of course, familiar with the research in this area by Henry Dale, the earlier work of J. N. Langley, and also the work of T. R. Elliott on the mimicry of neural responses by specific chemicals, most notably epinephrine (adrenaline).

Loewi's own account of the next stage of his research work brings in an element of mystery: in a dream he envisioned an experimental protocol to examine the possibility of a chemical neurotransmitter to the heart. The classic technique that he apparently dreamt and subsequently employed was to place two isolated frog's hearts in separate tissue baths. Stimulation of the vagus nerves to the first heart produced the well-known effect of slowing the heart beat; collection and transfer of its bathing fluid to the second heart produced the same effect. Similar stimulation of the sympathetic nerves of the first heart promoted its beating; again, transfer of its perfusate induced the same changes in the second heart. Obviously, some chemical released by neural stimulation of the first heart was effectively transferred to the second heart. There were, and still are, a number of technical difficulties with Loewi's experiment, and many contemporaries questioned Loewi's interpretation of his results. However, his demonstrations of the technique and his later work on establishing the chemical identities of the vagal transmitter (*Vagusstoff*) and the sympathetic transmitter (*Acceleranstoff*) provided convincing evidence of chemical mediation of nerve impulses. In 1926 Loewi and his collaborator E. Navratil suggested that the *Vagusstoff* was acetylcholine. The discovery by Dale and Dudley in 1929 that acetylcholine was a normal constituent of the animal body further increased the possibility that acetylcholine was indeed a neurotransmitter. Work on identifying the *Acceleranstoff* proceeded more slowly; useful accounts of the technical difficulties and debates surrounding this work have been published (Bacq 1975).

In 1938 the Nazis marched into Austria, and Loewi and his two younger sons were arrested as part of a general round-up of the male Jewish population of Graz. After much harassment and considerable private efforts by members of the international scientific community, Loewi was allowed to leave Austria. He was welcomed in England by Dale, who organized funding and facilities for him to continue his work in London, Brussels, and, Oxford. Meanwhile his wife was detained in Austria until the entire assets of the family, including Loewi's Nobel Prize money, had been transferred to Nazi banks. Eventually she was allowed to join her husband in exile. In 1940 he was offered, and accepted, a research professorship at the New York University School of Medicine.

At a time when, in the normal course of events, he could be expected to retire from research work, Loewi's career took a new direction. He resumed experimental work, and his friendly, enthusiastic personality attracted many invitations for lectures and articles. In particular he spent annual periods at the Wood's Hole Marine Biological Station, where he especially enjoyed the stimulating company of a wide variety of biologists.

He became an American citizen in 1946 and died on Christmas Day, 1961, having satisfied his love of fine food and wine with a lobster dinner on the previous evening.

E. M. TANSEY

Selected Bibliography

PRIMARY SOURCES

Loewi, O. 1935. "Problems Connected with the Principle of Humoral Transmission of Nervous Impulses." Ferrier Lecture. *Proceedings of the Royal Society of London* B 118:299–316.

———. 1936. "The Chemical Transmission of Nerve Action." Nobel Lecture. Reprinted in *Nobel Lectures, Physiology or Medicine*, vol. 2 (1922–1941), 416–32. Amsterdam: Elsevier, 1965.

———. 1945. "Aspects of the Transmission of Nervous Impulse: 1. Mediation in the Peripheral and Central Nervous System; 2. Theoretical and Clinical Implications." *Journal of the Mount Sinai Hospital* 12:803–6, 851–65.

———. 1954. "Reflections on the Study of Physiology." *Annual Review of Physiology* 16:1–10.

———. 1960. "An Autobiographic Sketch." *Perspectives in Biology and Medicine* 4:1–25.

SECONDARY SOURCES

Bacq, Z. M. 1975. *Chemical Transmission of Nerve Impulses.* Oxford: Pergamon Press.

Dale, H. H. 1962. "Otto Loewi." *Biographical Memoirs of Fellows of the Royal Society* 8:67–89.

Holmstedt, B., and G. Liljestrand. 1963. "Pharmacology of the Autonomic Nervous System." In *Readings in Pharmacology*, 169–201. Oxford: Pergamon Press.

Lembeck, F., and W. Giere. 1968. *Otto Loewi: ein Lebensbild in Dokumenten.* Berlin: Springer-Verlag.

KONRAD ZACHARIAS LORENZ
1973

Konrad Zacharias Lorenz was born on November 7, 1903, in Vienna. He received the Nobel Prize in 1973, jointly with Nikolaas Tinbergen and Karl von Frisch, for his comparative studies of the behavior of animals in nature, which laid the foundations of the field of ethology. Lorenz retired the same year as director of the Max Planck Institute for Behavioral Physiology in Seewiesen, Germany, but now, in his eighties, continues research and writing. He married his childhood playmate, Margarethe Gebhardt, in 1927; Frau Lorenz is a gynecologist. The couple have two daughters, Agnes and Dagmar, and a son, Thomas, who is a physicist.

Lorenz's parents were physicians: Adolf Lorenz was an orthopedic surgeon, and his wife Emma assisted in his practice. As a boy Konrad was fascinated by animals and spent much of his time playing with animals and watching and collecting birds, fish, and insects. He did well in science at school and wanted to study biology and evolution, but his father insisted on a medical education. He was sent to Columbia University Medical School in 1922 but spent much of his time at the New York Aquarium instead of at lectures. A difficult impasse was resolved when Konrad agreed to study medicine at the University of Vienna but was allowed to specialize in comparative anatomy, which enabled him to pursue his true passion. His first important paper, concerning the behavior of a pet jackdaw, was published in 1927.

After receiving his M.D. in 1928 Lorenz worked as an assistant at the University of Vienna's Anatomical Institute while completing his doctoral thesis in zoology under Oskar Heinroth. He also studied anatomy and psychology with Ferdinand Hochstetter and Karl Buhler. The Lorenz family had a summer home at Altenberg, a few miles outside of the city, and here he collected birds for observation and study—first jackdaws, then ducks and geese. His new wife, unlike his long-suffering but patient parents, adjusted happily to life in a menagerie. Living with the birds, feeding them by hand, treating them almost like children, Lorenz developed insights into their behavior and interactions impossible to discover in the laboratory or from standard field observations; these insights formed the basis of the science of ethology.

The most well known of these, the concept of imprinting, is permanently identified with his colony of greylag geese, although he observed the phenomenon in several species. Imprinting occurs early in the life of a young animal when it responds to the call of its mother, rapidly and permanently attaching itself to her. The animal's permanent concept of a parent, and later of a mate, is based on this early imprinting. Although the behavior itself appears to be genetically determined, the image of the mother apparently is not. Lorenz was able to imprint several families of young goslings on himself by making the appropriate calls at the appropriate time.

Imprinting was only one of many behaviors that Lorenz postulated was genetically determined but never enacted until triggered by an "innate releasing mechanism." For example, the tiny peeps of the goslings immediately released hereditary maternal behavior patterns in the goose mother. Lorenz argued for the evolutionary development of these complex determined social responses versus the rather limited individual learning patterns described by reflexologists and behaviorists, and the mystical "forces" postulated by the vitalists. His studies thus reintegrated science into the study of behavior in a meaningful and productive way (Marler and Griffin 1973, 465; *New York Times* 1973, 48).

Most of these observations and analyses were published between 1933, when Lorenz earned his doctorate, and 1938. He was appointed lecturer in comparative anatomy and animal psychology in 1937, but three years later left Vienna to accept the professorship in psychology at the University of Königsberg (now Kaliningrad). Although many other scientists had left Nazi Germany, Lorenz remained and offered no public challenge to Hitler's regime. In 1941 he was drafted into the German army medical service and subsequently served three years as a neurologist and field surgeon. Captured by the Russian army in 1944, he spent a further three and a half years in a prison camp in Armenia. Finally released in early 1948, he returned home to Altenburg.

The Max Planck Institute for the Advancement of Science in Germany offered him a small grant to resume his animal studies at his home. He reestablished his families of geese and ducks, and added an aquarium for tropical fish. The original research grew into the Department of Animal Sociology of the Institute of Comparative Anatomy, affiliated with the Austrian Academy of Science. Lorenz's first major effort after the war was a popular account of his work, *Er redete mit den Vieh, den Vogeln, und den Fischen* (1949), published in English as *King Solomon's Ring: New Light on Animal Ways*, which he illustrated with his own drawings. This delightful book, and its successor, *So kam der Mensch auf den Hund* (1950), or *Man Meets Dog*, made Lorenz world famous.

The Max Planck Society provided him with a formal research station at its Institute for Marine Biology in Buldern, Germany, in 1951. The Institute for Behavioral Physiology was established in 1955, with Lorenz, his fellow ethologist Gustav Kramer, and the physiologist Erich von Holst as codirectors. Here Lorenz devoted much of his time to advocating and developing the science he had created, through lectures and books. He was also in complete charge of the institute after 1961, for by then both Kramer and von Holst had died.

The most famous and controversial of his books, *Das sogenannte*

Böse: Zur naturgeschichte der Aggression (published in English as *On Aggression*), was published in 1963. Lorenz discussed animal aggression towards members of the same species as an essential behavior in maintaining territorial boundaries and ensuring evolutionary survival. His studies indicated, however, that most animals respond to certain submission behaviors from their own species by refraining from the kill. Lorenz then extended his analysis to humans, suggesting that man had not developed these evolutionary safeguards that inhibit intraspecies killing before he developed the weapons that made it possible; therefore, he has no instinctual protection against destruction of his own kind.

Lorenz's discussion of instinctual aggression, coupled with his advocacy of genetically determined behavior patterns, made him the focus of angry criticism. To some he seemed to be arguing for the inevitability of war and the hopeless enslavement of mankind to its biological heritage. Those who noted his failure to defy Nazi Germany saw his scientific views as part of a political or ideological position. His aggressive and rather doctrinaire personality added credence to these attacks. Supporters described Lorenz as single-mindedly dedicated to his field, with no interest in a political agenda, and noted his belief in man's eventual growth away from aggression, through natural evolution. He himself saw his opponents as "doctrinaires whose ideology has tabooed the recognition of this fact [genetic determination of behavior]."

"A very poor experimenter," as he describes himself, Lorenz championed the value of careful observation of natural behavior over experimental constructions and statistical descriptions. "It is an entirely erroneous assumption," he told a group of American medical students, "that you can attain any scientific result by quantification alone. If you feel that you only want to quantify, then please become mathematicians but for heaven's sake do not try to become doctors" (Marler and Griffin 1973, 465; Altman 1973, 48).

At the age of eighty-six, Lorenz remains the senior eminence of ethology. He still spends time regularly with his fish and geese. He is a member of the Austrian Academy of Sciences, the National Academy of Sciences (USA), the Royal Society of London, and many other national scientific societies. He has won many honors, including the Gold Medal of the Zoological Society of New York (1955); the City Prize of Vienna (1959); the Gold Bolsche Medal (1962); the Austrian Distinction for Science and Art (1964); the Prix Mondial of the Cino de Duca (1969); the Kalinga Prize from UNESCO (1970); the Grosse Verdienstkreuz (1974); and the Bayerischer Verdienstorden (1974).

MARCIA MELDRUM

Selected Bibliography

PRIMARY SOURCES

Lorenz, Konrad. 1966. *On Aggression*. New York: Harcourt Brace and World.

———. 1967. *Evolution and Modifica-*

tion of Behavior. Chicago: University of Chicago Press.

———. 1970–71. *Studies in Animal and Human Behavior*. Cambridge: Harvard University Press.

SECONDARY SOURCES

Altman, Lawrence K. 1973. "Birds and Bees." *New York Times* (October 12):48.

Marler, P., and D. R. Griffin. 1973. "The 1973 Nobel Prize for Physiology or Medicine." *Science* 182 (November 2):464–66.

1973. "Konrad Zacharias Lorenz." *New York Times* (October 12):48.

1973. "Three Behavioral Science Pioneers Win Nobel Prize for Medicine." *New York Times* (October 12):1, 48.

Evans, Richard. 1975. *Konrad Lorenz: The Man and His Ideas*. New York: Harcourt Brace Jovanovich.

Nisbett, Alec. 1976. *Konrad Lorenz*. London: Dent.

1977. "Lorenz, Konrad (Zacharias)." In *Current Biography Yearbook*, 247–77. New York: H. W. Wilson.

SALVADOR EDWARD LURIA
1969

Salvador Edward Luria was born in Turin, Italy, on August 13, 1913. He was the son of David and Ester (née Sacerdote) Luria. He received his M.D. degree in Turin in 1935. The rise of anti-Semitism in Mussolini's Italy forced Luria to leave his homeland after serving in the Italian army. He was a research fellow at the Curie Laboratory in Paris from 1938 to 1940; after the fall of France, Luria emigrated to the United States, working in the Medical Bacteriology Department at Columbia University (1940–42), and as a Guggenheim fellow at Vanderbilt University and Princeton University (1942–43). He joined the faculty at Indiana University (1944–50), moved on to the University of Illinois (1950–59), and finally settled at the Massachusetts Institute of Technology in 1959. Since 1978, he has been Emeritus Institute Professor of Biology at MIT. He shared the Nobel Prize in Physiology or Medicine in 1969 with A. D. Hershey and Max Delbrück for founding the "phage group" that helped establish molecular biology.

Luria first met Delbrück in 1940, at a physical society meeting in Philadelphia. Delbrück was a highly regarded physicist before he turned his attention to biology. Luria was a physics enthusiast but he had not met the standards that Enrico Fermi considered essential for doing well in graduate physics. Luria's initial interests in physics, however, led him to consider radiology and this in turn led him to work with Fermi in Rome and then at the radium laboratory in Paris. Luria chose microbiology as a field because he, like Delbrück, was attracted to the idea that microscopic organisms could provide a closer entry into the physics and chemistry of the gene and fundamental life processes. The association proved valuable for both Delbrück and Luria.

Delbrück had already worked out the life cycle of the bacteriophage virus. Luria and Delbrück decided to study mixed infections of two strains of this virus (later called T1 and T2). In the course of these experiments Luria encountered some strains of the host bacterium, *Escherichia coli*, that were resistant to infection. Did these bacteria acquire their resistance as a consequence of infection or did they arise as new mutations? Luria noted that resistant colonies of bacteria from any one sample of cells that he cultured arose in variable batches, much like the Poisson distributions around a mean. To test this possibility, Luria corresponded with Delbrück and the two worked out a more precise "fluctuation test" to see if these variable numbers reflected mutations arising before and after phage infection. They found this indeed to be the case. If a mutation in a bacterial culture arose shortly after inoculation, the batch size of resistant colonies was large. If the mutation in another culture arose just prior to plating, the batch size was very small. From the mathematics of the Poisson distributions that governs such events, Luria and Delbrück could then estimate the mutation rate to resistance to T1 or T2 in their strain of *E. coli.*

After this initial success with bacterial resistance to phage infection, Luria turned his attention to the possibility that the phage could also mutate. He chose host range as the trait to study because it was known that some T1 or T2 strains could infect more than one strain of *E. coli.* This study was also successful, and Luria detected host range mutants. As a side benefit of these experiments, Luria noted that some of the host range mutations arose as a portion of the viruses released from a single burst (lysis) of the infected bacterium. As in the fluctuation test for the origins of bacterial mutations, the partial bursts revealed late or early origins of the phage mutation during its logarthimic growth within the host cell.

In addition to the host range mutations found by Luria, other mutations were isolated by Luria, Hershey, and other phage workers. Of special value were morphological plaque mutations from phage plated on thickened overgrowths of *E. coli* host cells. These morphological mutations (such as particularly small or particularly large plaques, or turbid rather than the more typical clear plaques) Luria used with the multiple infection technique he and Delbrück had established earlier. The results of these experiments, independently carried out by Hershey, demonstrated recombination of the two traits in either double mutant (such as turbid and large) or fully normal plaque size and appearance.

The frequency of these recombinant plaques could then be used to map the genes and establish a formal phage genetics.

Luria also collaborated with T. F. Anderson to produce the first electron micrographs of bacteriophage; these micrographs showed a more complex structure than researchers had expected. Unlike the "naked genes" they were thought to be, bacteriophage viruses were actually complex organisms with a well-characterized protein coat and an inner core of nucleic acid.

The early Phage Group, stimulated by the association of Delbrück and Luria, was very small; the first meeting in 1947, in Nashville, Tennessee, consisted of Luria, Delbrück, Hershey, M. H. Adams, T. F. Anderson, S. S. Cohen, A. H. Doermann, and M. Zelle. Delbrück, Luria, and Hershey's success in establishing the key components of the bacteriophage life cycle and their advocacy for its use in genetic research had enormous influence on the development of modern molecular biology. Their work has been called the "transformation of the landscape of classical Mendelian genetics into the latter day molecular Crick-Watsonian scene" (Stent 1969); but it was within a long tradition of thought. From E. B. Wilson's chromosome theory, through the gene theory of Morgan's school, Muller's emphasis on the gene as the basis of life, and Luria's influence on his student Watson, researchers had narrowed in on the gene as the fundamental biological unit and its molecular structure and function as the key to our understanding of life.

Luria's influence on molecular biology has been extensive. He worked with Renato Dulbecco at Indiana University and supervised James Watson's dissertation on the reactivation of heavily X-irradiated phage. He established, with Hershey and Delbrück, a summer course in phage genetics that enabled hundreds of doctoral students from physics, chemistry, and biology to take up work on this remarkable system. He also wrote an influential text in virology that stressed the importance of viruses for revealing fundamental cell processes. Luria's years at MIT have stressed his administrative skills in building a department of talented research scholars in molecular biology. He also was the first to note the action of a class of enzymes that protected bacteria by attacking and cleaving the DNA of foreign viruses that penetrated through the bacterial cell membranes. These were the restriction enzymes, identified in the late 1960s by Daniel Nathans, Werner Arber, and H. O. Smith, that made possible modern techniques of genetic engineering.

Salvador Luria and his wife, Zella Hurwitz, whom he married in 1945, have one son, Daniel. He is a member of the National Academy of Sciences, the American Association for the Advancement of Science, and the American School of Microbiology. Among the other awards he has received for his work have been the Lepetit Prize (1935), the Lenghi Prize from the Italian Academy of Sciences (1965), and the Horowitz Prize from Columbia University (1969).

ELOF AXEL CARLSON

Selected Bibliography

PRIMARY SOURCES

Luria, S. E., and T. F. Anderson. 1942. "The Identification and Characterization of Bacteriophages with the Electron Microscope." *Proceedings of the National Academy of Sciences* 28:127–30.

Luria, S. E., and M. Delbrück. 1943. "Mutations of Bacteria from Virus Sensitivity to Virus Resistance." *Genetics* 28:463–470.

Luria, S. E. 1945. "Mutations of Bacterial Viruses Affecting Their Host Range." *Genetics* 30:84–99.

———. 1951. "The Frequency Distribution of Spontaneous Bacteriophage Mutants as Evidence for the Exponential Rate of Phage Reproduction." *Cold Spring Harbor Symposium in Quantitative Biology* 16:463–70.

———. 1966. "Mutations of Bacteria and Bacteriophage." In *Phage and the Origins of Molecular Biology*, edited by J. Cairns, G. S. Stent, and J. D. Watson, 173–79. Cold Spring Harbor, N.Y.: Cold Spring Harbor Laboratory of Quantitative Biology.

———. 1986. *A Slot Machine, A Broken Test Tube*. New York: Basic Books.

SECONDARY SOURCES

Carlson, Elof Axel. 1972. "An Unacknowledged Founding of Molecular Biology: H. J. Muller's Contribution to Gene Theory, 1910–1936." *Journal of the History of Biology* 4:149–70.

Judson, Horace Freeland. 1979. *The Eighth Day of Creation: The Makers of the Revolution in Biology*. New York: Simon and Schuster.

Olby, Robert. 1974. *The Path to the Double Helix*. Seattle, Wash.: University of Washington Press.

Stent, Gunther. 1969. "The 1969 Nobel Prize for Physiology or Medicine." *Science* 166:479–481.

ANDRÉ MICHEL LWOFF *1965*

André Michel Lwoff was born on May 8, 1902, at Ainay-le-Chateau, in central France. A microbiologist, Lwoff shared the 1965 Nobel Prize with Jacques Monod and François Jacob for their "discoveries concerning the genetic regulation of enzyme and viral synthesis." His parents, both Russian-born, were Marie Siminovitch Lwoff, a sculptress, and Salomon Lwoff, a French-trained medical director of a psychiatric hospital. Lwoff married his colleague, Margerite Bourdalieux, on December 5, 1925. They have no children.

Lwoff joined the Institut Pasteur in 1921, having completed studies for a bachelor of science and one year of medical school. He earned both his M.D. (1927) and his doctorate of science (1932) from the Université de Paris. He served in the French army in 1928. In 1938 he was appointed head of the Department of Physiologie Microbienne at the Institut Pasteur and, in 1959, professor of microbiologie at the Sorbonne. In 1968 he left the Institut Pasteur temporarily to become director of the C.N.R.S. Institut de Recherches Scientifiques sur le Cancer at Villejuif, south of Paris. He retired from the latter and returned to the Institut Pasteur in 1972.

Lwoff completed medical school at his father's wish, but his career and interests have centered on the research laboratory. He remembers that his special fascination with microbes was fostered by Elie Metchnikoff, a family friend. Lwoff's research interests are comprehensive, however, and his talents have enabled him to master the diverse fields of protistology, evolutionary theory, bacteriology, molecular biology, and virology. At age nineteen he began his research explorations with the zoologist Edouard Chatton. For the next fifteen years he spent most of his summers exploring the growth and behavior of "ciliates," microorganisms with mobile featherlike appendages, working at the marine biology laboratories at Roscoff, in western Brittany, or at Baynuls on the Mediterranean. He wrote his M.D. thesis on protozoa (Lwoff 1927). Chatton and Lwoff traced and compared the ciliates on two different crustacean hosts, demonstrating that these organisms "descended" from precursors in a pattern of genetic continuity (Chatton, Lwoff, and Lwoff 1927, 1935).

This concept of biochemical evolution became the theme of Lwoff's doctoral work. In the Institut Pasteur laboratory of Félix Mesnil, a former collaborator of C. L. Alphonse Laveran, Lwoff studied the growth and nutrition of various protozoa. He observed that their nutritional requirements changed from generation to generation in a manner that could be described as the loss of a series of biochemical functions. The idea of evolution as "loss of function" is now considered to be one aspect of a multifaceted type of evolutionary curve that also includes increasing diversity, but in the early 1930s it met with little acceptance. Nevertheless, André and Margerite Lwoff continued to study the evidence and refine their theory by an exhaustive analysis of growth factors in microorganisms.

In 1932–33 they spent a year in Heidelberg at the laboratory of Otto Meyerhof and, in 1936, some months with David Keilin in Cambridge. During the latter period the Lwoffs concluded that a little understood nutrient essential to the bacteria *Hemophilus influenzae*, called "Factor V," was a coenzyme that functioned like a vitamin. They were able to prove that this nutrient was identical with NAD, a biochemical coenzyme discovered by Otto Warburg shortly before. These results, which appeared in several articles in the *Proceedings of the Royal So-*

ciety of London during 1936–37, made it clear that, in spite of the unusual aspects of their theory, the Lwoffs were on the cutting edge of physiology. The culmination of Lwoff's investigations in physiological evolution was the publication of his book, *L'evolution Physiologique*, in 1944; this work received limited attention due to the exigencies of war and was not translated into English. By war's end, its author had moved on to lysogeny.

It was Lwoff's work on lysogenic bacteria that won him the Nobel Prize. Lysogenic bacteria are those that can be "lysed," or destroyed, by the appearance of rapidly dividing viruses called "bacteriophages." The bacteriophagic infection could disappear for a few generations, only to reappear mysteriously. Lwoff has used the analogy of recurrent cold sore infections (herpes virus) in the human organism. This phenomenon had been recognized since the early twentieth century and others had already concluded that the virus, somehow integrated into the host heredity, must replicate within the host cell, but the exact mechanism was unknown.

By meticulous study of bacteria, sometimes of individual, newly divided cells, Lwoff determined that all daughter cells were lysogenic; in other words, when exposed to the proper stimulus in some eventual, indeterminate generation, the latent virus would begin to multiply and cause lysis of the cell. He gave the name "prophage" to the viral genetic material, present but hidden. The future of research in this area would depend on the researcher's ability to demonstrate the presence of the virus by "inducing the prophage," that is, by provoking the virus to divide at a rate faster than that of the host cell.

Lwoff and his associates, Louis Siminovitch and Niels Kjeldgaard, accomplished this feat in early 1950 by exposing the bacterial culture to ultraviolet light. Thus, they paved the way for a host of successful experiments in molecular biology, including those of Jacob and Monod, whose insight linked induction of the prophage to stimulation of enzyme synthesis and ultimately to genetic control mechanisms. Lwoff ended his protozoa investigations by launching an authoritative text on bacterial physiology (2 vols., 1951–53). The second edition, appearing in 1979, was dedicated to him as "master craftsman" and "progenitor of the enterprise" (Levandowsky and Hutner, 1979, xiii).

Lwoff turned his attention in 1954 to disease as the metabolic relationship between virus and host with special attention to the poliovirus. He studied fever as a physiological response to infection. He envisaged a new concept of disease treatment and prevention in which the viral "infection" is kept under control by the persistence of "repressor," as theorized by Monod, rather than by an attempt to kill a virus that may be harmlessly integrated with host DNA. This idea is described in his 1965 Nobel Lecture. The interest in quiescent but persistent viruses led him naturally to the study of oncogenes, cancer-causing genes that most likely originate from viruses. His work with oncogenes led to his appointment as director of the Institut de Recherches Scientifiques sur le Cancer.

Now in his eighties and back at the Institut Pasteur, Lwoff continues to participate in the activities of the scientific community. Tall, aristocratic, and reserved, he has a passion for verbal precision and a brilliant, often sarcastic, wit. He created the nomenclature committee of the Institut to protect and enhance scientific language with exact and unencumbered terms, usually derived from Greek, to define the burgeoning discoveries of the Institut and other laboratories. His preoccupation with "evolution" and with metabolic relationships led to his appreciation of "order" as an evolutionary product and he readily applies social analogies to illustrate his views (Lwoff 1962). These philosophical preoccupations are evident in the communications he has sent to *Recherche* and to *Nature* in the 1980s. Lwoff's friends and colleagues frequently refer to him as an artist, not only for his talents in painting and sculpture, but for his ability to see the unseen and to shape the ideas of his time.

Lwoff has won the Charles-Leopold Mayer Prize and many other awards from the French Académie des Sciences and other international organizations. He is a member of numerous learned societies, including the American National Academy of Sciences (1955) and the Royal Society (1958). He holds honorary doctorates from the universities of Chicago (1959), Oxford (1959), Glasgow (1963), and Louvain (1966.)

JACKIE DUFFIN

Selected Bibliography

PRIMARY SOURCES

Chatton, E., A. Lwoff, and M. Lwoff. 1929. "Les infraciliatures et la continuitié génétique des systèmes ciliaires récessifs." *Comptes Rendues de l'Académie des Sciences* 188:1190–92.

Chatton, E., A. Lwoff, and M. Lwoff. 1935. "Les Ciliés Apostomes." *Archives Zoologie Experimentale et Gënetique* 77:1–453.

Lwoff, André. 1944. *L'evolution Physiologique. Etude des Pertes de Fonction chez les Microorganismes.* Paris: Hermann.

———. 1953. "Lysogeny." *Bacteriological Reviews* 17:269–337.

———. 1962. *Biological Order.* Cambridge, MIT Press.

———. 1965. "Virus Cell and Organism." Nobel Lecture. Reprinted in *Nobel Lectures in Physiology or Medicine*, vol. 4 (1963–70), 174–85. Amsterdam: Elsevier, 1972.

———. 1971. "From Protozoa to Bacteria and Viruses: Fifty Years with Microbes." *Annual Review of Microbiology* 25:1–26. Contains bibliography of ninety-three publications prior to 1969.

———. 1981. "Introduction au Vè Congrès International de Virologie (IAMS) 2–7 aout, Strasbourg." *Annales de Virologie (de l'Institut Pasteur)* 132E (April):121–34.

SECONDARY SOURCES

Jacob, François. 1988. *The Statue Within: An Autobiography*, 212–37. Translated by Franklin Philip. New York: Basic Books.

Levandowsky, M., and S. H. Hutner,

eds. 1979. *Biochemistry and Physiology of Protozoa.* New York: Academic Press.

Monod, Jacques. 1971. "Du Microbe de l'homme. In *Of Microbe and Life*, edited by Jacques Monod and Ernest Borek, 1–9. New York: Columbia University Press. This volume contains thirty-two essays by friends and colleagues dedicated "to André Lwoff for the Fiftieth Anniversary of his Immersion into Biology." Monod has also edited a "Bibiliographie résumé de l'oeuvre d'André Lwoff" with nineteen references, 10–13.

FEODOR LYNEN *1964*

Feodor Lynen was born on April 6, 1911, in Munich, Germany. He was a biochemist whose area of specialization was lipid metabolism. The 1964 Nobel Prize in Physiology or Medicine was awarded to Feodor Lynen and Konrad Bloch "for their discoveries concerning the mechanism and regulation of cholesterol and fatty acid metabolism." Lynen married Eva Wieland, the daughter of his mentor, Nobel laureate Heinrich Wieland, on May 14, 1937. They had five children. Feodor Lynen died August 6, 1979, in Munich.

His father, Wilhelm L. Lynen, was a distinguished professor of mechanical engineering at the Munich Technische Hochschule. His mother, Frieda Prym Lynen, was the daughter of the manufacturer Gustav Prym. Lynen completed his primary and secondary schooling in Munich and matriculated at the Chemistry Department of Munich University in 1930, where he studied with Heinrich Wieland, Otto Hönigschmidt, Kasimir Fajans, and Walter Gerlach. Heinrich Wieland, winner of the Nobel Prize for Chemistry in 1927, supervised his thesis research "On the Toxic Substances in Amanita" and introduced him to the new field of biochemistry. Lynen graduated in 1937. Maintaining his relationship with the University of Munich, Lynen became chemistry lecturer in 1942 and biochemistry professor in 1953. In 1954 he was named director of the Max-Planck-Institute für Zellchemie, an appointment that gave him outstanding opportunities for scientific research. Over the course of his career, Lynen studied the enzymatic steps of the fatty acid cycle, the role of biotin in fatty substance metabolism, fermentation, the citric acid cycle, biological phosphorylation and oxidation, and the regulatory mechanisms of metabolic processes.

In his Nobel Prize Presentation Speech, Professor S. Bergström, member of the Nobel Committee for Physiology or Medicine of the Royal Caroline Institute, pointed out that the word *cholesterol* meant "gallstone." The understanding of cholesterol has undergone a remarkable change since this substance was isolated from human gallstones some two hundred years ago. In the 1960s the correlation between atherosclerosis and the amount of cholesterol and other fats in the diet and the blood was already a lively topic. But the association between cholesterol and disease had obscured the fact that cholesterol is also a necessary constituent of all cells and has important functions in the body. Thus, the elucidation of its chemical structure and metabolism were significant achievements in organic chemistry and biochemistry. Moreover, these studies of the metabolism of lipids generated expectations that specific therapeutic tools would be discovered to aid in the battle against the diseases that had become the most common causes of death in the developed countries.

In his Nobel Lecture Lynen traced his own "pathway" from his first contact with dynamic biochemistry to the "exceedingly propitious" year 1937 when studies of the enzyme chain of respiration "had thrown the first rays of light on the chemical processes underlying the mystery of biological catalysis" (Lynen 1964, 103). Lynen's first independent investigations dealt with the metabolism of frozen yeast cells, the mechanisms of alcoholic fermentation, and the Pasteur effect. These research projects taught him to pay special attention to the permeability of cell membranes and alerted him to the importance of the adenosine polyphosphate system in energy transfer and the regulation of metabolic processes.

Working in Wieland's laboratory on the metabolism of acetic acid, Lynen made a fundamental discovery about the role of acetic acid as a building block for cholesterol. Lynen isolated the "activated acetic acid" that proved to be the precursor of the lipids and an essential constituent of various metabolic processes. In addition, Lynen was credited with two other very significant discoveries concerning the mechanisms of cellular metabolism: the elucidation of the mechanism of action of the vitamin biotin and the determination of the structure of cytohemin. Lynen recalled that during this period he first became totally concerned with the conversion of acetic acid into citric acid. This process had been made the focus of the aerobic degradation of carbohydrates when Hans Krebs formulated the citric acid cycle. However, Krebs regarded pyruvic acid as the condensation partner of acetic acid. In contrast, Lynen was firmly convinced, on the basis of his experiments with yeast, that pyruvic acid was first oxidized to acetic acid and only at that point could the condensation take place. His attempts to achieve the synthesis of citric acid from oxaloactic acid and acetic acid with the aid of yeast cells whose membranes had been made permeable to polybasic acids by freezing in liquid air were unsuccessful. These studies were interrupted for several years because during World War II basic research and scientific contact with the outside world became impossible.

After the war Lynen learned of advances that had been made in the study of "activated acetic acid." It was now known that the formation of "activated acetic acid" from acetate involved ATP as an energy source and the newly discovered coenzyme A (Lipmann 1953, 413–40). Lynen's group confirmed and extended these observations. Lynen recalled being "possessed" by the idea that the "activated acetic acid," which was probably an acetylated coenzyme A, must be a thio ester. He even remembered the moment when this idea first came to him. Thinking about the fact that Lippman had mentioned the content of disulfides in his publication on coenzyme A and the observation that every coenzyme-A-dependent enzyme reaction required the addition of cysteine or glutathione, he combined the two observations "in the assumption that sulphur was an essential constituent of coenzyme A and could affect the functions of the coenzyme only as a thiol group." Thus he was not surprised when "activated acetic acid" was purified and characterized as a thio ester. The next important step was proof that this "activated acetic acid" was indeed the long-sought acetyl donor. This discovery was fundamental to an understanding of the mechanism of the biosynthesis of both sterols and fatty acids. The solution to the "activated acetic acid" problem was also fundamental to appreciating the importance of "energy-rich" compounds in intermediate metabolism and the elucidation of the fatty acid cycle (Lynen 1964, 107). In addition to his fundamental studies of the biosynthesis of the fatty acids, Lynen and his group were also pioneers in elucidating the metabolic degradation of the fatty acids.

In 1964 Lynen optimistically predicted that practical, medicinal techniques for controlling fatty acid synthesis and thus directly attacking the problem of the circulatory diseases would soon result from basic research in fatty acid metabolism. Lynen also suggested that some of the problems of human beings could be ameliorated by indulgence in the simple joys. The basic research on lipid metabolism performed by Lynen and Bloch was taken very seriously by the medical community. Although no "magic bullet" was available, in June 1964 the American Heart Association recommended that the general public, as well as cardiac patients, reduce their fat intake. In the same year, from a study of five thousand persons, the National Heart Association concluded that people with high cholesterol levels in their blood were at increased risk of coronary disease.

Other honors awarded to Lynen include the Neuberg Medal (1954); the Justus von Liebig Medal, Gesellschaft Deutscher Chemiker (1955); the Carus Medal, Deutsche Akademie der Naturforscher Leopoldina (1961); the Otto Warburg Medal, Gesellschaft für Physiologische Chemie (1963): and the Normal Medaille, Deutsche Gesellschaft für Fettnissenschaft (1967).

LOIS N. MAGNER

Selected Bibliography

PRIMARY SOURCES

Lynen, Feodor. 1953. "Acetyl Coenzyme A and the Fatty Acid Cycle." *Harvey Lectures Series*, 48, 210–44.

———. 1955. "Der Fettsaurecyclus." *Angewandte Chemie* 67:463–70.

———. 1961. "Biosynthesis of Saturated Fatty Acids." *Federation Proceedings* 20:941–51.

———. 1964. "The Pathway from 'Activated Acetic Acid' to the Terpenes and Fatty Acids." Nobel Lecture, December 11, 1964. Reprinted in *Nobel Lectures, Physiology or Medicine*, vol. 4 (1963–1970), 103–40. Amsterdam: Elsevier, 1972.

———. 1976. "My Expeditions into Sulfur Biochemistry." In *Reflections on Biochemistry. In Honour of Severo Ochoa*, edited by A. Kornberg, B. L. Horecker, L. Cornudella, and J. Oro, 151–60. New York: Pergamon Press.

SECONDARY SOURCES

Boyer, P. D., H. Lardy, and K. Myrbäck, eds. 1980. *The Enzymes*, vol. 3. New York: Academic Press.

1967. *Current Biography Yearbook*, 263–65. New York: H. W. Wilson.

Fruton, Joseph S. 1982. *A Bio-Bibliography of the Biochemical Sciences Since 1800*. Philadelphia: American Philosophical Society.

Kennedy, E. P., and F. H. Westheimer. 1964. "Nobel Laureates: Bloch and Lynen Win Prize in Medicine and Physiology." *Science* 146:504–6.

Kornberg, A., B. L. Horecker, L. Cornudella, and J. Oro, eds. 1976. *Reflections on Biochemistry: In Honour of Severo Ochoa*. New York: Pergamon Press.

Lipmann, Fritz. 1953. "Development of the Acetylation Problem: A Personal Account." Nobel Lecture. Reprinted in *Nobel Lectures, Physiology or Medicine*, vol. 3 (1942–1962), 413–40. Amsterdam: Elsevier, 1964.

McElroy, W. D., and B. Glass, eds. 1952. *Phosphorus Metabolism*, vol. 2. Baltimore: Johns Hopkins University Press.

Sela, M., ed. 1964. *New Perspectives in Biology*. Amsterdam: Elsevier.

BARBARA McCLINTOCK *1983*

Barbara McClintock was born in Hartford, Connecticut, on June 16, 1902. Her father, Thomas Henry McClintock, was a physician and her mother Sara (née Handy) raised Barbara, her two older sisters, and a younger brother. They grew up in Brooklyn, New York, where Barbara developed an interest in science in high school. She attended Cornell University, starting in 1919, and eventually received her Ph.D. in

1927 in corn (maize) genetics. It is as a geneticist that she established the international reputation that earned her the Nobel Prize in 1983. She is one of only a few scientists to win an unshared award; the last unshared award in genetics went to H. J. Muller in 1946.

McClintock's contributions to genetics were based on annual breeding experiments with corn and cytological studies of the chromosomes of her plants. She pioneered the structural relation of plant chromosomes to their genetic effects and she worked out the interpretation of many complex chromosomal rearrangements that had not been described before. Independently of Curt Stern, she worked out a proof of the chromosomal basis of crossing over, the mechanism that enables individuals to combine the genetic traits from their father's sperm and from the mother's eggs to produce new combinations of those traits among their offspring. She also discovered a new phenomenon, transposable genetic elements, that remained a curiosity until they were discovered nearly twenty years later in bacteria and higher animals. Of major significance to geneticists was her analysis of the consequences of chromosome breakage to dividing cells, an interpretation that H. J. Muller used to explain radiation sickness.

McClintock worked alone throughout most of her career. She was a scientist in an era that rarely hired women for university positions and seldom granted them tenure. McClintock was a victim of sex discrimination that kept her from having her own graduate students, a first-rate facility, and the financial support that her male peers enjoyed in their careers.

McClintock remained at Cornell as an instructor until 1931, when she moved to the California Institute of Technology as a fellow of the National Research Council. She was an assistant professor at Cornell (1934–36) and at the University of Missouri (1936–41), but having failed to attain tenure at these institutions she joined the staff of the Carnegie Institution of Washington at Cold Spring Harbor, New York, where she remained for the rest of her career (1941–67) and where she continues today as a distinguished service member of the staff. She received a lifetime award, the first such given, from the MacArthur Foundation to continue her research.

McClintock studied the chromosomes of corn for her Ph.D. dissertation and identified each of the ten pairs with accuracy. These accurate cytological maps she later used to correlate with genetic abnormalities that arose from complex rearrangements of one or more of the individual chromosomes. With Harriet Creighton, in 1931, McClintock used the chromosome cytology and demonstrated its correlation to genetic crossovers involving genes associated with fragments of two chromosomes that had broken and joined in a new configuration. The correlation of the two approaches, one genetic and the other cytological, among the recombinant and nonrecombinant progeny receiving the distributed chromosomes and their fragments, was widely hailed.

McClintock examined many of

the induced rearrangements caused by X-rays, following up H. J. Muller's (and L. J. Stadler's) discovery from 1927 to 1929 that X-rays induce both gene mutations and altered chromosome structures. McClintock inferred that the loss of color factors, resulting in variegated streaks or spots on the corn kernels, may arise from ring chromosomes that are formed by radiation. Ring chromosomes, when mitotically replicating, interlock or produce unusual double-sized chromosomes that cannot successfully be distributed to the two cells formed by mitosis. This leads to loss of the factors controlled by the missing chromosome. McClintock photographed these rings in their normal and interlocked configurations to demonstrate her hypothesis.

Also induced by X-rays were chromosome breaks that did not immediately repair but instead replicated, leading to a delayed repair that formed one chromosome fragment that lacked a centromere (attachment point for a contractile fiber that moves chromosomes in cell division) and a second fragment with a centromere. The centromere-bearing fragment formed a chromosome bridge during cell division that either broke or prevented cell division. In either case the cell became abnormal and the genetic traits associated with the missing fragment or genes would become detectable, just as ring chromosomes were. McClintock called this occurrence a breakage-fusion-bridge cycle; it continues in corn plant tissue until the broken ends heal or the cell dies. In animal tissue, as H. J. Muller and his student, G. Pontecorvo, discovered in 1940, the breakage-fusion-bridge cycle does not lead to a healing of broken chromosome ends and eventually kills the cell line that has the defective chromosomes. The cycle accounted for the high mortality of embryos formed after fertilization from heavily X-rayed male fruit flies. After Hiroshima, Muller used McClintock's research to explain radiation sickness.

Although McClintock had achieved fame as a geneticist through these major contributions to cytogenetics, she made her most original and important discovery while studying a class of unstable mutant strains. The mutable genes that she followed were turned on or off by a regulatory element that McClintock inferred to be transposable from one chromosome to another. Some of her colleagues called them jumping genes, but McClintock saw them as regulators, transposable genetic segments that broke a chromosome at some destined site and inserted itself there, causing an adjacent gene either to cease or to start functioning. Although McClintock spent six years working out this pattern of transposable elements in maize, she did not publish her interpretation until 1948. The uniqueness of the system at the time, the complexity of corn genetics, and the turgid writing style McClintock used to present her data combined to make her work go unappreciated outside corn genetics for almost twenty years. In the mid-1960s, similar phenomena were noted in bacteria; transposable elements in those systems serve as a major means of transferring genetic material within and among related species. Transposable elements were also discovered in the 1970s in fruit flies, but their role there is less clear: some species of fruit flies do not have transposable elements, while other strains of a species are heavily infected with them. They do not seem to play a normal developmental role in fruit flies, but they may greatly accelerate the mutation rate among species that become infected with them—a substantial portion of spontaneously arising mutations in the best-known fruit fly species, *Drosophila melanogaster*, arise from insertions or departures of transposable elements.

McClintock is a short, thin, woman who speaks infrequently in public. Her lectures, especially for those not familiar with the complex genetic composition of corn kernels, frequently leave an audience bewildered. Her technical papers were so densely saturated with the details of her genetic crosses that they were often skimmed, misunderstood, or ignored. McClintock is, to her colleagues, a warm and caring person, eager to discuss her work and patient with students who ask questions. She is a private person, dedicated to her work, who shuns the public limelight often bestowed on Nobel laureates.

Elof Axel Carlson

Selected Bibliography

PRIMARY SOURCES

McClintock, Barbara. 1932. "A Correlation of Ring-Shaped Chromosomes with Variegation in *Zea mays.*" *Proceedings of the National Academy of Sciences* 18:677–81.

———. 1938. "The Fusion of Broken Ends of Sister Half-chromatids Following Chromatid Breakage at Meiotic Anaphases." *University of Missouri College of Agriculture Research Bulletin* 290:1–48.

———. 1942. "The Fusion of Broken Ends of Chromosomes of *Zea mays.*" *Proceedings of the National Academy of Sciences* 28:458–63.

———. 1948. "Mutable Loci in Maize." *Carnegie Institution of Washington Yearbook* 47:159.

———. 1950. "The Origin and Behavior of Mutable Loci in Maize." *Proceedings of the National Academy of Sciences* 36:344–55.

———. 1956. "Controlling Elements and the Gene." *Cold Spring Harbor Symposia on Quantitative Biology* 21:215

———. 1965. "The Control of Gene Action in Maize." *Brookhaven Symposia in Biology* 18:162–84.

SECONDARY SOURCES

Keller, Evelyn Fox. 1983. *A Feeling for the Organism: The Life and Work of Barbara McClintock.* San Francisco: Freeman.

JOHN JAMES RICKARD MACLEOD *1923*

John James Rickard Macleod was born in Cluny, Scotland, on September 6, 1876. A physiologist, Macleod shared the Nobel Prize in 1923 with Frederick Grant Banting for his sponsorship of Banting's work in isolating and purifying the pancreatic substance that regulates blood sugar, making possible its synthesis as insulin. At the time of the award, Macleod was professor of physiology at the University of Toronto. He married Mary Watson MacWalter in 1903; the couple had no children. He died March 16, 1935, in Aberdeen, Scotland.

Macleod's father, the Reverend Robert Macleod, answered a call to an Aberdeen church shortly after his son was born, and young John grew up in that city. He graduated from Marischal College at Aberdeen University in 1898 with degrees in both medicine and surgery, having won the Matthews Duncan and Fife Jameson medals. He was also awarded the Anderson traveling scholarship, enabling him to spend a year at the Physiological Institute in Leipzig, where he furthered his knowledge of biochemistry. On his return in 1902, he accepted an appointment as demonstrator in physiology at the London Hospital Medical College, working under Sir Leonard Hill.

Macleod's major interest was the respiratory system. Under Hill's guidance, he carried out experiments on intracranial circulation and on caisson disease, publishing a number of papers. Simultaneously, he did postgraduate work at Cambridge University and earned a diploma in public health. In 1902 he was appointed lecturer in biochemistry at the London Hospital and was named Mackinnon Research Scholar by the Royal Society.

In 1903 Macleod was the principal author of a textbook entitled *Practical Physiology*. His reputation had now spread to the United States, where several major medical schools were seeking to expand their curriculum in the basic sciences. He was offered the professorship of physiology at Western Reserve University in Cleveland, Ohio (now Case Western Reserve). Here he expanded his research to problems of protein and carbohydrate metabolism, including diabetes mellitus. Among other studies, he carried out a lengthy study of the breakdown of liver glycogen, which can be induced by a variety of experimental stimuli, including asphyxia or the injection of adrenalin. Macleod's hypothesis was that each of the various processes introduced a diastatic enzyme into the liver, which began the glycolytic process. He cowrote another book of physiology with Hill and also published *Diabetes: Its Pathological Physiology* in 1913.

In 1918 he became professor of physiology at the University of Toronto, where he continued his work on glucose metabolism and blood sugar levels. He also returned to his interest in respiration, studying the effects of anoxemia and of excess oxygen. His comprehensive and very successful textbook, *Physiology and Biochemistry in Modern Medicine*, written with Roy G. Pearce and others, was published in 1918 (Stevenson 1973, 614; Collip 1935, 1254).

In 1920 Macleod was concentrating on anoxemia but was recognized as the major Canadian authority on diabetes and on glucose metabolism. Although he was aware that the pancreas was often implicated in diabetic etiology, he was doubtful about suggestions that this digestive organ secreted a sugar metabolizing hormone.

Experiments with several animals had shown that ligation of the pancreatic ducts led after several weeks to almost total atrophy, leaving intact only the small section called the islets of Langerhans. Blockage of the ducts also resulted in the absence of glycosuria. These findings supported the theory that the pancreas, specifically the islets of Langerhans, secreted a hormone necessary for the normal metabolism of glucose by the body; and that diabetes mellitus, a disease characterized by inadequate glucose metabolism and consequent acidosis of blood and tissues, could therefore be traced to a malfunction or disorder of the pancreas.

Diabetes had been recognized as a discrete illness for centuries, but the process of glucose synthesis and metabolism was not understood until the work of Claude Bernard and others in the mid-nineteenth century. In 1889 Joseph von Mehring and Oscar Minkowski had demonstrated that the removal of the entire pancreas from dogs resulted in death, preceded by all the symptoms of severe diabetes. Minkowski and others had speculated that pancreatic extracts could be used to treat the illness, but an extract of the entire gland proved either ineffective or toxic. Several researchers had achieved partial successes but no clinically useful preparation had been found.

Lydia de Witt in 1906 had isolated and extracted only the islet tissue; this substance proved to be glycolytic (sugar producing), rather than digestive. Her findings suggested that the digestive secretions of the gland, such as the enzyme trypsin, were its major products, and that the special sugar metabolism hormone was generated only by the islets. However, de Witt had not been able to adapt her extract to clinical diabetes treatment.

In late 1920 a young surgeon named Frederick Banting approached Macleod with a research proposal. He would isolate the islets by ligation of the pancreatic ducts and then extract only this tissue for diabetic treatment. He hypothesized that extractions of the whole gland had been unsuccessful because the process would release the digestive enzymes, which would effectively destroy the glycolytic tissues. Banting was unaware of the many attempts that had been made; he was an idealistic and passionate young man who was convinced that he had found the solution to the grave problem of diabetes. Macleod was not unsympathetic but characteristically pointed out all the technical and theoretical problems with the proposal. Banting persisted, however, and Macleod finally agreed to help. He offered Banting a laboratory for eight weeks, an undergraduate assistant, and ten dogs. With this meager support, Banting left his private practice and moved to Toronto in April 1921 (Stevenson 1970, 440–41; Collip 1942, 401; 1935, 1256).

The undergraduate Macleod assigned was Charles H. Best, who in fact had just received his B.A. in physiology and chemistry when he began work with Banting in May, and who had already done a number of metabolism experiments. They were later assisted by C. H. Noble, another recent graduate. Macleod gave the young men some assistance in planning and designing their project and then left for a summer in Scotland.

The first stage of the work was surgical: performing ligation of the pancreatic ducts in one set of dogs and pancreatectomies in another set. There were many false starts and botched attempts. The initial ligations failed to result in the expected total atrophy and they had to operate again, this time applying several ligatures at different tensions. Pancreatectomy was attempted using the Hedon technique of removal in two stages but the available operating facilities were inadequate for this lengthy procedure. Banting therefore developed his own single-stage technique.

On July 27, the researchers finally had ready a dog with the necessary degree of pancreatic atrophy and another, depancreatized, animal, who was showing the symptoms of experimental diabetes. They prepared an extract of the remaining pancreatic tissue and injected it into the diabetic dog. Within two hours they observed a significant reduction in blood sugar and clinical improvement. By September, however, when Macleod returned, they had succeeded in developing an extract that would keep a diabetic animal alive indefinitely.

Banting and Best were elated but still faced the problem of developing a feasible method of hormone production for clinical use. It was hardly possible to sacrifice a gland-atrophied animal for every administration to a diabetic patient. They therefore spent the next several months searching for a method of obtaining a reliable supply of active "isletin."

Their strategies included stimulation of the pancreas to the point of exhaustion and extraction from whole fetal calf glands obtained from a local abattoir. The theory behind the latter was that the fetal gland might contain a higher proportion of islet and a lower proportion of digestive tissue than the mature pancreas. On November 17 Banting recorded a successful use of whole fetal gland "isletin." Some time passed before he and Best were able to find the right pH solution to repeat this result and still other possibilities were tested (Stevenson 1970, 441–42); Bliss (1982:91–92).

Neither Banting nor Best had received any stipend during the summer of 1921. Upon his return, however, Macleod arranged a formal appointment for Banting in the Department of Pharmacology. He put his own research on hold and concentrated his attention on the further purification of "isletin." At Banting's request, he enlisted James B. Collip, a young biochemist who had come to his department the previous spring. In January of 1922 Collip developed a fractional precipitation method that produced a whole gland extract pure enough for use with human patients. Macleod also suggested the name "insulin," which was used in the formal reports of the discovery.

Banting and Best first presented their research at the Physiological Journal Club of the University of Toronto in November. The following month, they made a joint report with Macleod to a meeting of the American Physiological Society, of which he was the president-elect (Stevenson 1970, 442; Collip 1942, 401; Best 1942, 400; 1959, 54).

On January 23, 1922, the first clinical trial of Collip's extract was conducted on a fourteen-year-old boy in Toronto General Hospital, who improved rapidly on daily doses. Throughout that year the two problems of commercial production and clinical guidelines were pursued simultaneously. Banting did some of the work on dosage determination. But he was neither a chemist nor a practiced clinician and was compelled to allow others to carry out most of these studies. Many researchers throughout the United States and Canada participated.

He had assigned his patent rights to the University of Toronto and the National Research Council of Canada. Collip's and Best's initial work was refined by themselves, Noble, E. L. Scott, J. Hepburn, and others in the university's Connaught Laboratories. An insulin product sufficiently concentrated to be mass-produced for clinical use was developed by the Eli Lilly Company and made commercially available by January 1923. Subsequent refinements were made by J. J. Abel of Baltimore, D. A. Scott of Toronto, and H. C. Hagedorn of Denmark.

Macleod concentrated his efforts on determining the mechanism of blood sugar reduction by insulin. He hypothesized that the significant action was increased oxidation and glycogen formation, an explanation later demonstrated experimentally by Best and others. Macleod's long-standing concern with respiration probably influenced his emphasis on oxygen and dismissal of the role of urinary dextrose/nitrogen ratio proposed by other authorities.

The clinical research on insulin was begun in Toronto by W. R. Campbell and A. A. Fletcher. Banting and Best had noted in their work with dogs that a large dose of the hormone resulted in hypoglycemia, which could be readjusted by glucose injections. Building on the studies of Frederick M. Allen, Campbell, Fletcher, and others soon determined that insulin was most effectively used in combination with diet therapy and careful monitoring of blood sugar levels, the approach still in use today (Stevenson 1970, 442–43; Best 1942, 399; Collip 1935, 1255).

Banting and Macleod were now international figures and were showered with honors. However, the role of others in the discovery was not clearly understood, a fact made clear when the 1923 Nobel Prize was awarded to them jointly, with no mention of Charles Best. Banting initially wanted to refuse the Nobel Prize but was convinced to accept it and to divide his share with Best. Macleod gave part of his award to Collip (Stevenson 1970, 443; 1973, 614–15; Best 1959, 54).

Macleod was made a Fellow of the Royal Society in 1923. He returned to Scotland in 1928 as Regius Professor of Physiology at Aberdeen University. He continued his researches at the university and the Rowett Institute, working on respiration, carbohydrate metabolism, and liver glycogen, until arthritis forced him to restrict his active involvement. He remained active guiding and directing students and colleagues until his death (Stevenson 1973, 615).

MARCIA MELDRUM

Selected Bibliography

PRIMARY SOURCES

Macleod, J. J. R., et al. 1902. *Practical Physiology*. London: E. Arnold.

Macleod, J. J. R., and Leonard Hill. 1906. *Recent Advances in Physiology*. New York: Longmans, Green.

Macleod, J. J. R. 1913. *Diabetes: Its Pathological Physiology*. New York: Longmans, Green.

Macleod, J. J. R., and R. G. Pearce. 1918. *Physiology and Biochemistry in Modern Medicine*. St. Louis: C. V. Mosby.

Macleod, J. J. R. 1926. *Carbohydrate Metabolism and Insulin*. New York: Longmans, Green.

SECONDARY SOURCES

Best, C. H. 1935. "The Late John James Rickard Macleod, M.B., Ch.B., LL.D., F.R.C.P." *Canadian Medical Association Journal* 32:556.

———. 1942. "Reminiscences of the Researches Which Led to the Discovery of Insulin." *Canadian Medical Association Journal* (November): 398–400.

———. 1959. "Sir Frederick Grant Banting." In *Dictionary of National Biography, 1941–1950*:53–55. London: Oxford University Press.

Bliss, Michael. 1982. *The Discovery of Insulin*. Chicago: University of Chicago Press.

Collip, J. B. 1935. "John James Rickard Macleod." *Biochemical Journal* 29:1253–56.

———. 1942. "Recollections of Sir Frederick Banting." *Canadian Medical Association Journal* 47 (November):401–403.

Harris, Seale. 1946. *Banting's Miracle: The Story of the Discoverer of Insulin*. Philadelphia: Lippincott.

Stevenson, Lloyd G. 1970. "Frederick Grant Banting." In *Dictionary of Scientific Biography*, I:440–443. New York: Scribners.

———. 1973. "John James Rickard Macleod." In *Dictionary of Scientific Biography*, VIII:614–615. New York: Scribners.

ILYA METCHNIKOFF *1908*

Ilya Ilyich Metchnikoff was born on May 16, 1845, near Ivanovka in the Russian Ukraine. The Nobel Prize in 1908 was awarded jointly to Metchnikoff and Paul Ehrlich "in recognition of their work on immunity." He died July 15, 1916, in Paris.

Metchnikoff's parents married around 1833 in St. Petersburg. Ilya Ivanovitch was an Imperial Guards officer from an aristocratic family. Emilia Lvovna was the daughter of Leo Nevahovitch, a Jewish writer who had converted to Christianity and held a government position. Discomfited by family responsibilities and the intolerant rule of Nicholas I (1825–55), Ilya Ivanovitch obtained a military sinecure and moved to a Ukrainian estate. A brother supervised stock raising, and Emilia directed the household. Ilya Ivanovitch became a remote personage submerged in provincial rounds—a "superfluous" man. An unwanted child, Ilya Ilyich entered this financially straitened home in 1845. Physically slight and vivacious like his mother, he became her favorite. The youngest of five children, he was neurotic but also charming, determined, and brilliant.

Ilya's thought was to be shadowed by the fates of three brothers. The eldest, Ivan Ilyich, rose to become a chief prosecutor but died at forty-five of stomach cancer—he was the subject of Tolstoy's tragic story, "The Death of Ivan Ilyich." Ilya's favorite, Leo, emigrated to the West, where he marched with Garibaldi and plotted revolution with Herzen and Bakunin; he died at age fifty of a heart attack. Ilya's "rival," Nicholas, a successful lawyer, died of a coronary at fifty-six. The cases of Ivan and Nicholas would be cited in Metchnikoff's philosophic writings.

A childhood tutor explained the plants and animals around the estate to Ilya, who determined to become a naturalist. At the Kharkov Lycée, his scientific precocity gained attention. With the advent of Alexander II in 1855, Western concepts—utilitarian, positivist, and materialist—swept the intelligentsia, preparing the way for the golden age of Russian science. Ilya eagerly read the daring books of Buckle, Büchner, and Vogt. Sympathetic to medicine and political reform, he nonetheless consecrated himself to furthering "positive" knowledge through basic science.

Graduating from the Lycée with highest honors in 1862, Metchnikoff set off for a German university but abruptly fled the strange surroundings. Chastened, he studied at Kharkov University, completing his courses in two years. Inspired by Darwin's theory, he published a paper on invertebrate morphology in 1863. In 1864 Metchnikoff went abroad for three years of research in Germany and Italy, where he met such leading biologists as Cohn, Henle, and Siebold. His bible was Fritz Müller's *Für Darwin* (1864), a work that heralded genetic connections between "lower" and "higher" animals. Allied views were elaborated by Haeckel in his "biogenetic principle" that individual development "recapitulates" earlier evolutionary stages. Working with Alexander Kavolevsky Metchnikoff mapped comparative embryology. Also, he found a patron in the physiologist, Sechenov.

Returning to Russia now aged twenty-two, Metchnikoff shared the Von Baer Prize with Kovlevsky and was appointed to Odessa University. Unbalanced by these triumphs, he willfully transferred to Petersburg University. Soon, a disappointing romance, zealous overwork, and poor laboratory facilities brought him close to breakdown. In 1869 he made a "rational" marriage to a sickly friend, Ludmilla Fédorovitch. The next years were a desperate struggle to rescue her from tuberculosis. Her death, in 1873, precipitated a suicide attempt.

Tormented by despair and poor health, Metchnikoff undertook travels through the steppe-lands to study the physical anthropology of the Kalmuck peoples. He returned to zoology at Odessa, and, in 1875, he married a young student, Olga Belokopitova. In 1879 his revered mother died, and in 1880 Olga endured severe typhoid fever. Meanwhile, the university's political atmosphere deteriorated, and Metchnikoff, an outspoken Darwinist, was labelled a "Red." The czar's assassination in 1881 unleashed the reactionaries and anti-Semites. Hopeless, Metchnikoff tried suicide again by injecting himself with relapsing-fever germs. Despite cardiac damage, he recovered; and the ordeal somehow restored his morale.

In 1882 Metchnikoff resigned from Odessa University and, providentially, became financially independent through an inheritance. He continued his research, looking for features in invertebrates he could correlate with vertebrate development. Metchnikoff was fascinated by amoebalike cells, of mesodermal origin, that digested food by absorption. He wanted to link such "wandering cells" with digestion in higher animals.

Metchnikoff's epochal discovery occurred in late 1882 in Messina, Sicily. He was watching (microscopically) "mobile cells of a transparent star-fish larva, when . . . suddenly . . . It struck me that similar cells might serve in the defence of the organism." He inserted tiny thorns into the larvae, and the next day observed mobile cells walling off the intrusions. This simple process he compared to accumulations of white blood cells in human inflammation. In an evolutionary context, he defined inflammation as "a reaction of the mesodermal cells against an external agent." He invented the term "Phago-cyte" (Gr. *phagein*, to eat), to connect defense with digestion. The pathologist Virchow encouraged him but warned that biomedical opinion generally would be hostile.

Metchnikoff extended his theory by studying the role of phagocytosis in metamorphosis and then in infectious disease. The fact that some infected animals succumbed, while others survived, brought up the question of "immunity." His paper on phagocytosis in anthrax (1884) aroused harsh criticism from the pathologist Baumgarten. At this time many scientists were seeking physicochemical explanations for biological phenomena. Ancient controversies reappeared: "solidism" (cells) against "humoralism" (sera); and "vitalism" versus "mechanism."

As director of the new Odessa Bacteriological Institute, Metchnikoff was able to investigate erysipelas, relapsing fever, and tuberculosis, and to publish (1887) a strong reply to Baumgarten. However, frustrated by the political and medical situation, he turned to the West for support of his ideas. Pasteur, who had battled for a cellular theory of fermentation, was sympathetic to phagocytosis and confided to Metchnikoff, "I at once placed myself on your side." In late 1888 he was installed (without salary) at the Pasteur Institute.

The first years in Paris were stressful, as new research bolstered humoralist immunology; and Behring's discovery of antitoxin and serotherapy won the limelight. Exhausted and depressed, Metchnikoff again considered suicide. Fortunately, he had steady reassurance from Pasteur, Roux, and Lister; and Cambridge University gave him an honorary degree (1891). Metchnikoff used his understanding of the natural history of immunology to deliver a powerful lecture series in 1891 on comparative pathology.

After 1895, immunologists increasingly reconciled elements from both the cellular and the humoral schools. As a senior director of the institute, Metchnikoff now felt more confident; students, among them Jules Bordet, helped expand his research to typhoid, typhus, and plague. In 1901 Metchnikoff published a comprehensive text on the immunology of infectious disease. The Nobel Prize was awarded in 1908. When he conferred with Leo Tolstoy in 1909, newspapers covered it like a summit of monarchs.

By the 1890s Metchnikoff himself was aging and experiencing cardiovascular symptoms. He went beyond these personal concerns to confront the larger social theme. Victories against infectious disease would benefit youth, only to reveal biomedicine's helplessness when faced with the "degenerative" diseases of middle and late life. Therefore, Metchnikoff began to elaborate militant philosophic schemes for scientific progress.

At the time, a cultural reaction was underway: the "revolt against positivism." Metchnikoff had much in common with French positivism, with its reliance on science and education and its desire for "order and progress." In 1903 he published the first of several books prophesying the scientific amelioration of human ills. Criticizing the upsurge of pessimism, he outlined an ideal life-pattern he termed "orthobiosis." Metchnikoff defended the chronically ill and handicapped from social-Darwinist views that they were "unfit" for expensive medical care. His "optimistic" writings reached a wide audience.

Independently of Freud, Metchnikoff focused on digestion, sex, and death as the major areas of "disharmony" between instinct and culture. Identifying sexuality as a pervasive force from childhood to advanced years, he challenged taboos and conventional interpretations. With Roux, he accomplished inoculation of syphilis into laboratory animals and also fashioned a preventative mercurous ointment.

To study and control senescence, Metchnikoff proposed the establishment of a new scientific discipline he named "gerontology." Observing age-related changes, he noted that phagocytes were removing certain cells, which he believed to be weakened, over time, by toxins. He speculated that the poisons originated in intestinal putrefaction, and he reported favorable results from ingestion of yogurt (lactobacilli).

In 1911 Metchnikoff returned to the Kalmuck people in Russia, leading an epidemiological investigation of tuberculosis. Appalled by conditions in the czarist empire, he felt drawn to the revolutionary intellectuals. Back in France, he sensed the threats of chauvinism and militarism. In his last writings, he inclined to a sort of positivist socialism.

Metchnikoff suffered a cardiac crisis in 1913; the next year, World War I broke out. He was dismayed by the virtual closing of the Pasteur Institute and considered the war to be a "criminal" relapse to "savagery." He had accepted his own life limits but had expected the next generations to advance to healthful, greatly prolonged life. On his seventieth birthday he wrote, "the powerlessness of medicine grieves me more and more, and . . . the war has interrupted all the work against disease." Moribund with congestive heart failure, it remained for him to set an example of uncompromising rationalism.

He died at age seventy-one in July 1916. It was the time of the Battle of Verdun, a holocaust of the young generation. After the war, the Pasteur Institute resumed its research; a revered urn contained the ashes of Metchnikoff. Revolutionary Russia named many biomedical facilities after Metchnikoff. In 1938 the first Congress on Aging convened in Kiev, and, in 1962, the USSR Institute of Gerontology was organized. In the United States, conferences in the 1930s led to formation of the Gerontological Society (1945) and eventually to the National Institute on Aging (1974). Immunology has expanded into virology, organ transplantation, and cancer research as well as gerontology and cardiology. And Metchnikoff's humanistic meliorism remains a vital philosophic theme.

GERALD J. GRUMAN

Selected Bibliography

PRIMARY SOURCES

Metchnikoff, Élie. 1892. *Leçons sur la pathologie comparée de l'inflammation, faites à l'institut Pasteur en 1891.* Paris: Masson, 1892. *Lectures on the Comparative Pathology of Inflammation, Delivered at the Pasteur Institute in 1891.* Translated by F. A. and E. H. Starling. London: Paul, 1893.

———. 1901. *L'immunité dans les maladies infectieuses.* Paris: Masson. *Immunity in Infective Diseases.* Translated by Francis G. Binnie. Cambridge: Cambridge University Press, 1905.

———. 1903. *Études sur la nature humaine, essai de philosophie optimiste.* Paris: Masson. *The Nature of Man: Studies in Optimistic Philosophy.* Translated and edited by P. Chalmers Mitchell. London: Heinemann, 1906.

———. 1906. *The New Hygiene: Three Lectures on the Prevention of Infectious Diseases.* Translated and edited by E. Ray Lankester. London: Heinemann, 1906.

———. 1907. *Essais optimistes.* Paris. *The Prolongation of Life: Optimistic Studies.* Translated and edited by P. Chalmers Mitchell. London: Heinemann, 1907.

SECONDARY SOURCES

Brieger, Gert H. 1974. "Élie Metchnikoff." In *Dictionary of Scientific Biography,* 9:331–35. New York: Charles Scribner's Sons.

Freeman, Joseph T. 1983. "Metchnikoff on Aging, 'Satiety of Life,' and Natural Death." Paper presented to 36th Annual Meeting of Gerontological Society of America (San Francisco, October 1983). In manuscript.

Karnovsky, Manfred L. 1981. "Metchnikoff in Messina: A Century of Studies on Phagocytosis." *New England Journal of Medicine* 304 (May 7):1178–80.

Metchnikoff, Olga. 1921. *Life of Élie Metchnikoff: 1845–1916.* Translated and edited by E. Ray Lankester. Boston: Houghton Mifflin. This book includes a useful bibliography.

Zeiss, Heinz. 1932. *Elias Metschnikow: Leben und Werk.* Jena: G. Fischer. This volume consists of an abridged translation of the above biography, plus many pages of excellent notes, correspondence, photographs, and a very thorough bibliography.

PETER BRIAN MEDAWAR *1960*

Peter Brian Medawar was born on February 28, 1915, in Rio de Janeiro, Brazil, to Nicholas Medawar, a Lebanese businessman, and his British wife, Edith Muriel Dowling. Trained as a zoologist, Medawar was a major force in establishing immunology as an independent discipline. Medawar's clinical and experimental work on skin transplantation led him to establish the laws of transplantation. He shared the Nobel prize in Physiology or Medicine with Sir Frank Macfarlane

Burnet in 1960 for his studies of "acquired immunological tolerance."

Medawar's family emigrated to England when he was four. The child received a quintessential upper-class British education, first at Marlborough College, the famous public school in Wiltshire, then at Magdalen College, Oxford University, where he graduated with a first-class honors degree in zoology in 1935. As an undergraduate Medawar had started some research on cellular cultures; after receiving his degree he was awarded two grants from Magdalen College to continue his work under Howard Florey, in the William Dunn School of Pathology at Oxford. Medawar early displayed his two poles of interest, experimentation and theoretical biology. At the same time he was working in the lab on embryo cell (mainly nervous) cultures, he embarked upon a study of the mathematical functions that might account for the patterns of cell growth, in the manner of D'Arcy Thompson, whose book, *Form and Function*, greatly influenced him.

Working with Florey, Medawar became involved in a program of research on lymph and lymphocytes, the function of which was still unknown. A new recruit in the laboratory was Jean Shinglewood Taylor, who was to become Mrs. Medawar in 1937; the couple eventually had two sons and two daughters. In 1938 Medawar received a prize for his work and became a fellow of Magdalen College. Though he retained his fellowship until 1944, he was recruited, during the war, to work with the surgeon Tom Gibson on the excruciating problem of tissue transplants at the Burns Unit of the Glasgow Royal Infirmary. Skin was almost valueless for covering wounds, as surgeons had long known that skin borrowed from another person sloughs off after a while.

In 1943, Medawar made an extensive review of the literature on transplantation. He classified the extant theories into three categories: those that explained rejection as "natural immunity," a consequence of the genetic make-up of individuals (blood groups); those that claimed that the graft was "toxic"; and those that explained rejection as an active immunization against foreign antigens (mainly through antibodies). At the same time, Medawar was studying the behavior of grafts in humans and in experimental models (mainly outbred rabbits). He introduced the term "second set" for the accelerated rejection seen in the recipient after a second graft from the same donor. Through analogy with active immunization against bacteria or other invaders, he acknowledged this phenomenon as immunological, since memory is the hallmark of the immune response.

Medawar was at first committed to the role of antibodies in rejection. Only in 1946 did he make it clear that the blood of rejecting rabbits does not display any antibody and that the capacity of rejection is not transferable with the serum. He came to oppose his compatriot Peter Gorer who, working in London on tumor transplantation in mice, believed antibodies to be the source of rejection. Moreover, Medawar developed the idea that graft rejection is analogous to delayed hypersensitivity reactions such as the response to the tuberculin test, an inflammatory reaction where lymphocytes are predominantly involved. This peculiar kind of immunity is transferable by cells and only by cells. Medawar argued that cellular immunity and antibody-mediated immunity were two sets of independent phenomena. This work led to his election as a fellow of the Royal Society in 1949.

In 1947 Medawar went to Birmingham University as Mason Professor of Zoology; four years later he moved to the University of London, to become Jodrell Professor of Zoology. In 1949, attending a congress in Stockholm, he was prompted by a Scottish geneticist, Dr. Donald, to solve a current issue in veterinary practice: distinguishing between dizygotic and monozygotic (identical) twins. According to the current knowledge, only the latter should accept skin or organ grafts. Surprisingly, working in the mud of a Staffordshire farm with R. E. Billingham, Medawar discovered that both categories of twin bulls could accept grafts. From Dr. Donald's and Macfarlane Burnet's book, *The Production of Antibodies*, Medawar learned about Ray Owen's observation of the existence of twin cattle chimeras, suggesting that blood exchange could induce an abnormal response of acceptance or tolerance. Burnet had hypothesized that the organism during its embryonic life learns to differentiate between its "biological self" and nonself. Medawar, Billingham, and Leslie Brent prepared a test of Burnet's idea, trying to reproduce the mutual tolerance they had observed in twin cattle by presenting moelcules (antigens) to an organism during embryo life. They injected fetal or newborn mice with tissue from a mouse of a different strain and were able to watch what Burnet had predicted a priori: "acquired immune tolerance." Once grown up, the mice would accept skin grafts from the previous donor. This tolerance was highly specific.

This kind of experimental tolerance was not immediately reproducible in humans, but the very idea of it fostered great expectations among physicians. The problem of transplantation, as Medawar had predicted in 1944, now belonged to the "art of the soluble;" indeed, it became "negotiable", again in Medawar's own terms (Medawar 1958). If tolerance was primarily a natural phenomenon, artificial tolerance could be induced in animals and possibly in man. Cortisone, for instance, was soon demonstrated to be highly effective in weakening a rabbit's capacity to reject grafts. Medawar's, Billingham's, and Brent's studies led to the current status of organ transplantation.

The immunology of transplantation was important not merely for its bearing on medical treatment but because it offered a royal pathway into biology's biggest problems. Tolerance was not limited to a lack of reactivity during neonatal life but was also a "general modality of the immune response" (Medawar 1956) that involved active cells. Immunology shifted to a central position in biology: "No other one property [incompatibility] discriminates so finely between an individual and another" (Medawar 1957).

In 1962 Medawar was appointed director of the National Institute for Medical Research at Mill Hill, London. There he supervised biomedical research projects, including studies on the antilymphocyte serum that, it was hoped, would help in delaying graft rejection. He conducted his own career in harmony with the advice he lavished on beginners in research (Medawar 1979). At this point, science administration seemed the best way he could contribute to the advancement of learning. Already a member of many scientific committees, Medawar became president of the British Association for the Advancement of Science in 1969.

At age fifty-four, at the peak of his career, Medawar suffered a cerebral hemorrhage. The stroke left him with a paralyzed left arm and leg. With the untiring support of his wife, who played an increasingly large role in his scientific life, Medawar fought adversity with great courage and returned to work. He resigned his directorship of the national Institute for Medical Research in 1971 (he was named director emeritus in 1975) but was able to pursue his research interests in the newly opened Clinical Research Center of the Medical Research Council in London; his work there bore mainly on tumor immunology. He used transplantation methods to investigate antigens shared by embryos and tumors, a still poorly understood phenomenon, thus returning to his first scientific love, embryology. In 1977 he became professor of experimental medicine at the Royal Institution. He received the Royal Medal in 1959 and the Copley Medal of the Royal Society in 1969. He was knighted in 1965. He was a member of the Royal Society and of the American Academy of Arts and Sciences.

In his later years Medawar wrote a number of books. *The Uniqueness of the Individual* (1957), a collection of essays, deals brilliantly with the issue of biological individuality, among other evolutionary problems. *Induction and Intuition in Scientific Thought* (1969) takes a scientific approach to philosophical issues. In *The Hope of Progress* (1972) Medawar predicted overpopulation in terms recalling Malthus, while at the same time dissecting the inconsistencies of social applications of Darwinian biology. *The Life Sciences: Current Ideas of Biology* (1976) provides students with a review of the whole field of biology. In *Memoir of a Thinking Radish* (1986) Medawar sketched his life and career. He died on October 2, 1987.

ANNE MARIE MOULIN

Selected Bibliography

PRIMARY SOURCES

Medawar, P. B. 1944. "The Behavior and Fate of Skin Autografts and Skin Homografts in Rabbits." *Journal of Anatomy* 78:176–199.

Medawar, P. B., R. E. Billingham, and L. Brent. 1953. "Actively Acquired Tolerance of Foreign Cells in Newborn Animals." *Nature* 172:603–606.

Medawar, P. B. 1956. "A Discussion on

Immunological Tolerance." *Proceedings of the Royal Society of London* 146:1–8.

———. 1957. *The Uniqueness of the Individual.* New York: Dover.

———. 1958. "The Immunology of Transplantation." *Harvey Lectures* 52:144–176.

———. 1960. *The Future of Man.* London: Methuen.

———. 1969. *Induction and Intuition in Scientific Thought.* London: Methuen.

———. 1972. *The Hope of Progress.* London: Methuen.

———. 1976. *The Life Sciences: Current Ideas of Biology.* New York: Harper and Row.

———. 1979. *Advice to a Young Scientist.* New York: Harper.

Medawar, P. B., and J. S. Medawar. 1983. *Aristotle to Zoos. A Philosophical Dictionary of Biology.* Cambridge, MA: Harvard University Press.

Medawar, P. B. 1986. *Memoir of a Thinking Radish. An Autobiography.* Oxford: Oxford University Press.

SECONDARY SOURCES

Billingham, R. E. 1974. "Reminiscences of a Transplanter." *Transplantation Proceedings* 6:5–17.

Lewin, R. 1981. "Lamarck Will Not Lie Down." *Science* 213:316–321.

Mitchison, N. A. 1987. "In Memoriam." *Immunogeuetica* 27:303.

Moulin, A. M., and I. Löwy, 1983. "La double nature de l'immunologie: histoire de la transplantation rénale." *Fundamenta scientiae* 3:201–218.

1987. Obituary. *British Medical Journal* 295:1072–1073.

OTTO FRITZ MEYERHOF *1922*

Otto Meyerhof was born in 1884, into a comfortable middle-class Jewish home in Hanover, Germany, the second child and first son of Felix Meyerhof, a merchant, and his wife Bettina (née May). In 1914, after completing medical studies, Meyerhof married Hedwig Schallenberg; the couple had two sons and one daughter. His research on cellular bioenergetics was focused for many years on the metabolic changes that occur during the contraction of voluntary muscle. He shared the Nobel Prize for 1922 with A. V. Hill, whose work focused on the biophysics of heat generation by voluntary muscle. In later years Meyerhof's interests encompassed a wide range of problems in physiological chemistry and enzyme regulation, to which he made substantial and lasting contributions. He left Germany in 1938 and eventually arrived in the United States at the end of 1940, where a position was created for him at the University of Pennsylvania. He died suddenly in Philadelphia in 1951.

Meyerhof's lifelong concern with philosophical and psychological questions began while he was still a young man. His initial research experience was in psychiatry, which he studied for his 1909 doctoral thesis at the University of Heidelberg. Shortly afterwards he moved to the Heidelberg Klinik where a slightly younger colleague, Otto Warburg, was pursuing the causes of cancer. Warburg's experimental approach was to explore the chemical reactions with the living cell and the changes that occurred when a normal cell became cancerous. Impressed by Warburg's ideas and energy, Meyerhof joined him in a study of cell respiration, working for a period at the world-famous Stazione Zoologica, in Naples, on biochemical changes in fertilized sea urchin eggs. This experience was to shape the rest of Meyerhof's career. His scientific contributions can be grouped under three main headings: 1) the bioenergetics of muscle contraction; 2) elucidation of the metabolic pathways involved in glycolysis; and 3) the discovery of energy-rich phosphorylated intermediates in metabolism.

After World War I, and following his move to the Department of Physiology at the University of Kiel, Meyerhof became totally absorbed in the experimental work on muscle biochemistry for which he was awarded a share of the Nobel Prize. Not surprisingly, that work was built on foundations created by other research. Previous work in the Physiological Laboratory, at Cambridge, had shown that muscle contraction was associated with the production of lactic acid, which then disappeared in the presence of oxygen. A. V. Hill had taken thermal measurements of muscle and determined that the heat produced was proportional to the rate of appearance of lactic acid. In 1918 Meyerhof started his own experiments on the biochemical phenomena associated with muscular contraction, greatly assisted by a new, faster microtechnique for the estimation of lactic acid. He amplified the earlier work, showing that lactic acid production was proportional to the mechanical work performed by the muscle and that the source of the lactic acid was the carbohydrate glycogen. He also showed, most importantly, that during the recovery period, oxygen consumption accounted for less than a third of the subsequent breakdown of the lactic acid into carbon dioxide and water. The remaining energy was utilized in regenerating glycogen from the lactic acid. This hypothesis, known as the Meyerhof cycle, provided a chemical explanation of A. V. Hill's thermodynamic results. While substantially correct, the cycle's precise details were not worked out for another twenty years. In essence the cycle begins with muscle carbohydrate (glycogen) being broken down to lactic acid, a process that generates energy. Excess lactic acid diffuses from the muscle into the blood stream and is carried to the liver, where it is used to synthesize glycogen, which in turn is metabolized into glucose. In this form it is transported by the blood back to the muscles. The glucose is reconverted into glycogen, which can then be broken down into lactic acid again, thus restarting what is now known as the Cori cycle (Kalckar 1983).

Both the bioenergetic work of Meyerhof and the thermodynamic experiments of Hill attempted to explain the cellular mechanisms of a physiological function in a living cell. This complementary work resulted in the joint award of the Nobel Prize in 1922. Shortly afterward Meyerhof was appointed to the Kaiser Wilhelm Institute for Biology in Berlin. In 1929 he became head of the Department of Physiology at the Kaiser Wilhelm Institute for Medical Research in Heidelberg.

During these years Meyerhof made some of his most important contributions. Several of his earlier results, particularly those that suggested that lactic acid itself played a central role in muscle contraction, were found to be incomplete, and work by a number of biochemists, including Meyerhof himself, further defined the steps of muscle metabolism. Other scientists had observed that cell-free yeast extracts could ferment glucose to alcohol. In 1925 he made a major breakthrough in isolating, from muscle cells, the enzymes responsible for the glycolytic pathway, thereby explaining how energy-rich glucose was broken down within the cell. These were two important steps in establishing that regulatory cell processes could occur in vitro if the required substrate was added. Meyerhof's discovery that such enzymes could be isolated from mammalian cells and therefore studied further, opened up a whole new phase in the study of cell bioenergetics. Not only Meyerhof but also many other biochemists were enabled to study the details of the multiple chemical reactions involved in cell metabolism.

A major promoter of this work was Meyerhof's countryman, Gustav Embden, who, by the early 1930s, proposed an outline for the complete sequence of reactions involved in the utilization of glucose by the cell. Mapping out the details of the metabolic pathways took a large number of people many years, but Meyerhof and his small group of associates, particularly Karl Lohmann, assisted in the diligent unravelling of the complex steps in the cycle, now known as the Embden-Meyerhof pathway. The understanding of these metabolic pathways is now regarded as a cornerstone of modern biochemistry.

Intimately associated with such work were experiments on high energy phosphorylated compounds, such as phosphocreatinine, and particularly the isolation by Lohmann of adenosine triphosphate (ATP). Their roles as "energy-carriers," able to release and accept free energy in the form of chemical bonding, elucidated the relationship between metabolic and mechanical events. In particular, it revealed that the utilization and subsequent resynthesis of ATP maintained the glycolytic cycle. After the discovery in 1930 by E. Lundgaard that muscle could contract without forming lactic acid, Meyerhof abandoned the hypothesis that lactic acid was necessary for muscle contraction. Further experiments showed that the splitting of ATP and its resynthesis in parallel with phosphocreatinine breakdown, with the subsequent production of lactic acid, was the critical chemical reaction associated with muscular contraction (Kalcker 1976, 28). This experimental work also showed that the basic biochemical mechanisms in a yeast cell were fundamentally similar to those in a mammalian cell. An important consequence of Meyerhof's approach was the demonstration of the similarity of biochemical processes in a wide variety of life-forms.

The rise of the Nazi party in Germany caused Meyerhof, like many Jewish scientists, to leave his homeland. He first sought asylum in France, then briefly in Spain, and finally came to the United States, where he became a citizen in 1946. Such personal disturbances seriously disrupted his professional work. By the time of his death he had reestablished his laboratory and was once more engaged in significant research. Many of his colleagues, not only in obituary notices and tributes to Meyerhof, but also in their own autobiographical accounts, remember him as a genial, encouraging man, whose particular inspiration was, by example, as an experimenter.

E. M. TANSEY

Selected Bibliography

PRIMARY SOURCES

Meyerhof, O. 1922. "Energy Conversions in Muscle." Nobel Lecture. Reprinted in *Nobel Lectures in Physiology or Medicine*, vol. 2 (1922–1941), 27–41. Amsterdam: Elsevier, 1965.

———. 1924. *Chemical Dynamics of Life Phenomena*. Monographs on Experimental Biology. Philadelphia: J. B. Lippincott.

SECONDARY SOURCES

Florkin, M., and E. H. Stotz. 1975. *Comprehensive Biochemistry*. Vol. 31, *A History of Biochemistry*, Part 3, "History of the Identification of Sources of Free Energy in Organisms." Amsterdam: Elsevier.

Hill, A. V. 1950. "A Challenge to Biochemists." *Biochimica et Biophysica Acta* 4:4–11. Meyerhof Commemoration Volume.

Kalckar, H. M. 1983. "The Isolation of Cori-ester, 'the Saint Louis Gateway' to a First Approach of a Dynamic Formulation of Macromolecular Biosynthesis." In *Comprehensive Biochemistry*. Vol. 35, *Selected Topics in the History of Biochemistry, Personal Recollections*, part 1, edited by A. Neuberger, L. L. M. van Deenen and G. Semenza, 1–24. Amsterdam: Elsevier.

———. 1976. "Origins of the Concept of Oxidative Phosphorylation: Retrospectives and Perspectives." In *Reflections on Biochemistry*, edited by A. Kornberg, B. L. Horecker, L. Cornudella, and J. Oro, 27–32. Oxford: Pergamon Press.

Nachmansohn, D. 1979. "Otto Meyerhof." In *German-Jewish Pioneers in Science, 1900–1933*, 268–311. Berlin: Springer-Verlag.

Peters, R. A. 1954. "Otto Meyerhof 1884–1951." *Obituary Notices of Fellows of the Royal Society* 9:175–200.

CESAR MILSTEIN 1984

The 1984 Nobel Prize in Physiology or Medicine was awarded to three immunologists: Cesar Milstein, Georges Köhler and Niels K. Jerne. Milstein and Köhler were cited for developing a successful technique of antibody production that had far-reaching applications in numerous areas of biology and medicine because it yielded well-defined, "pure" antibodies in unlimited amounts.

The Argentinian biochemist Cesar Milstein was born in Bahia Bianca, the second of three sons of Lazaro Milstein, a schoolteacher, and Maxima Milstein. He was educated at the Colegio Nacional of Bahia Bianca and took his degree in chemistry at the University of Buenos Aires in 1952. In 1953 Milstein married Celia Prilleltensky, now a distinguished biochemist in her own right. In order to make a living, he worked part-time at the Liebeschutz Laboratories as a technician in clinical biochemistry, remaining there until 1956. The situation in Argentina was not easy for apprentice scientists. Despite few opportunities for professional positions, Milstein decided to orient himself toward basic science, and worked toward a doctorate in biochemistry under A. O. Stoppani at the medical school of Buenos Aires. Milstein's first research was aimed at the elucidation of the function of certain sulfhydrile groups in aldehyde dehydrogenase, the enzyme that allows the oxidation of ethyl alcohol.

After receiving his doctorate in 1957, Milstein was hired by the Instituto Nacional de Microbiologia, but almost immediately he was awarded a fellowship from the British Council. He arrived in Cambridge just when Sanger was elucidating protein sequences by using radioactive markers. Milstein began studying the conditions of activity of some enzymes important in glucidic metabolism (phosphoglucomutase). Sanger pointed out to him the importance of sequencing the active site of the enzyme. Using radioactive labeling combined with other biochemical techniques, Milstein was able to establish the entire sequence of the enzyme. Consequently, he received a Ph.D. from Cambridge University in 1960. After briefly joining the staff of the Medical Research Council at the Department of Biochemistry, he took a position in Argentina as head of the newly created Division of Molecular Biology at the Instituto Nacional de Microbiologia.

This was a very promising time; the recently appointed director, Ignacio Pirosky, was developing the institute on a new basis, with the help of enthusiastic young scientists. Milstein pursued his work on the elucidation of enzymatic active sites. But after a military coup in Buenos Aires and the sudden dismissal of many scientists in the National Association of Scientists, including Pirosky himself, Milstein resigned in protest. Offered a job at Cambridge by Sanger, Milstein in 1963 returned to England, where he still lives.

Milstein shifted to the study of antibodies or immunoglobulins (molecules produced by lymphocytes when the organism is challenged by antigens, like vaccines). The enzyme-substrate interaction has been a model for antibodies and a source of inspiration for immunologists since Paul Ehrlich's early studies. Milstein compared the primary sequences of antibodies in order to understand differences in their specificity, or power of binding defined antigens. By 1965 he had become a member of the "Invisible College" of biologists trying to understand the molecular nature of antibody diversity. In the course of his research he became aware of the variability of certain antibody regions and came to support the hypothesis of a distinct genetic control for constant and variable parts of the antibody molecule. He found that the study of structural homologies in antibodies could provide clues for the evolution of a large group of molecules later named the immunoglobulin superfamily.

Typical for a biochemist, Milstein tried to link structure and function, applying this approach successively to all the fashionable molecules: enzymes, antibodies, nucleic acids like messenger RNA (mRNA turned out to be less rewarding than expected) and, finally, tumor antigens.

Myelomas are malignant tumors of the immune system. Their proliferating cells, derived from antibody-producing lymphocytes, produce large amounts of antibodies identical in their chemical structure. The antibodies are an invaluable source for the study of the byproducts of immunization, from both the chemical and genetic viewpoints. Myelomas yield huge quantities of "pure" antibodies, which permitted Edelman to sequence the first human immunoglobulin. Tumor cells are easy to cultivate, in contrast to normal cells like lymphocytes, which perish quickly. Milstein's research led him to become trained in the entirely new (for him) field of cell cultures.

The antibody response is not homogeneous. If an antigen, even a chemically pure one, is introduced into the body, the organism will respond with a mixture of antibodies directed against different patterns on the molecule and of variable affinity (forming very stable or easily-dissociated complexes). No "natural antisera" are the same; this situation makes experiments difficult to reproduce.

According to Macfarlane Burnet's theory, each lymphocyte, or clone, has a unique receptor specificity and is therefore precommitted to make only one antibody of defined specificity and affinity after antigenic stimulation. Milstein realized that the mass production of these clones would provide perfect pure reagents and would achieve the goal of early immunologists: absolute specificity.

The purpose of hybridoma technology is simple. Lymphocytes are not easily cultivated, in contrast with the easy growth of tumor cells. The problem can be solved by fusing myeloma cells (virtually immortal) and lymphocytes (sensitized against a given antigen) in order to establish a continuous line of antibody-producing cells. The technology itself resulted from advances in several unrelated fields of research: cell culture techniques, somatic cell genetics, and immunology.

During the 1950s, cell cultures were becoming routine laboratory procedures, setting the stage for the first hybridization attempts. In 1960 Barski had observed occasional spontaneous fusion of mouse tumor cells in culture. Okada and Tadokoro observed in 1962 that virus infection could increase considerably the number of fusions; the first virus widely utilized after 1965 was the Sendai virus, a paramyxovirus. Littlefield in 1964 provided a medium that made it easy to select hybrids by killing parental cells unable to survive unless complementing each other's deficiencies.

Milstein first studied the rate and nature of somatic mutation of myeloma cells in culture. He did not find evidence for a hypermutable segment. But his collaborator, Richard Cotton, prepared another experiment that involved the fusion of two myelomas from rats and mice. These hybrid cells produced both parental types of immunoglobulin, while usually only one type is produced (this phenomenon is named "allelic exclusion"). Working along these lines, Milstein was attracted to the possibility of realizing hybrids with myeloma cells and antibody-producing lymphocytes. These hybrids might help to provide the immunologist with his dream: tailor-made antibodies of a desired specificity, in infinite quantity. To Milstein, these hybrids seemed to be appropriate for the study of how somatic cells diversify in culture and how mutations modify the combining specificity of antibodies.

The stage was set for the final improvement by Georges Köhler, a young post-doctoral fellow who had come to Cambridge from Switzerland. Köhler immunized a mouse against sheep red blood cells. He then removed the spleen cells and fused them with a myeloma line. A fusion is a rare event; many hybrids perish. Out of 10^8 spleen cells, one might get about one hundred good hybrids against the selected antigen. And the surviving hybrids from colonies still have to be cloned, a tedious business, and tested for specificity. Milstein's and Köhler's work finally resulted in the obtainment of specific antibody-forming hybridomas, which they could store and dispatch to their friends and colleagues. They published their procedures for the production of the so-called monoclonal antibodies in 1975 (Milstein and Köhler 1975).

Within ten years, hybridoma technology had spawned a multimillion dollar industry. Antibodies could be raised *in vitro* against virtually any antigen, and these antibodies would be highly specific and capable of being produced in unlimited quantities. Milstein and Köhler in their seminal paper of 1975 had acknowledged that "such cultures would be valuable for medical and industrial use."

Monoclonal antibodies have been increasingly used as research reagents, for the purification of antigens, and for the detection or identification of antigens (e.g., tumor antigens). An interesting new area of study, originated by Milstein himself, was the dissection of subpopulations of lymphocytes according to the receptors on the surface (Milstein 1977), which was crucial to a new vision of the immune system and the understanding of the AIDS virus's pathogenicity against the lymphocyte. The technology continues to extend further into many areas of the biological sciences, with the medical developments the most well known. Therapeutic agents, especially in cancer, are being developed. This technology has attracted scientists and investors in biotechnology because monoclonal antibodies provide useful "kits," easily available in many medical fields, for quicker and more accurate diagnosis of diseases.

Köhler and Milstein did not patent their technique (Wade 1980). Milstein had asked the recipients of his hybrids to respect a gentlemen's agreement and reserve his position. A bitter polemic occurred between British and American researchers when, in 1979, a team from the Wistar Institute in Philadelphia successfully patented the basic hybridoma technology as it applied to tumor and viral antigens (Koprowski and Croce 1980). Milstein emphasized that the hybridoma technology was a by-product of basic research, in his case "messing about with isotopes and enzymes and antibodies" (Milstein 1982). He did not want to let the world of lawyers regulate science; he advocated intellectual freedom for scientists and complained about the perversity of a patenting system that impedes the flow of information and enforces the privileges of developed countries.

Milstein went on to develop hybridomas for various purposes, but eventually returned to his original project of immunogenetics. He invented a cascading procedure for obtaining antibodies against rare determinants. He investigated "hybrid" hybridomas expressing the two parental antibodies (Milstein 1982). However remote from "natural" antibodies that express antibodies of only one specificity, these far-fetched molecules provide fascinating insights into the genetic regulation of antibody production. With his collaborators, Milstein developed hybridomas raised against an artificial antigen as a system model for the study of the immune response and studied the variations of sequence and affinity of the corresponding messenger RNAs. In many ways, the immune response displays the features of "a Darwinian system," where adaptation (an improvement in antigen-binding) is the crucial feature.

Throughout his career, Milstein has been a very creative biologist; his intellectual leadership in the Cambridge circle played a major role in the unparalleled development of hybridoma technology in the United Kingdom. He also maintained a firm stand against the repeated infringements on human rights in Latin America and on many occasions joined the movement of protest against political repression in Argentina.

Since 1969 Milstein has been a

member of the governing board of the Laboratory of Molecular Biology. He was appointed head of the Protein and Nucleic Acid Chemistry Division at the Medical Research Council Laboratory in 1983.

Milstein is a foreign member of the American Academy of Science, a member of the Royal Society and of the Royal College of Physicians of London, and a member of the European Molecular Biology Organization. He has been awarded the Silver Jubilee Medal (1977), the Avery-Landsteiner Preis (1979), the Wolf Foundation Prize and the Louisa Gross-Horowitz Prize of Columbia University (1980), the Gardner Foundation Award (1981), the Gimenez Diaz Medal (1981), and the Royal Medal of the Royal Society (1982).

ANNE MARIE MOULIN

Selected Bibliography

PRIMARY SOURCES

Milstein, C., and G. K. Köhler. 1975. "Continuous Cultures of Fused Cells Producing Antibody of Predefined Specificity." *Nature* 256:495–97.

Milstein, C. 1980. "Monoclonal Antibodies." *Scientific American* 243: 66–74.

———. 1982. "Messing About with Isotypes and Enzymes and Antibodies." In *From Gene to Protein: Translation into Biotechnology*, edited by F. Ahmad et al. New York: Academic Press.

———. 1986. "From Antibody Structure to Immunological Diversification of Immune Response." *Science* 231:1261–68.

SECONDARY SOURCES

Cambrosio, A., and P. Keating. 1988. "Going Monoclonal: Art, Science, and Magic in the Day-to-Day Use of Hybridoma Technology." *Social Problems* 35:244–60.

Fazekas de St. Groth, S. 1985. "Monoclonal Antibody Production: Principles and Practice." In *Handbook of Monoclonal Antibodies: Applications in Biology and Medicine*, edited by S. Ferrone and M. P. Dierich, 1–10. Park Ridge, N.J.: Noyes Publications.

Koprowski H. and C. Croce. 1980. "Hybridomas Revisited." *Science* 210:248.

Shay, J. W. 1985. "Human Hybridomas and Monoclonal Antibodies." In *Human Hybridomas and Monoclonal Antibodies*, edited by E. G. Engleman, 5–20. New York: Plenum Press.

Wade, N. 1980. "Inventor of Hybridoma Technology Failed to File for a Patent." *Science* 208:693.

GEORGE RICHARDS MINOT
1934

Born into a prominent Brahmin family in Boston, Massachusetts, on December 2, 1885, Minot was the eldest son of the physician James Jackson Minot and Elizabeth Whitney Minot. He married Marian Linzee Weld on June 29, 1915, and fathered three children: Marian, Elizabeth, and Charles. An internist specializing in disorders of the blood, he received the 1934 Nobel Prize for "discoveries concerning liver therapy in cases of anemia." He died in Boston on February 25, 1950.

As a youth, Minot developed a strong interest in natural history. An avid lepidopterist, he published his first article when he was seventeen years old in the *Entomological News.* This early emphasis on careful observation and cataloging was excellent preparation for Minot's career as a clinical researcher.

Following in the Minot family tradition, George entered Harvard College and received a B.A. in 1908. He then matriculated at Harvard Medical School where he developed his interest in hematology under the tutelage of J. Homer Wright. Occasionally accompanying his father on rounds, Minot was exposed to a traditional clinical model that strongly emphasized diet and environment. After graduation in 1912, Minot worked at the Johns Hopkins Medical School, pursuing hematologic research in the laboratory of William H. Howell.

These early experiences equipped Minot with an intellectual framework that combined three key elements: 1) the natural historian's observation skills; 2) the physiologist's belief in laboratory-based experimental models; and 3) the clinician's traditional recognition of the importance of environmental influences on health and disease. This unique combination was a key element in Minot's extraordinarily successful career in clinical research.

Minot returned to Harvard in 1915 with the rank of assistant in medicine and found an environment increasingly supportive of clinical research. The opening of the Rockefeller Institute for Medical Research in 1910 provided a model of clinical research that many elite institutions sought to emulate. With the appointment of David Edsall as chief of medical services in 1912, the Massachusetts General Hospital (MGH) demonstrated its intention to bring scientific research to the bedside. Edsall, the first chief of medicine at the MGH from outside the Harvard sphere, firmly supported clinical research. Minot can be seen as an important transitional figure in the history of the MGH, with his family providing him with the social background so important for the "old" MGH and his scientific training providing him with the credentials critical to Edsall's "new" MGH.

Minot began to investigate

blood dyscrasias, initially studying alongside his old mentor, Wright. By fusing the descriptive techniques central to Wright's morphology with the new physiologic emphasis on function he had learned at Johns Hopkins, Minot became the first to recognize the fundamental importance of reticulocytes.

Reticulocytes are the earliest form of red blood cells that appear in the circulation. The number of reticulocytes in a blood smear provide a measure of bone marrow function. When Wright introduced Minot to a new staining technique that permitted the observation of these young cells, Minot rapidly grasped their significance. As an index of bone marrow function the number of reticulocytes could be used to classify anemias. Anemia associated with low reticulocyte counts stemmed from inadequate production of red blood cells. In contrast, anemias that were caused by the excessive destruction of red cells could be expected to have high reticulocyte counts as a patient's normal bone marrow sought to correct the anemia. In addition to this important diagnostic function, the reticulocyte count could also be used to monitor therapy with a change in the reticulocyte count serving as an indicator of therapeutic response well before the total blood count showed changes. The fusion of morphology and physiology by Minot helped create a new intellectual model for hematology, one that combined description with experimentation in an effort to determine the relationship between structure and function.

In 1915 Minot also began to seriously consider the role of diet in anemia. Research on nutrition became prominent during the early twentieth century, with studies by C. Eijkman, F. G. Hopkins, and E. McCollum revealing that dietary deficiencies had caused disease. Minot's early exposure to constitutional medicine at his father's side, combined with these new discoveries, prompted him to carefully examine the dietary habits of his anemic patients. His own battle with diabetes mellitus, which required Minot to follow a carefully prescribed diet, can only have reinforced his beliefs about the critical role diet plays in disease.

Although these elements had by 1916 provided the intellectual framework for Minot's ultimate discovery of the role of liver therapy in pernicious anemia, he would not turn to this problem until 1925. In the interim, Minot performed research on a wide variety of hematologic problems, including the anemias, leukemias, and hemostasis, continually emphasizing a physiologic approach. A brief foray into occupational medicine led to collaboration with Dr. Alice Hamilton and papers on diseases afflicting trinitrotoluene workers and the smokeless powder industry. As the years passed Minot's reputation as a clinical researcher grew, and in 1923 he was promoted to associate in medicine and chosen as the chief of the medical service at the Huntington Hospital, Harvard's cancer research center.

In 1925 Minot turned to the problem of pernicious anemia after he became intrigued when reading George H. Whipple's reports that dogs made anemic by repeated bleedings rapidly improved when fed liver. Here was clear experimental proof that diet was fundamental to anemia. The similarities between pernicious anemia and other diseases known to be influenced by diet, such as pellagra, sprue, and beri-beri, further strengthened Minot's belief that diet might be efficacious in pernicious anemia; Whipple's studies provided the specific diet.

Minot enlisted the services of a junior colleague, William P. Murphy, who had recently joined Minot's group practice. Together they decided to try a diet that required patients to consume huge amounts of liver, between 100 and 240 grams per day. The waxing and waning course that pernicious anemia typically followed had made previous efforts to assess the efficacy of dietary interventions difficult. However, by performing daily reticulocyte counts, Minot and Murphy realized that they had the ideal tool to evaluate their intervention, one that was quick, quantitative, scientifically sophisticated, and concordant with the growing emphasis on physiology. Shortly after initiating their experiment their highest hopes were realized. Within two weeks most patients showed marked clinical improvement. Laboratory studies revealed dramatic increases in the reticulocyte counts. After demonstrating this response in forty-five patients, Minot and Murphy presented their results at the 1926 meeting of the Association of American Physicians. Using state-of-the-art research methodology, they had discovered an effective treatment for a disease with a previously dismal prognosis; their announcement was received enthusiastically.

Following their dramatic announcement, Minot and colleagues sought to isolate the active ingredient of liver that reversed pernicious anemia. An interdisciplinary team of clinicians, physiologists, and biochemists created increasingly potent liver extracts. As demand or these extracts grew, it rapidly became clear that the research laboratory could not manufacture sufficiently large amounts of the extracts. A Committee on Pernicious Anemia was established to oversee the transformation of this research triumph into a therapy readily available to the medical community. A patent was obtained in the name of Harvard University, and a manufacturing license sold to Eli Lilly and Company. Soon thereafter liver extract was commercially available, an episode that provides an interesting early example of the growing links between the pharmaceutical industry and academic medicine during this era.

In 1928 Minot was promoted to professor of medicine and appointed the director of the Thorndike Memorial Laboratory at the Boston City Hospital, the focal point of much of Harvard's clinical research. With increasing administrative duties Minot's personal research production gradually declined. He continued, however, to remain central to the creation of hematology as an academic subspecialty by serving as the mentor for a generation of clinical scientists. His students vigorously pursued his research agenda with an ever increasing emphasis on physiology and biochemistry. Under Minot's direction, William B. Castle helped identify the absence of Intrinsic Factor as the underlying pathophysiology of pernicious anemia and laid the groundwork that would result in the 1948 demonstration of vitamin B-12 as the active ingredient supplied by liver therapy. Quick to adopt the team model of scientific enterprise that was becoming increasingly important for American science during the interwar period, Minot and colleagues at the Thorndike turned out an impressive array of papers; the Thorndike's influence on the development of hematology continues to be felt today.

By 1934, when he received the Nobel Prize for his work on pernicious anemia, Minot was already internationally prominent. Throughout his life he continued to actively pursue his interests in natural history, experimental physiology, and clinical medicine, and to promote an intellectual model of clinical research that combined morphology and physiology. A stroke forced Minot to retire in 1948, but in the final years of his life he was showered with awards and affection by his protégés.

STEVEN C. MARTIN

Selected Bibliography

PRIMARY SOURCES

Minot, G. R. 1926. "Treatment of Pernicious Anemia by a Special Diet." *Journal of the American Medical Association* 87:470.

Minot, G. R., and W. P. Murphy. 1927. "A Diet Rich in Liver in the Treatment of Pernicious Anemia—Study of One Hundred and Five Cases." *Journal of the American Medical Association* 89:759.

Minot, G. R. 1929. "Some Fundamental Clinical Aspects of Deficiencies." *Annals of Internal Medicine* 3:216–29.

———. 1935. "The Development of Liver Therapy in Pernicious Anemia: A Nobel Lecture." *Lancet* 1:361–64.

Minot, G. R., and W. B. Castle. 1935. "Interpretation of Reticulocyte Reactions: Their Value in Determining Potency of Therapeutic Materials, Especially in Pernicious Anemia." *Lancet* 2:319–30.

Minot, G. R. No date. Papers. Countway Library, Harvard Medical School, Boston, Massachusetts.

SECONDARY SOURCES

Castle, W. B. 1952. "The Contributions of George Richards Minot to Experimental Medicine." *New England Journal of Medicine* 247:585–91.

Kass, L. 1978. "William B. Castle and Intrinsic Factor." *Annals of Internal Medicine* 89:983.

Rackemann, F. M. 1956. *The Inquisitive Physician: The Life and Times of Georges Richards Minot, A.B., M.D., D.Sc.* Cambridge: Harvard University Press.

Wintrobe, Maxwell M., ed. 1980. *Blood, Pure and Eloquent: A Story of Discovery, People, and of Ideas.* New York: McGraw-Hill.

ANTONIO CAETANO DE ABREU FREIRE EGAS MONIZ *1949*

Antonio Caetano de Abreu Freire Egas Moniz was born in Avanca, Portugal, on November 29, 1874. A neurosurgeon, Egas Moniz received half the Nobel Prize in 1949 for his development of surgical frontal leucotomy for the treatment of psychosis, a pioneering if controversial technique; W. R. Hess was the other recipient. Moniz, a Renaissance man of wide interests and activities, also developed an effective method of diagnostic cerebral angiography. At the time of the award, he had been retired for four years from the chair of neurology at the University of Lisbon. He married Elvira de Macedo Dias in 1902; the couple had no children. He died on December 13, 1955, in Lisbon.

The son of Fernand de Pina Rezende Abreu and Maria do Rosario de Almeida e Sousa, Moniz received his early education in Pardilho, from his uncle, a priest. In 1891, at the age of sixteen, he entered the University of Coimbra. He was deeply interested in art, philosophy, literature, and engineering but finally selected medicine, completing his degree in 1899. He continued studies in neurology at Coimbra, and then in Paris and Bordeaux, where he worked with J. F. F. Babinski, J. A. Sicard, and other major French neurologists. From 1902 to 1911 Moniz was professor at Coimbra; he then became the first occupant of the Lisbon chair, where he was to remain until 1945.

For twenty years he pursued a second career as a liberal republican politician, not always a safe course in Portugal at that time. Moniz organized and led the Centrist party, serving in Parliament from 1900 to 1917. He was briefly ambassador to Spain in 1917, before becoming minister of foreign affairs and leading the Portuguese delegation at the Paris Peace Conference. However, his political career was also marred by imprisonment after the Revolution of 1908, an assassination attempt, and a political duel. Moniz retired from public life after the latter event in 1919. He remained involved in other spheres, writing history and literary criticism, composing, and patronizing the arts. Moniz, in all his work, exhibited a compassion and concern for others, combined with a conviction that problems could be solved by the right scientific application. He was also a proud and ambitious man, "dominated," as he said himself, "by the desire to reach something new in the scientific world" (Perino 1961).

Moniz began his work in cerebral angiography in the 1920s. He had suffered from gout since 1899 and could have accomplished little without the aid of his longtime collaborator, neurosurgeon Almeida Lima. Existing methods, including W. E. Dandy's use of air injections, were neither precise enough nor safe enough for regular clinical use.

Moniz sought to identify a radio-opaque dye that would not become diluted or toxic and that would pass through the capillaries without clotting the blood or blocking the vessels. He injected bromides, then iodides, into animals and cadavers for months before beginning experimentation on living human patients. His technique of dye injection and radiographic visualization enabled him to determine the normal pattern of arteries in the brain. He used this knowledge to develop a method of diagnosing and locating brain tumors by visualization of abnormalities in the arterial pattern. His results were announced in 1927 (Perino 1961, 266–67; Egas Moniz 1927).

Moniz now turned his attention to the problem of mental illness. As with his work on angiography, he was strongly motivated by a deep desire to relieve suffering and his belief that a workable scientific therapy could be found. He believed also that the solution would be medical or surgical, not psychoanalytic: "[O]nly by an organic orientation," he wrote: "can psychiatry make real progress" (quoted in Swazey 1971, 286–87). He was convinced that mental illness was a functional manifestation of a physical disorder of the neural system, possibly at the cellular level. In this, Moniz anticipated Roger Sperry and other recent investigators, but he lacked the skills to develop a methodology sophisticated enough to test these ideas in any depth (Perino 1961, 269).

His observations of psychotic patients led him to concentrate on their compulsive repetitions of thoughts and actions, sometimes meaningless, but nearly always causing deep anxiety in the patient. He theorized that these compulsions had an organic etiology in synaptic disease. The neural linkages somehow adhered to the surrounding tissues and otherwise lost their flexibility, thus trapping the patient's mind in a repetitive thought pattern.

While considering this problem, Moniz attended the Second International Neurological Congress in London in 1935, where he learned of animal experiments by Carlyle Jacobsen, John Fulton, and Margaret Kinnard. These American researchers had worked with chimpanzees who became markedly frustrated and discouraged, even violent, when confronted with problems they could not solve. After the neural connections between the frontal lobes and the rest of the brain were surgically severed, the animals appeared to recover with normal alertness and intelligence. They were still able to perform even complex tasks in visual discrimination and problem solving, but it was impossible for them to solve any problem involving extensive use of short-term memory or integration of data over time. For example, if the problem required that a chimpanzee open alternate doors in succession, he was apparently not able to remember which door he had last opened and would only perform the correct sequence by accident, never learning the solution. The animals' behavior when confronted with such a problem, however, was entirely different than before the surgery: they were quite docile and relaxed and made repeated attempts to perform any task given them without frustration or concern.

No definitely localized functions were ascribed to the prefrontal region (identified by Moniz as the region in front of the motor area of the brain). Accidents and operations for brain tumor in humans had indicated that injury to the frontal lobes resulted in personality change, but not in damage to any vital body process (Swazey 1971).

Moniz immediately perceived that frontal leucotomy might be the solution to the "synaptic fixation" he had hypothesized in compulsive psychosis. With old neural connections interrupted, the brain might be forced to form new and healthier thought patterns. Again with the assistance of Almeida Lima, Moniz devised an instrument, the encotome, and a technique, and operated on twenty seriously ill mental patients in 1935–36. His results, published in 1936, claimed a cure for seven patients, improvement of another seven, and no results in the remaining six cases. Moniz presented his new technique to the Medical Psychology Society in 1937 and performed several more operations before World War II began (Perino 1961, 269–70; Egas Moniz 1936).

Moniz's work was the first attempt to operate surgically to improve psychiatric illness. Several other frontal lobe operations were developed in the late 1940s, all variations of his basic model. Results were varied. In the severely psychotic, the operation does result in relief from compulsive and morbid anxieties. Although aberrant behavior may continue, the patient is no longer as deeply troubled and may be able to live outside an institutional setting. However, these changes are accompanied by a loss of imagination, foresight, and sensitivity, and some loss of individual personality. For these reasons, frontal leucotomy, which the Nobel Committee called "one of the most important discoveries ever made in psychiatric therapy," fell out of vogue quickly after the introduction of psychoactive drugs. Today many would consider Moniz's work in cerebral angiography, a method replicated for the localization and diagnosis of tumors and vascular disorders throughout the body, of more lasting value.

Moniz served as president of the Academia das Ciencias de Lisbon and was a member or honorary member of many national scientific societies, including the American Neurological Association, the Royal Society of Medicine, and the Academy of Medicine in Paris. In poor health by the end of the war, he retired in 1945 to Avanca, and was not well enough to attend the Nobel presentation.

MARCIA MELDRUM

Selected Bibliography

PRIMARY SOURCES

Egas Moniz, Antonio. 1927. "L'Encéphalographie Artérielle: Son Importance dans la Localization des Tumeurs Cérébrales." *Revue Neurologique* 2:72–90.

———. 1931. *Diagnostic des Tumeurs Cérébrales et Epreuve de l'Encéphalographie Artérielle*. Paris: Masson et Cie.

———. 1934. *L'Angiographie Cérébrale, Ses Applications et Résultats en Anatomie, Physiologie et Clinique*. Paris: Masson et Cie.

———. 1936. "Essai d'un Traitement Chirurgical des Certaines Psychoses." *Bulletin de l'Acádemie de Médecine*. 115:385–92.

———. 1936. *Tentatives Opératoires dans le Traitement de Certaines Psychoses*. Paris: Masson et Cie.

———. 1948. "Mein Weg zur Leukotomie." *Deutsche Medizinsche Wochenschrift* 73:581–83.

SECONDARY SOURCES

1980. "Moniz, Antonio Caetano de Abreau Freire Egas." *Modern Scientists and Engineers*, 2:319–20. New York: McGraw-Hill.

1955. "Obituary. Antonio Egas Moniz, M.D." *Lancet* 2:1345.

Perino, Francisco Ruben. 1961. "Egas Moniz: Founder of Psychosurgery, Creator of Angiography, Nobel Prize Winner, 1874–1958 (sic)." *Journal of the International College of Surgeons* 36 (August):261–71.

Swazey, Judith P. 1971. "Egas Moniz, Antonio Caetano de Abreu Freire." In *Dictionary of Scientific Biography*, 4:286–27. New York: Scribners.

Jacques Lucien Monod *1965*

Jacques Lucien Monod was born February 9, 1910, in Paris. A biochemist, he shared the 1965 Nobel Prize in Physiology or Medicine with André Lwoff and François Jacob for his contribution to "discoveries concerning the genetic regulation of enzyme and viral synthesis." His father, Lucien Monod, was a painter, engraver, and art historian, and his mother, Charlotte Todd MacGregor Monod, was an American, born in Milwaukee. In 1938 Monod married Odette Bruhl (d. 1972), archeologist, orientalist, and curator of the Musée Guimet. They had twin sons, Olivier and Philippe; one now a physicist, the other, a geologist. Monod died May 31, 1976, in Cannes.

Monod was educated in zoology at the Université de Paris (Sorbonne), completing his B.Sc. in 1931 and his doctorate in 1941. After a brief period with Edouard Chatton in Strasbourg in 1941, he became a professor at the Université de Paris, first with Maurice Caullery in the Laboratoire d'Evolution des Etres Organisés, and two years later in the laboratoire de Zoologie. In 1945 he joined the Institut Pasteur where he remained for the rest of his career as a researcher and administrator. He was appointed head of the Department of Cellular Biochemistry in 1953, and became director générale in 1971. From 1967 to 1971 he held the chair of molecular biology at the Collège de France.

Monod's family was Protestant and he was fluent in English. As a result, he was always at ease in the English-speaking scientific community and was particularly stimulated by his contact with American geneticists. In 1934 he went on a natural history expedition with the "Pourquoi Pas" to Greenland, and in 1936, influenced by Boris Ephrussi, he spent a few months with T. H. Morgan's genetics group at the California Institute of Technology. During World War II he was involved in the French Resistance and was arrested briefly by the Gestapo in December 1940. These activities meant he could no longer work at the Sorbonne. Undaunted, he continued in the Resistance until the liberation of Paris in 1944, when he enlisted in the army. At intervals during the war, he carried out clandestine research at the Institut Pasteur and was already familiar with its environment when he was able to join officially in 1945.

Monod helped elucidate the mechanisms of control and the communication of genetic information within the bacterial cell. He came to the study of molecular biology with a background in both zoology and biochemistry and a knowledge of microbiology that included techniques for growing living organisms in culture. When he began working in science, hereditary information was known to be associated with chromosomes, but the biochemical nature of this information and the means of communicating and expressing it were still a mystery. Monod was fascinated by genetics, but he had been working on what, at the time, seemed to be a different problem: growth. The fields soon merged.

Monod's doctoral dissertation was a biometric study of the factors governing the kinetics of growth in bacteria (Monod 1941). Among other things, he demonstrated that in some mixtures of two sugars, bacterial growth was regular and could be displayed by a smooth exponential curve; in other mixtures of two sugars, there was an initial growth spurt, followed by a lag, then a second spurt. Monod named this phenomenon, "idauxy." In December 1940 Lwoff suggested that "idauxy" might be the result of enzyme adaptation. Monod claimed that, at the time, he had never heard of enzyme adaptation, but from that moment on, it became his lifelong pursuit.

Monod's work on enzymes brought him much closer to the exciting advances in genetics. He had been intrigued by the potential of bacterial mutants as described by Luria and Delbrück. Using a mutant strain of bacteria isolated from the intestine of André Lwoff (ML or *Mutabile Lwoffi*), his team investigated the enzyme β-galactosidase. They were able to show that enzymes were stable in vivo under normal conditions and that adaptation actually meant, not a change in the enzyme, but the biosynthesis of an entirely new molecule.

Monod then turned his attention to the production of enzymes. In 1946 he extrapolated on his evidence and came to the prescient conclusion that a mutation in an enzyme's adaptive function was the result of a prior mutation in a gene. This reasoning bore similarities to the contemporary work of Gerti T. and Carl F. Cori on the inheritance of inborn metabolic defects. The adaptation of enzymes could be conceived as the result of a previously dormant but ever-present gene being stimulated to make its product. Since the 1944 work of Oswald Avery, genes were known to be associated with DNA, but exactly how they conveyed their message was unknown. In a series of experiments that took place before and after the Watson-Crick announcement of the structure of DNA (1953), Monod's team, with Melvin Cohn, demonstrated that enzymes were synthesized from amino acids in the presence of an "inducer," which was thought to be the substrate on which the enzyme acted.

The control of this production was the next consideration. Between 1958 and 1963, in collaboration with Jacob, Monod performed a series of classic experiments that led to an elegant theory of genetic control and to the Nobel Prize. Still using bacterial enzymes, they announced that the elaboration of an enzyme, also called the expression of a gene, takes place when an inhibition, called a "repressor," is removed. This famous experiment was dysorthographically nicknamed "PA-JA-MA(O)" for its authors (Pardee, Jacob, and Monod 1959).

Further studies concerning the origin and mechanism of action of the repressor resulted in the operon theory and messenger RNA (mRNA). The operon is a genetic unit, a group of adjacent genes on the same chromosome, consisting of the "structural" genes that code, in DNA, for the elaboration of enzymes or structural proteins via the intermediary of mRNA and an "operator" gene that can turn on the expression of the structural genes. The "repressor," a substance elaborated by a "regulator" gene elsewhere in the genetic material, acts on the operon to turn it off. Induction of enzyme production is the removal of the repressor, by the presence of substrate or other control action on the regulator gene, which itself can be subject to repression and derepression. When the repressor is removed, the structural gene is open to "transcription" by mRNA, which carries the coded message to ribosomes in cytoplasm where it is "translated" by other RNA into a chain of amino acids forming a protein (Monod and Jacob 1961). Watson and Crick had described how hereditary information was encoded in the structure of the DNA molecule; Monod and Jacob explained the dynamics of how that information was turned into anatomical structures and physiological functions.

Monod made one other major contribution, based on an idea that came to him suddenly in late 1961, an idea that he himself described as "la deuxième secret de la vie" (the second secret of life). He suggested and later found convincing proof that interactions between enzymes and other molecules (their activators, inhibitors, and substrates) depend on alterations in the shape of the enzyme molecule induced by the presence or absence of inhibitors and activators, resulting in varying affinity for the substrate. This shape-dependant control mechanism, Monod named "allostery" (Monod 1965).

Monod contributed "Forewords" to the French editions of works by both Ernst Mayer and Karl Popper. His own book, *Chance and Necessity*, is a philosophical essay on the origin of life and on heredity. Its main thesis is that life arose by chance, but the mechanisms of its perpetuation and its evolution are molecular events that can be known, studied, and predicted within reliable limits. Monod made controversial statements concerning dialectical materialism, which he called a "pseudoscience," and concerning the importance of "objectivity" as the essence and origin of modern science and as the distinguishing characteristic between scientific knowledge and ethics (see Stent 1971; Beigbeder 1972). His last book, to have been called, *L'Homme et le temps*, was never completed.

Monod thought of himself as Provençal (a southerner), rather than as a Parisian. He possessed a mercurial "double" personality: on the one hand, charming and courteous; on the other, hard, domineering, and incapable of accepting the slightest public opposition to his views (Lwoff, in Lwoff and Ullman 1979, p. 22). Gunther Stent has described how this intolerance led him to wound friends and admirers (in Lwoff and Ullman 1979, 231–37). The contrasting impressions he left ranged from exasperating conceit and arrogance to astonishing genius and virtue (M. Pollock, in Lwoff and Ullman 1979, 62). In spite of a slight polio disability in his left leg, he was a sailor and a rock-climber. Gifted in music, he learned cello as a child, founded and directed the Bach choir "La Cantate" (until 1948), and once was tempted by the offer to become conductor of an American orchestra. A self-avowed Communist until after the war, his political sympathies always leaned to the left and he was committed to social action. This was made manifest in his involvement with the French Underground during the war, but later, too, when he spoke out during the Lysenko affair against the use of fraudulent scientific statements in defense of injustices rooted in ideology. Monod was also a supporter of women's rights, especially on birth control issues. In 1968, during the Paris University uprisings, he was sympathetic to the student demands and made important contributions to the resultant reforms. His move from "the attic" of the Institut Pasteur, where the research labs were located, to its administration was a product of this social concern.

Monod was awarded many prizes, including the Prix Montyon in physiology from the Paris Académie des Sciences (1955), the Louis Rapkine Medal, London, England (1958), and the Chevalier de la Légion d'Honneur (1963).

JACALYN DUFFIN

Selected Bibliography

PRIMARY SOURCES

Monod, Jacques. 1941. "Recherches sur la croissance des cultures bactériennes." Thèse Doctorat ès Sciences. Paris: Hermann.

Pardee, Arthur B., François Jacob, and Jacques Monod. 1959. "The Genetic Control and Cytoplasmic Expression of 'Inducibility' in the Synthesis of β-Galactosidase by *E. coli.*" *Journal of Molecular Biology* 1:165–78.

Monod, Jacques, and François Jacob. 1961. "Genetic Regulatory Mechanisms in the Synthesis of Proteins." *Journal of Molecular Biology* 3:318–536.

Monod, Jacques, Jeffries Wyman, and Jean-Pierre Changeux. 1965. "On the Nature of Allosteric Transitions: A Plausible Model." *Journal of Molecular Biology* 12:88–118.

Monod, Jacques. 1965. "From Enzymatic Adaptation to Allosteric Transitions. Nobel Lecture, December 11, 1965. "Biography." In *Nobel Lectures in Molecular Biology*, 1933–75, 259–80, 281–82. New York: Elsevier, 1977.

———. 1970. *Chance and Necessity. An Essay on the Natural Philosophy of Modern Biology Le Hasard et la nécessité*, Paris, Seuil. Translated by Austryn Wainhouse. New York: Alfred A. Knopf, 1971.

———. 1978. *Selected Papers in Molecular Biology by Jacques Monod.* Edited by André Lwoff and Agnes Ullman. New York: Academic Press. [Reprints sixty-one of Monod's scientific papers and Lwoff's 1977 bibliography cited below].

SECONDARY SOURCES

Beigbeder, Marc. 1972. *Le Contre-Monod.* Paris: Bernard Grasset.

Jacob, François. 1988. *The Statue Within: An Autobiography*, 290–320. *La statue intérieure* 1987 Paris, Editions Odile Jacob. Translated by Franklin Philip. New York: Basic Books.

Judson, Horace Freeland. 1979. *The Eighth Day of Creation: Makers of the Revolution in Biology*, 352–58. New York: Simon and Schuster.

Lwoff, André. 1977. "Complete Bibliography of Scientific Papers." *Biographical Memoirs of the Fellows of the Royal Society* 23:405–415. Includes one hundred and thirty-one of Monod's scientific articles and other works.

Lwoff, André, and Agnes Ullman, eds. 1979. *Origins of Molecular Biology: A Tribute to Jacques Monod.* New York: Academic Press. Thirty-two essays on Monod by his friends and colleagues.

Mayer, Ernst. 1973. *Populations, espèces et évolution.* Paris: Hermann.

Popper, Karl. 1973. *La logique de la découverte scientifique.* Paris: Payot.

Stent, Gunther. 1971. "Ode to Objectivity. Does God Play at Dice?" *Atlantic Monthly* (November):125–30.

THOMAS HUNT MORGAN 1933

Thomas Hunt Morgan was awarded the Nobel Prize for Physiology or Medicine in 1933 "for his discoveries concerning the role played by the chromosomes in heredity." The eldest of three children, he was born in Lexington, Kentucky, on September 25, 1866, to Charles Hunt Morgan, and Ellen Kay Howard. In 1904 he married Lillian Vaughan Sampson; they had four children. He died in Pasadena, California, December 4, 1945.

Thomas Morgan inherited an ancestry of substantial achievement. His mother came from an old established Baltimore family, which included the composer of the national anthem; his paternal grandfather had reputedly been the first millionaire in Kentucky. His own father served in the 1860s as U.S. Consul in Messina, Italy, and was later principal administrator of the lunatic asylum *his* father had founded; his paternal uncle was the Confederate general John Hunt Morgan, of Morgan's Raiders' fame.

He grew up amidst the comforts of an elegant southern Georgian mansion, at a time when the labor of others was no longer free but could still be bought very cheap, and he enjoyed the sensual pleasures of the Kentucky countryside. His early education was rigidly disciplined, but academically entertaining and unthreatening. After completing a Ph.D. in zoology at Johns Hopkins University in 1890, Morgan succeeded E. B. Wilson, the United States' most distinguished biologist, as head of the Biology Department at Bryn Mawr, when Wilson moved to Columbia University. He traveled widely in Europe in the two decades around the turn of the century.

Out of these experiences would emerge one of those archetypal father-figures common in public life at the turn of the twentieth century; men who took for granted their position of authority and leadership, and who brought the liberal values of an international perspective to their scientific studies. Morgan would eschew formality in public and private life; he was discreetly generous, and he had a laconic sense of humor—he often referred to his four children as the F_1's, the common Mendelian notation for first generation offspring. He commanded great respect and a fierce loyalty from family, colleagues, and graduate students who enjoyed his patronage.

In 1904 Morgan joined Wilson at Columbia as professor of experimental zoology. He remained at Columbia for the next two decades, accomplishing there his most important work. He worked within an international community of Darwinian biologists deeply divided about evolutionary development. They had rejected descriptive morphology in favor of the more analytic experimental embryology, which used new cytological techniques to focus on discreet development in fertilization and egg maturation. Known in Europe as "developmental mechanics" or *Entwicklungsmechanik*, it was a mechanical approach to biology whose principal architect had been Wilhelm Roux. However, the new wine of "developmental mechanics" still came in two old bottles: scientists continued to argue about whether biological development was immanent or accidental, whether it emerged from a pre-existing form or evolved "epigenetically" from a general formless mass. Wilhelm Roux had startled experimental embryologists in 1888 with a theory that appeared to resurrect preformationism. Morgan was among those who favored the strongly materialistic theory of epigenesis.

This debate colored much of Morgan's early work. In 1895, on an extended visit to the zoological laboratory at Naples, Italy, where experimental embryology flourished, he collaborated with Roux's principal opponent, Hans Dreisch, whose experiments were giving substance to the epigenetic view that the cell is a "harmonious equipotential whole." (A complete bibliography of Morgan's work can be found in A. H. Sturtevant [1959]). And in the United States Morgan contributed to the controversial experiments in parthenogenesis conducted by his colleague and friend at Bryn Mawr, Jacques Loeb, one of the earliest pioneers in the study of external stimuli on plant and animal behavior. Morgan's first major book, *Regeneration* (1901), dwelt heavily on the theme that development was what he called a "physico-chemical" process involving the entire cell, and not any discreet part of it.

Opposition to the idea of immanence in biological development became an enduring theme in Morgan's work. In his first two texts on evolutionary theory, *Evolution & Adaption* (1903) and *Experimental Zoology* (1907), he rejected completely the idea of "selection" in natural selection and remained skeptical of it for most of his life.

By the time he moved to Columbia, in 1904, Morgan had turned his attention to the mechanism of inheritance. The principles governing the transmission of genetic traits had become generally known in 1900, when the work of Gregor Mendel, first published in 1865, was rediscovered. However, Mendel's laws were not immediately accepted by all biologists, including Morgan, who until 1910 considered Mendelian genetics a "particulate" theory, a form of preformationism (Morgan 1909).

Nor was he initially sympathetic with accumulating evidence, some contributed by his colleague and mentor E. B. Wilson, concerning the relation between Mendelian "factors" and the activity of the chromosomes in the nucleus. In 1905 Wilson and Nettie Stevens had identified chromosomes with the inheritance of sex, but five years later Morgan continued reluctant to accept the reductionism implicit in what was known as the "chromosome theory" of inheritance (Morgan 1910).

Rational and chance intervention finally converted him. In 1910 the argument of Wilhelm Johannsen, separating the ahistoric function of gene transmission (the genotype) and the historic development of gene expression (the phenotype), increased understanding of the significance and limitations of the concept of the gene, and finally dismissed epigenesis. In the same year the fly colony Morgan had recently begun to cultivate, to study inherited mutations, threw up a mutant displaying a relationship between sex and eye color. Accepting Wilson and Stevens's evidence of the relationship between sex inheritance and chromosomes enabled Morgan to see in his own discovery the likelihood that the Mendelian "factor" for eye color trait lay on the chromosome (Morgan 1910).

This discovery set Morgan's agenda for the next several years. Between 1910 and 1915 he and his associates, notably A. H. Sturtevant, H. J. Muller, and C. B. Bridges, made discoveries about the genetic behavior of the *Drosophila melanogaster*, (or common fruit fly), which silenced most skeptics of Mendelian laws and paved the way for their experimental, quantitative analysis. In their book *The Mechanism of Mendelian Heredity* (1915) the *Drosophila* group, as they became known, provided overwhelming confirmation that chromosomes were the site of the Mendelian unit of heredity (the gene); explained some previously inexplicable Mendelian anomolies; and, by means of combined cytological and morphological observations and experiments, produced chromosome "maps" showing genes to be units of inheritance (factors) distinct from formed traits or characters. This is the work for which Morgan was awarded the Nobel Prize, and it established what became known as the theory of the gene, or the classical gene concept (Morgan 1926).

In 1928 Morgan moved to California to become the first head of the Division of Biological Science at the California Institute of Technology, where he remained for the rest of his life. *Drosophila* genetics dominated the study of inheritance, and geneticists were increasingly studying the physical properties of the gene, particularly after H. J. Muller demonstrated gene mutation by radiation in 1927. During the 1930s Morgan actively encouraged the collaboration of physicists and biologists, and his laboratory at Caltech was the center of the world for a generation of classical geneticists now studying differential development by fusing classical with physical studies of the gene.

Morgan himself returned to the study of embryology, now looking for a genetic explanation of development. However, *Drosophila* was not well suited for this work, and he broke no new ground in his book *Embryology and Genetics* (1934). However, his work at Columbia had made him one of the most reknowned biologists in the world; his scientific honors included not only the Nobel Prize but also the Royal Society's Darwin and Copley Medals. From 1927 to 1931 he was president of the National Academy of Science, and in 1932 served as president of the 6th International Congress of Genetics.

ROSALIE STOTT

Selected Bibliography

PRIMARY SOURCES

Morgan, T. H. 1909. "What are 'Factors' in Mendelian Explanations?" *American Breeders' Association Report* 6:365–68.

Morgan, T. H. 1910. "Chromosomes and Heredity." *American Naturalist* 44:449–96.

Morgan, T. H. 1910. "Sex Limited Inheritance in Drosophila." *Science* 32:120–122. Reprinted in *Classic Papers in Genetics*, cited by A. Peters. Englewood Cliffs, N.J.: Prentice-Hall, 1959.

Morgan, T. H., A. H. Sturtevant, H. J., Muller, and C. B. Bridges. 1915. *The Mechanism of Mendelian Heredity*. New York: Henry Holt and Company. Reprinted 1972. N.Y.: Johnson Reprint Corporation.

Morgan, T. H. 1926. *The Theory of the Gene*. New Haven: Yale University Press.

SECONDARY SOURCES

Allen, G. E. 1975. *Life Science in the Twentieth Century*. Cambridge, England: Cambridge University Press.

———. 1978. *Thomas Hunt Morgan: The Man and His Science*. Princeton: Princeton University Press.

Blanc, M. 1985. "Darwin, Mendel, Morgan: The Beginnings of Genetics." *Diogenes* 131:101–13.

Carlson, E. A. 1974. "The Drosophila Group: The Transition from the Mendelian Unit to the Individual Gene." *Journal of the History of Biology* 7, no. 1:31–48.

———. 1966. *The Gene: A Critical History*. Philadelphia: Saunders.

Maienschein, J., R. Rainger, K. R. Benson, G. E. Allen, and F. B. Churchill. 1981. "Special Section on American Morphology at the Turn of the Century." *Journal of the History of Biology* 14, no. 1:83–191.

Roll-Hansen, N. 1978. "Drosophila Genetics: A Reductionist Research Program." *Journal of the History of Biology* 11, no. 1:159–210.

Sturtevant, A. H. 1959. "Thomas Hunt Morgan". In *Biographical Memoirs, National Academy of Sciences* 33:283–325.

PAUL HERMANN MÜLLER *1948*

P. H. Müller was born in Olten, Solothurn, Switzerland, on January 12, 1899, the son of Gottlieb Müller, an employee of the Swiss Federal Railway, and Fanny Leypoldt Müller. Müller's early childhood was spent in Lenzburg, Aargau, the birthplace of his father. When Müller was five years old, he and his family moved to Basel, where he attended primary school and Free Evangelical elementary and secondary schools. Müller married Friedel Rugsegger on 6 October 1927. They had two sons, Henry and Niklaus, and a daughter, Margaret. A chemist, Müller won the Nobel Prize in Physiology or Medicine in 1948 for his discovery of the high efficacy of DDT as a contact poison against several anthropods. He died on October 13, 1965, in Basel, Switzerland.

Müller became interested in chemistry in 1916, when he worked as a laboratory assistant in the chemical factory of Dreyfus and Company. In 1917 he was an assistant chemist in the scientific-industrial laboratories of Lonza A. G., where he gained practical knowledge in industrial chemistry. Desiring a career in this field, he enrolled at Basel University. He studied under Fichter and Rupe, and received his doctorate in 1925, with a thesis on the chemical and electrochemical oxidation of m-xylidine and its derivatives. In May 1925 Müller took a position as research chemist in the dye factory of J. R. Geigy A. G. His initial work at Geigy was done in association with Paul Lauger, who was interested in experimenting with methods for mothproofing textiles. By 1946, Müller had risen to the position of director of scientific research on substances for plant protection. He remained at Geigy until 1965.

Müller's work at Geigy centered on the study of plant pigments and natural tanning agents, which led him to use methods developed by botanists. Soon his work on preserving and disinfecting animal skins stimulated an interest in pesticides. He developed a mercury-free seed dressing. In 1935 Müller began to study contact insecticides. Others had been working in the field, but none had found an insecticide that could be used in agriculture. Müller drew up a number of ideals for contact insecticides, which included great toxicity for insects, rapid toxicity, little or no toxicity for plants and warm-blooded animals, no irritant effect or odor, long lasting effect, and low price.

Müller experimented with many different compounds on a variety of insects, bringing together the sciences of chemistry and biology. He learned that it would be possible to find safe and effective insecticides, since the absorption of the toxins by insects was physiologically different than that of warm-blooded animals. He worked with the group of chlorinated derivatives of phenyl ethane. In 1939 Müller began to experiment with 4,4′-dichloro-diphenyl-trichloroethane (DDT). DDT had been discovered by the Austrian Othmar Zeidler in 1873, but it was Müller who was able to demonstrate its properties as a contact insecticide. While experimenting with the Colorado beetle, which attacked potato plants, Müller noticed that larvae were also paralyzed by the poison. This finding showed that insects need not consume the poison in order to be affected by its properties. DDT, he asserted, was a contact poison, and therefore unique.

DDT met all of Müller's ideals. Minute amounts of DDT, which could be produced inexpensively, were highly toxic to insects, and the effects of spraying lasted several months. The insecticide, he showed, was effective against many different kinds of insects, and it seemed that it had very little effect on higher animals.

Müller patented DDT in 1940, and during the next few years he continued to study the relationship between the structure of the compound and its effects on insects. He also studied similar compounds, finding that none was as effective as the original. He concluded this set of experiments by stating that a "chemical compound is an individual whose characteristic action can be understood only from its totality, and the molecule means more in this case than the sum of its atoms" (Müller 1946).

DDT was introduced to the public in 1942, and was quickly appreciated for its efficacy against insects. It was widely used during World War II, especially to eliminate tropical insects that carried malaria and typhus. DDT's most important test took place in Naples, Italy, during early 1944, where it successfully checked a typhus epidemic and confirmed the work of another Nobel laureate, Charles Nicolle, who had discovered that typhus is caused by lice. At the height of the epidemic, sixty persons became ill each day. Authorities deloused 1,300,000 people, and within three weeks the epidemic was under control. This was the first time that such an epidemic had been stopped in winter. After the war, in occupied Japan, DDT was used to stop another such epidemic. Postwar Rockefeller Foundation-sponsored field trials of DDT in Greece helped to reduce the incidence of malaria dramatically. For this the University of Thessaloniki awarded Müller an honorary doctorate in 1963.

Although Müller understood the intense stability of the compound DDT he was only mildly concerned over the possibility of its accumulation in the body tissues of various species. He did not address this property in his ideals for contact insecticides, but he did mention in a 1946 article that synthetic DDT was unlike natural pyrethrum or rotenone, which are destroyed by light and oxidation. In the late 1960s, after widespread use, scientists realized the dangers of the accumulation of DDT in some animal species. Controversies then arose over the long-range effects of the compound.

VIRGINIA QUIROGA

Selected Bibliography

PRIMARY SOURCES

Müller, Paul Hermann. 1944. "Uber Konstitution und toxische Wirkung von naturlichen und neuen Synthetischen. Insektentotenden Stoffen." *Helvetica Chimica Acta* 27:899–928.

———. 1946. "Uber Zusammenhange Zwischen Konstitution und Insektizider Werdung." *Helvetica Chimica Acta* 29:1560–80.

———. 1948. "Dichlorodiphenyltrichoroathan und neuere Inzekticide." Nobel Lecture in *Les Prix Nobel en 1948*. 122–32. Stockholm: Elsevier.

SECONDARY SOURCES

1945. *Current Biography Yearbook.* 340–42. New York: H. W. Wilson.

1965. "Obituary." *Nature*, 208:1043–44.

1974. "Paul Hermann Müller." In *Dictionary of Scientific Biography*, 9:576–77. New York: Charles Scribner's Sons.

Schlessinger, Bernard S., and June Schlessinger. 1986. *The Who's Who of Nobel Prize Winners*, 95. Phoenix, AZ: Oryx Press.

Sourkes, Theodore L. 1966. *Nobel Prize Winners in Medicine and Physiology 1901–1965*, 261–65. London: Abelard-Schuman.

West, T. F., and G. A. Campbell. 1950. *D.D.T. and Newer Persistent Insecticides.* London: Chapman.

HERMANN JOSEPH MULLER
1946

Hermann Joseph Muller was born on December 21, 1890, in New York City. He is known primarily as a geneticist, the father of radiation genetics, and a major contributor to our understanding of mutation and the gene. His father, Hermann Muller, Sr., was the proprietor of an art metal works and his mother, Frances (née Lyons), raised him and his sister after the premature death of her husband. Muller married his first wife, Jessie Marie (née Jacobs), a mathematician, in 1922. They had one son, David, who is a professor of computer mathematics. Muller's second wife, Dorothea (née Kantorowicz), was a physician. They had one daughter, Helen, who is a professor of public health. Muller died April 5, 1967, in Indianapolis.

H. J. Muller, as he was known professionally, was a third-generation American who grew up in New York City in genteel poverty following the death of his father. Young Muller excelled in school and received a scholarship to attend Columbia University. He was attracted to natural science and fell under the influence of Edmund Beecher Wilson, whose courses in the cell and heredity reinforced his enthusiasm for studying evolution through heredity. After finishing his B.A. (1910), he began work on a M.A. in physiology at Cornell but quickly reestablished his Columbia connection when Thomas Hunt Morgan began work on fruit flies. With Calvin Blackman Bridges and Alfred Henry Sturtevant, Muller, Wilson, and Morgan established *Drosophila* genetics as preeminent in determining the theory of the gene and the mechanism of Mendelian heredity.

Muller completed the research for his Ph.D. under Morgan in 1915.

Muller was recruited by Julian Sorel Huxley to teach genetics at the Rice Institute. In 1919 Muller returned to Columbia for three years as an instructor and then joined the faculty at the University of Texas (1921–1932). These were the most productive years in his research program. As the economy collapsed after the 1929 financial panic, Muller turned his attention to social reform and was attracted to communism. He left the United States in 1932 for a year in Berlin; with the rise of nazism, he left Germany for the USSR, where he spent two years in Leningrad and four years in Moscow as a member of the USSR Academy of Sciences. Muller's clashes with the newly arising Lysenko movement and the arrest and execution of two of his students soured him on the Stalinist government. He left the USSR by volunteering to serve in the International Brigade during the Spanish Civil War. After the fall of Madrid, he found work at the University of Edinburgh (1937–1940). When World War II made his research impossible in Great Britain, he and his wife returned to the United States. He first took a position as an interim professor at Amherst College. In 1945 he was hired by Indiana University as a distinguished service professor; he stayed at Indiana until his retirement in 1974.

Muller's contributions are diverse and range through classical genetics, radiation genetics, theoretical genetics, human genetics, and evolution. He worked all his life with fruit flies to explore genetics experimentally, but he applied that knowledge to humans and other organisms. He established the existence of double crossovers and worked out measurements for correcting linkage maps. He analyzed complex and variable traits and showed, under constant environmental conditions, what the genetic components were that led to variations in expression of a Mendelian gene (he called this the theory of chief genes and modifiers and recognized that it was the basis for reduced penetrance and expressivity of hereditary traits in humans). He drew a distinction between gene mutations and all other forms of cytogenetic disturbances, and worked out the properties of normal and mutant genes, using the avalanche of experimental data from his laboratory to predict the artificial transformation of genes, to estimate the number of genes in a genome, and to develop a theory of the gene as the basis of life, extending Virchow's dictum, "all cells from preexisting cells," to the gene. He was convinced that the evolution of the gene was the basis for the origin of life.

In 1927 Muller completed experiments that proved without doubt that ionizing radiation induces gene mutations. Quick confirmation of Muller's results made radiation genetics a major branch of classical genetics. After World War II, Muller applied twenty years of research of radiation genetics to an interpretation of radiation sickness and to the estimates of spontaneous and induced mutation frequencies in humans. He became a voice of conscience in the radiation protection movement, pointing out abuses in industry, medicine, and the military. As a former communist sympathizer, he was distrusted during the early years of the cold war despite his intense criticism of the antigenetic Lysenko movement favored by the USSR under Stalin and Khrushchev.

Although Muller is best known for his induction of gene mutations with X-rays (for which he won the Nobel Prize), his working out of the laws of radiation genetics (the linearity of mutation frequency in response to dose of radiation received and the exponential increase in chromosome rearrangement frequency in relation to dose of radiation), Muller also discovered dosage compensation, coincidence and interference in recombination, modifier genes, variegated position effects, and the partial dominance of recessive genes. He proposed a theory of genetic load for human populations; worked out the mathematical laws for spread of recessive mutations in the population; and contributed to the neo-Darwinian conception of evolution by selection of the variations associated with individual gene mutation.

Muller was a founder of the American Society of Human Genetics and contributed to both human genetic studies and, independently of that society, to a eugenics movement that he felt was purged of the racism, spurious elitism, and sexism of the earlier eugenics movements that he had opposed in the 1930s. He hoped to establish sperm banks for fostering eugenic ideals, especially cooperativeness, intelligence, and longevity with good health. He abandoned attempts to launch such programs as his own health deteriorated. Although Muller failed to convince the postwar generation of the benefits of his eugenic views, he was successful in alerting his fellow scientists and the world's population to the hazards of radiation in the atomic age and he fought hard and thoroughly for those protections that would provide the least exposure of the population to chronic, low doses of radiation.

Muller was diminutive in size (five feet one inches) but physically strong, and enjoyed hiking in the mountains. He was a nervous, energetic speaker, at times eloquent and often tangential in his lectures, thinking aloud as he traced his ideas for his audience. He was considered by many to be "priority conscious" and troublesome as a colleague. Muller did not hesitate to lash out at those geneticists who minimized radiation hazards, who believed spontaneous mutations would lead to hybrid vigor, or who ignored the accumulation of mutations in the population. He was vilified by Stalinists in the USSR as a United States agent sent to stir up discontent, and equally vilified by the United States Atomic Energy Commission as a Soviet agent sent to inhibit development of nuclear armament. Muller's position confused those who saw complex problems in simplistic ways: he believed that fallout from nuclear weapons tests was a minor danger compared to the mutations arising spontaneously each generation, but he also believed that all unnecessary radiation introduced into the population leads to genetic deaths that do not have to occur. He was one of the rarer scientists of his generation, speaking out on public issues, often taking unpopular positions (such as his support of evolution and denunciation of racism in Texas in the 1930s), and jeopardizing his status in society. Like Socrates, he often found himself in the role of a gadfly.

ELOF AXEL CARLSON

Selected Bibliography

PRIMARY SOURCES

Muller, H. J. 1922. "Variation Due to Change in the Individual Gene." *American Naturalist* 56:32–50.

———. 1928. "The Problem of Genic Modification." *Proceedings of the Fifth International Congress of Genetics, Berlin, 1927. Zeitschrift fur induktive Abstammungs- und Vererbungslehre*, Supplement, 1:234–60.

———. 1929. "The Gene as the Basis of Life." *Proceedings of the International Congress of Plant Science* 1:897–921.

———. 1950. "Our Load of Mutations." *American Journal of Human Genetics* 2:11–176.

———. 1962. *Studies in Genetics: The Selected Papers of H. J. Muller.* Bloomington, Ind.: Indiana University Press.

———. 1973. *Man's Future Birthright: Social Essays of H. J. Muller.* Edited by E. A. Carlson. Albany, N.Y.: SUNY Press.

———. 1973. *The Modern Concept of Nature: Scientific Essays of H. J. Muller.* Edited by E. A. Carlson. Albany, N.Y.: SUNY Press.

SECONDARY SOURCES

Carlson, Elof Axel. 1982. *Genes, Radiation, and Society: The Life and Work of H. J. Muller.* Ithaca, N.Y.: Cornell University Press.

WILLIAM PARRY MURPHY
1934

Born on February 6, 1892, William P. Murphy was the son of Rose Anna Parry and Thomas Francis Murphy, a Congregationalist minister. He married Pearl Harriet Adams on September 10, 1919, and fathered two children, Priscilla and William. An internist, he received the Nobel Prize in 1934 for "discoveries concerning liver therapy in cases of anemia." He died on October 9, 1987, in Brookline, Massachusetts.

Unlike the other 1934 Nobel laureates, Minot and Whipple, Murphy was reared outside New England. Raised in Wisconsin and Oregon, he majored in math and physics at the University of Oregon and graduated with an A.B. in 1914. For a brief period of time he taught high-school physics before spending 1915 at the University of Oregon Medical School. His decision to transfer East and his application to only Harvard and Johns Hopkins Medical Schools suggest he was attracted by the growing emphasis on scientific medicine. He selected Harvard when he became the first recipient of a scholarship fund William Stanislaus Murphy (Harvard college 1885) had established for men named Murphy.

After receiving his M.D. in 1920, Murphy interned at the Rhode Island Hospital. He developed an interest in blood disorders during this time and became proficient at making and interpreting blood smears. He returned to Harvard for his residency at the Peter Bent Brigham Hospital in 1922. Attracted to clinical research, he actively participated in early studies on insulin under the direction of Reginald Fitz, and in 1923 was appointed an assistant in medicine at Harvard Medical School.

After he joined E. A. Locke's private group practice, he began to work closely with George R. Minot. Minot—the scion of a prominent Boston family—was developing a reputation as a first-rate diagnostician and an outstanding clinical researcher who specialized in blood disorders. As the junior partner, Murphy would initially see the patients, perform the history, physical, and necessary laboratory tests, and then present the information to Minot. Together they would then decide what their course of action should be. Minot was impressed with Murphy's hard work and dedication; their shared interest in hematology strengthened this relationship.

Minot had maintained an interest in the relationship between disease and diet since his medical school days. When Minot and Murphy became aware of George Whipple's 1925 studies that demonstrated liver could improve the anemia induced by repeatedly bleeding experimental dogs, they elected to try liver therapy in their patients with pernicious anemia. Although Murphy later claimed that he was responsible for suggesting the idea that they try liver therapy, it seems clear that Minot's long-standing belief that diet was intimately related to anemia was the foundation of their decision to pursue research. Minot's status was also critical in ensuring cooperation from potentially recalcitrant Harvard officials such as Henry A. Christian, the chief of service at the Brigham Hospital, who was skeptical about clinical research.

Murphy and Minot were able to accumulate a significant number of patients because they had close contacts at nearly all the Harvard hospitals, with Murphy working primarily at the Peter Bent Brigham and Minot at the Huntington and Massachusetts General hospitals. As the junior investigator, the clinical care of the patients and the primary data collection were Murphy's responsibility. By 1926 forty-five patients had been treated; the results were dramatic. Within two weeks patients experienced a marked improvement in their sense of well-being and their blood counts began to increase.

Minot presented these results at the 1926 meeting of the Association of American Physicians where the response was immediate and enthusiastic. Although it would take another twenty years before it became clear that vitamin B-12 was the key nutrient missing in pernicious anemia, the ability to effectively treat a condition that had previously been uniformly fatal brought widespread acclaim to Minot and Murphy.

Despite this success, the next several years were difficult for Murphy. It appears that he was never completely accepted as an equal by Minot. He never received a significant academic rank, remaining an assistant in medicine until 1928, when he was promoted to instructor. In 1935 he was promoted to associate in medicine and his final promotion was to the rank of lecturer in 1948. Initially a recipient of research support from Harvard's Proctor Fund, Murphy proved unable to establish himself as an independent investigator. Despite encouragement from Minot to pursue new paths, Murphy felt more comfortable attending to clinical details and concentrated his efforts on the important, but mundane, task of validating the potency of new forms of liver therapy.

Because the initial liver treatments were unwieldy, requiring that nearly half a pound of liver be ingested daily, the next several years were devoted to devising simpler treatments. Murphy himself attempted unsuccessfully to isolate an active liver fraction that could be used as an intramuscular injection. A more skilled chemist, Edwin Cohn of Harvard's Department of Physical Chemistry, succeeded in isolating increasingly potent liver extracts that resulted in the creation of acceptable oral, intramuscular, and intravenous solutions. Murphy's failure and Cohn's success suggest how difficult it had already become by the 1930s for physicians without laboratory training to compete with Ph.D. scientists in some areas. At Harvard, like many other institutions, interdisciplinary teams were created to minimize this problem, capitalizing on the complementary talents of diverse specialists. As events unfolded, Murphy's role would be almost exclusively clinical.

The development of therapeutic extracts created problems for the Harvard collaborators; Cohn's laboratory was unable and unwilling to mass-produce therapeutic products. To grapple with this problem, a Committee on Pernicious Anemia was established, a patent obatained for Harvard, and Eli Lilly and Company granted a manufacturing license. The committee was deeply concerned about assuring the purity and potency of this liver extract and insisted each batch be tested by the committee prior to its release. Murphy, now director of the Pernicious Anemia Clinic at the Peter Bent Brigham Hospital, supervised these tests.

Despite obvious practical importance, this emphasis on technical improvements in the therapy of pernicious anemia did not represent important new research. In the late 1920s Minot repeatedly warned Murphy that his funding would be discontinued if he did not develop new lines of research. As predicted, in 1931, the Proctor Fund ceased to support Murphy's research efforts. In the post-Flexnerian medical school purely clinical contributions were not sufficient to ensure academic success. Flexner's influential *Report* (1910) persuaded medical schools to reward research productivity above clinical work.

The cessation of funding proved particularly awkward to Murphy because he was suffering financially from the impact of the Great Depression. His private practice was not thriving and Murphy even had to borrow money from the wealthy Minot to sustain himself. The combination of Murphy's middle-class background, financial difficulties, and floundering research efforts starkly contrasted with Minot's wealth and scientific prominence. Tensions between the two gradually began to develop. When Minot and Whipple were awarded ten thousand dollars in 1930 by *Popular Science Monthly*, Murphy was incensed at his exclusion. Although eventually Minot reassured Murphy that the award was not specifically for their work on pernicious anemia but for more general research efforts—and even sent Murphy one thousand dollars from the prize money—a decided coolness had crept into their relationship. As this split widened, Murphy increasingly turned away from clinical research. Although he continued to work on pernicious anemia, he developed no other area of research interest. Instead, he created a consulting practice in hematology and developed ties to Lederle, a pharmaceutical concern.

Although the 1934 Nobel Prize was the crowning achievement of Murphy's scientific life, it did not significantly change his career path. After the award he continued to extend his practice and increased his lecturing around the country. He became somewhat of a gadfly, challenging the United States Pharmacopeia's initial work on the standardization of liver therapy in pernicious anemia and working with the Massachusetts Medical Society to evaluate chiropractic and osteopathy. In 1944 he established a Pernicious Anemia Research Fund; he was its sole trustee. Murphy eventually moved to Brookline, Massachusetts—a Boston suburb—and continued in private practice until he retired.

Ironically, the discovery that liver could treat pernicious anemia resulted from several flawed assumptions. First, Minot and Murphy believed that there was something intrinsic to liver that resulted in Whipple's successful treatment of his anemic dogs. It was only later that it was recognized that iron deficiency was the cause of these dogs' anemia. There was nothing specific about liver therapy, and any foodstuff rich in iron would have been equally effective. Second, although the fundamental pathology in pernicious anemia results from vitamin

B-12 deficiency, it appears that liver therapy contained inadequate amounts of vitamin B-12 to have reversed the disease process. It seems more likely that the large amounts of folate in liver were responsible for the clinical response of their initial patients.

Regardless of the inadequacies of Minot and Murphy's theoretical knowledge, they clearly demonstrated that pernicious anemia could effectively be treated with liver therapy. This triggered a research effort that ultimately pinpointed vitamin B-12 as the key problem in pernicious anemia and helped focus efforts on the relationship between nutrition and hematologic disorders.

STEVEN C. MARTIN

Selected Bibliography

PRIMARY SOURCE

Minot, G. R., and W. P. Murphy. 1926. "Treatment of Pernicious Anemia by a Special Diet." *Journal of the American Medical Association* 87:470–76.

———. 1927. "A Diet Rich in Liver in the Treatment of Pernicious Anemia." *Journal of the American Medical Association* 89:759–66.

Murphy, W. P., R. T. Monroe, and R. Fitz. 1927. "Changes in Composition of Blood in Pernicious Anemia." *Journal of the American Medical Association* 88:1211–14.

Minot, G. R., E. J. Cohn, W. P. Murphy, and H. A. Lawson. 1928. "Treatment of Pernicious Anemia with Liver Extract." *American Journal of Medical Sciences* 175, no. 5:599.

Murphy, W. P. 1933. "The Advantages of Intramuscular Injections of a Solution of Liver Extract in the Treatment of Pernicious Anemia." *American Journal of Medical Sciences* 186, no. 3:361.

———. No date. Papers. Countway Library, Harvard Medical School, Boston, Massachusetts.

SECONDARY SOURCES

Castle, W. B. 1952. "The Contributions of George Richards Minot to Experimental Medicine." *New England Journal of Medicine* 247:585–91.

Wintrobe, Maxwell M., ed. 1980. *Blood, Pure and Eloquent: A Story of Discovery, People, and of Ideas.* New York: McGraw-Hill.

DANIEL NATHANS *1978*

Daniel Nathans was born in Wilmington, Delaware, on October 30, 1928. A molecular biologist, Nathans shared the Nobel Prize in 1978 with Werner Arber and Hamilton O. Smith for his use of restriction enzymes to cleave, map, and analyze the structure of the simian virus SV40, following Arber's description of the restriction-modification model and Smith's isolation of the first restriction enzyme (known as Hind II) which cut DNA at specific identifiable sites. These three investigations led cumulatively to the techniques of DNA recombination and the potential breakthroughs of genetic engineering. Nathans is Boury Professor of Molecular Biology and Genetics at Johns Hopkins University, a title he has held since 1976. He has been director of the department since 1972. He married Joanne Gomberg in 1956; they have three sons: Eli, Jeremy, and Benjamin.

Nathans was the youngest of nine children of Samuel and Sarah Nathans, Russian Jewish immigrants, and grew up under considerable hardship during the Great Depression. He earned his baccalaureate at the University of Delaware (1950) and his medical degree at Washington University in St. Louis (1954). He had already developed an interest in research, and, following an internship at Columbia-Presbyterian Medical Center, he spent two years (1955–57) as clinical associate at the National Cancer Institute, where he studied protein synthesis in bone malignancy.

After completing his residency at Columbia-Presbyterian in 1959, he won a USPHS grant to do research at the Rockefeller Institute for Medical Research, where he worked with Fritz Lipmann and Norton Zinder. He continued his work on protein synthesis and became interested in the phenomenon of host-controlled variation among bacterial viruses. This process had been observed and described by Giuseppe Bertani, Salvador E. Luria, and Jean J. Weigle in the 1950s. A specific virus, or bacteriophage, is capable of infecting and rapidly destroying the cells of a specific strain of bacteria. However, the same virus, injected into a new bacterial culture, will be broken down into particles, or "restricted," by its host. A few phage particles, however, will survive within the bacterial culture, and will be reproduced (or "modified") as a new variant virus, capable of infecting the new host. The implications of this phenomenon for our understanding of the incidence and spread of viral infections are clearly of great interest (Linn 1978, 1070).

In 1962 Nathans became assistant professor of microbiology and director of genetics at Johns Hopkins. That same year, Werner Arber in Geneva had established the genetic basis of restriction-modification and proposed a model based on the recognition and cleavage of specific nucleotide sequences of the viral DNA by "restriction enzymes," or endonucleases, within the host bacterium. According to Arber's hypothesis, while the restriction enzyme effectively breaks down the viral DNA, a methylase enzyme acts to protect the bacterial DNA by identifying the identical sequences within the host and methylating them to shield them from attack. Some of the foreign sequences may also be methylated. The phage DNA, thus modified, will eventually generate a new variant virus.

Arber and his coworkers, by 1968, had isolated a Type 1 restriction enzyme, which recognized the specific nucleotide sequences of foreign DNA but cleaved the invader apparently at random. Although this discovery confirmed the model in part, the random activity of these enzymes had no potential for further investigation.

Nathans became associate professor in 1965 and full professor in 1967. He continued his research into the genetic development of bacteriophages and became interested as well in similar viruses that infect animals. By 1969 he had begun to concentrate on the simian tumor virus SV40, which causes tumors in monkeys. In that year, his colleague at Hopkins, Hamilton O. Smith, succeeded in isolating the first Type II restriction enzyme, which recognized and cleaved foreign DNA molecules at specific identifiable sites. Nathans immediately perceived the value of this enzyme as a "cutting tool" to use in the study of viral DNA (Linn 1978, 1071).

Working with Kathleen Danna, Nathans used the newly discovered enzyme, Hind II, to cut the double stranded SV40 DNA into eleven specific sections. They used these and other, larger fragments to determine the physical structure of DNA by identifying which pieces fit together, rather like a jigsaw puzzle. They then used radioactive labeling, enzyme cleavage, and tracking of the radioactivity in the fragments to determine the replication process of the DNA molecule. The replication process was found to be circular, two strands proceeding simultaneously in two directions from a unique point of origin and linking at a point 180 degrees opposite.

In subsequent experiments, Nathans and his coworkers accurately mapped and described the process of SV40 infection at the level of RNA production and hybridization. They were able to draw a detailed picture of the origin and direction of RNA activity at each stage of the infection and restriction processes. The methods they developed were later used to map and analyze a wide variety of complex DNA molecules and restriction nucleotide sequences (Nathans and Smith 1975, Linn 1978, 1071).

Smith's and Nathans's methods have been applied in several laboratories, including Herbert Boyer's and Howard Goodman's at UCSF, Paul Berg's and Stanley Cohen's at Stanford, and Kenneth and Noreen Murray's in Edinburgh, to cleave and recombine various DNA molecules, and then reproduce the resulting DNA in bacterial or other host cells. Boyer and his colleagues established that different DNA molecules cut by the same enzyme at identical sites will have "sticky edges" that "fit" with each other. The new technology makes possible the in vitro production of scarce enzymes and hormones, such as insulin. Research applications have included the mutation of tumor cells and the study of the control of genetic function.

However, experiments that combine eukaryotic with bacterial or viral DNA in a single replicable molecule have created fears of the creation of dangerous new pathogens. In 1974 Nathans joined other scientists in recommending that some types of recombinant DNA research be postponed until more was understood about the risks and requesting the NIH to establish specific guidelines for recombinant DNA research (Linn 1978, 1071).

Daniel Nathans is a member of the National Academy of Sciences, which honored him with the United States Steel Foundation Award in Molecular Biology in 1976, and a senior investigator of the Howard Hughes Medical Institute. He is also a member of the American Academy of Arts & Sciences.

MARCIA MELDRUM

Selected Bibliography

PRIMARY SOURCES

Nathans, Daniel. 1960. "Purification of a Supernatant Factor that Stimulates Amino Acid Transfer from Soluble Ribonucleic Acid to Protein." *Annals of the New York Academy of Sciences* 88:718–21.

———. 1965. "Cell-Free Protein Synthesis Directed by Coliphage MS2 RNA: Synthesis of Intact Viral Coat Protein and Other Products." *Journal of Molecular Biology* 13 (September):521–31.

———. 1968. "Natural RNA Coding of Bacterial Protein Synthesis." *Methods of Enzymology* 12:787–91.

Nathans, Daniel, and Kathleen J. Danna. 1972. "Studies of SV40 DNA. 3. Differences in DNA from Various Strains of SV40." *Journal of Molecular Biology* 64 (March): 515–18.

———. 1972. "Specific Origin in SV40 DNA Replication." *Nature* 236 (April 19):200–202.

Nathans, Daniel, S. P. Adler, W. W. Brockmann, et al. 1974. "Use of Restriction Endonucleases in Analyzing the Genome of Simian Virus 40." *Federal Proceedings* 33 (May): 1135–38.

Nathans, Daniel, and Hamilton O. Smith. 1975. "Restriction Endonucleases in the Analysis and Restructuring of DNA Molecules." *Annual Review of Biochemistry* 44:273–93.

SECONDARY SOURCES

Linn, Stuart. 1978. "The 1978 Nobel Prize in Physiology or Medicine." *Science* 202 (December 8):1069–71.

1982. "Nathans, Daniel." *Modern Scientists and Engineers*, 3:348–49. New York: McGraw-Hill.

Sylvester, Kathy. 1978 "Daniel Nathans." *New York Times* (October 13):60.

CHARLES JULES HENRI NICOLLE
1928

Charles Jules Henri Nicolle was born on September 21, 1866, in Rouen, France. A physician and bacteriologist, he won the Nobel Prize in Physiology or Medicine in 1928 for his work in determining the role of lice in the transmission of typhus. He died February 28, 1936, in Tunis, Tunisia.

Nicolle's early life was spent in Rouen. He was the second of three sons of Eugène Nicolle and Aline Louvrier. His father was a physician in Rouen with a position at the municipal hospital and also professor of natural history at the Ecole des Sciences et des Arts in the town. His mother was the daughter of a clockmaker. The Nicolles were destined to be a distinguished medical family. Both Charles and his elder brother Maurice became physicians of note. Charles's daughter and son Marcelle (b. 1896) and Pierre (b. 1898), from his marriage with Alice Avice of Rouen in 1895, became physicians, and so too did Maurice's son Jacques. The family was a close and devoted one.

After his secondary education at the Lycée Corneille in Rouen, Charles Nicolle studied medicine in Rouen and Paris. Literature had been his first love—and he later wrote several novels and collections of stories—but the wishes of his father that his sons become physicians prevailed in his career choice. His aptitude for medicine was shown in 1889 when he passed at his first attempt the competitive resident medical studentship examination in the Paris hospitals, and he became demonstrator at the Faculty of Medicine in the laboratory of Albert Gombault, an anatomophysiologist. But Charles was persuaded by his elder brother Maurice to enroll at the newly opened Institut Pasteur as Maurice himself had done. Charles Nicolle's discovery of the world of bacteriological research at the institute and the contacts he made there determined his future career and achievements. Nicolle studied with Emile Roux and Elie Metchnikoff and was influenced by the differing scientific styles of both men—Roux's insistence on exactitude and rigor in experimentation, and Metchnikoff's creative insights into the solution of research problems. In his own later work Nicolle's intuitive hypotheses about disease were always corroborated by careful experimentation.

In 1893 Nicolle wrote his doctoral thesis on the venereal disease soft chancre, caused by Ducrey's bacillus. He then returned to Rouen to a post as supplementary professor in the school of medicine, but, inspired by his Parisian experiences, he hoped to create in his native town a center of medical studies and laboratory research. His enthusiastic endeavors to achieve such a center over the next nine years were partly frustrated because his continuing work on venereal disease was unwelcome to potential bourgeois patrons of medical research in Rouen. His medical practice was also hampered by his increasing deafness, an affliction that had begun in his adolescence and which made social contacts difficult for the rest of his life.

The turning point in his career came in 1902. He decided to leave his beloved Normandy and accept Emile Roux's offer of a whole new life as director of the Institut Pasteur in Tunis. For the next thirty-three years, Nicolle devoted himself to the goal of understanding the uncharted bacteriology of diseases of the Mediterranean basin, especially those of North Africa. To accomplish this task he transformed a largely inactive and run-down laboratory for producing vaccines against rabies and providing yeasts for local winemakers into a well-financed, flourishing research laboratory housed in specially designed buildings, and also a center for chemical analyses and larger scale production of vaccines against smallpox, diphtheria, and tetanus. He also founded a journal to report results of research. Nicolle saw bacteriological research as a team activity and encouraged distinguished collaborators to come and work under his leadership. Once the significance of his work was recognized, researchers came from all over the world. His institute, of which he was the heart and soul, played an important part in enhancing France's eminence in bacteriology and extending French scientific culture to colonial territories. Nicolle's great personal charm and *politesse* were significant factors in the institute's success. His personality made him difficult to forget and his students and collaborators became devoted to him.

Nicolle's research was conducted in that exciting period in the early twentieth century when the explanatory power of the mature germ theory was leading to rapid discoveries about agents and vectors of disease by research terms throughout the world. Nicolle and his coworkers contributed to the understanding of a spectrum of diseases, including typhus, African infantile leishmaniasis, toxoplasmosis, Malta fever, and trachoma. Early work in Tunis led to the discovery by Nicolle that the dog was the reservoir of the parasite responsible for the African form of leishmaniasis and that it was a variety distinct from kala-azar, the form found in India (1908). A special culture medium that Nicolle developed helped in the investigation of all forms of leishmaniasis. The capture of Tunisian rodents led to the discovery with L. Manceaux of a new parasite he named *Toxoplasma gondii.* Parasites such as these were later found to cause both animal and human disease.

Nicolle is best known for his Nobel Prize–winning work on typhus, first announced in 1909 to the Academy of Sciences in Paris. Nicolle's insight that lice were the parasites involved in the transmission of the disease was based on recognition of the significance of the infection patterns of typhus in a local Tunisian hospital. Typhus was not communicated in the wards once the patients entering the hospital with the disease were washed and their clothes removed. His idea was substantiated by rigorous animal experimentation in association with Charles Comte and Ernest Conseil. A chimpanzee was injected with blood from a human typhus patient and then the disease was shown to be transmitted by lice to macaques. The discovery of the vector of typhus suggested effective means to control the disease. Systematic delousing campaigns largely eradicated typhus in Tunis, where the disease had recurred annually, and were of enormous significance in World War I in diminishing the extensive casualities from typhus that had accompanied the conflict of armies for centuries.

Nicolle's studies of typhus led him to the investigation of the complex role of a variety of vectors in other diseases. He showed the part played by lice in spreading the infection caused by Obermeier's spirillum, by flies in trachoma, and by ticks in diseases caused by spirochetes. The typhus work also helped direct his research to vaccines, a matter of great concern in the field of infectious diseases in the preantibiotic era. Knowledge of the preventive powers of the serum of convalescent typhus patients not only gave a means to protect attendants working with those suffering from the disease but also led Nicolle and Ernest Conseil to the development of a very successful vaccine for measles. Other areas of disease research to which Nicolle contributed were his recognition in 1918 that influenza by a virus, an issue undecided at the time, and later in 1931, the study of murine typhus.

The difficulties and expense of obtaining apes and monkeys as experimental animals fostered a search for other animals to use in typhus investigations. Nicolle's discovery with Charles Lebailly that guinea pigs were susceptible to typhus, although showing no apparent symptoms of the disease, was useful in solving these problems and assisting in the explication of exactly how lice carried and transmitted the disease. But what is more important, it led to Nicolle's major theoretical contribution to bacteriology, the concept of inapparent infections. The understanding that a disease could go through its entire life cycle in an apparently healthy individual, either human or animal, helped explain the continuing existence of infectious diseases and the generation of epidemics. Later work convinced Nicolle that such inapparent infection not only occurred in typhus but in other diseases as well, notably in measles and whooping cough.

Nicolle's accomplishments in bacteriological research were recognized in France by the award of the Osiris prize of the Institut de France in 1927, the year before his Nobel Prize, and by his appointment to the chair of experimental medicine at the Collège de France in 1932. Maintaining his post in Tunis, each year until his death he visited Paris to lecture at the Collège and conduct teaching on how to do research. Yet he did not set great store by such honors and saw his work at the Collège as a way to attract young minds to science.

The 1930s were an important period of literary production for him, and his books were much discussed in scientific and medical circles. He published his vision of the life spans and evolution of infectious diseases in *Naissance, vie et mort des maladies infectieuses* (1930), ideas followed up in 1933 in *Destin des maladies infectieuses*. He wrote two books on questions of biology, *Biologie de l'invention* (1932), in which he discussed creative thinking, and *La Nature, conception morale et biologique* (1934). These issues, and others relating to medical practice and the conduct of research, were the subject of his teaching at the Collège de France. His lectures on the latter topic were published as *Introduction à la carrière de la médecine expérimentale* (1932), *L'Expérimentation en médecine* (1934), and *Responsabilités de la médecine*, (2 vols., 1935 and 1936). His final work *La Destinée humaine* (1936), was on the future of mankind. Nicolle was ill for most of the last year of his life before dying from a heart attack. He was buried in the institute in Tunis according to his wishes.

CAROLINE HANNAWAY

Selected Bibliography

PRIMARY SOURCES

Nicolle, Charles, Charles Comte, and Ernest Conseil. 1909–11. "Transmission expérimentale du typhus exanthé-matique par le pou du corps." *Comptes Rendus de l'Académie des Sciences* 149:486.

[Nicolle, Charles]. 1930. "Conference du Docteur Charles Nicolle sur les travaux qui lui ont valu l'attribution du prix Nobel de Médecine." *Archives de l'Institut Pasteur de Tunis* 19:113–21.

Detailed accounts of the experiments on typhus transmission are:

Nicolle, Charles. 1910. "Recherches expérimentales sur le typhus exanthématique, enterprises à l'Institut Pasteur de Tunis pendant l'année 1909." *Annales de l'Institut Pasteur* 24:243–75.

———. 1911. "Recherches expérimentales sur le typhus exanthématique, enterprises à l'Institut Pasteur de Tunis pendant l'année 1910." *Annales de l'Institut Pasteur* 25:97–144.

Nicolle, Charles, Ernest, Conseil, and A. Conor. 1912. "Recherches expérimentales sur le typhus exanthématique, enterprises à l'Institut Pasteur de Tunis pendant l'année 1911." *Annales de l'Institut Pasteur* 26:250–80, 332–35.

Nicolle, Charles. 1930. *Naissance, vie et mort des maladies infectieuses.* Paris: F. Alcan.

———. 1932. *Biologie de l'invention.* Paris: F. Alcan.

———. 1933. *Destin des maladies infectieuses.* Paris: F. Alcan.

———. 1934. *La Nature, conception morale et biologique.* Paris: F. Alcan.

———. 1934. *L'Expérimentation en médecine.* Paris: F. Alcan.

———. 1935 and 1936, 2 vols. *Responsabilités de la médecine.* Paris and Tunis.

———. 1936. *La Destinée humaine.* Paris: F. Alcan.

SECONDARY SOURCES

A bibliography of Nicolle's numerous scientific papers is to be found in "Publications scientifiques de Charles Nicolle." *Archives de l'Institut Pasteur de Tunis* 25 (1936):209–48. There is no detailed scholarly biography of Nicolle.

1966. *Archives de l'Institut Pasteur de Tunis* 43. A special number devoted to commemoration of the hundredth anniversary of Nicolle's birth.

1986. *Bulletin de l'Académie Nationale de Médecine* 170, no. 2:271–304. A special number devoted to commemoration of the fiftieth anniversary of Nicolle's death.

Giroud, Paul. 1966. "Eloge de Charles Nicolle." *Bulletin de la Société de Pathologie Exotique* 59:442–53.

Lot, Germaine. 1961. *Charles Nicolle et la biologie conquérante.* Paris: Editions Seghers.

Mesnil, F. 1931. "Notice nécrologique sur M. Charles Nicolle (1866–1936)." *Bulletin de l'Académie de Médecine* 115:541–48.

Nicolle, Pierre. 1981. "Un événement capital dans la vie passionnée de Charles Nicolle: le prix Nobel de physiologie ou médecine." *Bulletin de la Société de Pathologie Exotique* 74:101–18.

MARSHALL WARREN NIRENBERG

1968

Born on April 10, 1927, in New York City, Marshall Warren Nirenberg grew up in Orlando, Florida, where his family moved when he was twelve years old. His father, Harry Nirenberg, was a land developer, and his mother, Minerva, a housewife. Nirenberg pursued an early interest in biology at the University of Florida, receiving his B.S. in zoology and chemistry in 1948 and his M.S. in zoology in 1952. While preparing his master's thesis, an ecological and taxonomic study of caddis flies (*Trichoptera*), Nirenberg became interested in biochemistry. Encouraged by faculty members at the University of Florida, he continued his studies in this field at the University of Michigan. He earned a Ph.D. in biological chemistry in 1957, working with James F. Hogg on the enzyme transport mechanism for hexose, a sugar, in ascites tumor cells. In 1961 he married Perola Zaltzman; they have no children.

In 1957 Nirenberg was recruited as a postdoctoral fellow for the National Institute of Arthritis and Metabolic Diseases (NIAMD), one of the National Institutes of Health

(NIH) in Bethesda, Maryland. A shy, quiet young man, Nirenberg studied enzymatic induction and bacterial adaptation in collaboration with William Jakoby. During this period Nirenberg took an evening course that stimulated his interest in the biochemistry of genetics. In 1960, when he moved to Gordon Thompkins's section of metabolic enzymes, NIAMD, as a permanent staff member, Nirenberg took up one of the most tantalizing scientific problems of that time, the genetic code. Specifically, he sought to describe on the molecular level the mechanism by which protein synthesis was directed in the cells of all living things.

Although people had observed for eons that certain traits were inherited, it was not until 1866 that Gregor Mendel, a Czech monk, demonstrated that inheritance was packaged into many independent units, now called genes. Observing the common pea plant, Mendel made careful counts of how a single, easily visible trait, such as round versus wrinkled seeds, was inherited. He showed that each parent transmitted one-half of his or her genes to an offspring and that the parental genes did not blend but remained segregated in transmission. Mendel's work was largely ignored until 1900, when it was rediscovered by agricultural investigators, who utilized the information to develop stronger, weed- and pest-resistant hybrids. Mendelian genetics also fostered a human "eugenics" movement to produce presumably healthier and more moral people. This attempt at social application of scientific knowledge, however, fell into disrepute during the 1930s, when its dark side was revealed in the Nazi efforts to create a super race and to eliminate those considered less desirable.

During the early decades of the twentieth century laboratory investigation of the genes themselves remained shackled by the limitations of technique. By 1913 investigators knew that genes were strung together on chromosomes in the nucleus of the cell and that chromosomes consisted of proteins and nucleic acids. Which of these materials comprised the genes, or, for that matter, what structure a gene might take, remained unknown. During the 1930s many investigators argued that genes were likely to be autocatalytic proteins. Near the end of World War II, however, Oswald Avery and Maclyn McCarty at the Rockefeller Institute of Medical Research demonstrated that nucleic acids, not proteins, transmitted genetic information and that deoxyribonucleic acid, or DNA, was the "molecule of heredity." This discovery stimulated an intensive period of study on DNA that culminated in 1953, when American James D. Watson and Briton Francis H. C. Crick, later Nobel Prize–winners themselves, announced that the structure of DNA assumed the shape of a double helix. They described two long, coiled, phosphate-sugar chains in the molecule that were joined by two sets of paired purine and pyrimidine bases.

The architecture of DNA suggested that the order of the bases in the molecule might represent a code for protein synthesis. Although millions of proteins are produced by living things, all are constituted of different arrangements of twenty amino acids. When Nirenberg took up the challenge of the genetic code, he and other investigators were seeking a method to demonstrate how genes coded for the placement of specific amino acids in proteins. Although the intermediate steps in the process then remained obscured, it shortly became clear that DNA itself was not directly involved in the process. Rather, in a process called transcription, the code was copied onto single-stranded messenger ribonucleic acid (mRNA), which interacted with other cell constituents to direct protein synthesis.

Nirenberg approached the problem by means of a cell-free system. Prepared with cell-sap from *Escherichia coli* bacteria, such a medium was essential to eliminate natural protein synthesis by intact cells. Nirenberg monitored the production of protein in the system and observed that the process could be stopped completely by the addition of the enzymes ribonuclease or deoxyribonuclease. Hoping to stimulate the production of a single protein from the inactive system, Nirenberg obtained from his NIH colleagues Leon Heppel and Maxine Singer synthetic RNA polymers containing a single repeating base. In a key series of experiments conducted with postdoctoral fellow Johann Heinrich Matthaei, polyuradylic acid, or poly-U, an mRNA polymer containing the repeating base uracil, was found to stimulate the production of an artificial protein comprised of the single amino acid phenylalanine. Subsequent experiments confirmed this result and showed that the code was composed of base triplets, known as *codons*. Thus was the first "word" of the genetic code deciphered: UUU coded for phenylalanine.

Although Nirenberg's method permitted rapid identification of the remaining triplets and their associated proteins, determining the sequence of bases within each triplet proved a stubborn problem. To overcome this obstacle, Nirenberg devised a technique based on the observation that a physically large complex was formed as protein synthesis took place. He used a filter of cellulose nitrate with pores less than half a micron in size, which trapped the protein-synthesizing complex while permitting other constituents to pass through. By radio-labeling one amino acid in a mixture of all twenty and by using mRNA polymers of carefully defined composition, Nirenberg utilized the filter to identify the radio-labeled amino acid for which the defined sequence of mRNA coded. Within five years of his initial publication on the first code word, all sixty-four triplet combinations of the four bases and their associated amino acids had been described. A molecular definition of the gene was also at hand: It was the series of bases that coded for the production of a single protein.

When his work on the genetic code was completed, Nirenberg turned his attention to problems of neurobiology as chief of the Laboratory of Biochemical Genetics in the National Heart, Lung, and Blood

Institute (NHLBI). Utilizing monoclonal antibodies and cultured cell systems, he and his colleagues investigated how neurons in the developing nervous system form synapses and distinguish appropriate from inappropriate synapses. One major finding from this work was that cyclic adenosine monophosphate, a nucleotide found among the hydrolysis products of all nucleic acids, regulates synaptogenesis by controlling the expression of voltage-sensitive calcium ion channels, which in turn are required for stimulus-dependent secretion of neurotransmitters at the synapses.

Nirenberg's work on the genetic code earned him numerous awards from organizations and institutions around the world. He was elected a fellow of the National Academy of Science (U.S.), a member of the American Academy of Arts and Sciences, a member of the American Society of Biological Chemists, a member of the American Chemical Society, and a member of many other professional societies. Among the many other honors he has received for his work are Molecular Biology Award, National Academy of Sciences, 1962; Paul Lewis Award in Enzyme Chemistry, American Chemical Society, 1964; National Medal of Science, President of the United States, 1965; Hildebrand Award, American Chemical Society, Washington, D.C., 1966; Research Corporation Award, 1966; American College of Physicians Award, 1967; Gairdner Foundation Award of Merit, Toronto, Canada, 1967; Prix Charles Leopold Meyer of the French Academy of Sciences, 1967; Franklin Medal, University of Pennsylvania, 1968; Distinguished Service Medal, U.S. Department of Health, Education and Welfare, 1968; Louisa Gross Horwitz Prize, Columbia University, 1968; Lasker Award, 1968. In 1968 he shared the Nobel Prize with Robert W. Holley and Har Gobind Khorana.

Deciphering the genetic code has permitted humans to understand for the first time how Nature governs life processes in all living things, for the code is essentially the same in plants, animals, and microorganisms. The importance of this code for biology has been compared to that of the periodic table of the elements for chemistry. Although Nirenberg's research was quite clearly an achievement in fundamental knowledge, its potential applications to medicine were clear. In the quarter century since the code was broken, a number of genetic markers for inherited diseases have been identified. A massive project to map the entire human genome is about to be launched. Research on genetic factors in cancer and in heart disease has expanded knowledge about these diseases and informed intervention strategies. Some investigators even speculate about the possibility of medical intervention at the cellular level to correct genetic problems. Nirenberg's contribution to the elucidation of the genetic code opened the way to such fruitful research, which may eventually produce effective strategies for dealing with inherited diseases.

VICTORIA A. HARDEN

Selected Bibliography

PRIMARY SOURCES

Nirenberg, Marshall W. 1963. "The Genetic Code: 2." *Scientific American* 208:80–94.

———. 1968. "The Genetic Code." Nobel Lecture. In *Les Prix Nobel en 1968*, 221–41. Stockholm: P. A. Norstedt and Söner, 1969.

———. 1983. "Modulation of Synapse Formation by Cyclic Adenosine Monophosphate." *Science* 222:794–99.

SECONDARY SOURCES

Judson, Horace Freeland. 1979. *The Eighth Day of Creation: Makers of the Revolution in Biology*, especially Chapter 8, "He Wasn't a Member of the Club." New York: Simon and Schuster.

Martin, Robert G. 1984. "A Revisionist View of the Breaking of the Genetic Code." In *NIH: An Account of Research in Its Laboratories and Clinics*, edited by DeWitt Stetten, Jr., and W. T. Carrigan, 282–96. New York: Academic Press.

SEVERO OCHOA *1959*

Severo Ochoa was born on September 24, 1905, in Luarca, Spain. His areas of scientific specialization within biochemistry include enzymology and the nucleic acids. He received the 1959 Nobel Prize in Physiology or Medicine jointly with Arthur Kornberg "for their discovery of the mechanisms in the biological synthesis of ribonucleic acid and deoxyribonucleic acid. Severo Ochoa and Carmen Garcia Cobian were married on July 8, 1931. They had no children.

His father, Severo Ochoa, was a lawyer and businessman. His mother was Carmen de Albornoz Ochoa. Severeo Ochoa was the youngest of seven children; his father died when he was only seven.

Ochoa received a B.A. from Malaga College, Spain, in 1921. His interest in biology was aroused by the work of the great Spanish neurologist Santiago Ramon y Cajal. He was awarded his M.D. with honors by the University of Madrid in 1929. While at the university he was assistant to Juan Negrin; during the summer of 1927 he worked with D. Noel Paton at the University of Glasgow. With support from the Spanish Council of Scientific Research, Ochoa began graduate work in 1929 with Otto Meyerhof at the Kaiser Wilhelm Institute für Medizinsiche Forschung at Heidelberg. Ochoa remembered Meyerhof as his most influential teacher. Under Meyerhof's direction he worked on the biochemistry and physiology of muscle. In 1931 he was appointed lecturer in physiology at the University of Madrid; he held this position until 1935. In 1932 he worked with Dr. H. W. Dudley on enzymology at the National Institute for Medical Research, London. In 1934 he returned to Madrid as lecturer in physiology and biochemistry and later became head of the Physiology Division of the Institute for Medical Research in Madrid. In 1936, with the Civil War turning the university into a battlefield, he returned to Meyerhof's laboratory at Heidelberg as guest research assistant to conduct research on some of the enzymatic steps of glycolysis and fermentation.

In 1937 Ochoa worked at the Plymouth Marine Biological Laboratory in England. In collaboration with his wife he investigated enzymatic phosphorylation in invertebrate muscle and the cozymase content of this tissue. From 1938 to 1941 he studied the biological function of vitamin B_1 with Rudolph A. Peters at Oxford University, with an appointment as demonstrator and Nuffield research assistant. During this period he became interested in the enzymatic mechanisms of oxidative metabolism.

His career in the United States began in 1941 with an appointment as instructor and research associate in pharmacology at Washington University, St. Louis, where he worked with Carl and Gerty Cori. In 1942 he obtained a position as research associate in medicine at the New York University School of Medicine. Remaining at New York University, he became assistant professor of biochemistry in 1945, professor of pharmacology in 1946, professor of biochemistry in 1954, and chairman of the Department of Biochemistry. He accepted a position as researcher with the Roche Institute of Molecular Biology, in New Jersey, in 1975.

Severo Ochoa's research on high-energy phosphates and their role in the body's energy processes resulted in the discovery and application of the enzyme polynucleotide phosphorylase, which catalyzes the synthesis of RNA. In his presentation speech for the 1959 Nobel Prize, H. Theorell stressed the importance of two principles necessary to life: proteins and nucleic acids. Because nucleic acids were divided into two different types, having very different functions, two prize winners had been selected: Arthur Kornberg for the synthesis of DNA, the hereditary substance in chromosomes, and Severo Ochoa for the synthesis of RNA, which assists in the synthesis of proteins. "It is to the everlasting credit of Ochoa and Kornberg," Theorell asserted, "to have clarified this fundamental mechanism by preparing proteins that build up nucleic acids in test tubes" (Theorell, 1959, 642). Theorell predicted that because of the work of Ochoa and Kornberg we would soon witness many important advances in biocehmistry, virus research, genetics, cancer research, and our fundamental understanding of the mechanism of life.

Ochoa's research has dealt primarily with enzymatic processes in biological oxidation and synthesis and the transfer of energy. This work has contributed significantly to knowledge of the basic steps in the metabolism of carbohydrates and fatty acids, the utilization of carbon dioxide, the biosynthesis of nucleic acids, the biological functions of vitamin B_1, oxidative phosphorylation, the reductive carboxylation of ketoglutaric and pyruvic acids, the photochemical reduction of pyridine nucleotides in photosynthesis, the enzymes of the Krebs cycle, polynucleotide phosphorylase, and the genetic code.

In 1955 Severo Ochoa and Marianne Grunberg-Manago announced the discovery of a new enzyme in *Azobacter vinelandii* that was capable of synthesizing RNA in the test tube from simple nucleotide units. At first they wanted to call the enzyme a synthetase, but because it produced random polymers they agreed to call it "polynucleotide phosphorylase." When highly purified, the enzyme requires an oligonucleotide to prime the reaction, but it does not require or copy a template. Some years later the polynucleotides synthesized in vitro were shown to be active as messengers in the biosynthesis of proteins. However, the precise biological significance of polynucleotide phosphorylase is still obscure. The enzyme had been found in several bacterial species and in plant tissues.

After an RNA polymerase that synthesized RNA under the direction of a DNA template was isolated from *Escherichia coli* in 1960, Ochoa isolated a similar enzyme from *Azobacter vinelandii* and proved that it was distinct from polynucleotide phosphorylase. Inevitably this work on the structure of synthetic polynucleotides, during the formative years of molecular biology, led Ochoa into experimental studies of the genetic code. Within a very short period the pioneering work of Marshall Nirenberg had been extended by Ochoa, Har Gobind Khorana, Charles Yanofsky, and others into a complete catalog of codons. Ochoa's next major research program involved the systematic investigation of the expression of the genetic message: 1) the replication of RNA viruses and 2) the expression of the nucleic acid message in protein synthesis in bacterial and developing eukaryotic systems.

In his Nobel Prize Lecture, Ochoa stressed the biological importance of RNA in the biosynthesis of proteins and as the genetic material of certain viruses. Cytoplasmic RNA was known to occur in two forms that differed in molecular weight and role in protein synthesis. RNA appeared to be synthesized in the nucleus and transported to the cytoplasm. Polynucleotide phosphorylase from the microorganism *Axobacter vinelandii* was capable of catalyzing the synthesis of high molecular weight polyribonucleotides from nucleoside diphosphates. The purified enzyme had the interesting property of catalyzing RNA synthesis not only from mixtures of the four naturally occurring ribonucleoside diphosphates, but also from any single nucleoside diphosphate, or from uncommon or unnatural nucleoside diphosphates. The incorporation of precursors into the macromolecule was found to be proportional to their concentration in the reaction mixture. However, the enzyme can synthesize polynucleotides of macromolecular size and the enzyme product was eventually shown to be as active as natural messenger RNA as a messenger in the biosynthesis of proteins.

Other honors awarded to Severo Ochoa include the Neuberg Medal Award, Society of European Chemists (1951), the Charles Meyer Price Award, Societé de Chimie Biologique (1955), the Borden Award, Association of American Medical Colleges (1958), the New York University Medal (1960), the Order of the Rising Sun, Second Class Gold Medal, Japan (1967), the Quevedo Gold Medal, Spain (1969), the Albert Gallatin Medal (1970), and the National Medal of Science (1979).

Ochoa holds honorary degrees from Oxford, Wesleyan, and the Universities of Glasgow, Salamanca, and Brazil and Washington University (St. Louis). He was honorary professor of the University of San Marcos, Lima, Peru. He has also been president of the International Union of Biochemistry (1961–67).

LOIS N. MAGNER

Selected Bibliography

PRIMARY SOURCES

Grunberg-Manago, Marianne, and S. Ochoa. 1955. "Enzymatic Synthesis and Breakdown of Polynucleotides; Polynucleotide Phosphorylase." *Journal of the American Chemical Society* 77:3165–66.

Grunberg-Manago, Marianne, P. J. Ortiz, and S. Ochoa. 1955. "Enzymatic Synthesis of Nucleic Acidlike Polynucleotides." *Science* 122:907–10.

Heppel, L. A., P. J. Ortiz, and S. Ochoa. 1956. "Small Polyribonucleotides with 5' Phosphomonoester End-Groups." *Science* 123:415–17.

Ochoa, Severo. 1959. "Enzymatic Synthesis of Ribonucleic Acid." Nobel Lecture, December 11, 1959. Reprinted in *Nobel Lectures, Physiology or Medicine*, vol. 3 (1942–62), 644–64. Amsterdam: Elsevier, 1964.

Sols, A., and C. Estevez, eds. 1976. *Collected Papers of Severo Ochoa, 1928–1975.* Madrid: Ministry of Education and Science.

SECONDARY SOURCES

1962. *Current Biography Yearbook*, 327–29. New York: H. W. Wilson.

Fruton, Joseph S. 1982. *A Bio-Bibliography for the History of the Biochemical Sciences Since 1800.* Philadelphia: American Philosophical Society.

———. 1972. *Molecules and Life. Historical Essays on the Interplay of Chemistry and Biology.* New York: Wiley-Interscience.

Grande, F. 1963. "Severo Ochoa." *ICSU Review of World Science* 5:147–58.

Kornberg, A., B. L. Horecker, L. Cornudella, and J. Oro, eds. 1976. *Reflections on Biochemistry In Honour of Severo Ochoa.* Oxford. Pergamon Press.

McElroy, W. D., and B. Glass, eds. 1957. *The Chemical Basis of Heredity.* Baltimore: Johns Hopkins Press.

1959. "Ochoa and Kornberg Win Nobel Prize." *Science* 130:1099–1100.

Theorell, H. 1959. "Presentation Speech." *Nobel Lectures, Physiology or Medicine*, vol. 3 (1942–62), pp. 642–644. Amsterdam: Elsevier, 1964.

GEORGE EMIL PALADE *1974*

George Emil Palade was born on November 19, 1912, in Jassy (or Iasi), Romania. A cellular biologist, Palade shared the 1974 Nobel Prize with Albert Claude and Christian R. de Duvé for their descriptions of the fine microscopic structure and functions of the cell, which laid the foundations of modern cell biology. Claude developed the pioneering techniques of centrifugal fractionation and electron microscopy that made the work possible and carried out the initial observations. Palade improved upon Claude's methods and conclusively established some of Claude's ideas but was himself responsible for drawing the map of the cell as we know it today. In particular, he described the mechanism of protein synthesis by the cellular ribosomes. De Duvé further extended the investigations and identified other particles and their functions. Although the three men worked separately for the most part, all were Europeans based for a part of their careers at the Rockefeller Institute for Medical Research (now Rockefeller University). Palade came to Rockefeller as a visiting investigator in 1946 but elected to remain in the United States after the communist takeover of Romania. At the time of the Nobel award, he was professor of cell biology at Yale University School of Medicine, a position he has held since 1972. Palade married his first wife, Irina Malaxa, in 1941; they had a son, Philip Theodore, and a daughter, Georgia Teodora. Irina Palade died in 1969. Palade married Marilyn Gist Farquhar, a cell biologist who worked with him at the Rockefeller Institute, the following year.

Palade's parents, Emil and Constanta Cantemir Palade, were both teachers; his father taught philosophy at the University of Jassy, and his mother taught elementary school. He entered the University of Bucharest to study medicine and received his degree in 1940 after six years of clinical internship in the Bucharest hospitals (1933–39) and four years as a research assistant and instructor in anatomy (1936–1940). During World War II his army assignment allowed him to continue teaching and research at the university, where he had attained the rank of associate professor by 1946.

Palade's particular interests were in histology and histophysiology. After the war he came to New York University to find out about recent work in the United States. He met Albert Claude at an NYU seminar on the electron microscopic research that Claude had pioneered. Palade introduced himself and quickly impressed the senior scientist, who arranged for a visiting appointment in James B. Murphy's laboratory at the Rockefeller Institute (Hicks 1974; Porter 1974, 517).

Claude had been working at Rockefeller since 1928 on his observations of the fine structures of the cytoplasm, that part of the cell outside the nucleus. He had used centrifugal fractionation, the high speed separation of masses of cells, to separate out the various particles; this method allowed him to identify large "secretory granules," smaller "mitochondria," and even smaller particles of ribonucleic acid, which Claude named "microsomes." He had also succeeded in preparing cells and tissues for the electron bombardment necessary for observation and photography with the electron microscope. Microphotography had revealed the "lacework" of strands and vesicles, called the "endoplasmic reticulum," that forms the infrastructure of the cell.

Palade's initial contribution was the use of buffered osmium tetroxide as an improved fixative for cells for electron microscopy. He worked with George Hogeboom and W. C. Schneider to improve fractionation methods. Using gradient sucrose solutions, the three were able to establish conclusively that the large "secretory granules" consisted primarily of masses of mitochondria, which oxidize fat and sugar to generate energy within the cell.

About the time this work was completed, Claude returned to Belgium. Palade also visited his homeland but decided not to stay under the new Communist government. He accepted a permanent appointment at Rockefeller, becoming a full professor of cytology in 1958. He applied for United States citizenship, and was naturalized in 1952. (Hicks 1974; Porter 1974, 517).

Palade now began with Keith R. Porter a complex series of observations and investigations of avian and mammalian cells with the electron microscope. The collaborators were the first to describe the individual structures of the "organelles," which was now the generic term for the microbodies inside the cell. They identified the double membrane that encloses the mitochondria and established that the endoplasmic reticulum is present in all cells except erythrocytes. The exact structure and connections of the network differ with cell type. It connects in some cells with the outer wall, and, in a few others, with the nuclear membrane. In muscle cells, it appears to play a role in contraction.

Palade noted as well that the microsomes, which were originally thought to be spare bits of mitochondria, were actually involved in some independent activity. In some cells, the microsomes were attached to the outer membranes of the endoplasmic reticulum; in others, they were floating freely. As Claude had earlier observed, they were rich in RNA, or nucleoprotein.

Palade has always believed that the cell holds the key to complex pathologies; that, for example, the degenerative diseases are the outcome of a breakdown of cellular processes, such as protein synthesis. With that in mind, he and Philip Siekevitz began a series of experiments on liver and pancreatic microsomes and on the pancreatic manufacture of proteins needed by the digestive system. (Hicks 1974; Rensberger 1974; Porter 1974, 518).

The researchers' technique involved morphological observation through the electron microscope, biochemical analysis of the fragments observed, and autoradiographic tracings of an amino acid injected into a guinea pig pancreas. By 1960 these innovative experiments had shown that the microsomes, now renamed "ribosomes," do in fact generate proteins, which are then transported through the strands, or "tubules," of the endoplasmic reticulum, and stored in large sacs, which Palade named "cisternae," before being carried to the outer cell wall for secretion (Palade and Siekevitz 1956; Palade and Siekevitz 1958).

Palade's team, including Lucien Caro, David Sabatini, C. Redman, Y. Tashiro, and J. D. Jamieson, further established that some larger ribosomes attached to the reticular membrane use amino acids to construct polypeptides and traced the transportation network, demonstrating the use of energy produced by the mitochondria, and the role of the Golgi complex, another internal structure, in sorting the proteins from other particles.

Palade continues his cellular studies in his laboratory at Yale. His later work with Marilyn Farquhar proposed a new model of cellular intake to replace the existing hypothesis that there were large pores within the cell membrane, which allowed the entry of nutrients and other molecular substances into the cell. In Palade's model, supported by electron micrography, sacs within the cell move to the surface and become part of the outer membrane to envelop and draw the molecule into the cytoplasm (Porter 1974, 518).

Palade's interest in his later work turned to the practical clinical applications of his discoveries. Reflecting de Duvé's statement that "We are sick because our cells are sick," he has sought to establish the link between defects or malfunctions of the cellular "protein factories" and various disorders. His work and that of his colleagues, he has said, "will help immensely . . . in the recognition and ultimately the control of a number of diseases, primarily the degenerative diseases" (Hicks 1974; Rensberger 1974).

In his leisure time, Palade enjoys reading, particularly history. He is a fellow of the American Academy of Arts and Sciences, a member of the National Academy of Sciences, and the founding editor of the *Journal of Cell Biology*. Among the many other awards he has received are the Passano Foundation Award (1964), the Albert Lasker Basic Medical Research Award (1966), the Gairdner Foundation Special Award (1967), and the Louisa G. Horowitz Prize (1970).

MARCIA MELDRUM

Selected Bibliography

PRIMARY SOURCES

Palade, George E., and Philip Siekevitz. 1956. "Liver Microsomes. An Integrated Morphological and Biochemical Study." *Journal of Biophysical and Biochemical Cytology* 2:171–200.

———. 1956. "Pancreatic Microsomes. An Integrated Morphological and Biochemical Study." *Journal of Biophysical and Biochemical Cytology* 2:671–90.

Palade, George E. 1958. "Functional Changes in the Structure of Cell Components." *Woods Hole Subcellular Particles Symposium*, 64–80.

Palade, George E., and Philip Siekevitz. 1958. "A Cytochemical Study on the Pancreas of the Guinea Pig. 1. Isolation and Enzymatic Activities of Cell Fractions." *Journal of Biophysical and Biochemical Cytology* 4 (March 25):203–18.

———. 1958. "A Cytochemical Study on the Pancreas of the Guinea Pig. 2. Functional Variations in the Enzymatic Activity of Microsomes." *Journal of Biophysical and Biochemical Cytology* 4 (May 25):309–18.

———. 1958. "A Cytochemical Study on the Pancreas of the Guinea Pig. 3. *In Vivo* Incorporation of Leucine-I-C14 into the Proteins of Cell Fractions." *Journal of Biophysical and Biochemical Cytology* 4 (September 25):557–66.

———. 1959. "A Cytochemical Study on the Pancreas of the Guinea Pig. 4. Chemical and Metabolic Investigations of the Ribonucleic Particles." *Journal of Biophysical and Biochemical Cytology* 5 (January 25): 1–10.

Palade, George E., and Marilyn Gist Farquhar. 1962. "Functional Evidence for the Existence of a Third Cell Type in the Renal Glomerulus. Phagocytosis of Filtration Residues by a Distinctive 'Third Cell.'" *Journal of Cell Biology* 13 (April):55–87.

Palade, George E. 1964. "The Organization of Living Matter." *Proceedings of the National Academy of Sciences* 52 (August):613–64.

SECONDARY SOURCES

Hicks, Nancy. 1974. "George Emil Palade." *New York Times* (October 11):22.

1967. "Palade, George Emil." In *Current Biography Yearbook* (July). New York: H. W. Wilson.

Porter, Keith R. 1974. "The 1974 Nobel Prize in Physiology or Medicine." *Science* 186 (November 8):516–20.

Rensberger, Boyce. 1974. "Three Cell Biologists Get Nobel Prize." *New York Times* (October 11):22.

IVAN PETROVICH PAVLOV *1904*

Ivan Petrovich Pavlov was born on September 14, 1849, in Ryazan, Russia. An experimental physiologist, he was awarded the Nobel Prize in 1904 for his work on digestive physiology. His stature as a scientist, however, also rests on his subsequent creation of the conditional reflex model for exploring behavioral neurophysiology. He married Serafima Karchevokaya in 1881; they had three children. Pavlov died on February 27, 1936, in Leningrad.

Pavlov was the oldest of eleven

children of Vavara Ivanova and Peter Dmitreivich Pavlov, a Russian Orthodox priest. Because Pavlov's early education was delayed by an accident, he entered a church school at age eleven. He subsequently attended the theological seminary in Ryazan. In 1870 Pavlov left the seminary without completing his studies and entered the University of St. Petersburg. While at the university he was particularly influenced by the physiologist Elie Cyon. In 1874, in his third year at the university, Pavlov became an active collaborator of Cyon and took up physiology as his major subject. His first scientific investigation, suggested to him by his mentor, concerned the pancreatic nerves, and for this he was awarded the gold medal of the university. Between 1875 and 1879 he completed a course of study at the Military Medical Academy. After qualifying as a doctor, he received a fellowship that enabled him to spend two more years in research at the academy. In 1883 he completed his dissertation for the degree of doctor of medicine. Having received the Wylie fellowship, Pavlov spent the years 1884–86 with two of the greatest physiologists of that time—Ludwig in Leipzig, and Heidenhain in Breslau. Upon returning to St. Petersburg he worked as an assistant to the noted clinician S. P. Botkin. In 1890 he was made professor of pharmacology at the Military Medical Academy and director of the physiological laboratory at the newly founded St. Petersburg Institute of Experimental Medicine. In 1895 he became professor of physiology at the academy, holding that position until 1924, when the Soviet Academy of Sciences established a special Institute of Physiology under his direction.

Although trained as a physician, Pavlov always worked as an experimental laboratory scientist, having contact with patients only at the end of his career. At the beginning of his career Cyon and Heidenhain directed his interest toward the physiology of the digestive tract. Under the influence of Botkin he developed a commitment to nervous, as opposed to humoral, explanations of bodily functions. As early as 1883 he expressed his preference for the theory of "nervism" which he defined as "a physiological theory which tries to prove that the nervous system controls the greatest possible number of bodily activities," (Babkin 1949, 225). With development of the germ theory and asceptic methods of surgery at that time, Pavlov was able to appreciate and develop surgical methods for research in physiology. Pavlov's skill as a surgeon allowed him to create experimental situations from which he systematically gathered a rich harvest of carefully controlled observations.

Pavlov always saw himself as a "pure" physiologist. Later in his career he reflected that this self-definition was established by the "deep and permanent though concealed" impression made upon him by his boyhood reading of a monograph by I. M. Schenov, "the father of Russian physiology," entitled *Cerebral Reflexes* (Pavlov 1928, 39). Early in his career this self-definition set a limit on and focused his interests. In his own words:

I would prefer to remain a pure physiologist, that is, an investigator who studies the functions of separate organs, the conditions of their activity, and the synthesis of their function in the total mechanism of a part or in the whole of the organism; and I am little interested in the ultimate, deep basis for the function of an organ or of its tissues, for which primarily chemical or physical analysis is required (quoted in Grigorian 1974, vol. 10, 432)

Later in his career this same self-definition influenced his rejection of psychological interpretations of his findings and prompted him to develop physiological models of higher mental processes. Pavlov was also committed to a positivist allegience to experimental observation. It was only later in his career that he began to speculate broadly about the implications of his work.

Pavlov's first independent work was on the physiology of the circulation of the blood. In one experiment, stimulated by Ludwig's work, he measured the blood pressure of a dog as it was influenced by variations in the volume of fluid in the circulatory system. This experiment is of interest because it employed the technique of experimenting on unanesthetized, neurologically intact dogs over time, which became the mainstay of Pavlov's methodology. In other studies he explored the nervous control of the heart, arguing that the rhythm and strength of the heart contractions were controlled by four kinds of nerves.

Pavlov's research on the physiology of digestion, for which he was awarded the Nobel Prize in 1904, began as early as 1879 but dominated his attention between 1890 and 1897. This work was an effort at accumulating observations on the nervous control of one organ system through his method of the chronic experiment. The rationale for this method, central to his approach to physiology, was:

that, in the ordinary method of the so-called "acute" experiment, carried out at one sitting, and complicated by free bleeding, many sources of error lie concealed. The crude damage done to the integrity of the organism sets up a number of inhibitory influences which react upon the functions of its different parts. The body as a whole, in which an enormous number of different organs are linked together in the most delicate fashion for the performance of a common and purposive work, cannot in the nature of things remain indifferent to forces calculated to destroy it. (Pavlov 1902, 15)

In order to observe digestion over time, Pavlov surgically opened several windows by creating fistulas through which the secretions of the salivary glands, the stomach, the pancreas, and the small intestine could be collected. His surgical success was particularly notable with the stomach. His teacher Heidenhain had succeeded in creating a method of studying gastric secretion through an exteriorized stomach pouch in 1879, but, unlike Pavlov, he had failed to maintain the nerve supply to this pouch. Other investigators had been able to collect gastric secretions, but these had been contaminated by the presence of food. Pavlov succeeded in collecting pure gastric secretions by establishing an esophagotomy, as well as a gastric pouch, in the same animal, thereby creating a "sham feeding" procedure.

Pavlov's results were dramatic. The intestinal enzyme enterokinase was discovered in his laboratory. The neural control of the pancreas was described as well as the composition of pancreatic secretions in response to different foods (Babkin 1949, 263). He demonstrated that the quantity and quality of the salivary secretions varied in accordance with the nature and strength of the stimulus acting on the mucosa of the mouth. In experiments utilizing sham feeding, conducted with Mme. Shumov-Simanovskaja, he showed that chewing and swallowing alone would provoke gastric secretion and he proved that the vagus nerve was the secretory nerve of the gastric glands. He also demonstrated the variations of the secretions of the stomach to different foods.

Of all of Pavlov's observations on digestion the one with the most far-reaching implications was the fact that the mere sight of food would stimulate salivary and gastric secretions. While Pavlov was aware that such "psychic excitation" had been previously observed and could be regarded as an artifact in certain experiments, he proceeded, in his characteristically systematic fashion, to explore this phenomenon. In doing this he shifted his focus from the study of digestive function to the study of "higher mental processes." This shift in focus resulted in an important crisis in his scientific development which he described as follows:

> I began to investigate the question of psychic secretion with my collaborators, Drs. Wolfson and Snarsky. Wolfson collected new and important facts for this subject; Snarsky, on the other hand, undertook to analyse the internal mechanism of the stimulation from the subjective point of view, i.e., he assumed that the internal world of the dog—the thoughts, feelings, and desires—is analogous to ours. We were now brought face to face with a situation which had no precedent in our laboratory. In our explanations of this internal world we diverged along two opposite paths. New experiments did not bring us into agreement nor produce conclusive results, and this in spite of the usual laboratory custom, according to which new experiments undertaken by mutual consent are generally decisive. Snarsky clung to his subjective explanation of the phenomena, but I, putting aside fantasy and seeing the scientific barrenness of such a solution, began to seek for another exit from this difficult position. After persistent deliberation, after a considerable mental conflict, I decided finally, in regard to the so-called psychical stimulation, to remain in the role of a pure physiologist, i.e., of an objective external observer and experimenter. (Pavlov 1928, 38–39)

According to Pavlov, the most important motive in his resolution of this crisis was the "unconscious" influence of Sechenov's efforts to "represent our subjective world from the standpoint of pure physiology" (Pavlov 1928, 39).

In the winter of 1901–2, with F. Tolochinov, he began to study the effects of the sight and smell of food on salivation. In his first report on these studies in 1903 he resisted temptations to leap from physiological to "psychic" interpretations by aggressively extending the physiological implications of his earlier work. He did this primarily by classifying all of the reactions of an animal to stimuli as either unconditional or conditional reflexes. In the first category he included the direct effects of stimuli such as food on the digestive process, while in the latter he included those indirect effects which to some suggested psychical explanations. He justified this assimilation of the "psychical" into the reflex paradigm by demonstrating the close functional dependence of conditioned reflexes on unconditioned reflexes. In his acceptance of the Nobel Prize for his work on digestive physiology in 1904, he chose to speak on this work on conditional reflexes. He extended the implications of his earlier physiological work by arguing that not only was the specific and variable response of the salivary glands to different unconditional stimuli an adaptation to the environment but that conditional stimuli acted as "signals" for the unconditional stimuli and consequently were "a further and more delicate adaptation of the salivary glands to the external world" (Pavlov 1928, 79).

Having switched his focus from the study of digestion to the study of conditional reflexes, Pavlov and his students applied the same systematic approach to the observation of functional relationships that they had used in the study of digestion. A number of these functional relationships have been accepted as classic and standard features of physiological and behavioral studies of animals and man. Among these functional relationships are, for example, extinction, the waning of a conditional reflex when it is no longer paired with an unconditional reflex; and generalization, the extension of a conditional reflex to new stimuli. These functional relationships were widely adopted and adapted, particularly by American behavioral psychologists. For Pavlov, the physiologist, however, conditioning always reflected the functioning of an organ, the brain; and he took exception to psychologists like Guthrie who he felt took "conditioning as the principle of learning," and did not "subject (this principle) to further analysis" (Pavlov 1941, 117).

Having established the conditional reflex model as a paradigm for understanding higher nervous processes, Pavlov further extended the sphere of his research interests to the psychophysiology and psychopathology of man. Here his work took on a more speculative cast than it had earlier. He extended the idea that conditional stimuli acted as signals to include human language as a secondary signal system. In 1920, drawing on general ideas of cortical excitation and inhibition, workers in his laboratory used his conditioning methods to produce experimental neuroses, that is, states of apparent conflict between excitation and inhibition. Observing the varied reactions of animals to such conflicts, Pavlov attempted to classify the types of higher nervous activity and compared these to Hippocrates's classification of temperaments. In the late 1920s he began to make observations on patients in a psychiatric hospital and attempted to explain the disorders he saw in terms of his work on conditioning.

Pavlov was committed above all to the idea that "for the natural scientist everything is in the method, in the opportunity to find a steadfast and reliable truth" (quoted in Kozulin 1984, 42). He pursued his early commitment to neurophysiology tenaciously and creatively, often rejecting the ideas of others when they threatened to deflect him from his own path. He adapted to the political regimes under which he worked because they let him pursue his scientific work. His reflections on psychiatry dominated Russian psychiatry after they were imposed on that field by the state. His influence was, however, international. Most, but not all, of his findings in digestive physiology still stand. His conditioning model had a powerful impact on western behavioral psychology, even when he could not accept the directions that psychology took. He has been praised for anticipating modern studies on behavioral neurophysiology. He was a tenacious and systematic experimentalist who produced methodological innovations in the study of physiological effects of nervous activity and created a powerful model for understanding the adaptive behavior of animals.

EDWARD M. BROWN

Selected Bibliography

PRIMARY SOURCES

Pavlov, I. P. (Russian Edition 1897) 1902. *The Work of the Digestive Glands*. Translated by W. H. Thompson. London: Charles Griffin and Company.

———. 1928. *Lectures on Conditioned Reflexes*. Translated by W. Horsley Gantt. New York: International Publishers.

———. 1941. *Conditioned Reflexes and Psychiatry*. Translated by W. Horsley Gantt. New York: International Publishers.

SECONDARY SOURCES

Babkin, B. P. 1949. *Pavlov: A Biography*. Chicago: University of Chicago Press.

Grigorian, N. A. 1974. "Pavlov, Ivan Petrovich." In *The Dictionary of Scientific Biography*. New York: Charles Scribner's Sons, v.10, 431–436.

Kozulin, Alex. 1984. "Personalities and Reflexes: The Legacies of Ivan Pavlov and Vladimir Bekterev." In *Psychology in Utopia: Toward a Social History of Soviet Psychology*. Cambridge: The MIT Press. 40–61.

Windholz, G. 1983. "Pavlov's Position toward American Behaviorism." *Journal of the History of the Behavioral Sciences* 19:394–407.

RODNEY ROY PORTER *1972*

Rodney Roy Porter was born in Liverpool, England, on October 8, 1917. A biochemist, Porter shared the 1972 Nobel Prize with Gerald M. Edelman for their independent, yet complementary, research on the chemical structure of antibodies. Porter began the work with his innovative cleavage of the antibody molecule. Edelman followed this lead to generate a remarkable period of creative structural analysis, in which he and Porter were the leaders. Porter was Whitley Professor of Biochemistry at Oxford University and chairman of the department from 1967 until his death. He married Julia Frances New in 1948; they had two sons, Nigel and Tim, and three daughters, Susan, Ruth, and Helen. He died in Winchester, England, on September 6, 1985.

Porter was the son of a railway clerk, Joseph L. Porter, and his wife, Isobel. He studied biochemistry at the University of Liverpool, graduating with honors in 1939. During World War II he served with the Royal Engineers and the Royal Army Signal Corps. Returning to his biochemical training, he began doctoral studies with Frederick Sanger in 1946. He became interested in immunology while studying Karl Landsteiner's work and learned from Sanger the techniques used in his sequencing of the fifty-one amino acids that make up insulin (Weinraub 1972).

Immunoglobulins are the antibody molecules in human blood that recognize and "capture," or bind, foreign antigens, including disease agents, and modify or degrade them. They appear to be very similar in structure; yet they vary sufficiently in the healthy body to successfully combat any of the millions of antigens encountered during a person's lifetime. Among other problems, it seemed impossible that the human genetic makeup could contain sufficient genes for each of the antibodies known to exist, each specific to a particular antigen.

Karl Landsteiner had advocated chemical analysis of antibody structure as the first step toward characterizing their action and discovering the secret of their antigenic specificity. The molecules, however, are large, complex, and cannot be purified. Porter wanted to try selective cleavage with enzymes to break the molecule into fragments for easier analysis. He obtained his first "pieces" with papain in 1948 and in that year also received his doctoral degree.

Porter spent another year with Sanger before accepting a position in microbiology research at the National Institute for Medical Research in London. He continued his antibody studies, but it was only in 1958 that he was able, using a purified form of papain, to recover three discrete and different fragments. Two of these (Fab) were very similar and active in attacking antigens; the third (Fc) clearly had a different, undetermined, function. Fc was also crystallizable, which meant it was fairly homogenous. With this work, he revolutionized immunology (Cebra 1972, 384).

Working with Henry Kunkel at the Rockefeller Institute, Gerald Edelman in 1960 used Porter's enzymatic cleavage techniques on human myeloma proteins to carry out further structural studies of human immunoglobulins. But he was not completely happy with his findings. Porter's method essentially broke the antibodies into bits of amino acids, allowing the assumption that the molecule was a single polypeptide chain. Edelman thought a more complex structure to be more likely and attempted analysis, using the reagent urea to reduce the disulfide bonds of the proteins. His results, published in 1959 and 1961, showed that in fact the immunoglobulin molecule consisted of at least two qualitatively different polypeptides, which he designated L (light) chains and H (heavy) chains. (The terms "light" and "heavy" refer to molecule weight.)

Edelman further demonstrated differences in L chains of guinea pig antibodies that indicated a relationship with the ability to bind different antigens. Finally, he suggested that immunoglobulin-related proteins, called Bence-Jones proteins, appeared very similar to the L chains and that the structural study of these compounds might prove fruitful.

The next step, immunologists realized, was the further detailed characterization of the antibody molecule. Porter had now moved to St. Mary's Hospital Medical School, an affiliate of London University. Here he and his colleagues began work on the L chains, while Edelman tackled "the whole molecule—a ghastly big job." Many researchers contributed, however, and this was a time of great excitement in the field. Informal meetings, called "antibody workshops," open to anyone working in the field, were held twice a year in locations "from California to Israel." Porter and Edelman were prominent at these meetings, encouraging and helping others (Altman 1972; Cebra 1972, 384–85).

In 1962–63, Porter, working with his long-term associate, Elizabeth Press, and with other colleagues, used controlled cleavage of the interchain bonds, followed by detailed molecular weight, protein, and antigenic analysis, to construct a four-chain model of immunoglobulin, which is now widely confirmed as the true picture. The model shows two pairs of H and L chains, which can be cleaved into Fab fragments; the fragments are the active antigen binding sites. They consist of a whole L chain, plus a nitrogen-hydrogen fragment (NH_2) of the H chain.

Additional discoveries were made throughout the 1960s. Edelman, supporting Frantiszek Franek of the Czech Academy of Sciences, found that the fragmented H and L chains worked together to bind antigens as effectively as the intact parent molecule. Norbert Hilschmann at Rockefeller and Frank Putnam at the University of Florida used Bence-Jones proteins to examine the amino acid sequences of the L chains. Their work indicated that the Ls consisted of a constant half (C_L) that never varied in structure and a variable (V_L) half. Porter and Robert Hill further contributed to mapping of these segments.

The segmented nature of the molecule was now apparent. Porter's group hypothesized that the H chain also contained a variable region that linked to the V_L segment to form the active antigen binding site. They used both human myeloma proteins and normal rabbit immunoglobulin, which is a mixed "pool" of antibodies. Both studies furnished evidence for a variable portion of the H chain (V_H), consisting of alternating amino acids, linked in different sequences (Cebra 1972, 385).

Edelman and his team meanwhile had pursued his quest to describe the complete molecule, using human myeloma protein. With the aid of William Konigsberg of Yale, they were able to publish complete data by 1969. These results for the first time compared the V_L and V_H segments and established that a single antigen-binding site is formed from these two different, and varying, polypeptides. The marked variation in the structure of these segments suggested a solution to the problem of antigenic specificity, which was eventually developed by Susumu Tonegawa.

The Edelman model also showed the now familiar repetition of the constant segments; Edelman suggested that each was responsible for secondary biologic functions of the molecule. Altogether, the model sequenced thirteen hundred amino acids in the complex protein.

Further research comparing sequences and attempting to bind "affinity labels" to the active sites to study their activity identified three short "hypervariable" segments within the V segments that were considered possible determinants of specific response to given antigens. Porter worked on the further characterization of the antibodies until his death. Edelman became interested in the process of their genetic synthesis, still attempting to clarify how the body is able to manufacture sufficient antibodies to meet most antigenic challenges. These investigations eventually led him to studies of brain development and a complex theory of genetic learning and variation throughout life (Cebra 1972, 385–86).

In Oxford, Porter and his family lived in a large farmhouse in Witney. On vacations, they enjoyed camping and climbing in the Swiss Alps. Porter also kept bees and often spent weekends alone fishing. He was killed in an automobile accident shortly before his scheduled retirement (Weinraub 1972, 24).

Porter was a Fellow of the Royal Society and a foreign member of the United States National Academy of Sciences. Among the many other honors he received for his work were the Gairdner Foundation Award (1966); the Karl Landsteiner Memorial Award from the American Association of Blood Banks (1968); and the Royal Medal of the Royal Society (1973).

MARCIA MELDRUM

Selected Bibliography

PRIMARY SOURCES

Porter, Rodney R. 1973. *Defence and Recognition*. Baltimore: University Park Press.

———. 1976. *Chemical Aspects of Immunology*. Burlington, North Carolina: Carolina Biological Supply.

Porter, Rodney R., and G. Ada. 1976. *Contemporary Topics in Molecular Immunology*. Vol. 6. New York: Plenum Press.

Porter, Rodney R. 1984. *Biochemistry and Genetics of Complement: A Discussion*. London: Royal Society.

SECONDARY SOURCES

Altman, Lawrence K. 1972. "Deciphering the Structure." *New York Times* (October 13):24.

Cebra, John J. 1972. "The 1972 Nobel Prize in Physiology or Medicine." *Science* 178 (October 27):384–86.

Weinraub, Bernard. 1972. "Pioneers in Immunology Research: Rodney Robert Porter." *New York Times* (October 13):24.

SANTIAGO RAMÓN Y CAJAL
1906

Santiago Ramón y Cajal was born on May 1, 1852, in Petilla de Aragon, a small and quite isolated village in the Spanish Pyrenees. His father, Justo Ramon Casassus, was a barber surgeon when Ramón was born, but he later completed a more formal education and graduated from the University of Zaragoza to become a country physician. The son of this struggling Aragonese doctor became one of the greatest histologists of all time. For his revealing and histologic studies of the brain and nervous system, Ramón y Cajal was awarded the Nobel Prize in Physiology or Medicine in 1906. He died on October 18, 1934.

As a child Cajal was considered to be indolent and quite lazy. Cajal initially served two apprenticeships, as was common in this period, to learn a trade; Fortunately for the history of medicine, he failed at both barbering and shoemaking. His father, in an effort to interest him in medicine, gave him some bones from a local graveyard. Cajal began by sketching these cemetery fragments, demonstrating a remarkable artistic talent. This early interest in osteology provided an impetus towards a career in medicine. Cajal matriculated at the University of Zaragoza, where he completed his studies in 1873. He was appointed professor of anatomy at the University of Zaragoza in 1877.

A man characterized early in life as indolent and lazy became one of the most energetic and ardent supporters of Spanish medicine and biology. Cajal remained an intensely loyal Spaniard and rapidly rose through the academic ranks, first at the University of Zaragoza, and then at the University of Valencia, where he was appointed professor of anatomy in 1884. He moved on to the University of Barcelona in 1887 and to the University of Madrid, the most prestigious university in Spain, in 1892. His major work was carried out at Madrid, where he formed the now famous Laboratorio de Investigaciones Biologicas.

Cajal's great contributions began with the refinement of the silver stain developed by Camillo Golgi. Using this silver stain, along with several of his own stain modifications, Cajal spent nearly fifty years unraveling the intricate anatomy and interconnecting dynamics of the central nervous system. Insights into this complex anatomical system led to his Nobel Prize award in 1906. Cajal's award was specifically based on his postulates for the "neuron theory" and his discovery of the anatomical connections of the central nervous system.

In the late 1880s Cajal began to study the nervous system of embryos. He outlined and accurately diagrammed the nerve cells and their processes. Cajal recognized early on, in contradistinction to Golgi's nerve net theory that postulated a "trellis" system of connections, that the neurons were independent units that communicated, by axon to dendrite. While Golgi's stain revealed the nerve cell body and its processes, Cajal's modifications of the stain enabled study of the intricate interconnections of the cells. Revealing these interconnections enabled Cajal to postulate that learning was acquired by a change in their richness and patterns; this theory challenged Golgi, who thought that learning was related to a decrease or increase in cells. Cajal published his results in the Continental journals, in French and German, which aroused the patriotic ire of his Spanish colleagues. But by publishing in French and German journals instead of obscure Spanish journals, Cajal promulgated his views throughout Europe.

An important point in Cajal's life came in 1889 when he presented his anatomical studies on the nervous system at the German Anatomical Congress in Berlin. Sitting in the audience during Cajal's presentation was Albrecht von Kölliker, the famous German anatomist, who immediately appreciated the significance of Cajal's work. Also in the audience was Charles Sherrington, who would later recommend that Cajal give the Croonian Lecture in London before the World Society in 1894. Cajal's total commitment to science is revealed in an anecdote by Sherrington. Cajal stayed with Sir Charles while in London, and during his stay in Sherrington's home would not allow the maid or anyone else into his bed chamber. His desire for such privacy was not understood until the maid was finally allowed in and discovered a histological laboratory complete with microscope—Cajal was continuing his laboratory investigations even while visiting London!

Using anatomical studies of the retina, olfactory bulb, cerebral cortex, and spinal cord, Cajal mapped out the static and dynamic interconnections of the central nervous system. The intricate layering and interconnection of the cerebral cortex neurons were all outlined and documented through Cajal's meticulous anatomical studies. He developed the concept of the cell body receiving information through dendrites and sending information through axons.

By the time Cajal died in 1934 at age eighty-two, he had published close to three hundred scientific papers, had received honorary degrees from Oxford and Cambridge, and had written several excellent texts, including a now rare work on color photography.

JAMES T. GOODRICH

Selected Bibliography

PRIMARY SOURCES

Ramón y Cajal, S. 1892. "Nuevo concepto de las histologia de los centros nerviosos." *Revista de Ciencias Médicas* 18:457.

———. 1894. *Die Retina der Wirbelthiere.* Wiesbaden: J. F. Bergmann.

———. 1899–1904. *Textura del sistema nervioso del hombre y de los vertebrados.* Madrid: Nicolas Moya.

———. 1907. "Die histogenischen Beweise der Neuroentheorie von His und Forel." *Anatomischer Anzeiger* 30:113.

———. 1909. *Manual de anatomia patologica general.* Madrid: N. Moya.

———. 1928. *Studies on Degeneration and Regeneration of the Nervous System.* Translated and edited by R. M. May. London: Oxford University Press.

———. 1937. *Recollections of My Life.* Translated by E. Horne Craigie and Juan Cano. Philadelphia: American Philosophical Society.

SECONDARY SOURCES

Cannon, D. F. 1949. *Explorers of the Human Brain. The Life of Santiago Ramón y Cajal.* New York: Schuman.

Haymaker, W., and F. Schiller. 1970. *The Founders of Neurology,* 147–151. Springfield: Thomas.

McHenry, L. 1969. *Garrison's History of Neurology,* 166–69. Springfield: Thomas.

Sprong, W. 1935. "Santiago Ramón y Cajal: 1852–1934." *Archives of Neurology and Psychiatry* 33:156–92.

TADEUS REICHSTEIN *1950*

Tadeus Reichstein was born in Wlocawek, Poland on July 20, 1897. He shared the Nobel Prize in 1950 with Philip S. Hench and Edward C. Kendall for their isolation and characterization of the hormones of the adrenal cortex. Reichstein and Kendall, working separately, investigated the cortical hormones for nearly twenty years; in 1949, Kendall's colleague Hench treated rheumatoid arthritis patients with one of the identified compounds and thus discovered the therapeutic effects of cortisone. At the time of his Nobel, Reichstein was Professor of Organic Chemistry at the University of Basel and was engaged in supervising the construction of a new Institute of Organic Chemistry, of which he later became Director.

Reichstein was the son of Gustava Brockmann and Isidor Reichstein, an engineer. His early childhood was spent in Kiev; he was sent to boarding school in Germany and later attended a technical high school in Zurich, where the family had moved in 1906. The Reichsteins became Swiss citizens in 1914. Young Tadeus entered the State Technical College in Zurich and received his degree in chemical engineering in 1920. After a year working in industry, he began graduate studies in organic chemistry at the University of Zurich. In 1927 he married Louise Henriette Quarls von Ufford, a native of the Netherlands. They had one daughter, Ruth.

At the University of Zurich, Reichstein's professor, Herman Staudinger, interested him in the identification of the substances that give coffee and chicory their distinctive aromas. After earning his doctorate, Reichstein began research on this problem under Staudinger's direction and then took it on independently with industrial funding. He continued with the project until 1931, not only identifying the complex aromatic composition of both foods but developing new chemical methods along the way.

In 1929, he was appointed Lecturer on Organic and Physiological Chemistry at the State Technical College. Two years later, having completed his aroma studies, he joined the laboratory of Leopold Ruzicka. From 1931 to 1934 Reichstein's research concentrated on identifying the structure of vitamin C. In 1933, he accomplished the first total synthesis of the vitamin in the laboratory and developed as well a commercially practical method of manufacture. By then he had become intrigued by the problem of the adrenal cortex.

The adrenal cortex is the outer layer of the adrenal gland, one of which rests on top of each kidney. The inner layer, the medulla, was known to secrete the hormone epinephrine, marketed as adrenalin, which initiated physiological response to emergencies. However, animals whose adrenal glands had been removed experimentally soon died. It was therefore believed that the adrenal gland secreted at least one additional hormone necessary to life. In 1928 G. N. Stewart and J. M. Rogoff in Cleveland had shown that a crude adrenal extract would sustain the life of an adrenalectomized dog (Rogoff and Stewart 1928).

Soon thereafter, several laboratories began efforts to isolate the new hormone, which was presumed to be a single substance secreted by the adrenal cortex and was called "cortin." Kendall and his colleagues, working at the Mayo Clinic in Minnesota, isolated a crystalline substance that they tentatively identified as cortin, in 1934. At Columbia University, O. Wintersteiner and J. J. Pfiffner reported in 1935 the discovery of five different cortical products, which they also prepared as crystals. In Zurich, meanwhile, Reichstein and his collaborator, Jacob von Euw, were at work and had identified four compounds by 1936 (Kendall *et al.* 1934, Wintersteiner and Pfiffner 1935, Reichstein 1936a).

Between 1936 and 1941, the researchers isolated either 28 or 29 different hormonal substances from adrenal cortical extracts. Only six were believed to be biologically active. The papers issuing from the several laboratories were confusing, since many compounds were reported and named by different teams almost simultaneously. Kendall's compound E, which he identified in 1936 and which was later to be known as coritsone, was isolated in the same year by both Reichstein, who designated it Fa, and the Columbia laboratory, which called it F. Two years later Kendall prepared his own compound F, which later became famous as hydrocortisone; Reichstein had already isolated this hormone and given it the designation M. Neither of these important discoveries were differentiated from the other substances found in the 1930s. (Reichstein 1937a, b; Reichstein and Shoppee 1943).

Reichstein and his associates identified more different cortical compounds than any of the other researchers. In 1936 he established the steroidal structure of these hormones by demonstrating their similarity to androgens (male sex hormones), whose structure was known. Kendall at least saw the Swiss scientist as his principal competitor in the race to identify the life-giving cortin, particularly as the Columbia team and other workers turned to different projects (Reichstein 1936b).

One of the most difficult problems with which all the researchers had to contend was obtaining an adequate supply of extract for analysis. Both Reichstein and Kendall began by using whole glands from slaughtered beef cattle. One thousand kilograms of glands would yield only a few grams of concentrated extract, two thirds of which appeared to be biologically inert. The preparation of a small cyrstalline sample of a single substance therefore required considerable effort and an enormous supply of glands. The tiny samples thus obtained were inadequate for physiological testing (Reichstein 1964).

It was therefore apparent that

methods of partial synthesis of the cortical steroids would have to be developed. (Total synthesis of a chemical compound is essentially "making it from scratch"; partial synthesis begins with another compound similar in structure and adds or removes the necessary atoms to create the desired substance.) Reichstein began experimenting with partial synthesis simultaneously with the analysis of cortical products. In 1937 he succeeded in preparing 11-desoxycorticosterone from desoxycholic (bile) acid, before this compound, which he named Q, had been isolated from gland extract. The following year he employed an improved extraction method and obtained both Q and 11-dehydrocortisone (identified by Kendall as Compound A in 1936). (Steiger and Reichstein 1937; Reichstein and von Euw 1938).

Reichstein was promoted to associate professor in 1937, but in 1938 he left Zurich to become Professor and Director of the Pharmaceutical Institute at the University of Basel, the institution which would be his professional home for the remainder of his career. There he continued his pursuit of better synthetic methods.

It appeared likely that the steroids that Reichstein had been able to synthesize, such as desoxycorticosterone, were qualitatively different from those that appeared to be important to carbohydrate metabolism. The latter are known as glucocorticoids; the former, now called mineralocorticoids, are involved in regulating electrolytes in the blood. The key functional difference between these two types of compounds appeared to be the presence of an oxygen atom on the eleventh carbon atom of the steroid skeleton. Oxygenating this position also was the most difficult step in the synthesis. Reichstein succeeded in completing this step and prepared the glucocorticoid 11-dehydrocorticosterone from desoxycholic acid in 1943, although by a very complicated low-yield procedure (Lardon and Reichstein 1943).

The suggestion was made in the late 1930s that the digitalis and/or the strophanthus plants were potential sources for a steroid compound oxygenated at the eleventh carbon atom. Reichstein was interested in this possibility but he quickly eliminated digitalis. Research on strophanthus, a West African vine, had to be put aside during World War II, as samples of the plant could not be obtained (Steiger and Reichstein 1938).

After the war Reichstein was appointed Chairman of the Department of Organic Chemistry and in 1948 he began the planning for the new Organic Chemistry Institute. These responsibilities forced him to relinquish the Directorship of the Pharmaceutical Institute in 1950, to gain more time for research.

Resumption of work on strophanthus led to the realization that there were chemical differences between some plant specimens that otherwise appeared identical. This observation directed Reichstein's curiosity to the chemical differentiation of plants, although cortiocosteriod research remained the primary occupation of his laboratory. Sarmentogenin, found in some strophanthus plants, was identified in 1948 as a practical starting point for the synthesis of adrenal steroids, but this finding was not followed by commercial development. Reichstein became sufficiently interested in botany to undertake the chemical analysis of the meadow saffron, the source of colchicine and related pharmaceuticals, in 1949. Unlike the strophanthus work, the saffron study had no relation to steroidal compounds. (von Euw *et al.* 1957; Santavy and Reichstein 1950; Uffer *et al.* 1954).

The announcement of the therapeutic action of cortisone in rheumatoid arthritis at the Mayo Clinic in 1949 generated worldwide acclaim for the men who had been painstakingly laboring with the cortical hormones for so long. In addition to the Nobel Prize, Reichstein received the Cameron Prize from the University of Edinburgh (1951) and was elected a Foreign Member of the Royal Society of London (1952). The Society later awarded him the Copley Medal (1968) for his continuing contributions.

In the early 1950s both Reichstein and Kendall undertook the problem of the "amorphous fraction," which was the material remaining after all known steroids had been separated from the adrenal extract by chemical methods. This fraction, however amorphous, was observed to have an effect on electrolyte metabolism similar to that of desoxycorticosterone. In 1948, S. A. Simpson and J. F. Tait at the Middlesex Hospital in London employed electrophoretic separation to determine the active constituents of the amorphous fraction. They devised a test that demonstrated in 1952 the unique and potent effect of one separated substance, which they called "electrocortin," on sodium-potassium homeostasis. Shortly afterward they began to collaborate with Reichstein. V. R. Mattox and M. L. Mason were pursuing the same substance in Kendall's laboratory.

In 1953 both groups succeeded independently in crystallizing the "new hormone," at first believed to be a variant of corticosterone. A few months later the Reichstein group established the correct structure and named it "aldosterone" (Grundy *et al.* 1952; Mattox *et al.* 1953; Simpson *et al.* 1954).

In his later years, Reichstein's main interest was the isolation and description of toxic substances from various plants, insects, and toads. These toxins had the steroid nucleus in common. He conducted these investigations, begun in 1948, through 1979 (Iseli *et al.* 1965, Reichstein *et al.* 1968, Brown *et al.* 1979).

In 1960 Reichstein retired from the Chairmanship to become Director of the Institute of Organic Chemistry. The following year, at the age of 64, he started a new project, studying the genetic and chemical taxonomy of ferns. This work led him to the thesis, earlier suggested by the strophanthus studies, that some plants can only be differentiated by their chemical constituents and the chemical-botanical taxonomies should be developed. (Widen *et al.* 1976). Reichstein became Professor and Director Emeritus in 1967 but has remained active in research and writing. He still lives in Basel. His most recent publication, on the chemistry of plant steroids, appeared in 1987, when he was ninety years old.

THOMAS G. BENEDEK

Selected Bibliography

PRIMARY SOURCES

Reichstein, Tadeus, and A. Grüsner. 1933. "Die Synthese der d-Ascorbinsaure (d-form des C-Vitamins)." *Helvetica Chimica Acta* 16:56–73.

Reichstein, Tadeus. 1936. "Über Cortin, das Hormon der Nebennieren-Rinde." *Helvetica Chimica Acta* 19:29–63.

———. 1936. "Über die Bestandteile der Nebennieren-Rinde. V. Chemischer Nachweis des Androstan-Skelettes." *Helvetica Chimica Acta* 19:979–87.

———. 1937. "Über Bestandteile der Nebennieren-Rinde. X. Zur Kenntnis des Cortico-Sterons." *Helvetica Chimica Acta* 20:953–69.

———. 1937. "Über Bestandteile der Nebennieren-Rinde. XI. Zur Konstruktion der C_{21} O_5 Gruppe." *Helvetica Chimica Acta* 20:978–91.

Steiger, M., and T. Reichstein. 1937. "Desoxy-cortico-steron (21-Oxy-progesteron) aus Δ^5-3-Oxy-ätiocholensäure." *Helvetica Chimica Acta* 20:1164–79.

———. 1938. "Ein Neuer Abbau des Digitoxigenins." *Helvetica Chimica Acta* 21:828–44.

Reichstein, Tadeus, and Jacob von Euw. 1938. "Isolierung des Substanzen Q (Desoxy-corticosteron) und R Sowie weitere Stoffe." *Helvetica Chimica Acta* 21:1197–1210.

Larden, A., and T. Reichstein. 1943. "Über Bestandteile der Nebennierenenrinde und Verwandte Stoffe. Teilsynthese des 11-Dehydro-corticosterons." *Helvetica Chimica Acta* 26:1197–1210.

Reichstein, Tadeus, and C. W. Shoppee. 1943. "The Hormones of the Adrenal Cortex," *Vitamins and Hormones.* R. S. Harris and K. V. Thimann, eds. 1:345–413.

Santavy, F., and T. Reichstein. 1950. "Isolierung neuer Stoffe aus den Samen der Herbstzeitlose Colchicum Autumnale L. Substanzen der Herbstzeitlose und Ihre Derivate." *Helvetica Chimica Acta* 33:1606–27.

Reichstein, Tadeus. 1950. "Chemistry of the Adrenal Hormones." Nobel Lecture. Reprinted in *Nobel Lectures in Physiology or Medicine.* Vol. 3 (1942–1962):292–308. Amsterdam: Elsevier, 1964.

Reichstein, T., *et al.* 1968. "Heart Poisons in the Monarch Butterfly." *Science* 161:861–66.

Brown, P., T. Reichstein, *et al.* 1979. "Cardenolides of Asclepias syriaca L., Probable Structure of Syrioside and Syribioside." *Helvetica Chimica Acta* 62:412–41.

Lardon, A., and T. Reichstein. 1987. "Chemical Degradation of Sarverogenin, Proof of the Presence of the Steroid Carbon Skeleton." *Helvetica Chimica Acta* 70: 894–928.

SECONDARY SOURCES

Grundy, H. M., *et al.* 1952. "Further Studies on the Properties of a Highly Active Mineralocorticoid." *Acta Endocrinologica* 11:199–220.

Iseli, E., *et al.* 1965. "Die Sterine und Bufalienolide der Haut von *Bufa formosus* Boulenger." *Helvetica Chimica Acta* 48:1093–1112.

Kendall, E. C., *et al.* 1934. "Isolation in Crystalline Form of the Hormone Essential for Life from the Supradrenal Cortex: Its Chemical Nature and Physiologic Properties." *Proceedings of the Staff Meetings of the Mayo Clinic* 9:245–50.

Mattox, V. R., H. L. Mason, and A. Albert. 1953. "Isolation of a Sodium-Retaining Substance from Beef Adrenal Extract." *Proceedings of the Staff Meetings of the Mayo Clinic* 28:569–76.

Reichstein, Tadeus. May 30, 1988. Personal communication to author.

Rogoff, J. M., and G. N. Stewart. 1928. "Studies on Adrenal Insufficiency in Dogs. V. The Influence of Adrenal Extracts on the Survival Period of Adrenalectomized Dogs." *Journal of Biological Chemistry* 84:660–674.

Simpson, S. A., *et al.* 1954. "Aldosteron. Isolierung und Eigenschaften. "Über Bestandteile der Nebennierenrinde und Verwandte Stoffe." 91. Mitteilung. *Helvetica Chimica Acta* 37: 1163–1200.

Uffer, A., *et al.* 1954. "3. Teilsynthese des Demecolcins und Einiger Anderer Colchicinderivate." *Helvetica Chimica Acta* 37:18–34.

Von Euw, J., *et al.* 1957. "Die Glykoside von Strophanthus Sarmentosus P. DC. 8. Untersuchung von Einzelpflanzen der 'Sarmentogenin-Produzierenden Variante b.'" *Helvetica Chimica Acta* 40:2079–2109.

Widen, C. J., *et al.* 1976. "Die Phloroglucide von Zwei Farnhybriden aus England und Schottland, von Authentischem Aspidium Remotum A. Braun und von Dryopteris aemula (Aiton) O. Kunze aus Irland." *Helvetica Chimica Acta* 59:1725–44.

Wintersteiner, O., and J. J. Pfiffner. 1935. "Chemical Studies on the Adrenal Cortex. II. Isolation of Several Physiologically Inactive Crystalline Compounds from Active Extracts." *Journal of Biological Chemistry* 111:599–612.

DICKINSON WOODRUFF RICHARDS, JR. *1956*

Dickinson Woodruff Richards, Jr., was born on October 30, 1895, in Orange, New Jersey. He was the son of Dickinson W. Richards, a lawyer, and Sally Lambert, whose father and three brothers were physicians. Dickinson Richards, Jr., received the Nobel Prize in Physiology or Medicine in 1956 for his work on heart catheterization and pathological changes in the circulatory system; he shared the award with André Frédéric Cournand and Werner Theodor Otto Forssmann. Richards died on February 23, 1973, in Lakeville, Connecticut.

Richards attended the Hotchkiss School in Connecticut. He entered Yale University in 1913, where he studied English and Greek, and received his A.B. degree in 1917. Richards was an outstanding student, recording the highest mark ever scored on the Greek entrance exam to Yale and leading his class in grades every year. He served in the U.S. Army during World War I, initially as an instructor in artillery and later as an artillery officer in France.

Richards then attended Columbia University College of Physicians and Surgeons, where he received an M.A. in physiology in 1922 and an M.D. in 1923. From 1923 to 1927 he was an intern and resident at Presbyterian Hospital in New York City. He worked in England for a year as a research fellow at the National Institute for Medical Research in London. He then returned to Presbyterian Hospital, where he started his studies of pulmonary and circulatory physiology with L. J. Henderson of Harvard University. From 1935 he was also medical adviser to the pharmaceutical company Merck and Company, a position from which he helped facilitate research on a wide range of drugs. In 1945 he became professor of medicine at Columbia University, and in 1947 he became Lambert Professor of Medicine, a position he held until he became emeritus Lambert Professor of Medicine in 1961. Richards was a member of many noted societies, including the National Academy of Sciences, and was president of the Harvey Society. He married Constance Burrell Riley in 1931; they had four daughters. Late in his career, he became interested in medical history, and coedited *Circulation of the Blood: Men and Ideas*, a book of essays on the history of the circulatory system.

Starting in 1929, Richards performed a series of experiments with A. L. Barach on the effects of oxygen therapy on diseases of the lung. These investigations led to the routine measurement of the concentration of the gases and the acidity of the blood in patients suffering from lung disease and eventually to the use of assisted ventilation for the treatment of these patients.

Richards started collaborating with Cournand on studies of the heart and circulation in 1932. They began with the explicit assumption that the heart, lung, and circulation form a single system for the exchange of gases between the environment and the organism. Their early work focused on the mechanical features of the lung. But Richards and Cournand were hindered in these early studies because they could not directly measure the gas content of blood as it was returning from the body to the lungs, with its oxygen content already delivered to the tissues. If they could only obtain samples of such blood from within the right atrium, the cardiac chamber that collects blood from the body before pumping the blood to the lungs to receive more oxygen, they would be able to calculate the cardiac output. That information would help them a great deal in understanding how the lungs were functioning. Forssmann had described passage of a catheter into his own right atrium in 1929, but little further investigation had been done using the technique. In 1936 Cournand returned to Paris to learn the technique of passing a tube into the right atrium. In New York, Cournand, Richards, and their colleagues practiced the technique on laboratory animals for four years, and found that the passage of catheters into animal's hearts did not significantly interfere with the functioning of these hearts.

Their first attempt to perform the procedure on a patient, in 1940, was unsuccessful. But they were encouraged to pursue this line of investigation by some senior investigators who were studying the heart's output using the ballistocardiogram, an instrument that recorded the motion of the body caused by the heart beat. These ballistocardiogram researchers wanted to compare their results with those from another method of determining the cardiac output. Cournand was able to insert a catheter into the heart and measure the cardiac output. He showed that the cardiac output as measured by the ballistocardiogram was too low, but, more importantly, he showed that it was practical and safe to routinely insert a catheter into the right side of the heart.

Over the next few years Richards, Cournand, and their colleagues made several technical advances. A new catheter was designed that was easier to maneuver than the old one, and a measuring device was constructed that enabled simultaneous recording of four different pressure tracings and the electrocardiogram. In 1942 they advanced the catheter into the right ventricle, and by 1944 they had advanced it as far as the pulmonary artery, thus enabling them to measure both the hemodynamic pressure and the amount of oxygen present in the blood at each stage of the blood's passage through the right side of the heart.

Early investigators had encountered a great deal of opposition from other physicians to the idea of passing catheters into the heart, because the procedure was thought to be extremely dangerous. Richards, Cournand, and their coworkers encountered much less opposition, perhaps because their research was performed as part of a study of various forms of shock, a subject of great importance for a country at war. Funded by the federal government through the Committee on Medical Research, from 1942 to 1944 Richards, Cournand, and their colleagues studied over one hundred critically ill patients suffering from all kinds of shock: traumatic shock, hemorrhagic shock, burn shock, shock caused by rupture of an internal organ. They outlined the profound effects of a reduction of circulating blood volume on cardiac output, particularly on the flow of blood to peripheral organs and to the kidney, and described how the condition could be reversed by appropriate volume replacement. Later, they applied the same technique to diagnose congenital cardiac defects, in which an abnormal opening between the cardiac chambers could be detected by means of pressure and oxygen measurements. In a similar fashion, measurement of the pressure in the cardiac chambers was found to be valuable for the diagnosis of acquired cardiac defects, particularly diseases of the heart valves. They also showed that elevated cardiac pressures could be a result of lung disease as well as of heart disease.

During his sixteen years as the chief of a large medical service, the Columbia University Medical Division at Bellevue Hospital, Richards was a subtle and inspiring leader who made the service one of the most popular in the country for internship applicants. He was also an advocate for the hospital, which he felt was being neglected by the New York City administration; in 1962 he founded the Better Bellevue Association. He spoke out on a variety of social issues, pressing for more health care for the aged and for hospital clinics to aid narcotic addicts. He was to the end a humanist and a social critic, characteristics evident in his essay collection *Medical Priesthoods and Other Essays*.

Richards and Cournand worked together from February 1932 until February 1973, a remarkably long period of collaboration. Together, using the insights of the third Nobel Prize winner of 1956, Werner Forssmann, Richards and Cournand demonstrated the feasibility of routinely measuring pressures and drawing blood samples from within the heart and the pulmonary circulation. Not long after the discovery that right-sided pressures could be measured, others extended the technique to measure pressures on the left side of the heart. Today, the passing of catheters into the heart for diagnosis is a routine procedure, one for which patients may not even spend the night in a hospital. But today's cardiologists do more than diagnose: they are using cardiac catheters to treat heart disease, both by instilling medicine directly into the heart and by using the catheters mechanically to expand a constricted blood vessel, or to ablate a diseased part of the heart. The techniques of Richards, Cournand, and Forssmann have been central to both the diagnosis and treatment of almost every type of heart disease.

JOEL D. HOWELL

Selected Bibliography

PRIMARY SOURCES

Richards, Dickinson W. 1943–44. "The Circulation in Traumatic Shock in Man." *Harvey Lectures*, Series 39, 217. New York: Academic Press.

———. 1956. "The Contributions of Right Heart Catheterization to Physiology and Medicine, with Some Observations on the Physiopathology of Pulmonary Heart Disease." Nobel Lecture. Reprinted in *Nobel Lectures, Physiology or Medicine*, vol. 3 (1942–1962), 513–26. Amsterdam: Elsevier, 1964.

Dickinson Richards. 1964. Biography. In *Nobel Lectures, Physiology or Medicine*, vol. 3 (1942–1962), 527–28.

Fishman, Alfred P., and Richards, Dickinson. 1964. *Circulation of the*

Blood: Men and Ideas. New York: Oxford University Press.

Richards, Dickinson W. 1970. *Medical Priesthoods and Other Essays*. N.P.: Connecticut Printers.

SECONDARY SOURCES

Cournand, André. 1975. "Cardiac Catheterization: Development of the Technique, Its Contributions to Experimental Medicine, and Its Initial Applications in Man." *Acta Medica Scandinavica*, Supplementum 579:7–32.

———. 1974. "Dickinson Woodruff Richards: 1895–1973. A Survey of His Contributions to the Physiology and Pathophysiology of Respiration in Man." *American Journal of Medicine* 57:312–328.

———. 1970. "Presentation of the Kober Medal for 1970 to Dickinson W. Richards." *Transactions of the Association of American Physicians* 83:36–42.

Galishoff, S. 1984. "Dickinson Woodruff Richards." I. *Dictionary of American Medical Biography*, edited by Martin Kaufman, Stuart Galishoff, and Todd L. Savitt, 2:633–34. Westport, Connecticut: Greenwood Press.

CHARLES ROBERT RICHET *1913*

Charles Robert Richet was born on August 25, 1850, in Paris. Although primarily a physiologist, Richet also won prominence as a psychologist, a bibliographer, a historian, a poet, a novelist, a playwright, and an aircraft designer. The Nobel Prize was awarded to him in 1913 for his discovery of anaphylaxis. He died December 4, 1935, in Paris.

His father, Alfred Richet, was professor of surgery in the Faculty of Medicine, Paris, and a member of the Academy of Sciences. His mother, Eugénie, was the daughter of a distinguished French jurist, Charles Renouard. Charles Richet married Amélie Aubry on August 27, 1878. They had seven children, one of whom, Charles, became professor of medicine in the Faculty of Medicine, Paris.

Richet wrote in his autobiographical note "Souvenirs d'un physiologiste," that although he would have preferred literature as a career, he had studied medicine to please his father (Richet 1933). As a medical student in Paris Richet became interested in hypnosis; this interest led to his first published paper, "Du Somnambulisme provoqué" (Richet 1875). His interest in hypnosis, and later in spiritualism, remained with him throughout his life. Charles Richet completed his studies for the M.D. in 1877, and for the *docteur ès science* (equivalent to a Ph.D.) in

1878. His theses for the two degrees, "Recherches Expérimentales et Cliniques sur la Sensibilité" and "Du suc gastrique chez l'homme et animaux, ses propriétés chimiques et physiologiques," were both based on a rare opportunity to study stomach function in a young man who had acquired a gastric fistula, a surgical opening into his stomach through the skin of his abdomen (Richet 1877; 1878). The fistula was required because his esophagus, or gullet, had been seared shut when he accidentally swallowed lye.

By 1878 Richet had qualified for a faculty position in basic science as *agrégé* in the Faculty of Medicine at Paris. The following year he published the first French translation of William Harvey's classical book, *De Motu Cordis*, which reported his discovery of the circulation of the blood (Richet 1879).

In his physiology laboratory Richet began to study body temperature regulation. In the course of his work on respiration, begun in 1883, he discovered that the dog, an animal not equipped with sweat glands, regulated his body temperature through panting, an act that caused evaporation of water through the upper respiratory passages (Richet 1886). Richet also discovered in 1885 that the fever that accompanies infection is induced from a small center in the brain that responds to bacterial toxins and foreign proteins (Richet 1885). In 1887 Richet discovered what is now known as passive immunity. He protected an animal against an infection by injecting it with blood from another animal that had recovered from the same infection (Richet 1888). Shortly thereafter Von Behring accomplished his Nobel Prize–winning development of a vaccine against diphtheria.

In 1888 Richet, with the engineer Tatin, began to work on the development of powered flight before the Wright brothers began their epoch-making experiments. Later Richet and Tatin were joined by two teenaged boys, Jaques and Louis Breguet. The Richet group lost the race to the Wright brothers by a few weeks, but the Breguet boys went on to found the first and, for many years, the largest aircraft factory in France, originally called Ateliers Breguet Richet and later just Breguet, as Richet became immersed in his other work.

During the years of experimentation with airplanes Richet wrote plays and in his laboratory studied the toxicity of metals. He discovered that antibacterial agents ultimately lose their effect on a microorganism when, after several generations, strains appear that are immune to the metallic poison (Richet 1881; 1883). The phenomenon is well recognized today as the development of bacterial resistance to antibiotics.

In 1894 Richet began a huge bibliographic undertaking, the *Bibliographica Physiologica* (Richet 1895). A year later he launched the multivolume *Dictionnaire de Physiologie*, designed to review the world literature on physiology. It was published each year until World War I (Richet 1895–1913). A further volume was published after the war, by which time the medical literature had become too vast to be reviewed by a single publication.

In 1902 Richet wrote a play, *Circé*, that was produced at the national theatre in Monte Carlo with Sarah Bernhardt in the lead. That same year Richet began the work on anaphylaxis that was to win him the Moscow Prize and a year later, in 1913, the Nobel Prize.

Richet and his collaborator Portier, with an interest in poisons, had found that injections of the fluid from the nematocysts of *Physalia*, the Portuguese Man-O-War, and the tentacles of the sea anemone, *Actinia*, were fatal to rabbits and other small animals but seemed to have little effect on dogs. But a second injection administered to a dog after an interval of three weeks caused an almost immediate violent death (Richet and Portier 1902). Richet and Portier then undertook a thorough study of this startling phenomenon, showing that the fatal outcome in dogs was not attributable to the nature of the poison but to the timing of a second injection of a foreign substance. Richet named the phenomenon "anaphylaxis" from a Greek root meaning "against protection." He later discovered that small doses administered at shorter intervals could immunize the animal. He further showed that susceptibility to anaphylaxis could be transferred from an animal that had received a poison injection to one that had not by injecting blood from the former into the latter (Richet 1909a). In addition, he found that mixing the blood serum from a sensitized animal with the substance that had produced the sensitivity caused anaphylaxis upon its injection into a new animal (Richet 1909b).

Not until he had won the Nobel Prize was Richet elected to the Academy of Sciences. That same year he was also awarded an entirely unrelated prize by the Académie Française for a poem about Pasteur (Richet 1922). He had also been honored earlier by the Académie for his poetry, a series of fables in verse called "Pour les Grands et les Petits."

Before World War I Richet was intensely active in the pacifistic movement, but after the war broke out he helped recruit Italy to the side of the Allies. Then, although already in his mid-sixties, Richet went into the trenches to treat soldiers with the anesthetic chloralose, which he had developed with Hanriot (Hanriot and Richet 1893). He also did pioneering work with blood plasma as a substitute for whole blood transfusions; transfusions were causing many deaths from red cell incompatibility because the blood types had not been discovered yet (Richet 1919a). For his wartime service Richet was awarded the Grand Cross of the Legion of Honor and the Croix de Guèrre. In 1919 Richet published his major work in history, *Histoire Générale*, which had been released two years earlier in German translation (Richet 1919b).

In 1925, at age seventy-five, Richet retired as a professor. He continued his interest in physiology and in the occult, holding that clairvoyance and other spiritualistic phenomena were simply aspects of physiology that had not been explained as yet. In 1935 Richet died of pneumonia.

Charles Richet was a complex man of many talents who had been born to wealth and position during a period of rapid social change in France. His personality was contradictory. Although versatile, sensitive, and open to new ideas, he was at times rigid and opinionated. He was restless and rebellious, yet loyal and dependable; he was also jealous of credit, vain, and sensitive to slights, yet generous and magnanimous with colleagues and even rivals. He was haughty and convinced of the superiority of the white race, yet gracious and concerned about suffering in all parts of the world. Alert and energetic, he seemed to view each of his many and varied pursuits as a game he was determined to win. His serious commitments were to the promotion of justice and the perfection of humanity, to ending war and to conquering diseases, especially cancer and tuberculosis. He aspired to these goals not as a religious believer but as what today might be called a liberal humanist. Because Richet's interests ranged so widely, he rarely pursued a new observation deeply and assiduously enough to exhaust the possibilities of inquiry and to test and firmly establish his inferences. Instead, his agile brain allowed him to leap from discovery to theory with unusually shrewd insights about significance, but only rarely did he mount a painstaking experimental challenge to his theory. Despite his intellectual peregrinations, Richet, through his remarkable sensitiveness to clues and his quick grasp of the significance of observations, was able to contribute substantially to a fruitful period in the development of medical science in Europe. His colleague, Emile Gley, in summing up Richet's career, wrote, "he sees the major functions of the organism as mechanisms of defense—based on evolutionary adaptation."

Richet's creative powers in science were recognized in a tribute by Nobel laureate Sir Charles Sherrington, considered by many as the father of neurophysiology. He wrote in 1912 for the celebration of Richet's twenty-five years as a professor: "To honor him is to honor the spirit of physiology in its most graceful, most eloquent and most inspiring presentment—physiology poetized so to say. May we not say that there is not one whose physiological writings and speaking display such imaginative power without allowing imagination to add or to subtract from scientific truth by one iota."

STEWART WOLF

Selected Bibliography

PRIMARY SOURCES

Richet, Charles. 1875. "Du somnambulisme provoqué." *J. de l'anatomie et de la physiologie normales et pathologiques de l'homme et des animaux* 11:343–78.

———. 1877. *Recherches experimentales et cliniques sur la sensibilité, par le Dr. Charles Richet.* Paris: G. Masson.

———. 1878. *Du suc gastrique chez l'homme et las animaux, ses propriétés chimiques et physiologiques.* Paris: G. Bailliere.

———. trans. 1879. William Harvey, *La Circulation du sang; des mouve-*

ments du coeur chez l'homme et chez les animaux; deux responses a Riolan. Paris: G. Masson.

———. 1881. "De la toxicité comparée des differents métaux." *Comptes rendus Académie des sciences* 93: 649–51.

———. 1883. "De l'action toxique comparée des métaux sur les microbes." *Comptes rendus Académie des sciences* 97:1004–6.

Hanriot, Maurice, and Charles Richet. 1883. "De l'action physiologique de chloralose." *Biologie Mémoires*, 1–7.

Richet, Charles. 1885. "Influence du systeme nerveux sur la calorification." *Comptes rendus Académie des sciences* 100:1021–24.

———. 1886. "Influence de la frequence de la respiration sur la chaleur chez le chien." *Comptes rendus Société de Biologie* 3:397–99.

Hericourt, Jules, and Charles Richet. 1888. "Sur un microbe pyogéne et septique (staphylococcus pyosepticus) et sur la vaccination contre ses effets." *Comptes rendus Académie des sciences* 107:690–92.

Richet, Charles. 1894–96. *Bibliographia Physiologica*, 1893–1894 (1895). *Repertoire des travaux de physiologie . . . classé d' après la classification decimale.* 2 vols. Paris: F. Alcan.

———. 1895–1913. *Dictionnaire de Physiologie*, 9 vols. Paris: Germer Baillière.

Richet, Charles, and Paul Portier. 1902. "De l'action anaphylactique de certains venins." *Bulletin de la Société de Biologie*, 170–72.

Richet, Charles. 1909a. "Role du systeme nerveux dans les phénomènes de la anaphylaxie aigué." *La Presse Medicale* (Mercredit) 7 Avril.

———. 1909b. "Etudes sur la crépitine (toxine de Hura Crepitans)." *Annales de l'Institut Pasteur* 23: 745–800.

———. 1919a. "Injections de gomme ou de plasma après hémorragie." *Comptes rendus Académie des sciences* 169:1072–74.

———. 1919b. "Abrégé d'histoire générale." In *Essai sur le passé de l'homme et des sociétés humaines*, 600. Paris: Hachette.

———. 1922. "La Gloire de Pasteur." *Paris Medical* (Annexe) 46:442–45.

———. 1933. *Souvenirs d'un physiologiste*. Joigny (Yonne): J. Peyronnet.

FREDERICK CHAPMAN ROBBINS
1954

Frederick Chapman Robbins was born in Auburn, Alabama, on August 25, 1916. A virologist and pediatrician, Robbins shared the Nobel Prize in 1954 with John Franklin Enders and Thomas Huckle Weller for their successful culturing of poliomyelitis virus in several types of human tissues. Their breakthrough not only laid the groundwork for the development of an effective polio vaccine but was also the prototype for modern methods of viral cultivation, diagnostic testing, and vaccine development. At the time of the award, Robbins, only five years out of residency, had just taken up an appointment as director of Pediatrics and Contagious Diseases at Cleveland Metropolitan General Hospital, the position he would occupy until 1965. His wife, whom he married in 1948, is Alice Havemeyer Northrup, daughter of John Northrup, the 1946 Nobel laureate in Chemistry. They have two daughters, Alice and Louise.

Robbins was the son of William Jacob Robbins, a plant physiologist who served for some years as director of the New York Botanical Garden, and Christine Chapman Robbins. He earned both a B.A. (1936) and a premedical B.S. (1938) from the University of Missouri before entering Harvard Medical School, where he completed his clinical training. While at Harvard, he met Thomas Weller, who became his roommate, and had the opportunity to study virology with John Enders. He had determined on pediatrics as a specialty and, after receiving his M.D. from Harvard in 1940, began an internship and residency at Children's Hospital in Boston.

World War II summoned Robbins to army service halfway through his residency. From 1942 to 1946 he was chief of the virus and rickettsial diseases section of the Fifteenth Medical General Laboratory, serving in North Africa and Italy. This assignment enabled him to conduct research on infectious hepatitis, typhus fever, and Q fever. He received the Bronze Star Medal for his wartime efforts.

After demobilization Robbins returned to Boston with a confirmed interest in research and in virology. He finished his residency at Children's Hospital in 1948 and was awarded a two-year National Research Council Senior Fellowship in Virus Diseases. This gave him the opportunity to work again with Enders, who was establishing a new program for viral research at Children's, and with Weller. Initially also a fellow, Weller was appointed assistant director of the Infectious Diseases Research Laboratory in 1949.

When Weller was still a medical

student in 1940, he and Enders, working with A. E. Feller, had achieved the first successful prolonged roller tube culture of a virus (Feller, Enders, and Weller 1940). During the war Enders had been working on the mumps virus, which often broke out among recruits and draftees. He and his team had developed diagnostic tests and a killed-virus vaccine for mumps. Robbins, Weller, and Enders now began a new series of viral studies. Robbins focused initially on the diagnosis of mumps infection with the antihemagglutinin test and the neutralization of mumps virus in tissue culture (Robbins et al. 1949).

In March 1948 Weller was growing the mumps virus in human embryonic tissue cultures with the addition of antibiotics to prevent bacterial contamination. At the end of one such experiment, he had a few extra tubes and decided to "try polio" to see if that virus would thrive in his system. His results with the embryo tissue encouraged him to attempt to culture poliovirus in other preparations. He was able to grow the virus in human foreskin cultures, the first time it had been successfully established in non-neural, nonembryonic cells.

Robbins, who had become interested in infant epidemic diarrhea, had developed a successful system of mouse intestinal tissue cultures, using antibiotics to inhibit bacterial overgrowth. He and Weller experimented with poliovirus in these cells but without success. They then developed a culture of human intestinal tissue that proved more hospitable: the poliovirus grew and throve. This was the first demonstration that polio could survive in the intestinal walls of infected individuals. The team also observed cellular changes in the cultures that provided clear evidence of viral replication. Enders coined the term "cytopathogenic" to describe the altered cells.

Over the next few months they were able to produce large quantities of the virus by refining their culture methods and to neutralize it with specific antibodies. The definitive report of their work appeared in *Science* in January 1949, less than a year after Weller had first introduced poliovirus into his spare tubes (Enders, Weller, and Robbins 1949). These classic experiments formed the basis for many diagnostic and vaccine applications, as well as contemporary methods of viral cultivation. The Nobel Committee voted to award John Enders the 1954 Nobel Prize for his significant contribution; he declined to accept unless Robbins and Weller shared the award, and the Nobel Committee complied with his wishes.

In 1950 Robbins was appointed instructor in pediatrics and associate director of the Isolation Service at Children's. He continued working with Enders on the cultivation of poliovirus and the application of the culturing techniques they had developed. Two years later he accepted the invitation from Cleveland Metropolitan and left Boston.

Robbins's subsequent career was notable for administrative and policy-making achievements, rather than research contributions, although he continued his investigations into pediatric virology and did major work on the parasite responsible for Q fever. He served as president of the Society for Pediatric Research in 1961–62. In 1965 he began a long and respected tenure as dean of the School of Medicine at Case Western Reserve. During this period he was active on many influential national committees, addressing the issues of human experimentation, abortion, vaccination programs, Third World health policies, and public food safety policy. He was also elected president of the American Pediatric Society for the 1973–74 term.

In 1980, upon retiring from Case Western as university professor and dean emeritus, he was named president of the Institute of Medicine of the National Academy of Sciences in Washington. Robbins took up this five-year appointment at age sixty-four, serving simultaneously as senior scholar in residence at the institute (1980–85) and as distinguished professor of the Department of Pediatrics at Georgetown University (1981–85). At the time of his selection colleagues described him as a capable leader willing to compromise; as a man widely respected in Washington; and as an individual who was not an innovator but one who would take a reasonable approach to innovation. These observations shed considerable light on Robbins the man and the administrator.

Among the many other awards he has won for his work are the Mead Johnson Prize from the American Academy of Pediatrics (1953), the Medical Mutual Honor Award (1969), and Ohio Governor's Award (1971).

MARCIA MELDRUM
JAMES J. POUPARD

Selected Bibliography

PRIMARY SOURCES

Feller, A. E., J. F. Enders, and T. H. Weller. 1940. "The Prolonged Coexistence of Vaccinia Virus in High Titre and Living Cells in Roller Tube Cultures of Chick Embryonic Tissues." *Journal of Experimental Medicine* 72:367–87.

Enders, J. F., T. H. Weller, and F. C. Robbins. 1949. "Cultivation of the Lansing Strain of Poliomyelitis Virus in Cultures of Various Human Embryonic Tissues." *Science* 109 (January 28):85–87.

Robbins, F. C., L. Kilham, J. H. Levens, and J. F. Enders. 1949. "An Evaluation of the Test for Antihemagglutinin in the Diagnosis of Infections by Mumps Virus." *Journal of Immunology* 61:235–42.

Weller, T. H., F. C. Robbins and J. F. Enders. 1949. "Cultivation of Poliomyelitis Virus in Cultures of Human Foreskin and Embryonic Tissues." *Proceedings of the Society for Experimental Biology* 72:153–55.

Robbins, F. C., and J. F. Enders. 1950. "Tissue Culture Techniques in the Study of Animal Viruses." *American Journal of Medical Science* 220:316–38.

SECONDARY SOURCES

1955. "Enders, John Franklin." In *Current Biography Yearbook*, 182–84. New York: H. W. Wilson.

Sun, Marjorie. 1980. "Institute of Medicine Gets New President." *Science* 210 (November 7):616–17.

Weller, T. H. 1989. "As It Was and As It Is: A Half-Century of Progress." *Journal of Infectious Diseases* 159 (March):378–83.

Williams, Greer. 1960. *Virus Hunters*. New York: Alfred A. Knopf.

RONALD ROSS *1902*

Ronald Ross's demonstration of the transmission of malaria by *Anopheles* mosquitoes—a discovery that required the detailed working out of the whole life history of the malarial parasite in both the mosquito and man—profoundly transformed the whole understanding of malarial fevers. Ross showed not only how and why malarial fevers occurred when and where they did, but how they might be prevented by eliminating the breeding places of *Anopheles* mosquitoes. Since malaria then afflicted many millions of people throughout the world, causing the deaths of untold multitudes and rendering many areas virtually uninhabitable, the discovery of its mode of transmission and means of prevention saved vast numbers of lives and removed a serious barrier to the economic development of warm temperate and tropical countries.

Ronald Ross was born at Almora, Nepal, on May 13, 1857, the first child of Major Campbell Claye Grant Ross, then attached to the Sixty-sixth Regiment of Bengal Native Infantry. In 1865, at the age of eight, he was sent to England for his education; he attended schools at Ryde, on the Isle of Wight, and at Springhill, near Southampton. In 1874, when he was seventeen, he entered St. Bartholomew's Hospital, London, to study medicine, but at that period in his life Ross was little interested in medicine and devoted much time to poetry and music. Nevertheless, the lectures by Sir James Paget and other distinguished Bart's teachers gave him an enduring respect for scientific medicine. While serving as an assistant house surgeon at Shrewsbury in 1877–78, Ross was impressed by the results of antiseptic surgery as conducted by one of Joseph Lister's students. In 1879 Ross passed the examination for membership in the Royal College of Surgeons, but he failed the examination for licentiate of the Society of Apothecaries, having devoted only one morning to study for it. Ashamed to continue accepting an allowance from his father, he became a ship's surgeon for the next year and a half.

Early in 1881 he successfully passed the examination of the Society of Apothecaries and entered the Indian Medical Service. In October 1881 Ross arrived at Bombay. He was stationed successively at various places in southern India, including Bangalore and Madras, and in Burma and the Andaman Islands. With little medical work to do, he devoted his abundant leisure to mathematics and poetry. In 1888 Ross returned on furlough to England, where he studied for the diploma in public health given jointly by the Royal College of Physicians and Surgeons. In April 1889 he married Rosa Bloxam. The following summer Ross took a course in bacteriology from Emanuel Klein at University College, London; this training acquainted him with microscopy and bacteriological technique.

On his return to India in the fall of 1889, Ross was sent on field service to Burma, where he encountered much malaria. In May 1890 he was appointed staff surgeon at Bangalore and began to study fevers. Although Bangalor had few cases of malaria, numerous cases of typhoid fever and other intestinal infections suggested to Ross that malaria might also be caused by an intestinal infection. In 1893, when he again became a regimental surgeon, he was stationed at Secunderabad. The rainy season brought much malaria, and Ross began to examine the blood of his patients for the malarial parasites that had been discovered by Alphonse Laveran in 1882. He failed to find them and began to doubt their existence.

When he returned to England on furlough the following year (1894), Ross called upon Dr. Patrick Manson, who showed him Laveran's crescent-shaped bodies in a stained specimen of malarial blood. Manson also showed Ross the other forms assumed by malarial parasites in the blood of a patient at Charing Cross Hospital. In China in 1877, Manson had found that the larvae of filaria worms, which caused elephantiasis, were sucked up with the blood of patients by mosquitoes and continued to develop within the mosquito. Manson thought that when the female mosquito died, after laying her eggs in water, the filaria worms would escape into the water, there to infect persons who might drink the water. In November 1894 Manson suggested to Ross that mosquitoes might transmit malaria in much the same manner. Manson said that at that time they knew the functions of the asexual forms of the malarial parasites, but they knew nothing of the sexual forms of the organisms, which Manson suspected the crescents and the long motile filaments (then mistakenly called flagella) to be. Since the malaria parasite could not be communicated directly from the blood of one person to that of another, it must have a second life outside the human body. Manson suggested that when a mosquito sucked malarial blood, the crescents entered its stomach where they emitted the motile filaments which, Manson thought, were flagellated spores. The filaments then, he surmised, passed through the stomach wall into the mosquito's tissues, where they underwent further development and were released into water when the mosquito died. On Manson's hypothesis, the mosquito served to provide a means of escape for the malaria parasite from the human body (Manson 1894). Since Manson did not think his hypothesis could be tested effecitvely in England, Ross resolved to study the question in India when both malaria patients and mosquitoes were plentiful.

After his return to India in 1895 Ross regularly examined the blood of fever patients for malaria parasites, and he began to breed mosquitoes to feed upon malaria patients. He was handicapped by his inability to obtain books on the classification and natural history of the various species of mosquitoes that he encountered. Nevertheless, his regiment was stationed near a small marsh where they suffered greatly from aestivo-autumnal (falciparum) and tertian malaria. In May 1895 Ross observed that the crescent forms of parasites gave rise to flagella much more abundantly in a mosquito's stomach than they did in fresh blood slides. After many frustrations, at Secunderabad on August 20, 1897, Ross found pigmented malarial parasites in the stomach wall of a brown dapple-winged mosquito that he later learned was a species of *Anopheles*. The next day Ross dissected a second mosquito, in which he found in the stomach wall the same cells only now much larger and more clearly defined (Ross 1897). Subsequently, he found that when the dappled-winged mosquitoes remained unfed, or when they were fed healthy blood, no such pigmented bodies appeared in their stomach walls (Ross 1898).

Ross was anxious to pursue his researches on the dapple-winged mosquitoes further, but a month after his discovery he was ordered to an isolated station at Kherwara in northern India where in autumn the weather was too cool for mosquitoes to be active. In February 1898, through Manson's intervention from London, Ross was assigned for six months to special duty at Calcutta, where he was given a small laboratory to investigate both malaria and kala-azar (later identified as leishmaniasis). At Calcutta, because of the difficulty of obtaining human malaria patients, Ross decided to study malaria (the blood parasite *Proteosoma*) in birds.

Meanwhile, at Johns Hopkins University, in November 1897, W. G. MacCallum had shown in bird malaria that the function of the flagellum was to impregnate certain large, round, pigmented cells. The flagella acted, therefore, as spermatozoa, and the round pigmented cells as ova. At Calcutta, Ross found the malarial parasites in the stomach wall of grey mosquitoes that had fed upon malaria-infected sparrows, larks, and crows, and by April 1898 he had traced the growth of the parasites up to seven days after they entered the mosquito. In June he observed that the pigmented cells in the mosquito stomach wall burst on the seventh or eight day to release multitudes of delicate threads, and early in July he found that the threads migrated into the mosquito's salivary gland. From the salivary gland the threadlike spores would pass in large numbers into the blood vessels of the bird when the mosquito secreted saliva into the wound made in the course of biting (Manson 1898, 1). On 25 June Ross had allowed infected mosquitoes to feed upon three healthy (i.e., malaria-free) sparrows and two weeks later he found multitudes of parasites in the sparrows' blood, whereas the blood of controls remained parasite-free (Manson 1898, 2).

In September 1898 Ross was compelled against his will to break off his malaria investigations to go to Nowgong in Assam to investigate kala-azar, a disease of then unknown cause that closely resembled severe malaria. His superiors understood neither the importance of his work on malaria nor the requirements of scientific investigation, and they repeatedly obstructed his work. In February 1899 Ross retired from the Indian Medical Service and returned to England. Shortly after his return he was appointed lecturer in the newly founded Liverpool School of Tropical Medicine. Ross immediately organized an expedition to Sierra Leone, where he traced the life history of human malaria in two species of *Anopheles* mosquitoes and worked out practical measures for the prevention of malaria by the elimination near human habitations of the pools of stagnant water in which *Anopheles* bred.

In 1900, influenced by Ross's demonstration of the transmission of malaria by *Anopheles* mosquitoes, Walter Reed and his coworkers found that yellow fever was similarly transmitted by the bite of *Stegomyia* mosquitoes. Early in 1901 at Havana, William C. Gorgas began a vigorous antimosquito campaign that eliminated yellow fever and greatly reduced malaria in the city. Later Gorgas used similar methods to prevent yellow fever and malaria during the building of the Panama Canal. Ross himself initiated and planned antimosquito programs for the prevention of malaria in many countries, including West Africa, the Suez Canal Zone, Mauritius, India, and Ceylon. Profoundly interested in mathematics, he developed mathematical models for the epidemiology of malaria that are still used in studying the epidemiology of insect-borne diseases.

In 1901 Ronald Ross was elected a Fellow of the Royal Society of London, and in 1902 he was awarded the Nobel Prize in Physiology or Medicine. In 1911 he was knighted. The following year Ross became physician for tropical diseases at King's College Hospital, London, and in 1926 he was appointed director of the Ross Institute and Hospital of Tropical Diseases founded at London in his honor. He died at the Ross Institute on September 16, 1932.

LEONARD G. WILSON

Selected Bibliography

PRIMARY SOURCES

Ross, Ronald. 1897. "On Some Peculiar Pigmented Cells Found in Two

Mosquitoes Fed on Malarial Blood." *British Medical Journal* ii:1786–1788.

———. 1898. "Pigmented Cells in Mosquitoes." *British Medical Journal* i:550–551.

———. 1902. "Researches on Malaria." Nobel Prize Lecture, December 12, 1902. Reprinted in *Nobel Lectures in Physiology or Medicine*. Vol. 1 (1901–21):25–119.

———. 1923. *Memoirs with a Full Account of the Great Malaria Problem and Its Solution*. London: J. Murray.

SECONDARY SOURCES

Manson, Patrick, 1898. "The Mosquito and the Malarial Parasite." *British Medical Journal* ii:849–853.

———. 1894. "On the Nature and Significance of the Crescentic and Flagellated Bodies in Malarial Blood." *British Medical Journal* ii:1306–1308.

———. 1898. "Surgeon-Major Ronald Ross's Recent Investigations on the Mosquito-Malaria Theory." *British Medical Journal* i:1575–1577.

Megroz, R. L. 1931. *Ronald Ross, Discoverer and Creator*. London: Allen and Unwin.

FRANCIS PEYTON ROUS *1966*

(Francis) Peyton Rous was born on October 5, 1879, in Baltimore, Maryland. He earned his bachelor's degree in 1900 and his medical degree in 1905, both at Johns Hopkins University in Baltimore, where he was trained in pathology, virology, and bacteriology. Between 1906 and 1909 he held an assistantship in pathology at the University of Michigan in Ann Arbor and studied pathology for a year in Dresden, Germany. Invited in 1909 to join the Rockefeller Institute (now Rockefeller University) in New York City by its president, Simon Flexner, Rous remained at Rockefeller for sixty years, officially retiring in 1945, but continuing to work in his laboratory until the December before his death. In 1915 he married Mary Eckford de Kay. They had three children, Ellen, Phoebe, and Marian (the last is the wife of Allen Hodgkin, winner of the Nobel Prize for Physiology or Medicine in 1963). Peyton Rous died on February 16, 1970, in New York City.

The award of the Nobel Prize to the octogenarian Rous was a late tribute to the meticulous and revolutionary work he initiated in 1909 when he began studies of a malignant tumor, a spindle-celled sarcoma (now named after him), found in the breast of a Plymouth Rock hen brought to the Rockefeller Institute by a local farmer. In his early experiments, Rous was able to propagate the sarcoma serially in close relatives of the index case, the first time an avian tumor had been successfully transplanted. By showing that the sarcoma could be successfully transplanted only in close kin within a purebred stock, Rous's work hastened the use of genetically homogenous laboratory animals in cancer research.

In 1911 Rous reported he was able to produce the spindle-celled sarcoma by inoculating fowl with the liquid remaining after tumor material had been passed through a Berkefeld filter impermeable to single cells but not to viruses. Although Rous did not invoke a specific agent, the work was the first to demonstrate that a malignant tumor might be transmitted by a virus.

The following year Rous described a new avian neoplasm, an osteochondrosarcoma which he produced by inoculating hens with a different cell-free filtrate potentiated by sterile earth or *Kieselguhr*. Rous showed that the tumor could be distinguished histologically from the spindle-celled sarcoma and that in all probability the two did not share the same causal agent. Two years later he reported on another sarcoma, distinctly dissimilar from the other two and caused by a third filterable agent. Without even specifying that any but the spindle-celled sarcoma was caused by a virus, he went on to conclude that the three neoplasms were due to agents of approximately similar size and "natural class" (Rous and Murphy 1914, 68). He inferred that these findings pointed to the existence of "a new group of entities" causing cancers in chickens (Rous and Murphy 1914, 68). He was careful, however, not to generalize beyond his data, nor to argue that viruses were the universal causal agents of cancer.

Rous's work was part of a continuum, a growing body of research that began in Europe in the 1890s when the virus was first recognized as a distinct biological entity. For most investigators of the period, viruses were pathogens distinguished from other microbes in that they were very much smaller, an inference drawn from virus' ability to pass through bacteriological filters and their invisibility under the light microscope. (The first images of viruses were obtained in the late thirties using the new electron microscope.) Viruses were also unusual in that they could not be cultured in artificial media. Little more was known of viruses, except that a growing number of animal, plant, and human diseases were recognized as virally caused, including hoof-and-mouth and tobacco mosaic diseases, rabies, and yellow fever. In 1908 two Danish investigators, Wilhelm Ellerman and Oluf Bang, showed that fowl leukemia was due to a filterable agent, but leukemia was not considered at the time a form of cancer. Consequently, Rous's work was the first to scientifically demonstrate to contemporaries that some neoplasms might have an infectious cause.

Although Rous had isolated several putative agents, transmitted those pathogens to a host, and carefully studied and described the neoplastic tissue that subsequently developed, his findings were not accepted by most cancer experts, either at the time or for the next forty years. Rous's viral hypothesis was at variance with contemporary theories of cancer causation, which held that tumor formation was a consequence of changes in cell physiology, possibly because of inherited cellular defects, physical degeneration attendant on aging, or tissue irritation (Patterson 1987, 56–63). Some critics dismissed Rous's work by arguing that his filtrates had not been free of cancerous cells, others that the chicken tumors were not true cancers, but inflammations. Damaging to Rous's hypothesis as well was that no tumors of viral origin had been isolated in mammals.

With the outbreak of World War I, Rous was drawn to other work that occupied him for the next two decades, specifically research on blood transfusion and the functions of the liver and gall bladder, and studies of living tissue and of vascular permeability. One of his most important discoveries concerned the preservation of blood cells.

In 1900 Karl Landsteiner had identified the four main blood groups, providing the basis for the safe transfusion of a donor's blood. Fourteen years later a Belgian, Albert Hustin, used sodium citrate to prevent blood from clotting. Rous's contribution to blood transfusion was to perfect, with his collaborators, methods of storing and preserving human blood cells; one of these preservatives, the Rous-Turner solution, is still in use. These procedures allowed the creation in 1917 of the first blood bank, established by O. H. Robertson, Rous's associate, behind the front lines in Belgium.

In 1931 the discovery by a colleague, Richard Shope, of a virally-caused mammalian tumor, a papilloma in wild cottontail rabbits, drew Rous back to cancer research. For the next two decades he investigated the Shope papilloma and the cancers associated with it. From this work he evolved important hypotheses regarding the natural history of cancer.

Rous began by establishing that the papillomata could develop into true neoplasms and that viruses could be recovered from these neoplastic growths in cottontails. He found, in addition, that benign papillomas, propagated by transmitting the virus from wild to domestic rabbits, gradually became malignant tumors. These findings appeared to corroborate the earlier results in fowl.

Rous also studied the role of coal tar and other chemicals as cancer agents and compared their effects on rabbits with that of the virus. He found that a chemical carcinogen like tar produced papillomas similar to those induced by the virus. These papillomas might progress to malignancy, but they normally regressed once tarring was discontinued. Rous discovered as well that a combination of tar and Shope papilloma virus behaved synergistically, increasing the variety of tumors and significantly reducing the time required for malignant tissue to appear.

From these investigations and from other experiments, Rous drew important inferences concerning "tumor progression," a term he coined. He distinguished between tumor initiators and tumor promoters. Some chemical carcinogens, for example, act primarily as initiators but promote neoplasms when they, the chemicals, are continually renewed. However, initiators can produce cells that, without being cancerous, have a neoplastic potential, one that becomes actualized in the presence of promoters. Some viruses serve as initiators only. Others are promoters as well and therefore act as continuing causes of neoplasms. Among such viruses are the oncogenic agents that Rous had originally identified as causing tumors in fowl.

During the years Peyton Rous researched the relationship of viruses to cancer, he headed one of the few laboratories engaged with the problem. Despite the general uninterest in his cancer work, Rous had faith in his research and felt that his discovery of the chicken sarcoma viruses was fundamentally important. After 1950 other scientists took up the investigation of tumor viruses, inspired perhaps by the isolation of leukemia viruses by Ludwik Gross and his colleagues in 1951 and by the successful typing of the polio viruses shortly before (Patterson 1987, 59). The discovery of new oncogenic viruses, proceeded rapidly, including the mouse parotid tumor virus (1953), the simian virus 40 (1960–62), cat leukemia (1964), and the murine leukemia viruses (1964–66). Not coincidentally, the first issue of a new journal, *Virology*, published in 1955, contained an article on Rous's investigation of the chicken sarcoma. These considerable discoveries served to redirect attention to Rous's pioneering work, so much so that one recent writer can claim that "few fields in modern biology and certainly no other field in cancer research can be traced back to the work of one man in the same way that the foundations in the field of viral oncology can be traced back to the work of Peyton Rous in 1911" (Klein 1980, v). Reassessments similar to this one led to the award of the Nobel Prize to Rous.

In addition to the Nobel Prize, which he shared with Charles Huggins, another cancer pioneer, Rous received other significant awards and honors, including the National Medal of Science, the Albert Lasker Award, the Kovalenko Award of the National Academy of Sciences, the Erich Darmstaedter Prize, and honorary degrees from the universities of Cambridge, Michigan, Yale, Birmingham, McGill, Chicago, and Zurich. He was the author or coauthor of almost two hundred articles published in the scientific press. Finally, for close to fifty years, he was first coeditor (with Simon Flexner), then editor, of the *Journal of Experimental Medicine*, published by Rockefeller University.

Gerald M. Oppenheimer

Selected Bibliography

PRIMARY SOURCES

Rous, Peyton. 1910. "A Transmissible Avian Neoplasm (Sarcoma of the

Common Fowl)." *Journal of Experimental Medicine* 12:696–705.

———. 1911. "Transmission of a Malignant New Growth by Means of a Cell-Free Filtrate." *Journal of the American Medical Association* 56: 198.

Rous, Peyton, James B. Murphy, and W. H. Tytler. 1912. "A Filterable Agent the Cause of a Second Chicken-Tumor, an Osteochondrosarcoma." *Journal of the American Medical Association* 59:1793–94.

Rous, Peyton, and James B. Murphy. 1914. "On the Causation by Filterable Agents of Three Distinct Chicken Tumors." *Journal of Experimental Medicine* 18:52–69.

Friedewald, William F., and Peyton Rous. 1944. "The Initiating and Promoting Elements in Tumor Production." *Journal of Experimental Medicine* 80:101–25.

Francis Peyton Rous Papers. No date. Philadelphia: American Philosophical Society.

SECONDARY SOURCES

Dulbecco, Renato. 1976. "Francis Peyton Rous." *National Academy of Sciences of the United States of America Biographical Memoirs*, vol. 48. Washington, D.C.: National Academy of Sciences.

Klein, George. 1980. "Introduction." In *Viral Oncology*, edited by George Klein. New York: Raven Press.

Patterson, James T. 1987. *The Dread Disease, Cancer and American Culture*. Cambridge: Harvard University Press.

Waterson, A. P., and Lise Wilkinson, 1978. *And Introduction to the History of Virology*. Cambridge, England: Cambridge University Press.

Bengt Ingemar Samuelsson
1982

Bengt Ingemar Samuelsson was born on May 21, 1934, in Halmstedt, Sweden. A biochemist, Samuelsson shared the 1982 Nobel Prize with Sune Bergström and John Robert Vane for their work in characterizing, differentiating, and describing the action of the prostaglandins, a field in which Bergström pioneered. Samuelsson was Bergström's protégé. His most important contribution was in determining and describing the biosynthesis of these compounds at the cellular level; he also discovered several new prostaglandins. At the time of the award, he was professor and chairman of the Department of Chemistry and dean of the Medical Faculty at the Karolinska Institute in Stockholm, having succeeded Bergström in both positions. That same year he became rector, or chief administrator, again following in his mentor's footsteps. He married Inga Karin Bergstein in 1958; they have one son, Bo, and two daughters, Elisabeth and Astrid.

Samuelsson's parents were Anders and Kristina Samuelsson. He began his medical studies at the University of Lund in southern Sweden, where he first met Sune Bergström. When the senior scientist returned to the Karolinska in 1958, his student followed, and the two began, with Jan Sjovalla and Ragnar Ryhage, to analyze the active lipids called prostaglandins.

The first interest in these compounds resulted from early artificial insemination procedures performed by Raphael Kurzrok, Charles Leib, and Sarah Ratner at Columbia University in 1930. The physicians noted that the injection of seminal plasma into the uterus caused the smooth muscle to contract and then to relax. Maurice Goldblatt in England and Ulf von Euler in Sweden undertook further experiments with seminal fluid from rams before World War II. They observed lowered blood pressure as well as smooth muscle responses in a number of animals. Von Euler identified the active compounds in the secretions of the prostate gland and gave them the name "prostaglandins."

Von Euler introduced Bergström to prostaglandins in 1945. The latter's interest was immediately stirred and he eagerly accepted a small quantity of the extracts von Euler had made from ram semen in the 1930s. Using the most advanced techniques available, he further purified the compounds and was astonished to observed that "after purification essentially to weightlessness, they retained extraordinary activity." Despite his fascination, Bergström's work on prostaglandins was delayed for almost a decade because of the technical difficulties involved and his own administrative commitments (Oates 1982, 765).

By 1958 several factors had made possible the isolation, analysis, and characterization of the mysterious compounds. Bergström, Samuelsson, and their colleagues, Jan Sjovall and Ragnar Ryhage, had collected a sufficient number of sheep seminal glands to prepare the extracts for intensive study. (Roughly 100 kilograms of sheep glands were required for each usable extract.) Bergström had developed the necessary methods of gas chromatography, and Ryhage had invented a method of interface between the chromatograph and the mass spectrometer that permitted the structural analysis of small quantities. The application of this technology to the study of the prostaglandins has now been replicated in many other scientific fields (Oates 1982).

The team soon isolated the first two compounds through 1964 they continued to describe the structure and activity of the prostaglandin group, including PGE_2, $PGF_{2\alpha}$, and PGD_2. The related compounds thromboxane A_2, prostacyclin, and the leukotrienes were discovered later. Prostaglandins are found throughout the human body. Each possesses the same twenty-carbon atom skeleton and fatty acid structure, but each is produced by different cells to perform different and highly specific functions. Thromboxane A_2, for example, is a product of platelets and stimulates platelet aggregation and vasoconstriction, whereas prostacyclin, metabolized by the endothelial cells, has the opposite action.

The new understanding of prostaglandin structure confirmed von Euler's hunch that these compounds were the result of lipid oxygenation. The logical candidate was arachidonic acid, a twenty-carbon polyunsaturated fatty acid. By 1965 Bergström, Samuelsson, and David Van Dorp at the Unilever Laboratories in Holland had demonstrated that arachidonic acid was indeed the common biosynthetic origin of all prostaglandins. This finding showed the way to their in vitro synthesis for research use and solved the supply problems (Oates 1982, 765–66).

Samuelsson meanwhile had received his doctorate in medical sciences in 1960 and his M.D. in 1961. From 1961 to 1962 he held a research fellowship in chemistry at Harvard University. Returning to Sweden, he took the position of assistant professor of chemistry at the Karolinska and began to investigate the production of prostaglandins in vivo. Using mass spectrometry to analyze the oxygenation of arachidonic acid, he identified an intermediate stage in the process, the formation of a cyclic endoperoxide. He and Mats Hamberg isolated two such endoperoxides, PGG_2 and PGH_2, which were intermediates in the synthesis of the D, E, and F prostaglandins discovered by Bergström's team. Their identification and description led to the search for other prostaglandins.

Samuelsson was appointed professor of chemistry at the Royal Veterinary College in Stockholm in 1967, returning to the Karolinska in 1972 as professor and chairman of the Chemistry Department. He had now become interested in the finding of John Vane in Britain that aspirin and some other drugs reduced pain and inflammation by inhibition of the biosynthesis of the prostaglandins from arachidonic acid. Aspirin also had the effect of blocking platelet aggregation, which was not known to be the result of prostaglandin action.

Samuelsson and Hamberg observed the effects of their endoperoxides on platelets and noted that these "intermediate" substances did act to aggregate the blood cells. By correlating their observations with the biochemical reactions in process, they found that the endoperoxides in platelets were synthesized to the hitherto unknown thromboxane A_2, which was very active in stimulating aggregation and also the contraction of vascular smooth muscle. Vane and his colleagues subsequently built on this research in their identification of prostacyclin, a prostaglandin compound with the reverse action. Knowledge of these two new substances added greatly to medical understanding of the body's blood clotting mechanisms and controls (Oates 1982, 766–67).

Aspirin and similar substances apparently block formation of prostaglandins from arachidonic acid by inhibiting the stimulus enzyme cyclooxygenase. However, corticosteroids have additional anti-inflammatory effects which aspirin does not. Samuelsson therefore theorized that the corticosteroids did not act on cyclooxygenase metabolism alone but on some related synthesis. Working with Pierre Borgeat, he observed the fate of arachidonic acid in polymorphonuclear leukocytes. The fatty acid was found to be oxygenated in these cells by a 5-lipoxygenase, into a new class of prostaglandins designated the leukotrienes. One of the intermediate products, an epoxide named LTA_4, was subsequently discovered, by Samuelsson, Robert Murphy, and E. J. Corey at Harvard, to react with glutathione to form several very powerful bronchoconstrictor compounds related to asthma and other anaphylactic reactions.

The multiple functions of the prostaglandins and their powerful activity have thus suggested a wide range of clinical applications, many still in the experimental stages. These include pain relief, induction of labor and of abortion, prevention of ulcers, correction of birth defects, vasodilation in heart surgery, and applications in asthma, cancer, and heart disease, among others (Oates 1982, 767–68; Altman 1982).

Serving as dean at the Karolinska from 1977 to 1982 and subsequently as rector, Samuelsson nevertheless has maintained a rigorous schedule of laboratory research. He is a member of the Royal Swedish Academy of Sciences and of the American Academy of Arts and Sciences. Among the many other awards he has received are the Anders Jahres Prize from Oslo University (1970), the Louisa G. Horowitz Prize from Columbia University (1975), and the Albert Lasker Basic Medical Research Award (1977).

MARCIA MELDRUM

Selected Bibliography

PRIMARY SOURCES

Bergström, Sune, and Bengt Samuelsson. 1967. *Prostaglandins. Proceedings of the Second Nobel Symposium, Stockholm, June 1966.* New York: Interscience Publishers.

Bergström, Sune, K. Green, and Bengt Samuelsson. 1972. *Third Conference on Prostaglandins in Fertility Control, January 17–20, 1972.* Stockholm: Karolinska Institute.

Bergström, Sune. 1973. *Report from the Meeting of the Prostaglandin Task Force Steering Committee, Chapel Hill, June 8–10, 1972, Stockholm, October 2–3, 1972, Geneva, February 26–28, 1973.* Stockholm: Karolinska Institute.

Bergström, Sune, and John R. Vane. 1979. *Prostacyclin.* New York: Raven Press.

SECONDARY SOURCES

Altman, Lawrence K. 1982. "Two Swedes and Briton Win Nobel for Clues to Body's Chemistry." *New York Times* (October 12):1, C3.

Oates, John A. 1982. "The 1982 Nobel Prize in Physiology or Medicine." *Science* 218 (November 19):765–68.

Wilford, John Noble. 1982. "Men in the News: Bengt Ingemar Samuelsson." *New York Times* (October 12):C3.

ANDREW VICTOR SCHALLY
1977

Andrew Victor Schally received the Nobel Prize in 1977 jointly with Roger Guillemin "for their discoveries concerning the peptide hormone production of the brain"; Rosalyn Yalow also shared the Nobel Prize that year for her development of the radioimmunoassay. Independently, Schally and Guillemin demonstrated hormonal activities in extracts of the hypothalamic region of the brain and then purified, isolated, and determined the structures of the hormones they had found. In doing so they made neuroendocrinology an accessible clinical science, with far-ranging implications for diagnostic testing and medical therapy.

Schally was born on November 30, 1926, in Wilno, Poland (now Vilnius, in the USSR). His parents were Major General Casimir Peter Schally, who had a distinguished military career, and Maria Lacka Schally. Little has been written of his early years, but Schally, ever mindful of the new life medical research had opened for him, wrote: "Having spent a harsh childhood during World War II in Nazi- and later Soviet-occupied countries of Europe, and having grown up in the atmosphere of necessary general national austerity in postwar England . . . I was perhaps more aware than others of the value of money and of the high cost of medical research" (Schally 1978, p. 348). Soon after the end of the war, Schally came to Great Britain, and received his diploma from the Bridge Allen School in Scotland in 1946. He next studied chemistry at the University of London and held research positions at the National Institute for Medical Research in Mill Hill, a leading center of biological research in England, from 1949 to 1952. He then emigrated to Montreal and received his B.Sc. degree in 1955 and his Ph.D. in 1957 from McGill University. He became attracted to hypothalamic endocrine research as early as 1954 while still an undergraduate, and it soon became his life's work.

In May 1956 Schally married Margaret Rachel White; they have a son and a daughter. After they were divorced, he married Ana Maria de Madeiros-Comaru, a doctor and endocrinologist from Brazil, in August 1976.

Schally became assistant professor of physiology at Baylor University School of Medicine, Houston, in 1957 and began to collaborate with Roger Guillemin. For five years they worked together in the elusive pursuit of the putative hypothalamic hormone that controlled secretion of ACTH by the anterior pituitary. In 1962 he moved to New Orleans to become head of the Endocrine and Polypeptide Laboratory at the Veterans Administration Hospital, as well as associate professor of medicine at Tulane University Medical School. "I was grateful for the opportunities I was given in the United States," he wrote later, "and I strongly wished to be useful to my new country, for which I felt a complete allegiance, having declared my intention to become a U.S. citizen in February 1959 and becoming naturalized in November 1962" (Schally 1978, 348). He became professor of medicine at Tulane in 1966, and in 1973 was named a senior medical investigator of the U.S. Public Health Service. Schally at present remains a professor at Tulane and head of the Endocrine and Polypeptide Laboratory at the New Orleans V.A. Hospital.

Like Roger Guillemin and others who entered the arena of hypothalamic endocrine research, Schally recalled that "a decisive stimulus was provided by the formulation by [Geoffrey W.] Harris and others of hypotheses relating to the hypothalamic control of secretion of the anterior pituitary gland. Harris and others postulated that neurohumoral substances might originate in the median eminence of the tuber cinereum [the floor of the hypothalamus to which the stalk leading to the pituitary is attached], reach the anterior lobe by way of the hypophysial portal system, and thus regulate pituitary secretion" (Schally 1977, 18). Schally recognized that the notion of hypothalamic control of the anterior pituitary and its many hormones would remain speculative until someone produced direct evidence of the existence of specific hypothalamic chemotransmitters that controlled release of these pituitary hormones.

Seven years of intensive effort to purify the presumed "corticotropin releasing factor" of the hypothalamus, two with Murray Saffran (his mentor at McGill) and five with Guillemin (his senior at Baylor), failed to produce enough material for identification and determination of its structure. The first hypothalamic hypophysiotropic factor was yet to be chemically characterized. But important progress had been made in research techniques in those years from 1955 to 1962. Investigators had developed new in vivo assays for hypothalamic hormones, using the radioimmunoassay techniques for which Rosalyn Yalow shared in the Nobel Prize in 1977. They also had developed new and powerful purification methods, particularly gel filtration on Sephadex columns, for separating different compounds dissolved in the same solution. Large quantities of hypothalami were now needed to allow researchers to purify sufficient quantities of material to permit characterization; Schally himself obtained hundreds of thousands of pig hypothalami from meat packing houses.

Now, in a reversal of the biblical progression, seven fat research years followed the seven lean years. Between 1962 and 1969 Schally and his colleagues in New Orleans devoted their efforts to isolating and identifying thyrotropin releasing hormone (TRH), the putative hormone of the hypothalamus that regulates secretion of thyroid stimulating hormone (TSH) of the anterior pituitary. The latter hormone in turn was known to govern activities of the thyroid gland, which plays a vital part in body (including brain) metabolism.

Between 1964 and 1966 Schally and his coworkers demonstrated the presence of TRH in partly purified fractions of pig and beef hypothalami using in vitro assays based mainly on release of TSH from rat pituitary glands. In 1966 they isolated 2.8 milligrams of TRH from 100,000 pig hypothalami using multiple techniques of gel filtration, phenol extraction, cellulose chromatography, counter current distribution, free-flow electrophoresis, and partition chromatography. They also reported that TRH was a small compound consisting of three amino acids: glutamic acid (glu), histidine (his), and proline (pro). This indicated that TRH was indeed a small protein, a peptide. It took three more years, from 1966 to 1969, to determine the precise structure of porcine TRH, to synthesize it, and to demonstrate unequivocally its biological activity.

At about the same time, Roger Burgus, Wylie Vale, and Roger Guillemin characterized ovine TRH as the same tripeptide in the same conformation, (pyro)Glu-His-Pro-NH_2. They also made a synthetic preparation that was biologically active. Before (and after) both groups had clearly demonstrated the structure of TRH there was much contention over priority of discovery—who presented which paper first, who was in the audience at the presentation, who submitted what papers for publication at an earlier date, even who first suggested the name "thyrotropin releasing hormone" (or "thyrotropin releasing factor," TRF).

A brief chronology of publication dates in the "TRF race" hints at the intensity of competition between the two groups. For simplicity the names Guillemin and Schally as used here stand for all the scientists in their groups, some of whom were the first authors of the research papers or presenters at national meetings:

May 1966, Guillemin: TRF contains only 5 to 8 percent amino acids; it therefore cannot be a peptide. October 1966, Schally: TRF contains glutamic acid, histidine, and proline, which account for only 30 percent of the compound; it cannot be a simple peptide. January 1969, Guillemin: these three amino acids make up 80 percent of the TRF molecule; perhaps it is a peptide. April 1969, Guillemin: Acetylation of the tripeptide Glu-His-Pro produces a substance with TRF-like biological activity. August 1969, Schally: Synthetic tripeptides of glu, his, and pro are inactive. September 1969, Schally: Two possible sequences of the three amino acids have TRF-like activity. November 1969, Guillemin and Schally (separately): (pyro)Glu-His-Pro-NH_2 is the chemical structure of TRF.

The race to purify and synthesize TRF ended in a draw. It was a victory for both sides but not what either side so palpably craved—a victory over the other. Guillemin claimed victory, writing in a letter (a copy of which went to Schally): "I simply cannot let Folkers, Bowers, & Schally go unchallenged when they claim *discovery* of an important observation indeed which is *at best* confirmation of what we have observed and demonstrated in this laboratory" (Wade 1981, 175). Schally responded, in part: "I cannot help feeling that your letters appear to reflect frustration at having come out second best in the race on TRH. Let me also remind you of your deliberate, repeated, personal, and scientific attacks against me as well as your constant failure to recognize our contributions" (Wade 1981, 176).

Much has been made of the ferocity of the Schally-Guillemin competition. The investigators themselves added fuel to the fire with public comments and reactions. By 1971 Schally, with Hisayuki Matsuo, Yoshihiko Baba, R. M. G. Nair, and Akira Arimura, had isolated and elucidated the structure of a new hypothalamic hormone. This was luteinizing hormone releasing hormone (LHRH), a decapeptide (small protein containing ten amino acids). It proved to be highly active in releasing in vivo the pituitary sex hormones that control ovarian and testicular function in humans as well as laboratory animals. Schally recalled his emotional state at the meeting of the Endocrine Society in June 1971 when he announced his group's success: "I listened with tension and suspense during the immediately preceding lecture and discussions, but Guillemin's group did not report the isolation and structure of ovine LHRH. When my time to speak came, I rose to my feet and presented our paper on isolation, structure, and synthesis of porcine LHRH. It was one of the most joyous moments in my life" (Schally 1978, 358).

In the end the elegant studies of the two men and the scientists who worked with them uncovered mechanisms by which information perceived by the brain was communicated to the anterior pituitary and, through it, to the tissues of the body. A rich scientific and medical harvest followed. In addition to the hypothalamic hormones controlling pituitary secretion of thyroid stimulating hormone and gonadotropins, those controlling secretion of growth hormones and ACTH have been chemically characterized, synthesized, and made available for further study and for medical diagnostic testing and treatment. Old disorders of the endocrine system became better understood and new ones were uncovered. Neuroendocrinology became immediately accessible to clinicians.

"The critical advantage that Guillemin and Schally held over their competitors lay in their motivation," wrote a science journalist. "The thirst for scientific glory, and the constant apprehension the other might win it all, gave a furious impetus to their efforts. Maybe they never faltered in their commitment to a researcher's formal goal, the better understanding of nature, but to this dry desire were added the human passions of ambition and rivalry" (Wade 1981, 281). In 1977 the selection committee in Stockholm wisely ended the duel of the neuroendocrine researchers by making Nobel laureates of both Andrew V. Schally and Roger Guillemin.

LAWRENCE SHERMAN

Selected Bibliography

PRIMARY SOURCES

Saffran, Murray, and A. V. Schally. 1955. "The Release of Corticotropin by Anterior Pituitary Tissue *In Vitro*." *Canadian Journal of Biochemistry and Physiology* 33:408–15.

Boler, J., F. Enzmann, K. Folkers, C. Y. Bowers, and A. V. Schally. 1969. "The Identity of Chemical and Hormonal Properties of Thyrotropin Releasing Hormone and Pyroglutamylhistidyl-proline Amide." *Biochemical and Biophysical Research Communications* 37:705–10.

Schally, Andrew V., A. Arimura, A. J. Kastin, H. Matsuo, Y. Baba, P. W. Redding, R. M. Nair, and L. Debeljuk. 1971. "Gonadotropin-releasing Hormone: One Polypeptide Regulates Secretion of Luteinizing and Follicle-stimulating Hormones." *Science* 173:1036–38.

Schally, Andrew V. 1977. "Aspects of Hypothalamic Regulation of the Pituitary Gland." Nobel Lecture. Reprinted in *Science* 202 (October 6):18–28.

———. 1978. "In the Pursuit of Hypothalamic Hormones." In *Pioneers in Neuroendocrinology II*, edited by Meites, B. T. Donovan, and S. M. McCann, 2:345–66. New York: Plenum Press.

SECONDARY SOURCES

McCann, S. M. 1988. "Saga of the Discovery of Hypothalamic Releasing and Inhibiting Hormones." In *Endocrinology: People and Ideas*, edited by S. M. McCann, 41–62. Bethesda, Md.: American Physiological Society.

Meites, Joseph. 1977. "The 1977 Nobel Prize in Physiology or Medicine." *Science* 198 (November 11):594–96.

Wade, Nicholas. 1981. *The Nobel Duel: Two Scientists' Twenty-one-Year Race to Win the World's Most Coveted Research Prize*. New York: Anchor Press/Doubleday.

SIR CHARLES SCOTT SHERRINGTON *1932*

Sir Charles Scott Sherrington was born on November 27, 1857, in London, England. A neurophysiologist, Sherrington shared the Nobel Prize in 1932 with Edgar Douglas Adrian for their pioneering investigations of the transmission of nerve impulses between the central nervous system and the muscles. Although Sherrington and Adrian never worked together, the work of each contributed to the other's endeavors throughout most of their highly productive careers. At the time of the award, Sherrington was Waynflete Professor of Physiology at Oxford and the senior eminence in British neurophysiology, only four years away from retirement. He had married Ethel Mary Wright in 1892; their only child, Carl E. R. Sherrington, became a railway economist. Sherrington died on March 4, 1952, in Eastbourne, England.

Sherrington's father, James Norton Sherrington, died when the boy was quite young. His mother, Anne Brookes, then married Dr. Caleb Rose of Ipswich, a classical scholar whose home was a rendezvous for artists of all kinds. Charles grew up in this stimulating environment, which shaped his catholic view of the universe and his broad interests. He pursued these as an adult, writing sociomedical studies in public health, works on the history of medicine, and even a volume of poetry, in addition to his many scientific papers. As one of his biographers has noted, "Sherrington [had a] pantheistic identification of himself with Nature . . . and his sense of wonder [led] to a poetic transcription of biological facts" (Granit 1966). He was also an excellent athlete, excelling in rugby and crew; in his later years, he was an early enthusiast for skiing at Grindelwald in the Alps.

Sherrington was educated at the Queen Elizabeth School in Ipswich. He matriculated at Gonville and Caius College, Cambridge, in 1881, where he worked under the great physiologist Sir Michael Foster. In Foster's laboratory he had the opportunity to meet many young scientists who would later become highly respected in their fields, including John Newport Langley, Newell Martin, Walter Gaskell, and Sheridan Lea. He co-wrote his first paper on the nervous system, on the effects of partial excision of the cortex in animals, with Langley in 1884.

After receiving his bachelor of medicine degree in 1884, he joined thousands of fellow medical students of the time who pursued further study in Germany. For three years he undertook training and research in physiology, histology, and pathology, working with Rudolf Virchow and Robert Koch, and taking part in a study of cholera in Spain and Italy. He returned to London in 1887 and was appointed a lecturer in systematic physiology at St. Thomas Hospital. After four years in this post, he succeeded Sir Victor Horsley as professor-superintendent of the Brown Institute for Advanced Physiological and Pathological Research, an animal facility. During this period he also made several visits to Strasbourg for work with the physiologist Friedrich Goltz on the functions of the central nervous system.

In 1895 he accepted the chair of physiology at the University of Liverpool, where he was to remain for eighteen years. He had already begun the work that would lead him to his fundamental concept of "the integrative action of the central nervous system."

Sherrington's work on the structure and operations of the nervous system built on the neuron theory of Ramón y Cajal, first proposed in

1889. Prior to Cajal, the dominant concept in neurophysiology had been the reticular theory, which postulated a continuous network of neural connections throughout the body. Cajal had used the silver nitrate preparation developed by Camillo Golgi as a staining mechanism for outlining nerve cells and fibers; he was thus able to define and trace specific limited pathways of impulse transmission at different points in neural and muscular action.

Sherrington initially studied the knee-jerk phenomenon but found that he could reach no conclusions on neural physiology until he had a better understanding of the neural anatomy. From 1887 to 1897 he painstakingly traced the sensory and motor fibers of the spinal cord, work he himself later described as "boring" and "pedestrian." But he succeeded in mapping the motor pathways of the lumbosacral plexus, identified sensory nerves within muscle tissue, and traced the distribution of the posterior spinal roots (Sherrington 1898, 45–186; Swazey 1975, 396).

As he followed these exacting trails, he developed an overriding conviction of integrated complexity, a sense that individual neural reflexes were not isolated responses but a linked series of inhibitory and excitory impulses coordinated and directed by the central nervous system into a single purposeful action. To comprehend this complexity, Sherrington needed to isolate and study simple single motor actions, correlating observed responses with his anatomical understanding. He worked with two types of animal experiments: the classic spinal animal, and the decerebrate rigid animal, which he named and established as an invaluable research preparation. Through extended studies of mundane acts, such as a dog scratching himself with his hind limb, he arrived at the fundamental principles of neural action (Sherrington 1898, 319–22).

These studies led to his formulation of "reciprocal innervation"—the coordination of concurrent inhibitory and excitory reflexes; his discovery of the interaction between higher (brain) and lower (motor nerve) level control over actions; and his most famous contribution, the idea of the synapse, the momentary contact of one nerve cell with another that is the basis of neural transmission. As Sherrington saw it, the brain-muscle pathway, the interplay of inhibition and excitation, the coordination of the central nervous system—all came together at the synapse, creating "the final common path," leading to the purposeful action. He presented these ideas in a series of seminal lectures, culminating in 1906 with his great work, *The Integrative Action of the Nervous System* (Sherrington 1904, 1–14; 1960; Swazey 1975, 396–98).

Sherrington was named to the Waynflete professorship in 1913. He was now occupied with refining and confirming the innovative concepts comprehended in "integrative action," but his research was interrupted by World War I, during which he served as chairman of the Industrial Fatigue Board. In 1915, to better understand this assignment, he disappeared from home and worked incognito for some weeks in a shell factory, putting in thirteen-hour shifts at the age of fifty-seven. During the war he also completed a classic textbook of physiology.

Sherrington returned to his full schedule of experiments in the 1920s, carrying out at least one each week, with the assistance of the "Sherrington School" of his students and assistants, including E. G. T. Liddell and John C. Eccles. He was able to use several new techniques, including isometric myography, for the measurement of muscular tension. His contributions during these years included a definitive analysis of the stretch reflex and his demonstration that inhibition is a distinct phenomenon, not merely the absence of, or reaction to, excitation. Edgar Adrian's work at Cambridge on the properties of the single nerve cell inspired Sherrington's further work on his ideas of the final common path, which finally culminated in his 1930 paper with Eccles on the motor unit. The motor unit, a spinal motoneuron, is a single cell that coordinates the actions of many muscle fibers. This fundamental concept represented the culmination of Sherrington's work, and, indeed, probably the culmination of the knowledge possible at the time without the use of electronics that were then just being introduced (Sherrington and Eccles 1930, 326–57; Swazey 1975, 399).

Sherrington retired in 1936 but remained active until nearly the end of his life. A generous, friendly man, Sherrington never lost his philosophical interests and spoke and wrote often on "the meaning of science." Pursuing this bent after leaving Oxford, he published two books, *Man on His Nature* and *The Endeavour of Jean Fernel*, about a sixteenth-century French physician who emphasized the need to study nature rather than written authority, and introduced the terms "pathology" and "physiology" to science.

Sherrington was elected a Fellow of the Royal Society in 1893. In addition to the Nobel Prize, Sherrington received many other honors, including the Royal Society's Royal Medal (1905); the Copley Medal (1927); the Order of Merit (1924); and a knighthood in 1922. In his last years he was in poor health but remained mentally active. He died of heart failure at Eastbourne in 1952, at the age of ninety-four.

ESTELLE BRODMAN
MARCIA MELDRUM

Selected Bibliography

PRIMARY SOURCES

Sherrington, Charles S. 1898. "Experiments in Examination of the Peripheral Distribution of the Fibres of the Posterior Roots of Some Spinal Nerves." *Philosophical Transactions of the Royal Society* 190B:45–186.

———. 1898. "Decerebrate Rigidity and Reflex Coordination of Movements." *Journal of Physiology* 33: 319–22.

———. 1904. "The Correlation of Reflexes and the Principle of the Common Path." *Report of the British Association for the Advancement of Science* 74:1–14.

———. 1906. *The Integrative Action of*

the Nervous System. New Haven: Yale University Press.

Sherrington, Charles S., and John C. Eccles. 1930. "Numbers and Contraction-Values of Individual Motor Units Examined in Some Muscles of the Limb." *Proceedings of the Royal Society* 106B:326–57.

Sherrington, Charles S. 1946. *The Endeavour of Jean Fernel*. Cambridge: Cambridge University Press.

SECONDARY SOURCES

Fulton, John F. 1952. "Sir Charles Scott Sherrington, O. M." *Journal of Neurophysiology* 15:167–90.

Granit, Ragnar. 1966. *Charles Scott Sherrington: An Appraisal*. London: Nelson.

Liddell, E. G. T. 1952. "Charles Scott Sherrington, 1856–1952." *Obituary Notices of Fellows of the Royal Society of London* 8:241–59.

Swazey, Judith P. 1975. "Sherrington, Charles Scott." In *Dictionary of Scientific Biography*, 12:395–403. New York: Scribners.

Viets, Henry. 1952. "Charles Scott Sherrington, 1857–1952." *New England Journal of Medicine* 246:981.

HAMILTON OTHANEL SMITH
1978

Hamilton Othanel Smith was born on August 23, 1931, in New York City. A molecular biologist, Smith shared the Nobel Prize in 1978 with Werner Arber and Daniel Nathans for his confirmation of Arber's model of host-controlled restriction-modification and his discovery and isolation of the first Type II restriction enzyme, Hind II, which cleaves DNA at the site of specific nucleotide sequences, exactly as predicted by the model. Nathans used the enzyme discovered by Smith to separate and map DNA molecules. These three investigations led cumulatively to the techniques of DNA recombination and the potential breakthroughs of genetic engineering. At the time of the award Smith was professor of microbiology at Johns Hopkins University, where he has been professor of molecular biology and genetics since 1981. He married Elizabeth Anne Bolton in 1957; they have four sons, Joel, Barry, Dirk, and Bryan, and a daughter, Kirsten.

Smith's father, Tommie Harkey Smith, was assistant professor of education at the University of Florida. In 1937 he accepted a position at the University of Illinois and he and his wife, Bunnie Othanel Smith, moved the family to Urbana. As a boy, Smith was interested in chemistry and electronics and enjoyed tinkering in a laboratory in the family basement. He began his college education at the University of Illinois in 1948 but transferred to the University of California at Berkeley two years later, graduating in biology in 1952. He completed his medical degree at Johns Hopkins in 1956, followed by an internship at Barnes Hospital in St. Louis, two years in the U.S. Navy Medical Corps, and a residency at Henry Ford Hospital in Detroit. During this ten-year period of career preparation, Smith was only able to pursue his research interest in biochemistry by reading in his rare free time.

In 1962, however, he won a National Institutes of Health fellowship to study molecular genetics at the University of Michigan. Here he became interested in the phenomenon of host-controlled variation among bacterial viruses. This process had been observed and described by Giuseppe Bertani, Salvador E. Luria, and Jean J. Weigle in the 1950s. A specific virus, or bacteriophage, is capable of infecting and rapidly destroying the cells of a specific strain of bacteria. However, the same virus, injected into a new bacterial culture, will be broken down into particles, or "restricted," by its host. A few phage particles, however, will survive within the bacterial culture, and will be reproduced or "modified") as a new variant virus, capable of infecting the new host. The implications of this phenomenon for our understanding of the incidence and spread of viral infections are clearly of great interest (Linn 1978, 1070).

In 1962 Arber and Daisy Dussoix had traced the mechanism of these processes to modification and degradation of the phage in DNA. Arber and his coworkers had subsequently developed a model based on the existence of bacterium-specific restriction enzymes or endonucleases. According to this theory, the enzyme recognizes specific sequences of nucleotides in the DNA of an invading phage and cleaves the DNA molecule at these specific sites. But the bacterium also contains a strain-specific modification enzyme that acts to protect the bacterial DNA by methylating the identical nucleotide sequences in the host; it may also act on the foreign DNA. The phage DNA, thus modified, eventually generates a variant virus.

Over the next few years, several workers carried out research that confirmed the model, including Arber, Urs Kuhnlein, and Stuart Linn in Arber's laboratory, and John Smith of the Medical Research Council at Cambridge, who were able to isolate mutated phages and modify DNA methylase; and Japanese investigators Toshiya Takano, Tsutomu Watanabe, and Toshio Fukasawa, who observed restriction activity in vitro but were unable to isolate the nuclease involved.

In 1968, however, Arber and Linn succeeded in partially isolating and describing the restriction endonuclease of *Esherichia coli B.* Mathew Meselson and Robert Yuan had similar success with the enzyme from *E. coli K.* These enzymes, now known as Type I, do in fact recognize specific nucleotide sequences in foreign DNA, exactly as Arber's model had predicted. However, they cut the DNA apparently at random, rather than at specific recognition sites (Linn 1978, 1070).

During Smith's five years as a research associate at Michigan, he studied the restriction-modification process extensively and spent some time in Geneva working with Arber. In 1967 he was appointed assistant professor of microbiology at Johns Hopkins, and in 1969 was promoted to associate professor.

In 1968 Smith, working with K. W. Wilcox, was observing the infection of the bacterium *Hemophilus influenzae* by the *Salmonella* bacteriophage P22. They noted that the bacterium degraded the phage DNA quite effectively and extensively but was unable to similarly break down DNA from *H. influenzae* itself. By 1969 they had extracted and isolated the responsible enzyme, which they named Hind II (Smith and Wilcox 1970).

Working with T. J. Kelley and B. Weiss, Smith demonstrated that Hind II was a true Type II restriction enzyme; that is, it both recognized a specific nucleotide sequence in a foreign DNA molecule and cleaved the molecule at that sequence site. The specific sequence recognized had a twofold rotational axis of symmetry; similar patterns have been found in all sequences that can be identified by the Type II enzymes (Smith 1970). Using the techniques developed by Smith to isolate restriction enzymes and identify the specific nucleotide sequences at the cleavage sites, researchers had identified over one hundred and fifty such enzymes by 1982 (Linn 1978, 1071).

Herbert Boyer and his colleagues at the University of California at San Francisco, including Daisy Dussoix, followed Smith's breakthrough with the discovery and characterization of several R factor restriction enzymes. Their work established the fact that different DNA molecules cleaved with identical enzymes at identical sites will have "sticky edges" that "fit" with each other—and can therefore be "recombined." In 1972 Daniel Nathans, using Hind II provided by Smith, perfected methods of DNA cleavage that enabled him to map and describe its structure with great precision and detail.

Smith's and Nathans's methods have been applied in several laboratories, including Boyer's and Howard Goodman's at UCSF, Paul Berg's and Stanley Cohen's at Stanford, and Kenneth and Noreen Murray's in Edinburgh, to cleave and recombine various DNA molecules, and then reproduce the resulting DNA in bacterial or other host cells. The technology makes possible the in vitro production of scarce enzymes and hormones, such as insulin. Research applications have included the study of tumor production and of the control of gene functions.

However, experiments that combine eukaryotic DNA with bacterial or viral DNA in a single, replicable molecule have created fears of the creation of dangerous new pathogens, leading the NIH to establish specific guidelines for recombinant DNA research (Linn 1978, 1071).

Smith is a member of the National Academy of Sciences, the American Society of Microbiology, the American Society of Biological Chemists, and the American Association for the Advancement of Science. He held a Guggenheim fellowship in 1975–76, and has been an editor of the journal *Gene* since 1976. An accomplished pianist, he enjoys playing and listening to classical music in his leisure time.

MARCIA MELDRUM

Selected Bibliography

PRIMARY SOURCES

Smith, H. O. 1968. "Deficient Phage Formation by Lysogens of Integration Deficient Phage P22 Mutants." *Virology* 34 (February):203–23.

Smith, H. O., and K. W. Wilcox. 1970. "A Restriction Enzyme from *Hemophilus Influenzae*: I. Purification and General Properties." *Journal of Molecular Biology* 51:379.

Smith, H. O. 1970. "A Restriction Enzyme from *Hemophilus Influenzae*: II. Base Sequence of the Restriction Site." *Journal of Molecular Biology* 51:393.

Smith, H. O., T. J. Kelley and P. H. Roy. 1974. "Enzymatic Methods for Sequence Analyses Applied to DNA Restriction and Methylation Sites." *Methods in Enzymology* 29:282–94.

Smith, H. O., and Daniel Nathans. 1975. "Restriction Endonucleases in the Analysis and Structuring of DNA Molecules." *Annual Review of Biochemistry* 44:273–93.

SECONDARY SOURCES

1978. Sylvester, Kathy. *New York Times* (October 13):59.

Linn, Stuart. 1978. "The 1978 Nobel Prize in Physiology or Medicine." *Science* 202 (December 3):1069–71.

1982. "Smith, Hamilton Othanel." *Modern Scientists and Engineers*, 3:130–31. New York: McGraw-Hill.

GEORGE DAVIS SNELL *1980*

The American immunogeneticist George Davis Snell received the Nobel Prize in Physiology or Medicine in 1980 jointly with Baruj Benacerraf and Jean Dausset. Called "the father of modern immunogenetics," he is "responsible for the recognition of the mouse analogue of the HLA system, known as H2, and for the development of appropriate strains of inbred mice."

George David Snell was born on December 19, 1903, in Bradford, Massachusetts. He was the youngest of three children. His parents, Cullen Bryant and Katharine Merrill (Davis) Snell, were New Englanders; although his father was born in Minnesota—where his own father had joined a frontier community after leaving Massachusetts—he had moved east as a young man. For a number of years, he was YMCA secretary in Haverhill. He invented a device for winding coils used in ignitors for motorboat engines. When Snell was four his parents moved to a home built by his great-grandfather in Brookline, Massachusetts.

He received his early education in the excellent Brookline public schools. He was attracted to science and mathematics, and liked to read books on astronomy and physics. But he also enjoyed sports, and often played touch football or scrub baseball with his friends. Imaginative stories and games played a major role in his childhood. Summers were spent at "the farm," a run-down farmhouse with seventy acres of land in South Woodstock, Vermont. Summers in Vermont stimulated a lifelong interest in gardening, farming, and forestry.

Snell entered Dartmouth College in 1922. A course in genetics taught by John Hiram Gerould especially influenced his choice of career. Snell received his B.S. in 1926. Following Gerould's advice, he went as a graduate student to Harvard University to work with William Ernest Castle, the first American biologist to look for Mendelian inheritance in mammals. He received a Sc.D. in genetics from Harvard University in 1930. His thesis on linkage in mice largely determined his later work.

While working under Castle, Snell spent parts of two summers at Woods Hole with Phineas Wescott Whiting, an earlier student of Castle, studying the genetics of the parasitic wasp, *Habrobacon*. This led to the publication of a paper on "The Role of Male Parthenogenesis in the Evolution of the Social Hymenoptera." He continued afterwards to show interest in the problems of social evolution, and has returned in a more active way to this area during his retirement.

Snell became an instructor at Dartmouth College in 1929, and an instructor at Brown University in 1930. As a National Research Council Fellow at the University of Texas from 1931 to 1933 he worked with Hermann Joseph Muller, who was conducting the research on X-rays and mutations that would later bring him a Nobel Prize. Snell showed that X-rays induce a high frequency of chromosomal translocations in mice. For the first time, induction by X-rays of mutational changes in mammals, had been demonstrated.

From 1933 to 1934 Snell was an assistant professor at Washington University, in St. Louis. As he later wrote, "Two years spent teaching and two years as a postdoctoral fellow under Hermann Muller studying the genetic effect of X-rays on mice served to convince me that research was my real love. If it was to be research, mouse genetics was the clear choice and the Jackson Laboratory, founded in 1929 by Dr. Clarence Cook Little, one of

Castle's earlier students, almost the inevitable selection as a place to work" (Snell, "Biographical Note, *Nobel Lectures*). In 1935 Snell decided to join the staff of seven at the Jackson Laboratory, in Bar Harbor, Maine. This lab would be home for the rest of his career. Under the leadership of Little and his successor, Earl Green, it grew from a small institution into the world center for studies in mammalian genetics. Snell later acknowledged: "I owe a great deal to it [the Jackson Laboratory] for providing the ideal home for my subsequent research" (Snell "Biographical Note," *Nobel Lectures*).

In Bar Harbor, Snell met Rhoda Beatrice Maude Carson. They were married on July 28, 1937. They have three sons: Thomas Carleton, Roy Carson, and Peter Garland.

From 1935 to 1957 Snell was a research associate at the Jackson Laboratory; he also briefly held the position of staff scientific director (1949–50). He spent his first few years following up the work begun with Muller. He worked especially on the detailed genetic analysis of two of the induced reciprocal translocations. In the late 1930s he became involved in problems of gene nomenclature in mice and in problems of strain nomenclature. At about the same time he was becoming interested in histocompatibility genetics, he carried out experiments that led to the discovery of immunological enhancement, i.e. "the curious inversion of the expected growth inhibition seen with certain tumors when transplanted to pre-injected mice" (Snell, "Biographical Note," *Nobel Lectures*). He soon found that he was not the first to have observed this phenomenon, and dropped the topic in favor of his genetic studies.

In 1944 Snell moved to the study of the genetics of immunology of tissue transplantation. For the next twenty-five years he concentrated almost exclusively on studies of histocompatibility genes and especially the H-2 complex. Multiple genes influence the success or failure of transplants in mice. Although it had been established that genes play a role in transplant success, individual loci remained to be identified. One locus was identified by Peter Alfred Gorer in London, when he discovered a blood group in mice that influenced the growth of transplants. Naming these transplant-influencing genes "histocompatibility genes," Snell outlined methods for their further analysis. The most important method was the production of congenic resistant strains. These are strains identical with established inbred strains except for the presence of a chromosome segment and accompanying histocompatibility gene introduced—by an appropriate series of crosses and test transplants—from some second strain. Snell's research led to the detection of a number of histocompatibility loci. One of these loci, later named his histocompatibility-2 or H-2, was shown in joint studies with Gorer to be the same as Gorer's blood group and histocompatibility locus. Gorer died in 1961, and Snell later observed "I just wish Peter Gorer were still alive to share the Prize" (Marx 1980).

Recombination and chemical studies showed that H-2 is actually not one locus but three closely linked polymorphic loci. Later, similar histocompatibility gene complexes were identified in other species, including man. These discoveries led to the concept that there is a major histocompatibility complex, probably characteristic of all vertebrates.

Besides studies of histocompatibility genes based on the use of transplants, Snell, Marianna Cherry, and P. Démant carried out serological studies of cellular alloantigens. This work contributed to the discovery of the last of the three known major histocompatibility loci in the H-2 complex and to a number of loci determining red cell and lymphocyte antigens.

Snell also discovered the phenomenon of hybrid resistance. When grafts of lymphoid tissue or tumor are made from one inbred organism to another produced by hybridization, or cross-breeding, of the original organism and a genetic variant, the graft will normally be rejected, despite the partial compatibility.

Snell carried out some of the early studies of immunological enhancement. Using inbred mice and transplantable tumors, he established the conditions that made this an easily reproducible phenomenon. Together with his collaborators, he showed that enhancement acts by reducing the barrier to transplants imposed by the H-2 complex. One mechanism of enhancement is the suppression of cellular immunity by induced antibody.

Much of Snell's work he himself notes, "was carried out on a collaborative basis." He said "I owe a great debt to the many wonderful people with whom it has been my privilege to work in these studies" (Snell, "Biographical Note," *Nobel Lectures*).

From 1957 to 1968 Snell was a senior staff scientist at the Jackson Laboratory. He became a senior staff scientist, emeritus, in 1968, and retired in 1973. From 1958 to 1962 he was a member of the NIH allergy and immunology study section. He went back to the University of Texas, as a Guggenheim Fellow, in 1953–54.

Snell became a member of the American Academy of Arts and Sciences in 1952. He was a corecipient of the Hekteon Silver Medal of the American Medical Association in 1955. He received the Griffin Award, Animal Care Panel, and the Bertner Foundation Award in 1962. He received the Career Award, National Cancer Institute, for 1964–68. He was given the Gregor Mendel Medal, Czechoslovak Academy of Sciences, in 1967. He was elected to the National Academy of Sciences in 1970. He received the Gairdner Foundation Award in 1976 and the Wolf Prize in Medicine in 1978. He became a foreign associate of the French Academy of Science in 1979, a member of the American Philosophical Society in 1982, and an honorary member of the British Society of Immunology in 1983.

He has received honorary degrees from Charles University (Prague), Dartmouth College, the University of Maine, Gustavus Adolphus College, Colby College, Bates College, and Ohio State University.

ELIE FEUERWERKER

Selected Bibliography

PRIMARY SOURCES

Snell, George D. 1933. "Genetic Changes in Mice Induced by X-Rays." *American Naturalist* 67:81.

———. 1954. "The Enhancing Effect (or Actively Acquired Tolerance) and the Histocompatibility-2 Locus in the Mouse." *Journal of the National Cancer Institute* 15:665–675.

———. 1956. "Histocompatibility Genes." *Science* 123:675–676.

———. 1970. "Immunological Enhancement." *Surgery Gynecology and Obstetrics* 130:1109–1119.

Snell, George D., Jean Dausset, and S. G. Nathenson. 1976. *Histocompatibility*. New York: Academic Press.

Snell, George D. 1980. "The Major Histocompatibility Complex: Its Evolution and Involvement in Cellular Immunity." *Harvey Lectures* ser. 74:49–80. New York: Academic Press.

SECONDARY SOURCES

Marx, Jean L. 1980. "1980 Nobel Prize in Physiology or Medicine." *Science* 210:621–623.

1980. "1980 Nobel Prizes." *Nature* 287: 671.

HANS SPEMANN *1935*

Hans Spemann was born on June 27, 1869, in Stuttgart, Germany. An anatomist and embryologist, Spemann received the Nobel Prize in 1935 for his studies of embryonic development, specifically his discovery of the "organizer effect" in the induction of embryo growth, which laid the foundation for further work in experimental embryology and morphology. His Nobel Prize came to him late in life, the same year that he retired as professor of zoology at the University of Freiburg-im-Breisgau. Spemann married Clara Binder in 1895; they had two sons, Fritz and Rudo. He died on September 12, 1941, in Freiburg-im-Breisgau.

Spemann's father, Johann Wilhelm Spemann, was a publisher and bookseller in Stuttgart. His mother, Lisinka Hoffman, came from a family of physicians. She died, however, when Hans was still a baby and his father later remarried. Hans grew up in prosperous and cultured surroundings. He received a classical gymnasium education; there was little science instruction and he performed poorly in his zoology classes. He left school in 1888 and became an apprentice in his father's business.

After a year's military service (1889–90), Spemann returned to bookselling. It was then that his reading of the works of the poet Goethe and the Darwinian zoologist Ernst Haeckel inspired him to study biology. He entered the University of Heidelberg in 1891 as a medical student and passed his preliminary examination in 1893. He was beginning his career during a period of great German achievement in cell biology.

At Heidelberg, under the tutelage of Carl Gegenbaur, Spemann became interested in the study of comparative anatomy. He also knew Gustav Wolff, who would discover the regeneration of the lens in the newt's eye in 1894. From Heidelberg, he went to the University of Munich for the winter of 1893–94, where he became acquainted with August Pauly, the pseudo-Lamarckian zoologist.

These men and their ideas encouraged Spemann to give up medicine for research into "general biological problems." He therefore elected to study at the Zoological Institute of the University of Würzburg, where Theodor Boveri and Oskar Schultze were pioneering experimental approaches. Boveri set him to work on descriptive embryology of fixed specimens of the nematode *Strongylus paradoxus*; nematodes were then a popular subject for studies of chromosomes and cleavage. This was Spemann's introduction to the amphibian embryo, which would become his own favorite model.

At Würzburg Spemann had the opportunity to work with Julius Sachs in botany and Wilhelm Röntgen in physics, as well as in zoology. In 1895 he received his degree in all three disciplines. He then began work on another of Boveri's interests, the common basic structures (homologies) underlying head evolution.

During the winter of 1896–97 Spemann was convalescing in the Alps following a chest infection. To pass the time, he studied August Weismann's *Das Keimplasma*, which refuted Lamarckian theories of evolutionary adaptation. Lamarck's theory, which was a forerunner of Darwin's *Origin of Species*, asserted that an organism acquires new traits or characteristics in response to its environment, and that these new traits are then passed on to its progeny, resulting in gradual modifications in the organism over time. Weismann disputed the idea that such acquired characteristics could be inherited and instead developed a hypothesis based on transmission of heredity through the reproductive cells or germ plasma. According to this theory, the fertilized egg contained a number of specific factors, each of which would generate specific characteristics of the new organism.

Wilhelm Roux had attempted to verify Weismann's theory by destroying some of the blastomeres (cells formed in the first few divisions after fertilization) in the frog's egg. He had not, however, then been able to generate a viable embryo from the altered egg, leading him to the partial conclusion that, up to a certain point, each part of the embryo is essential to the development of the whole.

Returning to his research in 1897, Spemann began a similar series of experiments on salamander eggs. Rather than killing the blastomeres, however, he separated them and heated them at different temperatures. He then found it necessary to insert the resulting embryo into a cooling tube, which necessitated use of a hair loop. His experimental rearrangement of the cells in this purely technical maneuver led, in June 1897, to the development of double-headed embryos. Spemann published the results of these "hair-loop" experiments between 1901 and 1903.

He qualified as a lecturer in zoology at Würzburg in 1898 and continued his studies of embryonic development. While looking at a frog embryo at the neurula stage (when the layer of cells that will become the nervous system develops), he noticed structures that he guessed were rudimentary preforms of the lens of the eye. He realized that it would be possible to destroy the eye while leaving the lens rudiments unaffected, and in this way test the interdependence of the development of the two structures. Using an eclectrocautery needle, he destroyed the rudiment of a single eye on the neural plate. He then observed the side of the embroyonic head where the eye had been destroyed, and noted that the lens failed to form. Spemann therefore proposed a theory of lens induction: induction of the formation of the lens will not occur if the eye fails to form, even if the lens rudiment itself is present.

In 1906 he transplanted ectodermal cells (cells that will form skin, feathers, scales, and so forth, formed in the same layer as the neural cells) from the embryonic head and flank to the lens site. He also experimented with transplantation of the optic cup (the rudimentary retina) to other areas of the epidermis. In this way he demonstrated that the presence of the optic cup will induce the formation of a lens, complete with transparent cornea, from cells that do not normally take this form, and in various unrelated parts of the embryo.

Spemann continued to pioneer new techniques and approaches to the study of embryology, still an undeveloped field within anatomy, and his reputation grew. In 1908, at age thirty-nine, he was appointed professor of zoology and comparative anatomy at the Zoological Institute at Rostock, and, in 1914, he was asked to head a division of the newly founded Kaiser Wilhelm Institute for Biology in Berlin-Dahlem. By 1918, after many years' work, he proposed the concept of the "organization-center"; according to this concept, embryonic development is dependent upon the interactions of different types of cells, and certain "organizer" cells determine the orderly development of the entire organism. Finally, in 1919, he moved to the even more prestigious Department of Zoology at the University of Freiburg-im-Breisgau, the chair once occupied by August Weismann himself.

He attracted many research students to Freiburg and a "Spemann school" arose. Twenty-three graduated under his supervision between 1920 and 1935. It was one of his students, Hilde Pröscholdt, who in 1921 began the critical work with the gastrular embryo of the newt *Triton taeniatus*. The gastrula stage of embryonic development consists of a double layer of cells arranged around a central cavity with an opening at one end; this opening is called the blastopore. Pröscholdt transplanted the dorsal (outer) blastopore lip into the ventral (inner) area of a second gastrula. The transplantation induced the development of a "twin" embryo, which began to develop within the ventral cells. Spemann and his student had found the cells responsible for the organizer effect.

By 1922 they had obtained five additional specimens that formed the basis for the definitive paper published in 1924. Tragically, by the time the paper appeared, Hilde Pröscholdt, who had married the embryologist Otto Mangold, had been killed in an accident.

After 1923 Spemann demonstrated that different cells of the organizer tissue will induce the production of different parts of the embryo. But he found also that the responding cells appeared to play a role of their own. The tail, or posterior portion of the organizer, tended to produce embryonic tails, but, grafted onto the head area of another embryo, the tail organizer may produce another embryonic head.

In 1931 questions about the nature of the organizer stimulus acquired a sudden new prominence. Following Marx's demonstration that organizers do not lose their activity when anesthetized, Spemann attempted to block activity by killing or squashing the organizer cells. In 1932 Spemann, in a paper written with Mangold and Johannes Holtfreter, established that a killed organizer retained its inductive properties.

There followed a massive outpouring of work, directed primarily by Holtfreter. Particularly influential was his surprising finding that ventral ectoderm, the very cells that respond to the organizer, appear to acquire oganizer activity themselves when the organizer is killed. The researchers hypothesized that organizer factors were latent in the responding cells and could be unmasked by "indirect induction." Many new workers were now attracted to the field to identify and isolate these organizer factors, which were now recognized to be chemical in nature. Ultimately, their work led to the modern science of morphogenesis, the study of the genetic and biochemical factors that influence the development of the embryo into a complete organism, with significant implications for the study of birth defects and teratologic disorders in humans.

Spemann himself, although his research led to these mechanistic investigations, remained an organicist. His own work emphasized supracellular explanations in terms of processes involving the whole embryo, in preference to cellular interpretations of development. Thus, he often used anthropomorphic terminology, referring to the "learning powers" of cells and to the "destiny" of the embryonic tissues. The concept of the organizer, a kind of authoritarian cellular mastermind, coincided with widespread interest in the idea of formative fields and with the yearning for social order among the German bourgeosie in the chaos following World War I. Spemann continued to write and speak in these terms even as the later experiments pointed his colleagues in other directions.

He was a rigorous and intent experimentalist and a pioneer of new techniques; these qualities and his highly focused approach enabled him to open new approaches to the fundamental question of development. He retired with the title of emeritus professor in 1935 and published the definitive account of his research, *Embryonic Development and Induction*, in 1936. He died in 1941 at age seventy-two.

PAUL WEINDLING

Selected Bibliography

PRIMARY SOURCES

Spemann, Hans. 1938. *Embryonic Development and Induction*. New Haven: Yale University Press.

———. 1943. *Forschung und Leben, Erinnerungen*. Stuttgart: Englehorns.

SECONDARY SOURCES

Hamburger, Victor. 1988. *The Heritage of Experimental Embryology. Hans Spemann and the Organizer*. Oxford. Oxford University Press.

Horder, Timothy, and Paul Weindling. 1986. "Hans Spemann and the Organizer." In *A History of Embryology*, edited by Timothy Horder, Jan A. Witkowski, and C. Wylie, 183–242. Cambridge: Cambridge University Press.

Mangold, Otto. 1982. *Hans Spemann, Ein Meister der Entwicklungsphysiologie, Sein Leben und Sein Werk*. Stuttgart: Wissenschaftliche Verlagsgesellschaft.

Waddington, C. H. 1975. "Spemann, Hans." In *Dictionary of Scientific Biography*, 12:567–69. New York: Scribners.

ROGER WOLCOTT SPERRY *1981*

Roger Wolcott Sperry was born on August 20, 1913, in Hartford, Connecticut. A neurobiologist, Sperry shared the Nobel Prize in 1981 for his contributions to our understanding of the human brain, specifically for his "split-brain" studies, which focused on the respective functions of the left and right hemispheres. Sperry's body of work laid the foundations of modern neurobiology and opened up the possibility of the incorporation of humanistic concepts such as consciousness and values into psychological theory. The other half of the 1981 Nobel Prize was awarded jointly to David H. Hubel and Torsten N. Wiesel. At the time of his award, Sperry was Hixon Professor of Psychobiology at the California Institute of Technology, where he has been professor emeritus since 1984. Sperry married Norma Deupree in 1949; they have two children, Glenn Tad and Janeth Hope.

Sperry's father, Francis Bushnell Sperry, a Hartford banker, died when he was eleven years old; his mother, Florence Kraemer Sperry, thereafter worked in a local high school to support the family. Sperry attended Oberlin College in Ohio, where he studied English literature and was active in sports; his psychology teacher, R. H. Stetson, interested him in the application of physiology to psychological study. He received an M.A. in psychology from Oberlin in 1937 and then entered the doctoral degree at the University of Chicago to study with Paul Alfred Weiss.

Weiss had conducted experiments that seemed to indicate that specific nerves were not genetically linked to specific behavioral functions but rather acquired control of those functions through experience, governed by the brain; thus a specific nerve could be connected to any part of the body and "learn" to control the functioning of that part.

Sperry's doctoral dissertation, based on repeated stimulation of crossed nerves in the hind legs of a rat, effectively demolished this theory by demonstrating that, in fact, the left foot nerve continued to stimulate the left foot, even when surgically reconnected to the right foot. This work earned him a Ph.D. in zoology in 1941.

Further work with amphibians, whose nerves regenerate themselves, supported Sperry's concept of "chemoaffinity," or the differentiation of neural functions based on genetically determined chemical composition. Further, the concept described similar chemical differentiation of organ cells, so that each neuron links with the specific organ or structure, with the specific *cell*, that carries the same genetic chemical code. In support of his concept, Sperry demonstrated repeatedly that each nerve has its own unalterable function; thus a nerve controlling the frog's left eye, even if severed and repositioned, will reconnect itself and resume control of the left eye (Sperry 1973). Sperry's chemoaffinity model is still "at the center" of the field of neurobiology (Gazzaniga 1981, 518).

During 1941–42 Sperry did postdoctoral research with Karl S. Lashley at Harvard and the Yerkes Primate Laboratories. He remained at Yerkes through the war years, when he worked for the Office of Scientific Research and Development on the surgical repair of neural injuries. At Yerkes, working with graduate students N. Miner and R. Myers, he developed new techniques for delicate brain surgery in cats and monkeys, using the stereomicroscope. With these methods, he successfully challenged the cortical functioning theories of Lashley and others by demonstrating the central role of selectively organized fiber circuitry within the brain.

In 1946 Sperry returned to the University of Chicago as assistant professor of anatomy, becoming an associate professor of psychology in 1952. He and Ronald Myers still faced a major challenge to their fiber circuitry model in the anomalous results of surgical procedures sectioning the corpus callosum, the major cable of fibers connecting the left and right hemispheres of the brain. Severance of the connection in laboratory animals produced no apparent change in the animals' behavior or ability to function.

Sperry and Myers demonstrated that a cat trained to distinguish shapes with one eye would remember and transfer the knowledge to the other eye, even if the optical connections were severed. However, a cat with a severed corpus callosum, or "split brain," would not be able to make the transference. In an extended series of animal experiments throughout the 1950s, they were able to create situations in which animals behaved as if they had "two entirely separate brains" (Sperry 1964). However, split-brain animals allowed to behave normally showed no signs of their condition, since each side of the brain controlled one half of the body and the two sides functioned symmetrically.

Sperry had made the move to Cal Tech in 1954 and, in 1961, he was given the opportunity to pursue human split-brain research at White Memorial Medical Center in Los Angeles. Joseph Bogen and Philip Vogel had performed commissurotomies, or severance of the corpus callosum, on several epileptic patients to prevent uncontrollable seizures. The surgeons and the patients agreed to cooperate with Sperry and his graduate students, including Colwyn Trevarthen, Jerre Levy, Michael S. Gazzaniga, Robert Nebes, Charles Hamilton, and Eran Zaidel.

The commissurotomy patients had learned how to coordinate the visual, aural, and other perceptions of left and right hemispheres and were therefore able to function at an apparently normal level, like the laboratory animals. But when one half of a patient's perceptual apparatus was blocked—by covering one eye, for example—his internal fission became apparent. The left brain, controlling the right side of the body, was easily able to respond to written and verbal stimuli; the right brain, controlling the left side, appeared completely unable to do so. However, a patient who saw a picture of an object with his left eye was able to select the object from others with his left hand, even without seeing it. Verbally, the same patient would insist he could not recognize the picture and that his selection of the correct object was completely random (Gazzaniga, Bogen, and Sperry 1962).

With experiments like these, Sperry and Gazzaniga were able to establish that each hemisphere possesses specific higher abilities crucial to human functioning. The left hemisphere, as had long been suspected, controls verbal activity; more fundamentally, it handles processes that proceed in a logical, sequential fashion, such as writing, mathematics, reasoning, and judgment. But the right brain is necessary for the grasp of more complex, simultaneous processes, such as artistic and musical composition, face and voice recognition, and "intuition." Each hemisphere, moreover, possesses its own consciousness and self-awareness (Sperry 1966).

Sperry's work laid the foundation for much new research in neurobiology, psychiatry, and psychology. Clinicians perceived exciting applications in the treatment of mental and psychosomatic illness and of learning disorders such as dyslexia.

Sperry himself believes that the implications of his hemispheric specialization studies are far richer and more profound. His new model supersedes his earlier emphasis on fiber circuitry, instead incorporating the role of consciousness as an interactive property of mind that both influences and is influenced by physical and chemical processes of the brain. This concept of "mentalism" offers a potential basis for understanding on a psychophysiological level humanistic ideas such as affection, free will, and value formation. Sperry foresees that the traditional barriers between science and the humanities will be replaced by a new common ground (Sperry 1983).

Among the many other honors Sperry has received for his work are the Howard Crosby Warren Medal of the Society for Experimental Psychology (1971), California Scientist of the Year (1972), the William Thomas Wakeman Research Award of the National Paraplegic Foundation (1972), the Karl S. Lashley Award of the American Philosophical Society (1976), and the Albert Lasker Basic Medical Research Award (1979). He and his wife enjoy camping and fossil hunting and were in fact camping in a remote area of Baja California on the day the Nobel Prize was announced. He also devotes leisure time to artistic hobbies such as drawing, sculpting, and ceramics.

MARCIA MELDRUM

Selected Bibliography

PRIMARY SOURCES

Sperry, Roger W. 1952. "Neurology and the Mind-Brain Problem." *American Scientist* 40:291.

———. 1955. "On the Neural Basis of the Conditioned Response." *British Journal of Animal Behaviour* 3:41.

———. 1961. "Cerebral Organization and Behavior." *Science* 133 (June): 1749–57.

Gazzaniga, Michael S., Joseph Bogen, and Roger W. Sperry. 1962. "Some Functional Effects of Sectioning the Cerebral Commissure in Man." *Proceedings of the National Academy of Sciences* 48 (October 15): 1765–69.

Sperry, Roger W. 1964. "The Great Cerebral Commissure." *Scientific American* 210 (January):42–52.

———. 1966. "Lateral Specialization in the Surgically Separated Hemispheres." *The Neurosciences: Third Study Program*, edited by O. Schmitt and F. G. Worden, 161–86. New York: Holt, Rinehart and Winston.

———. 1968. "Mental Unity Following Surgical Disconnection of the Cerebral Hemispheres." *Harvey Lectures*, Series 62, 293–322. New York: Academic Press.

———. 1969. "A Modified Concept of Consciousness." *Psychological Reviews* 76 (November):532–36.

———. 1973. "Chemoaffinity in the Orderly Growth of Nerve Fiber Patterns of Connection." *Proceedings of the National Academy of Sciences* 50:703–10.

———. 1981. "Changing Priorities." *Annual Review of Neuroscience*, 1–15.

———. 1983. *Science and Moral Priority: Merging Mind, Brain, and Human Values*. New York: Columbia University.

SECONDARY SOURCES

Altman, Lawrence K. 1981. "Studies Advance Work on Brain, Eye Disorders." *New York Times* (October 10):50.

Cousins, Norman. 1985. *Nobel Prize Conversations with Sir John Eccles, Roger Sperry, Ilya Prigogine and Brian Josephson*. New York: Saybrook.

Gazzaniga, Michael S. 1981. "The 1981 Nobel Prize in Physiology or Medicine." *Science* 214 (October 30): 517–18.

1981. "Roger Wolcott Sperry." *New York Times* (October 10):50.

Schmeck, Harold M., Jr. 1981. "Three Scientists Share Nobel Prize for Studies of the Brain." *New York Times* (October 10):1.

1986. "Sperry, Roger Wolcott." In *Current Biography Yearbook*, 53–56. New York: H. W. Wilson.

EARL WILBUR SUTHERLAND, JR.

1971

Earl Wilbur Sutherland, Jr., received the Nobel Prize in 1971 "for discoveries concerning the mechanism of action of hormones." The fifth of six children, he was born November 19, 1915, in Burlingame, Kansas. His father, Earl Wilbur Sutherland, had farmed in the southwest before becoming a drygoods store owner in the Kansas town. His mother, Edith M. Hartshorn Sutherland, co-owned and managed the store with her husband. Sutherland attended Washburn College, Topeka, Kansas, from 1933 to 1937, and was awarded the B.S. degree. He then attended Washington University School of Medicine, St. Louis, from 1937 to 1942, and was awarded the M.D. degree. He was to write later that "as a student I was intrigued and puzzled by the actions of hormones. I'm still fascinated by the complex manifestations which occur when a small amount of one of the chemicals is omitted or injected. . . . The hormones appear to regulate existing functions—to accelerate or inhibit intrinsic activities—and often we know little of the basic physiology or biochemistry at the molecular level"

(Sutherland, *Cyclic AMP* 1971, chapter 1).

After interning at Barnes Hospital, St. Louis (1942–1943), Sutherland entered the army, serving as battalion surgeon, U.S. Third Army, from 1943 to 1945 and as staff physician at a military hospital in Germany in 1945. Upon re-entering civilian life, Sutherland returned to Washington University, where he served as instructor and then associate professor in biochemistry from 1945 to 1953. He accepted appointment as director of the Department of Pharmacology at Case Western Reserve University, Cleveland, Ohio, in 1953 and remained there for ten years.

His marriage to his first wife, Mildred Rice, lasted from 1937 to 1962, when they were divorced. He married his second wife, Claudia Sebeste Smith, in 1963; together they had two sons and two daughters.

Sutherland was next professor of physiology at Vanderbilt University, Nashville, Tennessee, from 1963 to 1973. He moved on to Miami, Florida, to become professor of medicine at the University of Miami from 1973 to 1974. He died in Miami on March 9, 1974, after suffering a massive esophageal hemorrhage.

Returning to St. Louis from his work as army physician in Europe during World War II Earl Sutherland joined the Washington University laboratory of Carl Cori. To some coworkers Sutherland appeared as a balding, gregarious, easygoing man. But Cori noted other attributes that helped to describe Sutherland's success in scientific investigation: the gift of intuition, a remarkable degree of tenacity generated by that intuition, excellent laboratory work habits, and singularity of purpose in his experimentation. Carl and Gerty Cori had completed their work on identification of the enzymes involved in the breakdown of glycogen (the storage form of glucose) for which they won the Nobel Prize. Sutherland concentrated his research on two closely related questions: how the hormones epinephrine (adrenalin), produced in the medullary portion of the adrenal gland, and glucagon, secreted by certain islet cells in the pancreas, acted in the liver to stimulate the degradation of glycogen to glucose; and how phosphorylase, and enzyme, acted to initiate the breakdown of glycogen in liver and muscle. By measuring levels of intermediates in the glycogen degradative pathway, Sutherland established in live extracts that it was the first step in glycogen degradation that was affected by epinephrine or by glucagon. This initial step was catalyzed by the enzyme phosphorylase.

Undertaking a detailed examination of phosphorylase at his new laboratory at Case Western Reserve University, Sutherland found that two other enzymes involved in glycogen breakdown were also present in liver extracts. One converted active phosphorylase to an inactive form, releasing inorganic phosphate in the process. The other reactivated the inactive form once again, incorporating the inorganic phosphate into the phosphorylase molecule. Once Sutherland demonstrated that phosphorylase could be activated and deactivated, it was clear that degradation of glycogen was controlled by the relative amounts of active/inactive enzyme.

The liver slices used by Sutherland and his coworkers were readily prepared in large quantities: this was one of the original advantages of using this system to study the effects of the hormones epinephrine and glucagon. Now Sutherland and coworkers studied the activation of phosphorylase by these hormones in a preparation of liver homogenates (broken liver cells). They discovered that in cell-free extracts containing cell membranes both epinephrine and glucagon promoted the accumulation of the active form of phosphorylase. This observation of significant hormone action in a cell-free extract was a landmark finding which overcame the major barrier to understanding how hormones act. Never before had specific hormone effects been observed in cell-free systems. It had been assumed that hormones operated only on whole cells. Now it appeared that a particulate fraction was the site of hormone action and that a signal of some kind was generated as a consequence of the interaction of hormone and membrane. Sutherland and coworkers hypothesized that hormonal action was a molecular process—that the binding of a hormone to the plasma membrane of a cell led to production of a substance that stimulated phosphorylation of the phosphorylase. What was this substance?

Accumulating in the cell-free extracts of liver after epinephrine treatment was a small heat-stable nucleotide (a molecule that consists of a nitrogenous base, a sugar, and one or more phosphate groups). This molecule promoted the conversion of inactive phosphorylase to the active form, and carried out the task of releasing glucose within the cell. The molecule turned out to be adenosine 3′, 5′-monophosphate, now commonly known as cyclic AMP (cAMP). Cyclic AMP proved to be the common intermediate in the action of a number of hormones that control the activity of animal cells. It accumulated in extracts only when the cell membrane fraction was present, suggesting that certain hormones (including epinephrine and glucagon) acted on the outside of the cell membrane to promote synthesis of cyclic AMP.

Further investigations showed that cyclic AMP was formed from adenosine triphosphate (ATP), which plays a central role in energy exchanges in biological systems. Cyclic AMP is formed from ATP by the action of adenylate cyclase, an enzyme that is an integral membrane protein. Cyclic AMP then exerts its effects in animal cells by activating specific intracellular enzymes (cyclic-AMP-dependent protein kinases) that catalyze the transfer of a phosphate group from ATP to a small group of proteins in the target cell. The activation of these specific protein kinases thus leads to the cellular activity characteristic of the hormone that initiates this cascade.

Sutherland's discoveries made possible a unifying concept of the mechanism of hormone action. Hormones may be considered as first messengers, leaving their site of synthesis and secretion to circulate in the blood stream to their target tissues. These are tissues that contain receptors for the hormones. Sutherland suggested that after the hormone combines with its specific receptor there is an increase in the activity of adenylate cyclase present in the cell membrane. This increase in turn increases the level of cyclic AMP within the cell. Cyclic AMP then acts to stimulate certain enzymes (protein kinases) already present in the tissue to alter the rate of one or more specialized functions. Thus cyclic AMP is considered a second messenger in the scheme of hormone activity. An important feature of this second messenger model is that the hormone, the first messenger, need not enter the cell to have its metabolic effects. Further experiments by many investigators have revealed that cyclic AMP is a second messenger for many other hormones in addition to epinephrine and glucagon. Cyclic AMP has been shown to affect a myriad of cellular processes, including degradation of storage fuels (such as glycogen), increasing secretion of acid by gastric mucosal lining, dispersion of melanin pigment granules in the skin, and inhibition of blood platelet aggregation. Of special importance is the fact that cyclic-AMP-dependent protein kinases are found in all animal cells, where they probably account for all of the effects of cyclic AMP. The substrates for these protein kinases differ in different cell types, explaining why the effects of cyclic AMP vary according to the target cell. There are many different protein kinases in cells; only a small number are regulated by cyclic AMP.

It was soon realized that Earl Sutherland had discovered a new biological principle and had made possible a unifying concept of the mechanism of hormone action. It is now known that most hormones bind to cell surface receptors and trigger cascades of enzymatic reactions within the cell. The adenylate cyclase cascade, leading to an increased level of intracellular cyclic AMP, was the first pathway to be elucidated. In addition, cyclic AMP also plays an important role in nonendocrine regulatory mechanisms. It acts at the gene level in *Escherichia coli* and other bacteria to regulate bacterial metabolism; it is a signal for amoebas and certain slime molds to aggregate; and it is involved in immune responses and the activity of brain cells.

Earl Sutherland spent his entire investigative life following up his youthful work in determining how two hormones, epinephrine and glucagon, individually elicited the breakdown of glycogen by the liver. The existence of hormones was known for many decades before he began his work: Sutherland revealed their mechanisms of action. As one scientist noted, with the discovery of adenylate cyclase and cAMP, Sutherland "provided a distinct permanent separation between the hormone and the cellular component that produces the biological effect of the hormone," a necessary condition to generate the modern cell receptor concept (Roth "Receptors," in *Endocrinology: People and Ideas,*

1988, 379). In retrospect, he added, "Sutherland's work of the middle and late 1950's was remarkably slow in having effects on the field because it was so revolutionary and because the assay system (activation of phosphorylase to promote glycogenolysis) was so difficult." This sentiment was shared by another scientist who wrote an appreciation in 1971 (Pastan, "The 1971 Nobel Prize for Physiology of Medicine," 393) at the time of the awarding of the Nobel Prize: "One of the most impressive aspects of Sutherland's contribution is that it is truly unique. Today important discoveries are often made simultaneously in different laboratories. In the case of Earl Sutherland, the rest of us were years behind."

LAWRENCE SHERMAN

Selected Bibliography

PRIMARY SOURCES

Sutherland, Earl W., and T. W. Rall. 1960. "The Relation of Adenosine-3′, 5′-Phosphate and Phosphorylase to the Actions of Calecholamines and Other Hormones." *Pharmacological Reviews* 12:265–99.

Sutherland, Earl W., T. W. Rall, and T. Mermon. 1963. "Adenylcyclase I: Distribution, Preparation and Properties." *Journal of Biological Chemistry* 237:1220–27.

Krishna, G., B. Weiss, and B. B. Brodie. 1968. "A Simple Sensitive Method for the Assay of Adenylcyclase." *Journal of Pharmacology and Experimental Therapeutics* 163:379–85.

Sutherland, Earl W. 1971. "Studies on the Mechanism of Hormone Action." Nobel Lecture. Reprinted in *Science* 177 (August 4, 1972):401–7.

Robison, G. Alan, Reginald W. Butcher, and Earl W. Sutherland, eds. 1971. *Cyclic AMP*. New York: Academic Press.

Robison, G. A., and E. W. Sutherland. 1971. "Cyclic AMP and the Function of Eukaryotic Cells: An Introduction." In *Cyclic AMP and Cell Function*, Annals of the New York Academy of Sciences, vol. 185, edited by G. Alan Robison, Gabriel G. Nabas, and Lubos Triner, 5–9.

SECONDARY SOURCES

Pastan, Ira H. 1971. "The 1971 Nobel Prize for Physiology or Medicine." *Science* 174 (October 22):392–93.

Roth, Jesse. 1988. "Receptors: Birth, Eclipse, and Rediscovery." In *Endocrinology: People and Ideas*, edited by S. M. McCann, 369–96. Bethesda, MD: American Physiological Society.

Stryer, Lubert. 1988. "Hormone Action." In *Biochemistry*, Lubert Stryer, 975–83. 3d ed. New York: W. H. Freeman.

ALBERT SZENT-GYÖRGYI 1937

Albert Szent-Györgyi von Nagyrapolt was born in Budapest on September 16, 1893. His father, Nicolaus, belonged to a family of wealthy landowners, while his mother's family had distinguished itself by producing three generations of scientists. Despite the protests of his uncle, the histologist Mihaly Lenhossek, who felt that his nephew lacked scientific talent, Albert von Szent-Györgyi followed this family tradition by becoming a chemist. His enormous talents earned him the Nobel Prize in 1937 "for his discoveries in connection with the biological combustion processes, with especial reference to vitamin C and the catalysis of fumaric acid." He died at Woods Hole, Massachusetts, on October 22, 1986.

After receiving his primary education in Budapest, Szent-Györgyi entered the university there to study medicine in 1911. Under his uncle's guidance, he studied histology and physiology. The outbreak of World War I interrupted Szent-Györgyi's medical studies and he was sent to the front. Thoroughly disgusted with the immorality of war, he wounded himself with his own gun and returned gladly to his studies. He obtained his medical degree in 1917 and returned to service in an army bacteriological laboratory. Even this laboratory proved hazardous to Szent-Györgyi, who objected to dangerous experiments being conducted on Italian prisoners of war. As punishment, he was sent to the malaria-infested swamps of northern Italy, where only the end of the war averted a perilous fate.

After the war Szent-Györgyi embarked on an intellectual pilgrimage. His first destination was Pozsony, where he served as assistant to the pharmacologist G. Mansfeld. After briefly studying electrophysiology with Armin von Tschermak in Prague and learning about pH with Leonor Michaelis in Berlin, Szent-Györgyi spent two years in Hamburg studying physical chemistry at the Institute for Tropical Hygiene. From there he journeyed to Leyden, where he worked for two years as an assistant in the Pharmacological Institute. Finally, he settled in Groningen at the Physiological Institute where he served as assistant to H. J. Hamburger.

The work that led to the Nobel Prize began at Groningen in the area of respiration. It was generally understood that the oxidation of carbohydrates was the major source of enegy in the cells and that the crucial reaction in this process was the production of water from hydrogen and oxygen. A controversy arose, however, between the Otto Warburg school, which argued for the preliminary activation of oxygen by respiratory enzymes, and the Heinrich Wieland school, which opted for the preliminary activation of hydrogen. Szent-Györgyi devised an experiment in which he knocked out oxygen activation in tissue by cyanide. This stopped respiration, proving that oxygen activation was necessary. When he added methylene blue to the minced tissue, however, the dye restored respiration, which meant that it first reacted with activated hydrogen enabling the latter to be subsequently oxidized. He concluded that both oxygen and hydrogen activation were prerequisite for respiration. During these experiments he became fascinated by succino-dehydrogenase and citroco-dehydrogenase (enzymes that activate hydrogen), which seemed particularly important in the economy of the cell because they were so closely associated with its structural elements (now known to be the mitochondria). He proved the catalytic activity of succino-dehydrogenase by showing that once it was inhibited by malonic acid, respiration stopped. This discovery of C_4-dicarboxylic acid comprised part of the work honored by the Nobel Prize.

Although Krebs' later work proved that Szent-Györgyi's understanding of the functions of C_4-dicarboxylic acids such as fumaric acid was incorrect, Krebs acknowledged Szent-Györgyi's pioneering role in establishing the field. Krebs also expressed personal gratitude and affection for Szent-Györgyi's help in difficult times.

The main area of Szent-Györgyi's research honored by the Nobel Prize—the isolation of vitamin C—also started in the area of oxidation. He was interested in the adrenal cortex since the suppression of the functions of this organ led to Addison's disease. He theorized that the brown pigmentation that appears in man before life is extinguished might be due to the damaged oxidation mechanism, as is the case with plants. Hence, he undertook studies of plants that turned brown upon withering, such as the potato. He figured out that the pigmentation was the result of damage to the reduction mechanism, which could not provide hydrogen at a rapid enough rate to prevent oxidation. Since this system did not yield any understanding of adrenal function, he turned to plants that did not turn brown on withering, such as oranges. In this system, the coloring can be induced only in the presence of peroxidase which accelerates the oxidation process. On substituting juices squeezed from these plants for pure peroxidase, he noticed a slight delay of about a second in the reaction, which he traced to the presence of a reducing substance that counteracted the oxidation process. He then discovered with great excitement that the adrenal cortex contained an analogous reducing substance in relatively large amounts.

The death of Hamburger in 1927 occasioned Szent-Györgyi's move to Cambridge University as a Rockefeller Fellow. There he earned a Ph.D. degree by isolating this reducing substance, which he named "hexuronic acid." In order to obtain the large amount of this substance that was necessary for constitutional analysis, he accepted the invitation of E. C. Kendall and went to the Mayo Clinic in Rochester, Minnesota. He returned to Cambridge with twenty-five grams of "hexuronic acid," which he divided up between W. N. Haworth and himself. Haworth's constitutional analysis failed due to insufficient amount, but Szent-Györgyi's functional study showed that even though it could not take the place of the adrenal glands, it overcame the pigmentation of Addison's disease.

In 1930 Szent-Györgyi finally returned to Hungary, as professor of medical chemistry at the University of Szeged. He went back to elucidating intermediate steps of the oxidation process and discovered a new catalyst, cytoflave, which was soon identified with vitamin B2, or riboflavin, by another group of scientists. The arrival of a young American-born Hungarian, J. L. Svirbely, who was experienced with vitamin research, enabled Szent-Györgyi to confirm his suspicion that "hexuronic acid" was identical with vitamin C by demonstrating that it had an antiscorbutic effect (preventing and counteracting scurvy) and that this effect of the juices of plants corresponded with their hexuronic acid content. With this confirmation, Szent-Györgyi and Haworth rebaptized hexuronic acid as "ascorbic acid." While searching for ways to obtain this substance in large quantity, he took the paprika from his own dinner to the lab since it was practically the last foodstuff that he had not analysed: the paprika turned out to be a rich source of ascorbic acid. Taking advantage of the last season of the paprika industry for which Szeged was the center, Szent-Györgyi prepared three kilograms of the substance with the support of the American Josiah Macy, Jr., Foundation. Constitutional analysis and functional studies proved conclusively that ascorbic acid was identical with vitamin C and that the activity of the substance was not dependent on impurities. Within two years of his work vitamin C was synthesized and its therapeutic effects were being intensely investigated.

Szent-Györgyi had turned his attention to the problem of muscle contraction when politics intervened in his life once again. During World War II he successfully carried out a spy mission to Istanbul to establish a contact with the Allies. When word of his mission leaked out, Hitler was enraged and ordered Szent-Györgyi's capture. He and his entire family immediately went into hiding. He was treated with utmost respect and favor when the Soviets liberated Budapest, but the brutal acts of the Stalin regime in Hungary ultimately caused Szent-Györgyi to seek refuge in Switzerland. He later emigrated to the United States, where he found his haven in Woods Hole, Massachusetts. For many years, Szent-Györgyi served as director of the Institute for Muscle Research at the Woods Hole Marine Biological Station, while conducting his own research in the cellular biology of cancer. During the American phase of his career, Szent-Györgyi has gained the admiration and affection of his American colleagues and students and has continually spoken forcefully against the war industry and for the peaceful application of science. "The road to peace," he insists, "does not lead over bombs and dead bodies."

Szent-Györgyi married Cornelia Demeny in 1917; they had one daughter, also named Cornelia. After his first wife died, he married Marta Borbiro, a coworker, during the war. That marriage later ended in divorce, and he married Marcia Houston, an American, in 1975. Szent-Györgyi was a member of the National Academy of Sciences, the American Academy of Arts and Sciences, and the Budapest Academy of Sciences. Among the many other honors he received for his work were the Cameron Prize from the University of Edinburgh (1946) and the Lasker Award (1954).

MI GYUNG KIM

Selected Bibliography

PRIMARY SOURCES

Szent-Györgyi, Albert. 1932. "Lost in the Twentieth-Century," *Annual Review of Biochemistry*, 32, 1–14.

———. 1937. "Nobel Lecture". Reprinted in *Les Prix Nobel en 1937*, Stockholm: Imprimerie Royale P. A., Norsted & Söner, 1938, 1–11.

———. 1975. "Interview. A talk with Albert Szent-Györgyi," *The New Hungarian Quarterly*, 16, no. 57, 136-150.

SECONDARY SOURCES

Benjamin Kaminer, ed. 1977. *Search and Discovery: A Tribute to Albert Szent-Györgyi*, New York: Academic Press.

EDWARD LAWRIE TATUM 1958

Edward Lawrie Tatum was born on December 14, 1909, in Boulder, Colorado. He received half the Nobel Prize in Physiology or Medicine in 1958 jointly with George W. Beadle for their work establishing the "one gene, one enzyme" theory that genes regulate cellular processes chemically. The other half was awarded to Joshua Lederberg. Edward Tatum was the oldest of three children of Arthur Lawrie Tatum, physician and pharmacologist at the University of Wisconsin, and Mabel Webb, one of the earliest woman graduates of the University of Colorado. On July 28, 1934, he married June Alton; they had two children. They were divorced in 1956 and later that same year he married Viola Kantor, a dentist. She died in 1974 and in the same year he married Elsie Bergland. He died on November 5, 1975, at his home in New York City.

Edward Tatum completed a Ph.D. in biochemistry at Wisconsin

in 1934 and spent another year there as a research assistant. He went to the University of Utrecht in the Netherlands in 1936 on a General Education Board Fellowship. The following year he moved to Stanford as a research associate to George Beadle, professor of biology, and in 1941 he was promoted to assistant professor. He served as a civilian staff member of the U.S. Office of Scientific Research and Development in 1944. At the end of the war he moved to Yale as associate professor of botany, becoming professor of microbiology the following year. He returned to Stanford in 1948 as professor of biology. In 1956 he was appointed professor and head of the department of biochemistry at Stanford. In 1957 he moved east again, to become a member and professor of the Rockefeller Institute, later Rockefeller University, where he remained until his death.

The science of genetics had come of age by the twenties, by which time T. H. Morgan and associates, particularly H. J. Muller, had established a considerable platform of experimental proof, via the genetics of *Drosophila melangoster*, or common fruit fly, of the particulate nature of the gene. However, genetics alone could not describe its physical form or chemical expression. Considerable work had been done on the genetics of plant and animal pigments by the twenties, for example, but there was "widespread reluctance to draw conclusions about direct gene action" (Sturtevant 1965, 100). And answers from other disciplines came only slowly. Archibald Garrod, an English physician, had shown in 1909 that certain diseases traceable to enzyme-deficiency were heritable, but his work was overlooked. The English scientist J. B. S. Haldane was one of only a few biochemists who took seriously suggestions of a relationship between genes and enzymes.

When George Beadle and Boris Ephrussi, an embryologist, transplanted embryonic *Drosophila* eye tissue in Paris in 1935 to show the genetic basis of the synthesis of eye pigment, the idea that a gene controlled an enzyme was thus already present. So that when Edward Tatum, the biochemist, went to Stanford in 1937, to assist the geneticist George Beadle to identify the enzymes responsible for eye pigmentation in *Drosophila*, the collaboration was uncommon but not unprecedented. The singularity of their work was Beadle's decision to dispense with *Drosophila* and use instead *Neurospora*, or common bread mold. This decision made experimental proof of the gene-enzyme theory possible.

George Beadle was familiar with *Neurospora*'s utility as a genetic tool because it had been pioneered by B. O. Dodge in the twenties and developed in the thirties by Carl C. Lindegren in the laboratories of T. H. Morgan at Caltech, where Beadle had worked. *Neurospora* had a brief life cycle and it could reproduce both sexually and asexually, thus providing both pure strains and Mendelian inheritance patterns through which a mutant could be traced. *Neurospora* was also a biochemical tool Tatum had come to understand well. At Wisconsin and Utrecht he had learned how to track the biochemical pathways of the nutritional requirements of bacteria and fungi. At Utrecht, he had worked with F. Kögl, the discoverer of the growth factor biotin, in the laboratory of Nils Fries, who had written on the nutritional requirements of a number of fungi related to *Neurospora*.

At Stanford Tatum used Fries's work to establish that the nutritional requirements of *Neurospora* were minimal. It had a sophisticated mechanism of enzyme systems that enabled it to synthesize for itself most of the amino acids and vitamins needed for growth, lacking only a few basic salts and sugars and the recently discovered vitamin biotin. The subsequent experiments were extensive but basically simple. Selecting through irradiation a stock of nutritional mutants (those that could not grow on a minimal medium but could grow on a medium containing all nutritional requirements), they then grew them on a minimal medium to which individual amino acids and vitamins were added, thus identifying particular mutant deficients. A mutant that grew on a medium supplemented with vitamin B_6 was shown to inherit in Mendelian sequence.

Tatum's work identifying the biochemical nutritional requirements of fungi helped speed up the production of penicillin during World War II, and he also helped develop new methods of testing the purity of vitamins and amino acids in foods and tissues. After the war Tatum developed his techniques for identifying nutritional mutants so as to include bacteria. He was thus able to supply Joshua Lederberg in 1946 with the clear-cut genetic markers he needed to detect the rare incidence of bacterial genetic recombination, the experiments for which Lederberg was awarded the other half of the Nobel Prize.

It is difficult now to grasp the concern expressed by Tatum's father to George Beadle in 1938, about the future professional value to a biochemist of collaborative work with a geneticist (Beadle 1974, 7–8). And Edward Tatum was appointed professor of biology at Stanford in 1941 only in the face of "substantial opposition to the concept that a chemist had a place in a department of biology" (Lederberg 1979, 3). Yet he pioneered the methodology that enabled *Neurospora* to be used most effectively to pursue the chemical nature of the gene. The singular importance, then, of the work of this biochemist in the transformation of modern biology, lies perhaps in the reflection Joshua Lederberg made on Tatum's death, that his work gave "impetus and morale" to scientists who were not inclined to accept the view "widely held by biologists that the living cell's processes were too complicated to understand" [*New York Times*, November 7, 1975].

Tatum received the Remsen Award of the American Chemical Society in 1953. He was a member of numerous scientific societies, including the American Society of Biological Chemists, the American Association for the Advancement of Science, and the Harvard Society.

He was elected to the National Academy of Sciences in 1952. He served on the advisory committee of the National Foundation, the Committee of the National Resource Council on Growth, and the American Cancer Society. He was a founder member of the *Annual Review of Genetics* and served on the editorial board of *Science*.

ROSALIE STOTT

Selected Bibliography

PRIMARY SOURCES

Beadle, George W., and E. L. Tatum. 1941. "Genetic Control of Biochemical Reactions in Neurospora." *Proceedings of the National Academy of Sciences* 27: 499–506. Reprinted in *Classic Papers in Genetics*, edited by James A. Peters, 166–73. N.J.: Prentice-Hall.

Tatum, E. L. 1958. "A Case History in Biological Search." Nobel Lecture. Reprinted in *Nobel Lectures in Molecular Biology 1933–1974*. Amsterdam: Elsevier, 1977.

SECONDARY SOURCES

1975. "Obituary." *New York Times*, (November 7):40.

Beadle, George W. 1973. "Recollections." *Annual Review of Biochemistry* 43:1–13.

Horowitz, N. H. 1979. "Genetics and the Synthesis of Proteins." *Annals of the New York Academy of Science*, 253–66.

Kopp, C. 1982. "The Edward Lawrie Tatum Papers at the Rockefeller University Archives." *Journal of the History of Biology* 15, no. 1 (Spring):153–54.

Lederberg, J. 1979. "Edward Lawrie Tatum." *Annual Review of Genetics* 13:1–5.

Olby, Robert C. 1974. *The Path to the Double Helix*. Seattle: University of Washington Press.

Portugal, F. H., and J. S. Cohen. 1977. *A Century of DNA*. Cambridge: M.I.T. Press.

Sturtevant, A. H. 1965. *A History of Genetics*. New York: Harper and Row.

Wagner, R. P., and H. K. Mitchell. 1955. *Genetics and Metabolism*. New York: John Wiley.

HOWARD MARTIN TEMIN 1975

The 1975 Nobel Prize in Physiology or Medicine was awarded jointly to Howard Temin, Renato Dulbecco, and David Baltimore for their "discoveries concerning the interaction between tumor viruses and the genetic material of the cell." Temin is a biochemist who has specialized in the molecular biology of tumor viruses. He proposed the controversial "provirus hypothesis" to explain the replication of RNA tumor viruses like Rous sarcoma virus and had demonstrated the validity of his model by demonstrating the existence of the enzyme known as reverse transcriptase; this enzyme carries out RNA-dependent DNA synthesis.

Howard Temin was born on December 10, 1934, in Philadelphia, Pennsylvania. His father, Henry Temin, was an attorney and his mother, Annette Lehmann Temin, was active in civic affairs, especially problems related to education. Temin married Rayla Greenberg, a population geneticist, on May 27, 1962. They have two daughters.

Temin earned his B.A. from Swarthmore College, where he majored in biology. At the California Institute of Technology, he originally majored in experimental embryology, but decided to study animal virology in Renato Dulbecco's laboratory. Temin's doctoral thesis involved research on Rous sarcoma virus (RSV). He received his Ph.D. in 1959. Much of Temin's early work on Rous sarcoma virus (RSV) was performed in collaboration with Harry Rubin, a postdoctoral fellow in Dulbecco's laboratory. While at Caltech, Temin also came under the influence of Max Delbrück and Matthew Meselson. Remaining at Caltech as a postdoctoral researcher in 1959–1960, Temin began the series of experiments that led to the formulation of the "provirus hypothesis."

In 1960 Temin became assistant professor in the McArdle Laboratory for Cancer Research, Department of Oncology, in the Medical School of the University of Wisconsin at Madison. Temin advanced to associate professor in 1964 and full professor in 1969. Remaining at the University of Wisconsin, he became, successively, Wisconsin Alumni Research Foundation Professor of Cancer Research (1971–1980); American Cancer Society Professor of Viral Oncology and Cell Biology (1974–present); Harold P. Rusch Professor of Cancer Research (1980–present); and Steenbock Professor of Biological Sciences (1982–present). From 1964 to 1974 he also held a Research Career Development Award from the National Cancer Institute. In 1987 Temin was Braund Distinguished Visiting Professor at the University of Tennessee and First Wilmot Visiting Professor at the University of Rochester.

During his first years at Wisconsin, Temin worked in a basement laboratory with two technicians. He acquired a postdoctoral fellow in

1963 and a graduate student in 1965. Until about 1968 his research group generally consisted of only two or three postdoctoral fellows and graduate students. Studies of the control of the multiplication of uninfected and Rous sarcoma virus-infected cells in culture during the late 1960s led to an appreciation of the role of specific serum factors in the control of cell multiplication in vitro and the identification of a chicken fibroblast multiplication-stimulating factor in calf serum.

In 1958 Temin and Harry Rubin had developed the first reproducible in vitro assay for a tumor virus. Refining his studies of RSV at the University of Wisconsin, Temin proposed in 1964 that a DNA intermediate is involved in RSV infection. According to the provirus hypothesis, after a cell was infected by an RNA virus a DNA provirus was synthesized from the RNA viral genome. Progeny viral RNA would then be synthesized from the DNA provirus that contained all the genetic information of the RNA virus. This hypothesis explained the known sensitivity of infection to inhibitors of both DNA synthesis and DNA-dependent RNA synthesis. The provirus hypothesis also accounted for the stable inheritance of RSV in transformed cells by postulating that the DNA provirus could integrate itself into the genome of the host cell.

The provirus hypothesis remained controversial for some years, partly because much of the evidence was indirect and depended on the use of inhibitors that might themselves have produced artifacts. Perhaps the suspicions about artifacts were exaggerated by the pervasive influence of "the central dogma of molecular biology," which taught that genetic information always flowed from DNA to RNA and then into proteins. RNA viruses had been incorporated into the central dogma in terms of experiments using the antibiotic actinomycin D, which suggested that RNA viruses had lost the DNA to RNA step and were simply reduced to transferring information from RNA to protein. Attempting to use actinomycin D to isolate the RSV provirus, Temin discovered that the antibiotic inhibited virus production when added to RSV-producing cells. Temin concluded that the RSV provirus was DNA. Further experiments demonstrated that new DNA synthesis was required for RSV infection.

The provirus hypothesis requires information to flow in the "wrong" direction, that is from RNA to DNA. Temin continued to accumulate additional evidence implicating DNA synthesis in RSV infection, without overcoming the prevailing skepticism of other molecular biologists until 1970, when Temin and Satoshi Mizutani proved that the virions of RSV contain an enzyme that can transcribe the single-stranded RSV RNA into DNA. By providing a mechanism for the information of a DNA intermediate during RNA tumor virus infection and transformation, this experiment converted skeptics into true believers. The term "reverse transcriptase" was coined by an anonymous correspondent for the British journal *Nature*.

Interestingly, within a few weeks of the announcements by Baltimore and Temin of the demonstration of reverse transcriptase, Sol Spiegelman, the director of Columbia University's Institute of Cancer Research and one of Temin's main critics, confirmed the existence of reverse transcription in his own laboratories in eight additional RNA cancer viruses. Moreover, Francis Crick, one of the architects of the central dogma, soon published a paper in *Nature* showing that reverse transcription could be incorporated into central dogma.

In his Nobel Lecture, Temin discussed the establishment of the DNA provirus hypothesis and the implications of RNA-directed DNA synthesis. This work had been accomplished with avian RNA tumor viruses. Rous sarcoma virus, originally described by Peyton Rous in 1911, may be considered the prototype RNA tumor virus. To understand the behavior of RSV scientists had to understand that genetic information was encoded in and transferred by nucleic acids and that viral genomes could be incorporated into cell genomes. They also needed the technical tools of quantitative virology and methods of studying animal viruses in cell culture. Temin was introduced to RSV while a graduate student in 1956 by Harry Rubin, a postdoctoral fellow in Renato Dulbecco's laboratory. Temin and Rubin developed better techniques for the assay of RSV in tissue culture. With this assay system it was possible to demonstrate that the genome of RSV was RNA and that viral genes controlled the morphology of transformed cells. These experiments supported the hypothesis that transformation of the host cell was the result of the action of viral genes.

Studies of the kinetics of mutation of RSV genes and the inheritance of viral genes in cells infected with two different Rous sarcoma viruses demonstrated a high rate of mutation in viral genes. Moreover, cells infected by mutant viruses underwent a change in morphology. From considerations of RSV infection, replication, and transformation, Temin was led to his provirus hypothesis. At first the hypothesis was strictly genetic and provided no explanation for the molecular nature of the provirus, but considerations of the stable inheritance of the provirus suggested that the provirus was integrated with the cell genome.

Experiments performed by Satoshi Mizutani in Temin's laboratory suggested that RSV contained a DNA polymerase. RSV endogenous RNA-directed DNA polymerase was characterized in 1970. Avian RNA tumor virus DNA polymerases proved to be stable and were relatively easy to study and purify. Within a few years, these DNA polymerases have become one of the standard tools of molecular biology. Although the discovery of reverse transcriptase substantiated Temin's hypothesis, further proof was eventually added by experiments involving nucleic acid hybridization and infectious DNA.

In describing the relationship between the provirus hypothesis and attempts to understand the origin of genes for cancer, Temin concluded that "I do not believe that infectious viruses cause most human cancers, but I do believe that viruses provide models of the processes involved in the etiology of human cancer" (Temin, "Provirus Hypothesis," *Nobel Lectures*, 523). Temin had demonstrated that the genetic information in RNA is transferred to DNA during the replication of some viruses, including some cancer causing viruses, but he has been cautious in his interpretation of this work.

Other honors awarded to Howard Temin include the Pap Award, Papanicolaou Institute (1972), the Waksman Award, Theobald Smith Society (1972), the Award in Enzyme Chemistry, American Chemical Society (1973), the Gairdner Foundation International Award (1974), the Albert Lasker Award (1974), the Lucy Wortham James Award, Society of Surgical Oncologists (1976), and the Gruber Award, American Academy of Dermatology (1981). Temin has received honorary degrees from Swarthmore College (1972), New York Medical College (1972), the University of Pennsylvania (1976), Lawrence University (1976), Temple University (1979), the Medical College of Wisconsin (1981), Colorado State University (1987), and the Université Pierre et Marie Curie (1988). In 1988 Temin was Ochoa Lecturer, International Congress of Biochemistry, and Prague and Muller Lecturer, International Congress of Genetics, Toronto.

Temin serves on the editorial boards of several journals, including the *Journal of Cellular Physiology*, the *Journal of Virology*, and the *Proceedings of the National Academy of Sciences*. He has been a member of the Virology Study Section of the National Institutes of Health, a fellow of the American Academy of Arts and Sciences, and a member of the National Academy of Sciences.

LOIS N. MAGNER

Selected Bibliography

PRIMARY SOURCES

Temin, H. M. 1963. "The Effects of Actinomycin D on Growth of Rous Sarcoma Virus *in Vitro*." *Virology* 20:577–82.

———. 1964. "The Participation of DNA in Rous Sarcoma Virus Production." *Virology* 23:486–94.

———. 1964. "Nature of the Provirus of Rous Sarcoma." *National Cancer Institute Monograph* 17:557–70.

Temin, H. M., and D. Baltimore. 1972. "RNA-directed DNA Synthesis and RNS Tumor Viruses." *Advances in Virus Research* 17:129–86.

Temin, H. M. 1972. *RNA-Directed DNA Synthesis*. San Francisco: W. H. Freeman.

———. 1975. "The DNA Provirus Hypothesis. The Establishment and Implications of RNA-directed DNA Synthesis." Nobel Lecture. Reprinted in *Nobel Lectures in Molecular Biology 1933–1975*, 509–29. Amsterdam: Elsevier, 1977.

SECONDARY SOURCES

Barry, R. D., and B. W. J. Mahy, eds. 1970. *The Biology of Large RNA Viruses*. New York: Academic Press.

Burnet, F. M., and W. M. Stanley, eds. 1959. *The Viruses*, vol. I. New York: Academic Press.

Eckhart, Walter. 1975. "The 1975 Nobel Prize for Physiology or Medicine." *Science* 190:650, 712, 714.

Gross, L. (1972). *Oncogenic Viruses*. New York: Pergamon Press.

Mahy, B. W. J., and R. D. Barry, eds. 1975. *Negative Strand Viruses*, vol. 1. New York: Academic Press.

Smith, K. M., M. A. Lauffer, and Bang, eds. 1972. *Advances in Virus Research*, vol. 17. New York: Academic Press.

Tooze, J., ed. 1973. *The Molecular Biology of Tumor Viruses*. New York: Cold Spring Harbor Laboratory.

MAX THEILER *1951*

Max Theiler was born on January 30, 1899, in Pretoria, South Africa. A virologist, Theiler won the Nobel Prize in 1951 for this demonstration that a virus, not a bacteria, was the etiologic agent of yellow fever and for his development of a safe and effective vaccine for this deadly disease. At the time of the award, he had been newly appointed director of laboratories of the Rockefeller Foundation's Division of Medicine and Public Health, having previously served on the staff of the International Health Division since 1930. Theiler and his wife, Lillian Graham, whom he married in 1928, had one daughter, Elizabeth. He died on August 11, 1972, in New Haven, Connecticut.

Theiler's family was of Swiss background. His father, Sir Arnold Theiler, was director of the Institute of Veterinary Research at Onderstepoort, South Africa; his mother was the former Emma Jegge. Theiler attended Rhodes University College in Grahamstown before enrolling at age eighteen in a two-year premedical program at the University of Capetown. In 1919 he traveled to England to complete his training, but the University of London refused to recognize the courses he had taken in South Africa. Rather than repeat these studies, Theiler decided to prepare for the medical licensing examination by taking clinical training at St. Thomas' Hospital. This plan would not lead to a medical degree but would qualify him as a medical practitioner.

He passed the examination in 1922 and then enrolled in a four-month course offered by the London School of Tropical Medicine and Hygiene. Here his interest in yellow fever was first aroused. He met Dr. Oscar Teague at the London School; Teague recognized the young man's ability and arranged for him to obtain an assistantship at the School of Tropical Medicine at Harvard. Theiler arrived in Boston in 1922 to begin work with Dr. Andrew Sellards.

At Harvard he began studies of amoebic dysentery and rat-bite fever; he also renewed his interest in yellow fever, which soon became his major preoccupation. This highly virulent infection had been a major cause of mortality in tropical countries for centuries. Walter Reed and William Gorgas, during the Spanish American War and the occupation of Cuba, had established its transmission via the mosquito *Aedes aegypti*; effective mosquito control measures had since virtually eliminated the disease in the United States, Panama, Mexico, and other areas of the Western Hemisphere. But yellow fever remained endemic in the animal populations of jungles and rain forests; travelers in these areas might pick up the infection and act as carriers to infect others. Tropical disease specialists therefore continued to investigate the etiology and search for a possible cure of yellow fever. Gorgas had become the head of the Rockefeller Foundation Yellow Fever Commission, charged with eradication of the disease.

A major question was whether the pathogenic agent was a bacterium, as argued by Dr. H. Noguchi of the Rockefeller Foundation, or a "filtrable virus." In 1927 Sellards, Theiler, and their colleagues presented proof of the viral etiology. The following year, Adrian Stokes, J. H. Bauer, and N. P. Hudson of the Rockefeller African Unit at Accra isolated and successfully infected rhesus monkeys with a yellow fever virus they named the Asibi strain. Their work confirmed the viral cause but also pointed to the potential dangers of infection from carriers other than *Aedes aegypti*.

Later in 1928 Sellards travelled to Dakar in French West Africa and isolated a second strain, which was designated the French strain. He brought back to Harvard the frozen liver of an infected monkey. Theiler determined to use this material to attempt the experimental induction of yellow fever in white mice.

Inoculation of laboratory mice with the standard methods had failed to induce the infection. Theiler therefore injected his suspension of infected tissue directly into the brain. He succeeded in inducing encephalomyelitis, or infection of the brain and spinal cord, without concurrent involvement of other organs—the heart, liver, and kidneys—as was observed in yellow fever in man and monkeys. However, he was able to reisolate the viral strain from the infected mice; the animals had definitely contracted yellow fever.

Theiler also noted that when rhesus monkeys were inoculated with the strain taken from the mice, its effects appeared weaker and less virulent than the original virus. These results were important for two reasons: first, the laboratory mouse was a much more convenient and less expensive research model than the rhesus monkey; second, the attenuation of the virus after passage through the mouse suggested the potential for development of a successful clinical vaccine.

The study of this virulent disease was highly dangerous in these years; courage as well as skill was required. Five investigators, including Noguchi, died of yellow fever between 1928 and 1930; Theiler himself contracted the infection from his mouse tissues in June 1929 but survived.

Theiler's first report of his infected mice, appearing in *Science* in 1930, was greeted with harsh criticism. Even his mentor, Sellards, was very skeptical. After others had replicated his work, however, the unknown virologist was acclaimed. Later in the year he was offered the opportunity to join the intensive yellow fever research work at the Rockefeller Foundation, working under Dr. W. Sawyer. Here his first project was the demonstration that mice could be immunized against the disease by inoculation with serum from human survivors who had developed natural immunity.

Two different approaches were now employed towards development of a vaccine from Theiler's mouse-adapted virus. Inoculation of humans with the mouse preparation alone, attempted by Sellards and others, produced unfortunate results; the virus was still too powerful. French workers, however, developed in 1939 a method of applying the mouse-adapted virus externally to the scarified skin. This technique, the "Dakar scratch vaccine," was quite effective and widely used in French Africa, often in combination with smallpox vaccine.

Sawyer and his colleagues, meanwhile, were able to immunize monkeys safely using a preparation of mouse virus and human immune serum. Their vaccine was then introduced for the protection of the researchers and health care workers exposed to yellow fever. Although it appeared to be both effective and reasonably safe, it required large amounts of human immune serum, which were simply unavailable.

Theiler undertook to develop a "hyperimmune" serum, using a variety of animal models, including horses, rabbits, goats, and monkeys. He developed sera that provided adequate protection when very small amounts were added to the mouse virus. Nevertheless, the production of such sera was sufficiently expensive and complex to make this vaccine infeasible for large-scale use. The only permanent solution was to produce a more attenuated form of the mouse-adapted yellow fever virus.

In 1934 Theiler set up a series of experiments, using chick and mouse embryo cultures, to grow both Asibi and French strains. Soon after he began these studies, an Asibi culture, which had gone through a series of 176 passages, suddenly and spontaneously mutated within a chick embryo from which most of the neural tissue had been removed. The mutant strain, named 17D, appeared much weaker and less active than its parent; injected into monkeys' brains, it induced a mild, generally nonfatal, encephalitis, with little or no involvement of other organs.

Clinical tests of a human vaccine derived from 17D began in Brazil in 1937 and established its safety and efficacy within three years. The vaccine has been in worldwide use ever since; millions of doses have been distributed by the Rockefeller Institute alone. To fully appreciate the impact of Theiler's discovery, it is necessary to realize the extent to which yellow fever control today is taken for granted by physicians and laymen alike.

Theiler remained at the Rockefeller Foundation for thirty-four years. After the development of 17D, he turned his attention to a variety of other infections, including Weil's disease, dengue fever, and Japanese encephalitis. He became particularly interested in poliomyelitis and identified a virtually identical encephalomyelitis in mice, which is now often called Theiler's disease.

In 1964 Theiler was appointed professor of microbiology at Yale, thus achieving the distinction of a Nobel Prize and association with three of the most prestigious institutions in American medicine without an earned academic degree. Among the many other honors he received for his work were the Chalmers Medal from the Royal Society of Tropical Medicine and Hygiene (1939), the Flattery Medal from Harvard (1945), and the Albert Lasker Award from the American Public Health Association (1949). He retired from Yale in 1967, and died five years later at age seventy-three.

MARCIA MELDRUM
JAMES J. POUPARD

Selected Bibliography

PRIMARY SOURCES

Theiler, Max. 1930. "Susceptibility of White Mice to Virus and Yellow Fever." *Science* 71:367.

———. 1930. "Studies on Action of Yellow Fever Virus in Mice." *Annals of Tropical Medicine* 24:249–72.

Theiler, Max, and H. H. Smith. 1936. "Use of Hyperimmune Monkey Serum in Human Vaccination against Yellow Fever." *Bulletin de l'Office Internationale d'Hygenie* 28:2354–57.

Theiler, Max. 1959. "Yellow Fever." In *Viral and Rickettsial Infections of Man*, edited by Thomas Rivers and Frank Horsfall, 343–60. Philadelphia: Lippincott.

SECONDARY SOURCES

Strode, George, ed. 1951. *Yellow Fever.* New York: McGraw-Hill.

1952. "Theiler, Max." In *Current Biography Yearbook*, 586–87. New York: H. W. Wilson.

Williams, Greer. 1960. *Virus Hunters.* New York: Alfred A. Knopf.

AXEL HUGO THEODOR THEORELL
1955

A. H. T. Theorell was born in Linkoping, Sweden, on July 6, 1903, the son of Thure Theorell and Armida Bill. Theorell's father practiced medicine in Linkoping as surgeon-major to the First Life Grenadiers. In 1931 Theorell married Elin Margit Elizabeth Alenius. They had one daughter, Eva Kristina, who died in 1935, and three sons: Klas Thure Gabriel, Henning Hugo and Per Gunnar Tores. A research biochemist specializing in enzymology, Theorell won the Nobel Prize in Physiology or Medicine in 1955 for his discoveries concerning the nature and mode of action of oxidation enzymes. He died on August 15, 1982, in Stockholm.

Theorell's early schooling began at a state secondary school in his hometown of Linkoping. He passed his matriculation examination there in May 1921. That fall he went to the Karolinska Institute to study medicine. Even before he graduated in 1924 with a bachelor of medicine degree, he was appointed to the staff of the institute. Immediately after graduation, he spent three months at the Pasteur Institute in Paris, where he studied bacteriology.

From 1924 to 1930 Theorell worked at the Karolinska Institute under Einar Hammersten on plasma lipids and their influence on the sedimentation of red blood cells. In 1930 he was awarded the research degree of M.D. with a thesis on the lipids of the blood plasma and was then appointed lecturer in physiological chemistry.

Theorell served on the faculty of Uppsala University from 1930 to 1936. During the years 1933 to 1935 he held a Rockefeller Fellowship that enabled him to work with Otto Warburg, a pioneer in enzyme research, in Berlin. During this period Theorell became interested in oxidation enzymes, the subject that became his life's work.

Theorell returned to Sweden from Germany in 1935, and in 1936 he was appointed head of the newly established Biochemical Department of the Nobel Medical Institute. There, as professor and administrator, he continued his work in enzymology until he retired in 1970.

Theorell discussed the history of enzymology when he accepted the Nobel Prize in Physiology or Medicine in 1955. Since at least the time of the ancient Greeks, he said, men had observed enzymatic reactions, such as fermentation and decay. During the nineteenth century Jons Jacob Berzelius—a fellow Swede who had also attended Linkoping High School—tried to explain such changes, rather than simply observe them. In 1835 he developed the concept of catalysis by saying that there is a force in organic as well as inorganic nature that has the ability to produce certain kinds of chemical activity. Theorell agreed with Berzelius' "far-sighted and prophetic" theory, declaring that enzymes were the catalyzers of the organic world.

In 1926, nearly one hundred years after Berzelius, German chemist Richard Willstätter attempted to produce pure enzymes. Willstätter conducted various adsorption experiments, removing impurities from selected enzymes, until little actual substance was left. He found that when he tested for protein, sugar or iron, the solutions gave negative results, even though they still revealed the catalytic enzyme effect. Willstätter reached the controversial conclusion that enzymes did not belong to any class of known substances.

During the 1920s J. B. Sumner and J. H. Northrop conducted similar purification experiments. Sumner produced the colorless crystals known as the enzyme urease. Northrop and his collaborators crystallized out pepsin, trypsin, and chymotrypsin. All of these substances were proteins, which challenged Willstätter's findings, yet none of the experimenters could prove conclusively that what they had produced were pure enzymes. Willstätter contended that the proteins were just inert carriers of small catalytic molecules.

Theorell's contribution to this work began in 1933 at Warburg's institute in Berlin. Warburg had been working on respiratory enzymes for decades. In 1914 he outlined the main structural aspects of the respiratory enzymes present in all cells. Later, when experimenting with crushed sea urchin eggs, he showed that absorption of oxygen could be increased when ferro-salts were added. Between 1921 and 1926 Warburg had convinced the scientific world that the respiratory enzyme contained iron.

Theorell added to this knowledge when he proved that enzymes were made up of proteins, putting to rest Willstätter's theory that had left enzymes unclassified. One year before Theorell arrived in Berlin, Warburg and his collaborator Christian had produced a yellow-colored preparation of an oxidation enzyme from yeast. Theorell showed that protein was a necessary component of the enzyme. He showed that the yellow enzyme isolated from yeast consisted of two parts, in a simple molecular relation of 1:1. The first was an enzyme of vitamin B_2 plus a phosphate group, and the second was a protein apoenzyme. He proved that neither part of the enzyme worked without the other, and that one part was a pure protein. For his work in the reversible splitting of the coenzyme from the yellow enzyme, Theorell was called the "'Master of Enzyme Research" by Warburg.

After 1935 Theorell continued work in enzymology, contributing especially to our knowledge of several oxidation enzymes, for which he won the Nobel Prize. He furthered understanding of the mechanism by which the coenzyme oxidizes glucose. He studied cytochrome C, peroxidases, catalases, flavoproteins, and pyridine protiens. He isolated crystalline myoglobin, and researched alcohol dehydrogenase, which led to the development of blood tests for alcohol levels.

Theorell was active in many scientific organizations. He was a member of learned societies in Sweden, Denmark, Norway, Finland, the United States, France, Italy, Poland, Belgium, and India. He was Secretary of the Swedish Medical Society from 1940 to 1946, and Chairman from 1947 to 1948 and from 1957 to 1958. He was a member of the Swedish Society for Medical Research from 1942 to 1950, the State Research Council for the Natural Sciences from 1950 to 1954, and the State Medical Research Council from 1958. Theorell was chairman of the Association of Swedish Chemists from 1947 to 1949. From 1954 to 1964 he was Chief Editor of the journal *Nordisk Medicin.* He served on many government committees and was chairman of the Swedish National Committee for Biochemistry.

VIRGINIA QUIROGA

Selected Bibliography

PRIMARY SOURCES

Theorell, Axel Hugo Teodor. 1943. "The Heme-Protein Linkage in Hemoglobin and in Horseradish Peroxidase." *Arkiv Kemi Mineral. Geol.* 16A:1–18.

———. 1951. "Catalases and Peroxidases." In *The Enzymes: Chemistry and Mechanism of Action*, 397–427. New York: Academic Press.

———. 1967. "Function and Structure of Liver Alcohol Dehydrogenase." *Harvey Lectures*, vol. 2, part 1. Series 61, 17–41. New York: Academic Press.

———. 1970. "Introduction to Mechanisms of Enzyme Actions." In *Metabolic Regulation and Enzyme Action*. A. Sols and S. Grisolia, eds. London: Academic Press.

———. 1975. "My Life with Proteins and Prosthetic Groups." In *Proteolysis and Physiological Regulation*, 1–27. D. W. Ribbons and K. Brew, eds. New York: Academic Press.

SECONDARY SOURCES

1964. *Nobel Lectures Including Presentation Speeches and Laureates' Biographies: Physiology or Medicine 1942–1962*, 480–97. Amsterdam: Elsevier Publishing Company.

Schlessinger, Bernard S. and June H. 1986. *The Who's Who of Nobel Prize Winners*, 99–100. Phoenix: Oryx Press.

Sourkes, Theodore L. 1971. *Nobel Prize Winners in Medicine and Physiology 1901–1965*, 323–29. London: Abelard-Schuman.

Taton, Rene, ed. 1964. *History of Science in the Twentieth Century*, 382–83. New York: Basic Books.

NIKOLAAS TINBERGEN 1973

Nikolaas Tinbergen was born on April 15, 1907, in the Hague, the Netherlands. A zoologist, he was awarded the Nobel Prize in 1973, jointly with Karl von Frisch and Konrad Lorenz, for his contributions to ethological research. He is most noted for his experimental elucidation of many theoretical problems, and in particular for the isolation of the stimulus that triggers a particular response and the measurement of the costs and benefits of evolutionary adaptation. At the time of the award, Tinbergen had just retired from his position as professor of animal behavior in the Animal Behavior Department he himself had organized at Oxford University. He and his wife, Elisabeth Amelie Rutten, a chemist whom he married in 1932, have two sons, Jacob and Dirk, and three daughters, Catharina, Jannetje, and Gerardina.

Tinbergen's parents were Dirk Cornelis and Jeannet van Eek Tinbergen. His older brother Jan became an economist and won the first Nobel Prize awarded in that field in 1969. Niko spent hours during his childhood watching birds and fish, and collecting plants and shells, at his parents' summer home, a cottage in Hulshorst near the sea. He enrolled at the State University of Leiden to study biology. Although as a boy he had been afraid of stinging insects, he wrote his doctoral thesis on the bee-killers, a species of digger wasps he was able to observe at Hulshorst. He confirmed experimentally that these insects used visual discrimination to locate their nests; this project earned him his Ph.D. in 1932.

He and his wife then participated in an expedition to Greenland (1931–32), where he observed the behaviors of snow buntings, phalaropes, sled dogs, and Eskimos. On their return, Tinbergen was appointed to the faculty at Leiden. For the next ten years he studied and experimented with wasps, sticklebacks (fish), and hobby falcons. His ability to test hypotheses drawn from observation by "comprehensive, careful, and quite ingenious experiments" distinguished him among the pioneers of ethology and made him a valuable collaborator of Konrad Lorenz, a self-described "poor experimenter." After meeting the older man in 1936, Tinbergen visited Lorenz's summer home at Altenberg for six months, where he and Lorenz studied the egg-rolling and retrieving behavior of the greylag goose. This joint project initiated a lifelong correspondence (Marler and Griffin 1973, 465; *New York Times*, 1973, 48).

The outbreak of World War II and the German occupation of the Netherlands interrupted their friendship. After he protested the treatment of Jewish professors at Leiden, Tinbergen was arrested and sent to a German prison camp for two years. In 1947 he returned to the university and was appointed professor of experimental biology. His studies at this time concentrated on the evolutionary processes leading to camouflage and other coloring adaptations. In 1949 he was invited to join the faculty at Oxford University to inaugurate animal behavior studies.

Tinbergen's pathbreaking work of the 1950s focused primarily on the behavior of seagulls, observed on the Farne Islands and at Scolt Head and Ravenglass. With his associates—Esther Cullen, Martin Moynihan, and Rita and Uli Weidman—he studied the attack, nest-building, chick-feeding, and mating behaviors of the birds, and the stimuli that elicited the behaviors. In the laboratory, he and his collaborators then used inanimate surrogates to separate the elements of each stimulus and study the response. These methods enabled the researchers to identify the particular element that triggers a particular evolved response. Further studies made clear the complex social and ecological trade-offs that influenced the equally complex behaviors. The research of this period confirmed hypotheses formulated by Tinbergen in Leiden in the 1940s (Marler and Griffin 1973, 465–66).

Eventually, Tinbergen extended these ideas to the problem of autism in children. He drew an analogy between the children's behavior and that of the gull caught between fear of other birds and the desire for companionship. Assisted by his wife, he achieved some success with therapy based on this analogy, but was heavily criticized by physicians who supported an organic etiology.

In another extension of his work to human behavior, he has supported the contention of his colleague Lorenz that humans' power to kill their own species has outrun their inhibition against doing so in response to submissive signals, and that we are consequently at great risk of destruction at our own hands.

Tinbergen was appointed to a full professorship at Oxford in 1968. His several fascinating books have attracted many lay readers, including children who enjoy his stories, *Kleew* and *The Tale of John Stickle*, originally published as letters to his own children while he was a German prisoner. Although retired since 1973, he continues to write and to observe gulls at his country home in Cumberland. An active ice skater and hockey player in his youth, he enjoys outdoor activity, combined with drawing and photography (*New York Times*, 1973, 48).

A BBC docmentary about his work, *Signals for Survival*, won the Italia Prize in 1969. He has received many honors, including the Bolsche Medal (1969), the Salvin Medal from the British Ornithology Union (1969), and the Jan Swammerdam Medal (1973).

MARCIA MELDRUM

Selected Bibliography

PRIMARY SOURCES

Tinbergen, Nikolaas. 1958. *Curious Naturalists.* New York: Basic Books.

———. 1960. *The Herring Gull's World: A Study of the Social Behavior of Birds.* New York: Basic Books.

———. 1962. *Social Behavior in Animals, with Special Reference to Vertebrates.* New York: John Wiley.

———. 1972–73. *The Animal in Its World: Explorations of an Ethologist, 1932–72.* Cambridge: Harvard University Press.

Tinbergen, Nikolaas, and Elisabeth A. Tinbergen. 1972. *Childhood Autism: An Ethological Approach.* Berlin: Parry.

SECONDARY SOURCES

Altman, Lawrence K. 1973. "Birds and Bees." *New York Times* (October 12):48.

Hall, Elizabeth. 1974. *Psychology Today* 7 (March):68–71.

Marler, P., and D. R. Griffin. 1973. "The 1973 Nobel Prize for Physiology or Medicine." *Science* 182 (November 2):464–66.

1973. "Nikolaas Tinbergen." *New York Times* (October 12):48.

1975. "Tinbergen, Niko(laas)." In *Current Biography Yearbook*, 414–16. New York: H. W. Wilson.

SUSUMU TONEGAWA *1987*

Susumu Tonegawa was born on September 5, 1939, in Nagoya, Japan. An immunobiologist, Tonegawa was the sole recipient of the Nobel Prize in 1987 for his demonstration of the mechanism of antibody production within the human body. An aggressive, determined researcher, he conducted experiments over a period of years that revealed a surprising, "unprecedented" model of genetic activity. Tonegawa has been a full professor at the Massachusetts Institute of Technology since 1981. In 1985 he married his second wife, Mayumi Toshinari, a former television reporter in Japan. Mrs. Tonegawa is now pursuing graduate studies in cognitive science at MIT. The couple have one son, Hidde.

Tonegawa received his undergraduate education at Kyoto University, completing his B.S. in chemistry in 1963. He came to the United States for graduate study, earning a Ph.D. in biology from the University of California at San Diego in 1969, and continuing as a research fellow at UCSD and the Salk Institute. In 1971 he joined the staff of the Basel Institute for Immunology, where he began the experiments that led to his prizewinning discovery.

The question Tonegawa undertook to answer was described by Thomas Waldmann of the National Cancer Institute as "the preeminent immunology problem" of the past thirty years: how cells are able to generate antibodies against any of the possible infections threatening the human body. The number of bacteria, viruses, and other infectious agents are virtually unlimited—and frequently mutate into new variations. When the body is threatened by such an invader, the cells have only a short time to identify the danger and manufacture appropriate antibodies. Yet the healthy individual is able to successfully resist hundreds of infections during his lifetime (Marx 1987, 484; Kolata 1987).

The earliest theories of antibody manufacture assumed that the sperm and egg cells contain all the genetic material needed to make any possible antibody. But, accurate knowledge of the structure and makeup of the germ cells made it clear that there is simply not enough room for all the genes that might potentially be needed. An alternate hypothesis, the "somatic mutation" theory, assumed a limited number of antibody genes that could mutate rapidly and with great flexibility to build the body's defenses.

Antibody molecules consist of two heavy protein chains and two smaller, light protein chains, organized in a symmetrical Y shape. Human antibodies are divided into five types, based on the components of the constant, or "C" segments, of the chains, which are the same for each antibody within a class. The constant segments form the base of the Y. The outer ends of the Y, however, vary significantly from one antibody to another; these are named the variable, or "V" segments.

In 1965 William Dreyer of the California Institute of Technology and J. C. Bennett of the University of Alabama suggested that the V and C segments are DNA-encoded separately within the germ cells and then combined during the process of development; thus, only one gene would be needed to encode the constant region, but each of the different V segments would have to be represented individually (Marx 1987, 484; Altman 1987).

Tonegawa followed up on this idea in experiments from 1974 to 1978 in Basel, working with Nobumichi Hozumi and other colleagues. They studied DNA from mouse embryos and then from mouse tumor cells that produced antibodies. They were able to establish that the genes encoding the V and C regions were initially widely separated in the embryo cells and then apparently joined together in the tumor cells. In collaboration with Walter Gilbert and Allan Maxam of Harvard University, Tonegawa then analyzed the nucleotide sequences of the DNA, using the new techniques originated by Daniel Nathans. The analysis revealed an unsuspected new region of 1250 uncoded base pairs of DNA separating the V and C segments, which was named the intron.

He next sequenced an embryonic gene segment encoded for the V region of a light protein chain and found that it lacked the full coding necessary for the complete chain of 110 amino acids; only 98 acids were represented. Philip Leder of the National Institute of Child Health and

Human Development reported a similar finding. The clear implication was that the V segment is actually genetically encoded as two or more segments. Leroy Hood of Caltech and Martin Weigert of the Fox Chase Institute in Philadelphia corroborated these findings in independent analyses of the amino acids in the light chains (Marx 1987).

Tonegawa and the Basel team found the missing piece, named the joining, or "J" segment, in the embryonic DNA, separated by 1250 base pairs from the gene encoding the C region. A light chain consists of the C-J-V sequence. However, both Tonegawa and Hood found in studying the formation of the heavy protein chains that still another segment is needed to complete the variable part of these chains; this is the diversity, or D, segment.

The new model of antibody production demonstrated by Tonegawa and the other researchers is based on several hundred different V segments, and also several J and D variations. Any of the possible V-J combinations, forming the light chains, may combine with any of the V-D-J combinations, forming the heavy chains; thus from the basic genetic components, several hundred million antibodies can be constructed.

The V-J and V-D-J combinations form during the development of the antibody producing cell; but the full antibody only emerges when the intron is cut out and the C and J segments joined directly. Hood and others have identified further variations based on slightly "incorrect" joinings or on somatic mutation, as earlier suggested. The possibilities therefore are literally endless, making possible a strong defense against the multiple infectious agents that threaten the body (Marx 1987, 485).

Applications of the model in clinical medicine include the improvement of vaccines and other therapies and the avoidance of rejection in organ transplants. But probably the most significant implication is for the study of the failure of immune defenses in lymphomas and leukemias, autoimmune disorders, and AIDS. In Burkitt's lymphoma, for example, the cancer cells grow from B lymphocytes, which are normally immune cells. Leder and other investigators have discovered that these cells in Burkitt's patients show heavy chain chromosomal abnormalities; when the segments begin to combine to form antibodies, some parts of the chain become weak and fragile, while in others DNA "control" is lost, allowing the development of irregular mutations, or tumors.

At MIT, Tonegawa has continued his research on the genetic basis of immunology. Among other findings, he has discovered that T cell receptors, which identify antigens and stimulate antibody production by B cells, are similar to antibody proteins in their genetic structure and assembly of several DNA segments. He has also identified an "enhancer," a fragment of the intron of the heavy-chain gene, which apparently plays an important role in gene function.

Described by his colleagues as "a very private man" and "not very interactive," he works in his own small laboratory, often on his own and late into the night, and has participated only minimally in teaching. But his single-minded and intent approach to his work has obviously brought results. Although many colleagues were working on the problem of antibody diversity at the same time, Tonegawa was the first to devise and carry out the very difficult experiments that led to the solution (Altman 1987; Marx 1987, 485; Kolata 1987).

He is the first Japanese to win the Nobel Prize in Physiology or Medicine. Among the other awards he has received are the Albert Lasker Medical Research Award (jointly with Hood and Leder), and the Bristol-Myers Award, both in 1987. He is a member of the American Association of Immunologists and a foreign associate of the National Academy of Sciences.

MARCIA MELDRUM

Selected Bibliography

PRIMARY SOURCES

Tonegawa, S., and M. Hayashi. 1968. "Genetic Transcription Directed by the B2 Region of Lambda Bacteriophage." *Proceedings of the National Academy of Sciences USA* 61 (December):1320–27.

Tonegawa, S., C. Steinberg, S. Duke *et al.* 1974. "Evidence for Somatic Generation of Antibody Diversity." *Proceedings of the National Academy of Sciences* 71 (October):4027–31.

Tonegawa, S. 1976. "Reiteration Frequency of Immunoglobulin Light Chain Genes; Further Evidence for Somatic Generation of Antibody Diversity." *Proceedings of the National Academy of Sciences* 73 (January):203–7.

Tonegawa, S., N. Hozumi, G. Mathhyssens *et al.* 1977. "Somatic Changes in the Content and Context of Immunoglobulin Genes." *Cold Spring Harbor Symposium on Quantitative Biology*, 41, no. 2: 877–89.

Tonegawa, S., C. Brack, N. Hozumi, and V. Pirotta. 1977. "Organization of Immunoglobulin Genes." *Cold Spring Harbor Symposium on Quantitative Biology* 42, no. 2:921–31.

Tonegawa, S., C. Brack, N. Hozumi *et al.* 1977. "Dynamics of Immunoglobulin Genes." *Immunological Review* 36:73–94.

Tonegawa, S., C. Brack, M. Hirama, and R. Lenhard-Schuller. 1979. "Somatic Recombination and Structure of an Immunoglobulin Gene." In *Cells of Immunoglobulin Synthesis*, edited by B. Pernis and H. S. Vogel, New York: Academic Press:15–32.

SECONDARY SOURCES

Altman, Lawrence K. 1987. "MIT Scientist Wins Nobel Prize for Medicine." *New York Times* (October 13):C1, C3.

Kolata, Gina. 1987. "An Aggressive, Brilliant Researcher." *New York Times* (October 13):C3.

Marx, Jean L. 1987. "Antibody Research Garners Nobel Prize." *Science* 238 (October 23):484–85.

JOHN ROBERT VANE 1982

John Robert Vane was born on March 29, 1927, in Tardebigg, Worcestershire, England. A biochemist and pharmacologist, Vane won the Nobel Prize in 1982 jointly with Sune Bergström and Bengt Samuelsson, for their work in characterizing, differentiating, and describing the action of the prostaglandins, a field in which Bergström pioneered. Vane developed the dynamic bioassay method that he then used to investigate the behaviors of the various prostaglandins in the body. His hypothesis that aspirin's analgesic and anti-inflammatory effects were a result of its inhibition of prostaglandin synthesis was not only a pharmacologic breakthrough but encouraged research into the influence of these highly active compounds on all physiologic functions. Vane is group research and development director at the Wellcome Research Laboratories in Kent, the position he held at the time of the Nobel award. He married Elizabeth Daphne Page, a family counselor, in 1948; they have two daughters, Nicola and Miranda.

Vane grew up in Birmingham with his parents, Maurice and Frances Florence Fisher Vane; his father was a businessman. He received a chemistry set for Christmas when he was twelve and as a teenager conducted many experiments in the kitchen and backyard, not always to the delight of his family. After he began to study at the University of Birmingham, however, his interests matured and changed, and he eagerly accepted a suggestion from a professor that he study pharmacology at Oxford with J. H. Burn. During his work with Burn he learned the creative methods of bioassay (measurement of a substance's effects in a living biological system) developed by the British scientists Sir Henry Dale and Sir John Gaddum. Vane received his B.S. in chemistry from Birmingham in 1946, his B.S. in pharmacology from Oxford in 1949, and his Ph.D. from Oxford in 1953. During his last two years at Oxford, he held a Stothert Research Fellowship from the Royal Society (*Current Biography* 1986, 576; Oates 1982, 765).

Vane taught from 1953 to 1955 at Yale University before accepting an appointment as senior lecturer in the Department of Pharmacology at the Institute of Basic Medical Sciences, of the University of London and the Royal College of Physicians. In the early 1960s he developed his dynamic bioassay method to study the metabolism of the angiotensins in the blood. Using a group of isolated organs known to contract in response to certain substances, he bathed each with a "cascade" of blood or other fluid. By comparing the responses of the organs with those already determined and with each other, he was able simultaneously to measure the presence and level of the substances in the fluids. He was promoted to professor of experimental pharmacology in 1966.

By that time, he had learned of Bergström and Samuelsson's work and was preparing to adapt his bioassay to the study of the prostaglandins (Oates 1982, 765).

The first interest in these highly active lipid compounds resulted from early artificial insemination procedures performed by Raphael Kurzrok, Charles Leib, and Sarah Ratner at Columbia University in 1930. The physicians noted that the injection of seminal plasma into the uterus caused the smooth muscle to contract and then to relax. Maurice Goldblatt in England and Ulf von Euler in Sweden undertook further experiments with seminal fluid from rams before World War II. They observed lowered blood pressure as well as smooth muscle responses in a number of animals. Von Euler identified the active compounds in the secretions of the prostate gland and gave them the name "prostaglandins."

Von Euler introduced Sune Bergström to prostaglandins in 1945. The latter's interest was immediately stirred and he eagerly accepted a small quantity of the extracts von Euler had made from ram semen in the 1930s. Using the most advanced techniques available, he further purified the compounds and was astonished to observe that "after purification essentially to weightlessness, they retained extraordinary activity." Despite his fascination, Bergström's work on prostaglandins was delayed for almost a decade because of the technical difficulties involved and his own administrative commitments (Oates 1982, 765).

By 1958 several factors had made possible the isolation, analysis, and characterization of the mysterious compounds. Bergström and his colleagues, Jan Sjovall, Bengt Samuelsson, and Ragnar Ryhage, had collected a sufficient number of sheep seminal glands to prepare the extracts for intensive study. (Roughly 100 kilograms of sheep glands were required for each usable extract.) Bergström had developed the necessary methods of gas chromatography, and Ryhage had invented a method of interface between the chromatograph and the mass spectrometer that permitted the structural analysis of small quantities. The application of this technology to the study of the prostaglandins has now been replicated in many other scientific fields (Oates 1982, 765–66).

The team soon isolated the first two compounds; through 1964 they continued to describe the structure and activity of the prostaglandin group, including PGE_2, $PGF_{2\alpha}$, and PGD_2. The related compounds thromboxane A_2, prostacyclin, and the leukotrienes were discovered later. Prostaglandins are found throughout the human body. Each possesses the same twenty-carbon atom skeleton and fatty acid structure, but different ones are produced by different cells to perform different and highly specific functions. Thromboxane A_2, for example, is a product of platelets and stimulates platelet aggregation and vasoconstriction, whereas prostacyclin, metabolized by the endothelial cells, has the opposite action.

The new understanding of prostaglandin structure confirmed von

Euler's hunch that these compounds were the result of lipid oxygenation. The logical candidate was arachidonic acid, a twenty-carbon polyunsaturated fatty acid. By 1965 Bergstrom, Samuelsson, and David Van Dorp at the Unilever Laboratories in Holland demonstrated that arachidonic acid was indeed the common biosynthetic origin of all prostaglandins. This finding showed the way to in vitro prostaglandins synthesis for research use and solved the supply problems (Oates 1982, 765–66).

In England, John Vane and his colleague, Priscilla Piper, obtained some prostaglandins for testing from the Upjohn Company and used the cascade method to differentiate their actions. In the course of their initial assays of lung tissue, they observed a strong, transient contraction of a rabbit aorta, in response to an unknown substance, which they named RCS (rabbit aorta contracting substance). They soon demonstrated that aspirin and other anti-inflammatory drugs inhibited the action of RCS.

Over a weekend in 1971 Vane wondered if the synthesis of prostaglandins from arachidonic acid and the effects of the anti-inflammatory drugs were related, and then quickly designed an experiment to test the hypothesis. By Monday he had completed the experiment, which was confirmed by further trials. Aspirin, indomethacin, and several other drugs were shown to inhibit the production of PGE_2 and $PGF_{2\alpha}$. Vane then proposed that this inhibition accounted for the drugs' ability to alleviate pain and reduce inflammation (Oates 1982, 766–67).

Samuelsson was interested in Vane's findings. The logical assumption was that the mysterious RCS was in fact a new prostaglandin. However, aspirin also had the effect of blocking platelet aggregation, an effect not known to be the result of prostaglandin action.

Samuelsson had been investigating the production of prostaglandins in vivo. Using mass spectrometry to analyze the oxygenation of arachidonic acid, he had identified an intermediate stage in the process, the formation of a cyclic endoperoxide. Samuelsson and Mats Hamberg observed the effects of their endoperoxides on platelets and noted that these "intermediate" substances did act to aggregate the blood cells. By correlating their observations with the biochemical reactions in process, they found that the endoperoxides in platelets and in lung tissue were synthesized to a hitherto unknown substance which they named thromboxane A_2. This compound, Vane's RCS, was very active in stimulating aggregation and also the contraction of vascular smooth muscle (Oates 1982, 766–67).

Vane had joined the Wellcome Foundation in 1973. Working with Salvador Moncado, Richard Gryglewski, and Stuart Bunting, he applied his bioassay techniques to other tissues to determine which were the sites of prostaglandin synthesis. While testing vascular tissue in 1976, they observed vasodilation and the inhibition of platelet aggregation: in other words, precisely the opposite effects to those observed with thromboxane A_2. Vane's team worked with the Upjohn research staff to characterize this new prostaglandin, which is produced primarily in the vascular endothelium by metabolism of the same endoperoxide that produces thromboxane. It was given the name prostacyclin. Knowledge of these new compounds clarified and extended medical understanding of the body's blood clotting mechanisms and controls (Oates 1982, 767).

Aspirin and similar substances apparently block formation of prostaglandins from arachidonic acid by inhibiting the stimulus enzyme cyclooxygenase. However, corticosteroids have additional anti-inflammatory effects that aspirin does not. Samuelsson therefore theorized that the corticosteroids did not act on cyclooxygenase metabolism alone, but on some related synthesis. Working with Pierre Borgeat, he observed the fate of arachidonic acid in polymorphonuclear leukocytes. The fatty acid was found to be oxygenated in these cells by a 5-lipoxygenase, into a new class of prostaglandins designated the leukotrienes. One of the intermediate products, an epoxide named LTA_4, was subsequently discovered, by Samuelsson, Robert Murphy, and E. J. Corey at Harvard, to react with glutathione to form several very powerful bronchoconstrictor compounds related to asthma and other anaphylactic reactions.

The multiple functions of the prostaglandins and their powerful activity has thus suggested a wide range of clinical applications, many still in the experimental stages. These include pain relief, induction of labor and of abortion, prevention of ulcers, correction of birth defects, vasodilation in surgery, and applications in asthma, cancer, and heart disease, among others (Oates 1982, 767–68; Altman 1982).

John Vane was elected to the Royal Society in 1974. He is active in the British Pharmacological Society and the Society for Drug Research. Although he enjoys water-skiing, snorkeling, and scuba diving, "he works 99 percent of the time," according to his wife, because "he enjoys his work so much." Among the many other honors he has received are the Baly Medal from the Royal College of Physicians (1977), the Albert Lasker Basic Medical Research Award (1977), the Peter Debye Prize from the University of Maastricht (1980), the Galen Medal from the Apothecaries' Society, and the Louis Pasteur Foundation Prize (1984) (Wilford 1982).

MARCIA MELDRUM

Selected Bibliography

PRIMARY SOURCES

Vane, John R., and Harry Robinson. 1974. *Prostaglandin Synthetase Inhibitors—Their Effects on Physiological Functions and Pathological States*. New York: Raven Press.

Vane, John R., and Y. S. Bakhle. 1977. *Metabolic Functions of the Lung*. New York: Dekker.

Vane, John R., and S. H. Ferreira. 1979. *Inflammation*. New York: Springer-Verlag.

Vane, John R., and S. K. Bergström. 1979. *Prostacyclin*. New York: Raven Press.

Vane, John R., and G. V. R. Bonn. 1981. *Interactions Between Platelets and Vessel Walls.* Great Neck, N.Y.: Scholium International.

Vane, John R. 1982. *Prostacyclin in Health and Disease.* Edinburgh: Royal College of Physicians.

SECONDARY SOURCES

Altman, Lawrence K. 1982. "Two Swedes and Briton Win Nobel for Clues to Body's Chemistry. *New York Times* (October 12):1, C3.

Oates, John A. 1982. "The 1982 Nobel Prize in Physiology or Medicine." *Science* 218 (November 19):765–68.

1986. "Vane, John R(obert)." In *Current Biography Yearbook*, 575–78. New York: H. W. Wilson.

Wilford, John Noble. 1982. "Men in the News: John Robert Vane." *New York Times* (October 12):C3.

HAROLD ELLIOT VARMUS *1989*

Harold Elliot Varmus, molecular virologist, was born December 18, 1939, in Oceanside, New York. He shared the 1989 Nobel Prize with J. Michael Bishop for their pathbreaking discovery that normal cellular genes can malfunction and trigger the abnormal cell growth of cancer. Varmus is currently professor of biochemistry and biophysics at the University of California at San Francisco.

Varmus's father was a general practitioner. Varmus earned his B.A. in English literature at Amherst College in Massachusetts in 1961 and continued on to graduate school at Harvard, specializing in seventeenth century prose. In 1962, however, he decided he wanted "to have more to do with contemporary life" and began the study of medicine at Columbia University. After receiving his M.D. in 1966, he spent four years as a research fellow, working with Ira Pastan at the National Cancer Institute on bacterial production of proteins. At NCI he confirmed his preference for research over clinical medicine (Kolata 1989).

In 1970, Varmus accepted a postdoctoral fellowship at UCSF and "ran into Mike Bishop almost by accident. . . . Mike and I hit it off right away." The two began investigating the behavior of retroviruses, which can cause cancer to develop in animals, and oncogenes, the carcinogenic genes found in the viruses. Rous sarcoma virus, for example, produced sarcoma, or cancers of the connective tissues, in chickens, and could also "infect" cells in laboratory cultures with remarkable virulence. In the 1970s, a single gene, called *src* for sarcoma, had been identified as the oncogene in Rous sarcoma virus. However, no human cancer had ever been traced to Rous sarcoma or to any other retrovirus (Marx 1989a).

Robert Huebner and George Todaro of the National Cancer Institute had suggested that all cells might contain potential oncogenes, in the form of viral DNA left over from some ancient infection of early life forms. Through many evolutionary generations, the hypothesis said, the DNA lay dormant, merely replicating itself with the normal cellular DNA. But certain stimuli, such as radiation, would cause the viral material, which Huebner and Todaro called "proviruses," to become active and to produce malignant cell growth (Marx 1989a).

Bishop and Varmus set up a series of experiments to test this oncogene hypothesis. Their idea was to find *src* gene DNA material in normal chicken cells. Lacking the techniques of gene cleavage and sequencing that have since been developed, they found the work "brutally difficult." Bishop has said that he "personally did not think the experiments would work" (Kolata 1989).

The painstaking efforts of the UCSF team, including C. T. Deng, Ramareddy Guntaka, Deborah Spector, Dominique Stehelin and P. K. Vogt, did indeed uncover *src* gene DNA, not only in chicken cells but in those of several other birds and some mammals. The guilty gene was found not to be an ancient viral invader, however, but a normal cellular gene. This observation "turned the oncogene hypothesis on its head" and was doubted by many scientists when first reported in 1976, but since then nearly 50 normal cellular genes have been identified as "proto-oncogenes" (Marx 1989a; Kolata 1989).

The work of Bishop, Varmus, and others has shown that these genes assist in the regulation of normal cell growth and division. Radiation, chemical toxins, or other carcinogens may produce a mutation of the gene, which will then initiate abnormal cell division, resulting in malignant growth. Carcinogenesis by a retrovirus is not caused by the viral genes; rather, the virus picks up a normal gene from a cell during infection and then carries it to another cell, where the gene becomes an abnormal component of the DNA and again triggers malignancy.

The discovery of the proto-oncogene, while overturning ideas of viral origin, strongly supported researchers' convictions that "there is a final common pathway in causing cancer" and has led to much new and creative investigation. It has been important as well for clinical diagnosis, prognosis and treatment. If particular types of oncogenes are detected in cancerous cells, the physician gains a better understanding of the history and probable course of the disease and is able to plan therapy accordingly (Marx 1989a; Kolata 1989).

Harold Varmus was appointed assistant professor of microbiology in 1972 and full professor in 1982. In 1988, he spent a year's sabbatical working with David Baltimore at MIT. Baltimore commended his "very long-range perspective. . . . [he] can see what it would mean if his experiments are successful" (Kolata 1989). Varmus is a member of the National Academy of Sciences, the American Society of Microbiologists, and the American Society of Virologists. He serves as an associate editor for *Cell and Virology* and as a consultant for the American Cancer Society.

For Varmus, winning the Nobel Prize was a pleasant shock, slightly marred by the protest of Dominique Stehelin, now with the Institut Pasteur in Lille, France, that the prize should have been shared with him for carrying out some of the crucial experiments. His claim was rejected, however, by the Nobel Committee, which reiterated its view that Bishop and Varmus were the "key persons in the discovery" (Marx 1989b; Kolata 1989).

MARCIA MELDRUM

Selected Bibliography

PRIMARY SOURCES

Varmus, H. E., J. M. Bishop, and P. K. Vogt. 1973. "Appearance of Virus-Specific DNA in Mammalian Cells Following Transformation by Rous Sarcoma Virus." *Journal of Molecular Biology* 74 (March 15):613–626.

Varmus, H. E., J. Stavneser, E. Medeiros, *et al.* 1975. "Detection and Characterization of RNA Tumor Virus-Specific DNA in Cells." *Bibliotheca Haematologica* 40:451–461.

Stehelin, D., H. E. Varmus, and J. M. Bishop. 1975. "Detection of Nucleotide Sequences Associated with Transformation by Avian Sarcoma Viruses." *Bibliotheca Haematologica* 43 (October):539–541.

Stehelin, D., H. E. Varmus, and J. M. Bishop, *et al.* 1976. "DNA Related to the Transforming Gene(s) of Avian Sarcoma Virus is Present in Normal Avian DNA." *Nature* 260 (March 11):170–173.

Stehelin, D., R. V. Guntaka, H. E. Varmus, *et al.* 1976. "Purification of DNA Complementary to Nucleotide Sequences Required for Neoplastic Transformation of Fibroblasts by Avian Sarcoma Viruses." *Journal of Molecular Biology* 101 (March):349–365.

Bishop, J. M., B. Baker, D. Fujita, P. McCombe, D. Sheiness, K. Smith, D. H. Spector, D. Stehelin, and H. E. Varmus. 1978. "Genesis of a Virus-Transforming Gene." *National Cancer Institute Monographs* 48 (May):219–223.

SECONDARY SOURCES

Kolata, Gina. 1989. "2 Doctors Share Nobel Prize for Work with Cancer Genes." *New York Times* (October 10):C3.

Marx, Jean L. 1989. "Cancer Gene Research Wins Medicine Nobel." *Science* 246 (October 20):326–327.

———. 1989. "Controversy Over Nobel." *Science* 246 (October 20):326–327.

JULIUS WAGNER-JAUREGG
1927

Julius Wagner-Jauregg was born on March 7, 1857, in Wels, Austria. A psychiatrist, Wagner-Jauregg received the Nobel Prize in 1927 for his use of malaria inoculation to induce fever in patients with dementia paralytica, or syphilitic paresis. He had retired as extraordinary professor of psychiatry and nervous diseases the year before winning the award. Wagner-Jauregg married Anna Koch in 1899; they had two children, a daughter, Julia, and a son, Theodor, who became a professor of chemistry. Wagner-Jauregg died on September 27, 1940, in Vienna.

He was born Julius Wagner, the son of Ludovika Ranzoni and Adolf Johann Wagner, an Austrian government official. He was educated at the famous and elite Schottengymnasium in Vienna and began his medical studies at the University of Vienna in 1874. His career was rooted in the new fields of microscopy and experimental biology, which he acquired at the Institute of General and Experimental Pathology. Here, as assistant to Salomon Stricker from 1874 to 1882, he became familiar with the use of experimental animal models. He also met the young Sigmund Freud, and the two became lifelong friends. Wagner earned a Ph.D. in 1880 with a thesis on the accelerated heart. Shortly thereafter, in 1883, his father was granted the title "Ritter von Jauregg" and he became Wagner von Jauregg. He took the hyphenated name "Wagner-Jauregg" when titles of nobility were abolished after the dissolution of the Hapsburg Empire in 1918.

For a short time after leaving the institute, he worked in the Department of Internal Diseases at the University of Vienna but was apparently unable to find a permanent position in internal medicine. In 1883, therefore, he accepted a job as Max von Leidesdorf's assistant in the Psychiatric Clinic, although he had no training in neurology or psychiatry. He became greatly interested in the field, however, qualifying to teach neurology in 1885 and psychiatry three years later. In 1887 Wagner von Jauregg acted as director of the clinic while Leidesdorf was ill.

His first research concerned the problem of stimulating respiration after strangulation and led him to studies of the functions of the accelerant and vagal nerves. He attempted shock therapy using large doses of chemical agents and physical stimuli. His ideas about shock interested him in the possibilities of treating mental illness by fever induction.

His first paper on the effects of febrile illness on psychosis appeared in 1887; he noted that the patients' mental state appeared to improve after the fever subsided. In particular, paresis, or dementia paralytica, the progressive paralytic infection of the brain and meninges associated with tertiary syphilis, was remitted, sometimes for years, following high fever. As likely candidates for fever induction, he named malaria and erysipelas.

From 1889 to 1893 Wagner von Jauregg succeeded Richard von Krafft-Ebing as professor of psychiatry and neurology and director of the Neuro-Psychiatric Clinic at the University of Graz. At Graz, he became interested in the relationship between cretinism and goiter, which he attributed to a failure of thyroid function. He endeavored to develop therapies based on a glandular extract and on the addition of minimal doses of iodine to table salt. In 1923 the Austrian government finally implemented the sale of iodized salt.

Wagner von Jauregg also continued his work with fever therapy on paresis patients at Graz. He was reluctant to try malaria at this time, even though it could be treated successfully with quinine. Instead, he used tuberculin, newly discovered by Robert Koch, to safely induce a fever without actually infecting the patient with a deadly disease. After the tuberculin injections did lead to remissions in several trial patients, he began systematic treatments, combined with an iodine-mercury antisyphilitic compound and then with Salvarsan. However, although remissions were often observed, nearly all the patients eventually relapsed. When tuberculin was later found to be more dangerous than at first thought, the experiments were discontinued.

He also became interested at this time in forensic medicine and the legal process of certification of the insane. He served on the Austrian Board of Health as advisor on psychiatric issues and assisted in formulating the law on certification, which remained in effect for many years.

In 1892 Wagner von Jauregg was appointed to the staff of the Landesirrenstalt (the State Asylum); and the following year returned to Vienna as extraordinary professor of psychiatry and nervous diseases and director of the university clinic. In 1902, seeking more varied and interesting cases, he transferred his clinical base to the Vienna General Hospital, where he served as director of the Psychiatry Clinic. In 1911, however, the Landesirrenstalt and the University Clinic were moved to a new and larger facility in suburban Steinhof. Wagner von Jauregg returned to his old position, where he presided over a thriving and theoretically diverse school of psychiatry.

In 1917, his earlier experiments with tuberculosis and other pyretics having failed to produce permanent results, he finally determined to act on his thirty-year-old idea of experimental malaria induction for syphilitic paresis. The admission of a malaria patient to one of his wards appeared to be the prompting of fate. He inoculated a series of nine cases; six soon demonstrated impressive remissions. Of these six, three were successfully arrested for ten years. After observation of these patients over a two-year period, he was sufficiently encouraged to publish his results and to extend the study.

Induction of malaria to produce fever was the treatment of choice for syphilitic paresis until penicillin came into general use after World War II. The disease is easy to control and the mortality is low. The results are generally excellent, with 30 to 40 percent of the patients showing complete recovery; most of these are in the early stages, since it is impossible to reverse the damage once the paralysis has progressed to the central nervous system.

Wagner von Jauregg's ideas about nonspecific process therapies, to shock the body's natural defenses and increase its powers of resistance, were in conflict with the "magic bullet" concept advanced by Paul Ehrlich. Salvarsan, Ehrlich's discovery, was not effective against tertiary syphilis, although Wagner von Jauregg used it with his tuberculin treatment and later combined malarial fever therapy with neoarsphenamine, an improved form of Salvarsan. In the case of syphilis, penicillin, a broad-spectrum antibiotic, proved more effective than either model, but nonspecific and stress treatments still have an influence in modern psychiatry.

Malarial fever induction as a treatment for a progressive neurologic disease also has to be understood in the context of the clinical emphasis of the Vienna Medical School and the transfer of experimental interventive techniques from general medicine. Wagner von Jauregg approached psychiatry as an experimental biologist.

His many students found him aloof and reserved but fair and conscientious. He was dedicated to his work at the university and the Landesirrenstalt until his retirement in 1928, at age seventy-one.

In his last years, Wagner-Jauregg enjoyed good health and remained active, publishing eighty scientific papers. He was further honored for his therapeutic discovery by the Cameron Prize from the University of Edinburgh (1935) and the Gold Medal of the American Committee for Research on Syphilis (1937). He died in 1940, at age eighty-three.

PAUL WEINDLING

Selected Bibliography

PRIMARY SOURCES

Wagner von Jauregg, Julius. 1887. "Über den Einwirkung Fieberhafter Erkrankungen auf Psychosen." *Jahrbuch für Psychiatrie und Neurologie* 7:94–131.

———. 1901. "Zur Reform des Irrenwesens." *Viennaer Klinische Wochenschrift* 14:293–96.

———. 1915. *Myoxödem und Kretinismus.* Leipzig, Germany: F. Deuticke.

———. 1918–1919. "Über den Einwirkung der Malaria die Progressive Paralyse." *Psychiatrisch-Neurologische Wochenschrift* 20:132–34.

———. 1936. *Fieber und Infektionstherapie. Ausgewahlten Beitrage 1887–1935.* Vienna: Verlag fur Medizin, Weidmann.

SECONDARY SOURCES

Dattner, B. 1970. "Julius Wagner, von Jauregg." In W. Haymaker and F. Schiller, *The Founders of Neurology*, 528–31. Springfield, Illinois: C. C. Thomas.

Lesky, Erna. 1976. *The Vienna Medical School of the Nineteenth Century*, 350–64. Baltimore: Johns Hopkins University Press.

———. 1976. "Wagner von Jauregg, Julius." In *Dictionary of Scientific Biography*, 14:114–16. New York: Scribners.

SELMAN ABRAHAM WAKSMAN
1952

Selman Abraham Waksman was born on July 22, 1888, in Priluka, Russia. A soil microbiologist, Waksman was awarded the 1952 Nobel Prize in Physiology or Medicine in recognition of his "ingenious, systematic and successful studies of the soil microbes that have led to the discovery of streptomycin, the first antibiotic effective against tuberculosis." The isolation of streptomycin by Waksman and his coworkers in 1943 represented the first major success of a project that Waksman had instituted four years earlier to methodically screen thousands of actinomycetes for their antimicrobial activity. The actinomycetes, soil microorganisms displaying morphological characteristics of both bacteria and fungi, had been a research interest of Waksman's for decades and the discovery of streptomycin was a logical, if unforeseeable, culmination to his career as a microbiologist strongly committed to pursuing practical applications for his science. Waksman died on August 16, 1973, in Hyannis, Massachusetts.

The son of Jacob Waksman, a modest property owner, and his wife Fradia London, Waksman spent his youth within the Jewish community of the small Ukrainian village of Priluka. Early in his life, as he struggled to obtain a secondary education, the young Waksman personally experienced the legal and social restrictions that limited the lives of Jews in czarist Russia. Therefore, even after successfully sitting for the university matriculation examinations as an extern at an Odessa *gymnasium* in 1910, Waksman decided to emigrate to the United States. He became a naturalized citizen six years later. Although Waksman fervently embraced his new homeland, he maintained through his life the cosmopolitan outlook and broad cultural interests characteristic of the Russian-Jewish intelligentsia. Waksman maintained his ties to his past in another way as well: his wife, Deborah B. Mitnik, was also a native of Priluka. The couple was married August 5, 1916, and had one son, Byron H. Waksman.

A brief sojourn with relatives on a farm in New Jersey and the award of a scholarship led Waksman to continue his education at nearby Rutgers College. There, the direction of Waksman's scientific interests was decisively shaped under the influence of bacteriologist Jacob G. Lipman. While still an undergraduate, Waksman began a study of microbial soil populations under Lipman's direction, becoming particularly interested in the then little-known actinomycetes. After receiving his B.S. in agricultural science in 1915, Waksman stayed on as a research assistant to Lipman at the New Jersey Agricultural Experimental Station, completing his master's degree in soil bacteriology in 1916. Waksman then left Rutgers to continue graduate studies in biochemistry at the University of California at Berkeley, where he completed his doctoral research into the biochemistry of microbial processes with T. B. Robertson in 1918.

Waksman's separation from Rutgers proved to be brief, he returned in 1918 to accept a position as microbiologist at the New Jersey Agricultural Experimental Station and lecturer in soil microbiology in the College of Agriculture. Waksman remained on the faculty at Rutgers for the rest of his career, becoming a full professor in 1930, head of the Department of Microbiology from 1940 to 1954, and director of the Institute of Microbiology (founded by Rutgers University with the royalties from streptomycin) from 1949 until his retirement in 1958.

During the first two decades of his scientific activity Waksman established a distinguished reputation in his field as a microbiologist primarily, but not exclusively, concerned with the study of soil microorganisms. Waksman also played an important role in the development of soil microbiology as a scientific discipline in the United States. He trained dozens of students in his laboratory at Rutgers, influenced thousands of others through his treatise *Principles of Soil Microbiology* (1927), and also labored to strengthen ties with the international community of soil microbiologists.

Waksman himself assessed his own scientific contributions from this period as "fruitful if not revolutionary" (*My Life with Microbes*, 1954). From his early interest in actinomycetes, Waksman moved on to tackle a host of other topics in soil microbiology. These included the isolation and investigation of *Thiobacillus thiooxidans*, a sulfur-oxidizing soil microbe; study of the relation of microbes to soil fertility and work on development of a microbial index of soil fertility; research into the role of microbes in organic decomposition; and work on the origin and nature of humus. His work on humus led Waksman to the study of marine microbes and a position as marine bacteriologist at the Woods Hole Oceanographic Institution from 1931 to 1942. Always eager to find practical outlets for his research, Waksman also worked as a consultant to government and industry on a number of problems, from a survey of New Jersey peat bog resources to methods for large-scale production of microbial enzymes and fermentation products. The scores of publications that issued from the Rutgers lab on these diverse topics were possible due only to Waksman's strong organizational abilities and tight control over the research projects of his students and associates.

During the 1930s Waksman was gradually drawn to a new area for application of his knowledge of soil microbes: the investigation of their potential use against the pathogenic microbes that cause disease. While Waksman's own previous research on the antagonistic and associative effects of microorganisms had pointed in this direction, the decisive factor in drawing his attention to his field seems to have been the work of a former student, René Dubos, who had been investigating soil bacteria for their antibiotic activity since the late 1920s. Dubos's isolation of the highly toxic antibiotic gramicidin from a soil bacteria in 1939 helped convince Waksman that a systematic search of soil microbes would be a fruitful way to uncover other, more usable antimicrobial substances.

That same year, Waksman initiated a systematic and intensive research program for isolating, identifying, and testing potential antibiotics derived from soil microbes, devoting much of the personnel and resources of his laboratory to the project. For financial assistance he turned to private sources, including Merck and Company of New Jersey, a pharmaceutical firm for which Waksman had been a consultant for some time. In addition to funding a fellowship in Waksman's laboratory, Merck agreed to provide research and development assistance for any promising antibiotics in exchange for exclusive assignment of patent rights to the company.

Waksman's conviction that the actinomycetes would prove to be a particularly good source of antimicrobial substances was borne out by the isolation of actinomycin in 1940 and streptothricin in 1942—both were highly toxic but promising antimicrobial agents. The enormous work of identifying and testing thousands of strains of actinomycetes was finally rewarded with success in August 1943 when one of Waksman's graduate students, Albert Schatz, isolated streptomycin from a strain of actinomycete that Waksman himself had first studied twenty-five years earlier. The Rutgers team quickly found that this newest antibiotic was both relatively nontoxic and effective against a number of pathogenic bacteria *in vitro*. By the time the first notice of the discovery of streptomycin appeared six months later, the clinical and commercial potentialities of streptomycin were being intensively studied not only at Rutgers and at Merck but also by William H. Feldman and H. Corwin Hinshaw, clinicians at the Mayo Clinic who had been carrying out their own search for an antituberculosis drug for some years. It was the success of the Mayo trials of streptomycin against tuberculosis in animals and humans that dramatically brought the drug to the forefront of medical and public attention.

In the resulting avalanche of publicity and acclaim, much of the public attention focused on Waksman as the discoverer of the world's newest "miracle drug." Thus began a new and unexpected public life for the scientist, characterized by extensive international travel, lectures, and tours of medical facilities. Everywhere Waksman was met by outporings of gratitude by former tuberculosis patients and their families. Official acknowledgment of the importance of streptomycin was not long delayed, and Waksman began to accumulate an impressive list of awards and honorary degrees.

But the success of streptomycin also brought problems in its wake. Waksman and Rutgers University soon felt that the great demand for streptomycin rendered their agreement with Merck both impractical and inequitable, and they persuaded the company to return the patent to Rutgers and agree to a nonexclusive licensing arrangement instead. The royalties from the eight companies that eventually produced the antibiotic proved to be an unexpected financial windfall for the university and Waksman personally.

This in turn sparked another difficulty: a law suit brought by Albert Schatz in 1950 demanding formal recognition as codiscoverer of streptomycin and a share of the royalties from its sale. This widely publicized case, of a kind hitherto virtually unknown within the American scientific community, evidently deeply shocked and embarrassed Waksman. The suit was eventually resolved in an out-of-court settlement in which Schatz's role was acknowledged and a formula for the distribution of royalties among Waksman, Schatz, and the other scientists and technicians involved in the project was agreed upon. Waksman later reduced his personal share of the royalties still further, devoting the remainder to the establishment of the philanthropic Foundation for Microbiology.

After the trauma of the Schatz lawsuit, Waksman was to some extent vindicated two years later when he became the sole recipient of the Nobel Prize in Physiology or Medicine for 1952. But the award of the prize to Waksman alone does raise the issue of whether the contributions of Dubos, Feldman, and Hinshaw to the search for, and application of, streptomycin were adequately acknowledged. An additional irony was that by the early 1950s the initial euphoria over streptomycin had faded as significant problems and limitations to the use of streptomycin in the treatment of tuberculosis became apparent. In fact, 1952 was the year of the introduction into clinical practice of the chemical isoniazid, a significantly more effective treatment for tuberculosis.

In the postwar period Waksman's scientific work continued to focus on the actinomycetes and their antibiotic products. The screening program at Rutgers continued unabated, and a number of other promising substances were isolated, two of which—neomycin (1949) and candicidin (1953)—found significant medical applications. In addition to directing this work, Waksman completed an extensive study and review of the literature on the actinomycetes which was collected in a three-volume monograph, *The Actinomycetes* (1959–62). Waksman also devoted much energy to the planning and development of the new Institute of Microbiology at Rutgers, where he was able to establish a broad-based program of basic and applied research. After retirement in 1958, Waksman continued to lead a productive life of travel, lecturing, and writing. He died of a cerebral hemorrhage at his home on Cape Cod, Massachusetts, in 1973 at age eighty-five.

ELIZABETH A. HACHTEN

Selected Bibliography

PRIMARY SOURCES

Waksman, Selman A. 1927. *Principles of Soil Microbiology*. Baltimore: Williams and Wilkins.

———. 1954. *My Life with Microbes*. New York: Simon and Schuster.

———. 1959. 1961. 1962. *The Actinomycetes*. Vol. 1, *Nature, Occurence and Activities*. Vol. 2, *Classification, Identification, and Descriptions of Genera and Species*. Vol. 3, *The Antibiotics of Actinomycetes* (with H. A. Lechevalier). Baltimore: Williams and Williams.

———. 1965. *The Conquest of Tuberculosis*. Berkeley and Los Angeles: University of California Press.

SECONDARY SOURCES

Dowling, Harry F. 1977. *Fighting Infection: Conquests of the Twentieth Century*. Cambridge: Harvard University Press.

Parascandola, John, ed. 1980. *The History of Antibiotics: A Symposium*. Madison, Wis.: American Institute of the History of Pharmacy.

1973. *Selman Abraham Waksman: 1888–1973*. New Brunswick, N.J.: Institute for Microbiology. Addresses delivered at a memorial service at the Institute of Microbiology, Rutgers University, October 13, 1973.

Swann, John P. 1986. *American Scientists and the Pharmaceutical Industry: Cooperative Research in Twentieth-Century America*. Baltimore: Johns Hopkins University Press.

Woodruff, H. Boyd, ed. 1968. *Scientific Contributions of Selman A. Waksman*. New Brunswick, N.J.: Rutgers University Press. Includes complete bibliography of Waksman's publications.

GEORGE WALD 1967

George Wald was born on November 18, 1906, in New York City. A biochemist, Wald shared the 1967 Nobel Prize with Ragnar Granit and H. K. Hartline for his work on the biochemistry of vision, in particular his description of the critical role of vitamin A in the synthesis of the visual pigments in the retinal receptor cells. At the time of the award, he was professor of biology and biochemistry at Harvard, the position he held until his retirement. Wald and Frances Kingsley were married in 1931; that marriage ended in divorce in 1957. The following year, he married Ruth Hubbard, a former student who became a researcher in her own right and a collaborator in her husband's work. Wald has two sons from his first marriage, Michael and David, and two children with his present wife, Elijah and Deborah.

Wald's father, Isaac Wald, was a Jewish immigrant from Poland; his mother, Ernestine Rosenmann, came from Germany. The elder Wald worked as a tailor and the family was quite poor. They saved for years to send George to Washington Square College of New York University, where he received his bachelor of science degree in 1927. He then began graduate study at Columbia under Selig Hecht, a pioneer in visual physiology, who became the young biologist's mentor. Years later, Wald said of their relationship, "I felt his presence always. What I did or said or wrote was in a sense always addressed to him" (Dowling 1967, 468).

He earned his master's degree in 1928 and his Ph.D. in 1932. A National Research Council fellowship enabled him to spend the following year in Europe, working first with Otto Warburg in Berlin-Dahlem at the Kaiser-Wilhelm Institute. Here he studied the pigment "visual purple," now called rhodopsin, first discovered by Wilhelm Kuhne in the rod receptor cells of the retina. The rods "see" shapes and light variances at night but cannot respond to colors. Rhodopsin had the interesting property of "bleaching" to white when exposed to light, then returning to its normal hue in darkness. Hecht had suggested to Wald that the pigment was composed of two elements, which were separated by light. In Berlin he succeeded in breaking rhodopsin into two components as predicted. One was a protein, which he called opsin; the other appeared to be vitamin A.

Wald then spent four months in Zurich with Paul Karrer, who had described the vitamin's chemical structure the year before; Wald assisted him in verifying this discovery. He planned then to carry out a different project under Otto Meyerhof, but while in Heidelberg he investigated some frog retinae and isolated retinene, a yellowish carotenoid, that appeared to be the "bleached" element of rhodopsin. Wald returned to the United States in 1933 and took the second year of his fellowship at the University of Chicago. He was now firmly committed to "the life with molecules" (Wald, 1967, 292–93).

Wald was recruited by the Department of Biology at Harvard, where he was appointed tutor in biochemical sciences in 1934, rising to faculty instructor in 1939. At Harvard, he continued his investigations of rhodopsin. He confirmed that vitamin A in the eye is oxidized to retinene which combines with opsin to form rhodopsin.

In the 1940s he studied the vision of cataract patients who had received artificial lens grafts. This work led him to the realization in 1945 that the normal human lens is a yellow filter, which allows the differential focusing of blue and violet from yellow and green. Without such a filter, a person's vision is blurred. The yellow lens also blocks ultraviolet light.

Wald was promoted to associate professor in 1944 and to full professor in 1948. By 1950 he had synthesized rhodopsin in the laboratory. He and Ruth Hubbard then made a preparation of rod cells and exposed the mixture successively to light and to dark. In the light the rhodopsin rapidly broke down into opsin and retinene and the retinene returned to its vitamin A form. In the dark the reaction reversed itself and rhodopsin reformed. These converse processes are the reason the eye takes a minute to "adjust" when suddenly exposed to light or to darkness.

Wald's and Hubbard's attempts to repeat the reaction with different forms (molecular configurations or isomers) of vitamin A, however, failed, leading them to the realization that retinene was actually a highly unstable form of the compound. Its instability assisted it to combine tightly with opsin. The action of light was to force the molecules to take a more stable form, which then broke the opsin bond. This experiment was the first demonstration of the involvement of molecular transformations in a biological function (Wald 1967, 299–03; Dowling 1967, 468).

Throughout the 1950s Wald worked with Hubbard and Paul K. Brown to identify the pigments in the cone receptor cells, which react to light and recognize colors. They identified red, yellow-green, and blue pigments as different forms of opsin combined with the unstable form of retinene. These are porphyropsin and cyanopsin in the cone cells and iodopsin in the rods. While the red and yellow-green forms were found together, the blue pigment, located only after examination with a microspectromphotometer, is found only in specific cells, which react to the shorter focus of blue light through the yellow lens filter. Three investigators at Johns Hopkins, Edward F. MacNichol, William B. Marks, and William Dobelle, independently confirmed these findings.

Wald's work explained that the color pigments in the eye are actually synthesized from vitamin A only in darkness; the process stops when the eye is exposed to light. He established the vital importance of vitamin A to normal vision. Without sufficient dietary intake of this vitamin, a person loses visual sensitivity and becomes "night blind." His was the first specific description of the biochemical function of a fat-soluble vitamin (Wald 1967, 295; Dowling 1969, 469).

A witty and enthusiastic man, Wald was a popular and inspiring teacher at Harvard until his retirement in 1977. His biological research often led him into general scientific and philosophical thought. In 1960 he developed a new course in introductory biology which, rather than emphasizing classification and distinctions between life forms, discussed the common elements and processes of all organisms: atoms, molecules, fermentation, respiration, and photosynthesis. He has also written extensively on scientific education and biochemical evolution and developed two famous lectures, "The Origin of Life" and "The Origin of Death." Wald is also a collector and connoisseur of art, including both Rembrandt etchings and primitive pottery. His interest in the latter has taken him to Mexico to join archaeological digs. He is politically active as well, particularly in antinuclear protests (Dowling 1969, 469).

George Wald is a member of the National Academy of Sciences, the American Academy of Arts and Sciences, the Optical Society of America, the American Society of Biological Chemists, and the American Association for the Advancement of Science, among other organizations. He has received many honors for his work, including the Eli Lilly Research Award (1939), the Albert Lasker Award from the American Public Health Association (1953), the Proctor Medal from the Association for Research in Ophthalmology (1955), the Rumford Medal from the American Academy of Arts and Sciences (1959), the Ives Medal from the Optical Society (1966), and the T. Duckett Jones Award from the Helen Hay Whitney Foundation (1968). In 1967 he was awarded the Paul Karrer Medal from the University of Zurich jointly with Ruth Wald.

MARCIA MELDRUM

Selected Bibliography

PRIMARY SOURCES

Wald, George. 1934. "Carotenoids and Vitamin A Cycle in Vision." *Nature* 134 (July 14,.):65.

———. 1945. *General Education in a Free Society*. Cambridge: Harvard University Press.

———. 1947. "Chemical Evolution of Vision." *Harvey Lectures*, series 41, 117–60.

Wald, George, and Paul Brown. 1950. "Synthesis of Rhodopsin from Retinene." *Proceedings of the National Academy of Science* 36 (February). 84–92.

Wald, George, and Ruth Hubbard. 1950. "Synthesis of Rhodopsin from Vitamin A." *Proceedings of the National Academy of Science* 36 (February): 92–102.

Hubbard, Ruth, and George Wald. 1952. "Cis-Trans Isomers of Vitamin A and Retinene in Vision." *Science* 115 (January 18): 60–63.

Wald, George. 1966. *Twenty-Six Afternoons of Biology*. Reading, Mass: Addison-Wesley.

Wald, George. 1967. "The Molecular Basis of Visual Excitation." Nobel Lecture, December 12, 1967. Reprinted in *Nobel Lectures in Physiology or Medicine*, Vol. 4 (1963–1979), 292–317. Amsterdam: Elsevier, 1972.

———. 1974. *Visual Pigments and Photoreceptors: Review and Outlook.* New York: Academic Press.

SECONDARY SOURCES

Brody, Jane E. 1967. "Work of the Laureates Has Contributed to Grasp of the Visual Process." *New York Times* (October 19):40.

Dowling, John E. 1967. "Nobel Prize: Three Named for Medicine, Physiology Award. George Wald." *Science* 158 (October 27):468–69.

Todd, Richard. 1969. "George Wald, the Man, the Speech." *New York Times Magazine* (August 17):28–29+.

1968. "Wald, George." In *Current Biography Yearbook*, 412–14. New York: H. W. Wilson.

Wiskari, Werner. 1967. "Three Scientists Given Nobel Prize for Research on Eye." *New York Times* (October 19):1, 40.

OTTO HEINRICH WARBURG
1931

Otto Heinrich Warburg was born on October 8, 1893, in Freiburg im Breisgau, Germany. He was the scion of a distinguished old family of bankers, public servants, and savants. His father, Emil Warburg, one of Germany's foremost scientists, held the chair in physics at the University of Berlin, among the most coveted professorships in the field. His mother, Elisabeth Gaertner, came from a prominent South German family. Frequent visitors to their home included individuals who deeply influenced the younger Warburg: Emil Fischer and Walther Nernst, for example, respectively the leading organic and physical chemists of the day, and Albert Einstein.

Fischer directed Otto Warburg's doctoral thesis, which he completed in 1906 at the University of Berlin, following earlier training at the University of Freiburg. Next, Warburg studied medicine at Heidelberg, receiving his M.D. in 1911. He stayed on at the university until 1914, by which time he was already involved in important research and the author of thirty major articles. In April of that year Warburg was appointed head of a research department at the prestigious Kaiser Wilhelm Gesellschaft in Berlin, a post he relinquished soon thereafter to serve as a lieutenant in the Prussian Garde Ulanen, a cavalry regiment that fought on the Russian front. Following the war, Warburg returned to the Kaiser Wilhelm Institut für Biologie in Berlin Dahlem. He remained there until 1931, when, with funding from the Rockefeller Foundation, he set up the Kaiser Wilhelm Institut für Zellphysiologie. Warburg and his team were able to continue their work during the Hilter years, although after 1942 they had to remove themselves to an estate outside Berlin to avoid the Allied bombings. When the Russian army captured the area, they confiscated Warburg's equipment, leaving him without a laboratory until 1950, when his old institute, temporarily the United States military headquarters of the Berlin High Command, again became the Kaiser Wilhelm Institut für Zellphysiologie. (It was renamed the Max Planck Institut in 1953.) Because of Warburg's eminence and his productivity, the governors of the Institut excused him from its mandatory retirement rule, so that he continued to work until close to the end of his life. Otto Warburg died at home in Berlin on August 1, 1970. He never married, but lived with Jacob Heiss, his longstanding companion.

Warburg's life was entirely devoted to his career as a research scientist. This singlemindedness of purpose, harnessed to a severe sense of order and discipline and an exceptional intelligence, allowed him to make an extraordinary number of significant contributions to his field, the biochemical study of the cell. (His productivity and originality may be superficially measured by the fact that he was nominated for a second Nobel Prize in 1944, one he could not accept because Hitler forbad the award to German citizens.) He had, in addition, a superb talent for developing new laboratory techniques (including tissue slicing and his adaptation of the manometer) and for devising ingenious approaches to studying scientific problems. He was also able to work closely and supportively with his few students, three of whom, Otto Meyerhof, Hans Adolf Krebs, and Hugo Theorell, themselves won Nobel Prizes in Physiology or Medicine. His standing as a scientist was marred, however, by a tendency toward vituperative polemics with competitors and colleagues, especially when he felt his interpretations or his status slighted. He was also criticized for remaining in Germany during the Hitler period, particularly since the Warburg family was Jewish. Hermann Goering had Warburg's ancestral line redefined to make him a "quarter-Jew," and other highly placed Nazi officials lent Warburg their protection. Warburg's own defense was that he was a talented and productive scientist whose work depended upon the laboratory and the team of technicians he had fashioned at Berlin Dahlem (Krebs 1981, 60).

Warburg's work centered on cell respiration, seriate catalytic actions that result in the liberation and transfer of chemical energy within living cells. This highly complex process was little understood when Warburg began his studies. He set out, in particular, to discover and describe the catalysts that enabled cell respiration to occur.

In research he performed before

World War I, Warburg established that small concentrations of cyanide inhibit cell oxidation. From this he inferred that catalysts containing a heavy metal must play a role in respiration, since cyanide forms complexes with such metals. Further work led him to hypothesize that the element involved was iron. This supposition was strengthened in 1926, when Warburg found that carbon monoxide also inhibited cell respiration, with inhibition increasing as oxygen pressure decreased. Carbon monoxide, it was known, joins with iron porphyrins like hemoglobin in the red blood cells, replacing the oxygen that normally binds to the heme and is transported by it.

Acting on a suggestion by Archibald Hill, Warburg then tested whether the inhibiting action of carbon monoxide on cell respiration was reversed by light, which occurs when carbon monoxide is bound to hemoglobin. Using yeast cells in suspension, Warburg found that cell respiration in the presence of carbon monoxide increased when light was switched on for some time and decreased in the dark. Moreover, by bombarding the yeast cells with light of the same intensity but of varying wave lengths, Warburg was able to measure the absorption spectrum of the unknown, clearly iron-containing catalyst. The spectrum he obtained was similar but not identical to that of hemoglobin and other subcellular iron porphyrins. Warburg named his catalyst the "iron-transferring enzyme."

For the discovery of the enzyme, its nature, and action, Warburg received the Nobel Prize in 1931. Other workers, David Keilin in particular, established in the late thirties that Warburg's enzyme was a newly isolated cytochrome, labelled a_3, a subsystem that catalyzes the oxidation of hydrogen in the final state of the cell's respiratory process.

During the 1930s Warburg's focus shifted to another area of cell respiration, that of the dehydrogenases, the enzymes that remove hydrogen from a substrate. Work performed between 1912 and 1925, particularly by Wieland and Thumberg, indicated that dehydrogenases alter molecules so that some of their hydrogen atoms are easily removed and transferred to a hydrogen acceptor like oxygen or methanol blue (Keilin 1966, 125–26). Initially critical of these findings (and a proponent of an opposing theory of biological oxidation), Warburg became impressed by further evidence and began his own experiments, using methanol blue as an oxidizing agent. In experiments performed between 1931 and 1933, he showed that the hydrogen transferring process involved an enzyme or *Ferment* and a coenzyme or *Co-ferment*. Using yeast as the source of his *Ferment*, Warburg found that it contained a yellow component that he labelled "yellow enzyme" and from which he derived luminoflavin. Other laboratories demonstrated that luminoflavin was produced from riboflavin and that the latter was a vitamin, B_2. Hugo Theorell, a fellow in Warburg's laboratory, showed that it was the phosphorylated riboflavin in the *Ferment* that alternately underwent oxidation and reduction.

The discovery of the first yellow enzyme was important, both because it established the existence of an oxidation-reduction system in cell respiration in addition to the iron porphyrins, and because it opened the way to the isolation of many other yellow enzymes (or flavoproteins), some of which were found by Warburg and his colleagues in the late 1930s.

During the same period, Warburg analyzed the *Co-ferment*. By 1935–36 he could report that it contained nicotinamide (derived from niacin, or vitamin B_3), which served the coenzyme as its catalytically active principle, allowing it to undergo reversible reduction in hydrogen transfer. Subsequent work by Warburg and his colleagues demonstrated that the nicotinamide-containing enzymes could be separated into two groups distinguished by the number of phosphates they contained. Following Warburg's work, many other coenzymes were found that have nicotinamide as a hydrogen carrier. Currently, more than 150 of them have been identified.

Warburg's investigation of the dehydrogenases proved very fruitful. His work defined and explained crucial catalytic actions that occur during cell respiration. It elucidated the central function of vitamins in those catalytic processes and led to an understanding of the role of niacin in the etiology of pellagra. And it opened the way to a rapid accumulation of further knowledge concerning the dehydrogenating enzymes. For his work on the flavins and on nicotinamide-containing coenzymes, Warburg was nominated for a second Nobel Prize, referred to earlier.

In addition to the work described, Warburg made many other important contributions, only some of which can be cited. Beginning in the twenties, he undertook fundamental investigations of the metabolism of cancer cells, studies he continued through the 1960s. Starting in 1914, he also attempted, building on the work of Einstein and of Emil Warburg, to measure the maximum thermodynamic efficiency of photosynthesis (studying in this instance the transformation of energy *into* living compounds). Finally, with collaborators, Warburg succeeded in crystallizing nine of the catalysts of cellular fermentation, an accomplishment that led to more detailed study of anaerobic processes and of cell constituents, and which allowed the mass production by commercial manufacturing of pure enzymes, coenzymes, and substrates.

Otto Warburg received many other honors in addition to the Nobel Prize. These included the German Order of Merit, the Freedom of the City of Berlin, Foreign Membership in the Royal Society, and an honorary doctorate from Oxford University. In 1963, to memorialize his eightieth birthday, the German Society for Physiological Chemistry created an "Otto Warburg Medal." Many other honors were offered to Warburg but he chose not to accept them, mainly because he preferred to invest the personal time such honors required in his scientific work.

GERALD M. OPPENHEIMER

Selected Bibliography

PRIMARY SOURCES

Warburg, Otto. 1930. *The Metabolism of Tumors*. London: Constable and Company.

———. 1949. *Heavy Metal Prosthetic Groups and Enzyme Action*. Translated by Alexander Lawson, Oxford: Clarendon Press.

———. 1962. *New Methods of Cell Physiology*. New York: Interscience Publishers.

SECONDARY SOURCES

Keilin, David. 1966. *The History of Cell Respiration and Cytochrome*. Cambridge: Cambridge University Press.

Krebs, Hans. 1981. *Otto Warburg, Cell Physiologist, Biochemist and Eccentric*. Oxford: Clarendon Press.

JAMES DEWEY WATSON *1962*

James Dewey Watson was born in Chicago, Illinois, on April 6, 1928, the son of a physician, James Dewey Watson, Sr., and Jean Mitchell Watson. At an early age Watson showed his precocity and appeared as a Quiz Kid on a national radio show. He entered the University of Chicago at the age of fifteen and took an interest in natural sciences, especially ornithology and genetics. He was turned down by his first-choice graduate schools, the California Institute of Technology and Harvard, and accepted a fellowship at Indiana University, which had several first-rate geneticists, including H. J. Muller, T. M. Sonneborn, and S. Luria, but no ornithologists on its faculty. At age nineteen Watson began his graduate education and early identified the gene as the subject he would pursue.

Watson felt less than enthusiastic about fruit flies and paramecia, the organisms chosen by his elders for gene research; he himself was intrigued by the idea of using bacteriophages to study the gene. Viruses were closer to genes, biochemically, than were the enormously more complex cells and chromosomes of eukaryotic organisms. At age twenty Watson completed a Ph.D. dissertation on heavily irradiated bacteriophages and the attempts to recover them. Luria, his advisor, then advised him to go to Europe to study biochemistry. While on a National Research Council fellowship (1950–51), he began studies which proved a disappointment because they did not provide any insights into the structure of DNA (deoxyribonucleic acid) by then thought to be the hereditary material by most bacteriophage geneticists.

Watson arranged, through Luria, to have his fellowship transferred to Cambridge where he hoped to work on the x-ray crystallography of DNA and there joined F. H. C. Crick, 12 years his senior, but still lacking a Ph.D. Watson was not especially qualified for such a project since he had not worked in this field before, considered himself inept in mathematics, and still had only the vaguest ideas about the biochemistry of nucleic acids. Watson, however, was intensely interested in molecular biology, learned quickly, and knew how to think in original ways when confronted with complex problems.

The association proved fruitful. After several false leads Watson and Crick proposed a structure of DNA based on their interpretation of x-ray diffraction photographs which they and M. Wilkins had independently prepared. The DNA was a double helical molecule of complementary chains of nucleotides, each strand moving in an opposite direction. The complementary association was highly specific, the purine adenine pairing with the pyrimidine thymine and the purine guanine pairing with the pyrimidine cytosine (or, in abbreviated form, with only AT or GC pairing permissable). The doubling, the internal location of the bases, and the helical organization were all inferred from the x-ray diffraction patterns on the photographs. The principle of complementary base pairs, however, was not derived from the x-ray crystallography but from a "goodness of fit" that Watson inferred from the physical structures of the individual bases and confirmed by making cardboard and metal cutout representations that he pieced together. Nor was the sequence of bases, which they recognized could be aperiodic or nonrepetitive, based on these approaches. This was a biological implication popularized earlier by Erwin Schrödinger, who referred to genes as "aperiodic crystals." Watson and Crick published their structure in a brief note to *Nature* and followed with another brief note on the biological significance of their structure. The double helix model of DNA permitted geneticists to interpret gene replication or chromosome replication at a molecular level. It also implied that mutations could arise from changes in the base sequence within a gene by copying errors or other mechanisms. They did not propose any specific way by which the information encoded in the genes or DNA might be chemically passed into the cell so as to produce the products of those genes.

The double helix model of DNA was profoundly influential and stimulated interest in the genetic code, the extension of genetic replication to prokaryotic and eukaryotic cells, and the role of genes in producing their products. Watson returned to the United States as a senior research fellow at the California Institute of Technology from 1953 to 1955 and then moved to Harvard (1956–68), where he actively studied the role of DNA in protein synthesis. Watson had inferred in 1952 what was later to be called the genetic dogma (also called the central dogma by Crick): that DNA makes RNA, and RNA makes protein. But it was not until the RNA virus called tobacco mosaic virus (TMV) was successfully separated into its RNA and protein components (in 1956) that this dogma was seriously accepted as a useful model. The RNA, but not the protein of TMV, when introduced into tobacco leaf cells, caused infectious lesions with myriads of new virus particles. This action implied that RNA did indeed carry genetic information, and was indeed involved in protein synthesis. Watson sought, and successfully demonstrated, the existence of adaptor molecules, proposed by Crick, as soluble RNA molecules that carried amino acids to a form of RNA (later called messenger RNA) that is copied off the gene. In this conception of the function of the gene at the molecular level, the sequence of nucleotides in the gene is transcribed or copied as messenger RNA, which then enters the cell machinery for protein synthesis. Such units are called ribosomes. The ribosomes are like tape recorders that receive the messenger RNA and translate the nucleotide sequence into a corresponding sequence of amino acids in a protein which subsequently peels off the ribosome. The transfer RNA molecules transport the amino acids at one end of the molecule and have a coding region at another locus that matches a complementary sequence in the messenger RNA.

Since 1968, Watson has been the director of the Cold Spring Harbor Laboratories, under his leadership the laboratory has shifted its efforts in the direction of tumor biology. The contributions of the scholars working at Cold Spring Harbor are substantial and the annual gatherings of molecular biologists who present their ideas and findings have enriched the molecular approaches to understanding many aspects of life. Watson is also the director of the "human genome project," a massive international effort funded substantially by the United States Congress to map every gene in the human genome and to determine the nucleotide sequence in each of the genes mapped. Most of the project is expected to be completed by the start of the twenty-first century.

Watson's account of his discovery of the structure of DNA with Crick, and of the roles of M. Wilkins and R. Franklin in preparing the X-ray diffraction photographs that were essential for their successful interpretation, was published in 1968. *The Double Helix* was an international best-seller which provided readers with the portrait of a young, naive, ambitious, and opinionated scientist whose success depended on luck, intense work, original insights, and a conviction that the structure of DNA would provide the clues to its major biological functions. Although Watson was criticized for presenting such an unconventional portrait of a scientist, his honest self-appraisal made science more comprehensible and accessible in its historical and personal dimensions. Watson also synthesized the prevailing views of molecular biologists and in a clear prose developed a leading text, *The Molecular Biology of the Gene*, that has shaped the thinking of a generation of undergraduate biology students.

James Watson married Elizabeth Lewis in 1968; they have two sons. He is a member of the National Academy of Sciences, the

American Society of Biological Research, the American Philosophical Society, and the American Academy of Arts and Sciences. Among the many honors he has received for his work are the Warren Triennial Prize (1959), the Eli Lilly Biochemistry Award (1960), the Lasker Prize (1960), the John J. Carty Medal from the National Academy of Sciences (1971), and the Presidential Medal of Freedom (1977).

ELOF AXEL CARLSON

Selected Bibliography

PRIMARY SOURCES

Watson, J. D., and F. H. C. Crick. 1953. "Molecular Structure of Nucleic Acids. A Structure for Deoxyribose Nucleic Acid." *Nature* 171: 737–38.

———. 1953. "Genetical Implications of the Structure of deoxyribonucleic Acid." *Nature* 171:964–67.

Watson, J. D. 1963. "The Involvement of RNA in the Synthesis of Proteins." *Science* 140:17–26.

———. 1965. *The Molecular Biology of the Gene.* New York: W. A. Benjamin.

———. 1966. "Growing Up in the Phage Group." In *Phage and the Origins of Molecular Biology*, edited by J. Cairns, G. S. Stent, and J. D. Watson, Cold Spring Harbor, N.Y.: 239–245. Cold Spring Harbor Laboratory of Quantitative Biology.

———. 1968. *The Double Helix.* New York: Atheneum.

Alberts, Bruce, Dennis Bray, Julian Lewis, Martin Raff, Keith Roberts, and James D. Watson. 1983. *Molecular Biology of the Cell.* New York: Garland.

SECONDARY SOURCES

Fraenkel-Conrat, H., 1956. "The Role of the Nucleic Acid in the Reconstitution of Active Tobacco Mosaic Virus." *Journal of the American Chemical Society* 78:882–883.

Judson, Horace Freeland. 1979. *The Eighth Day of Creation: The Makers of the Revolution in Biology.* New York: Simon and Schuster.

Olby, R. C. 1974. *The Path to the Double Helix.* Seattle, Wash.: University of Washington Press.

THOMAS HUCKLE WELLER *1954*

Thomas Huckle Weller was born on June 15, 1915, in Ann Arbor, Michigan. A virologist and public health specialist, Weller won the Nobel Prize in 1954 jointly with John Franklin Enders and Frederick Chapman Roberts for their successful culturing of poliomyelitis virus in several types of human tissues. Their breakthrough not only laid the groundwork for the development of an effective polio vaccine but was also the prototype for modern methods of viral cultivation, diagnostic testing, and vaccine development. At the time of the award, Weller had just been made professor of Tropical Public Health and chairman of the Department of Public Health at Harvard, positions he occupied until his retirement in 1985. Weller married Kathleen R. Fahey in August 1945. They have two sons, Peter Fahey and Robert Andrew, and two daughters, Nancy Kathleen and Janet Louise.

Weller's parents were Carl V. Weller and the former Elsie A. Huckle. His early interest in tropical and viral diseases was developed at the University of Michigan, where he received his A.B. in 1936 and his M.A. in 1937. While attending medical school at Harvard, he won a traveling fellowship from the Rockefeller Foundation to study malaria in Florida and public health in Tennessee. His graduation from Harvard in 1940 was wreathed with laurels: magna cum laude honors in parasitology, a fellowship in tropical medicine, and a teaching fellowship in bacteriology.

Weller completed an internship in bacteriology and pathology at Children's Hospital in Boston, but the outbreak of World War II interrupted his academic career. Enlisting in the U.S. Army Medical Corps in 1942, he taught courses in tropical medicine and malariology, then became officer-in-charge of bacteriology and virology in San Juan, Puerto Rico. He was later assigned to the Army Medical School in Washington. After his discharge in 1945, he returned to Boston to complete his residency at Children's Hospital, followed by a year's postdoctoral fellowship, working with John Enders, who was establishing a new laboratory for viral research at Children's. In 1949 he was named assistant director of the Research Division of Infectious Diseases.

When Weller was still a medical student in 1940, he and Enders, working with A. E. Feller, had achieved the first successful prolonged roller tube culture of a virus (Feller, Enders, and Weller 1940). During the war Enders had been working on the mumps virus, which often broke out among recruits and drafteees. He and his team had developed diagnostic tests and a killed-virus vaccine for mumps. Weller and Enders now began a new series of viral studies; they were joined by Frederick Robbins, Weller's Harvard roommate, now a National Research Council senior fellow.

In March 1948 Weller was growing the mumps virus in human embryonic tissue cultures with the addition of antibiotics to prevent bacterial contamination. At the end of one such experiment, he had a few extra tubes and decided to "try polio" to see if that virus would thrive in his system. His results with the embryo tissue encouraged him to attempt to culture poliovirus in other preparations. He was able to grow the virus in human foreskin cultures, the first time it had been successfully established in non-neural, nonembryonic cells.

Robbins, who had been working with infant epidemic diarrhea, had developed a successful system of mouse intestinal tissue cultures. He and Weller experimented with poliovirus in these cells, but without success. They then developed a culture of human intestinal tissue which proved more hospitable: the poliovirus grew and throve. This was the first demonstration that polio could survive in the intestinal walls of infected individuals. The team also observed cellular changes in the cultures that offered clear evidence of viral replication. Enders coined the term "cytopathogenic" to describe the altered cells.

Over the next few months they were able to produce large quantities of the virus by refining their culture methods and to neutralize it with specific antibodies. The definitive report of their work appeared in *Science* in January 1949, less than a year after Weller had first introduced polio into his spare tubes (Enders, Weller, and Robbins 1949). These classic experiments formed the basis for many diagnostic and vaccine applications, as well as contemporary viral culture techniques. The Nobel Committee voted to award John Enders the 1954 Nobel Prize for his significant contribution; he declined to accept unless Robbins and Weller shared the award and the committee complied with his wishes.

Weller could have devoted his subsequent career to elaboration of his success and development of a polio vaccine. However, his drive and wide-ranging curiosity were already leading him into other investigations. His reaction to the Nobel Prize award was typical. He learned of the honor shortly after his appointment at chairman of the Department of Public Health in 1954. Returning to his office from the inevitable series of interviews and meetings, he slumped into a chair and remarked drily, "Now I guess we'll have to show them that wasn't a flash in the pan" (Chernin 1985). Under Weller's leadership, the department grew to national prominence.

In virology, he had already pioneered in culturing rubella (1952) and the etiologic viruses of chickenpox and shingles (1953). He went on to establish that varicella and zoster were the same virus (1954). From 1957 to 1973 he established most of the basic information on cytomegalovirus.

In parasitology, Weller made significant contributions to our understanding of helminths with his extensive research on schistosomiasis over a period of years (1945–82), including diagnostic and immunologic studies as well as work on the basic biology of these organisms. In protozoology, he was the first to culture *Toxoplasma gondii* in cells (1954, 1957) and to demonstrate the airborne transmission of *Pneumocystis carinii* (1971).

Weller's career spanned the modern era of molecular biology. His work and that of the team he assembled at Harvard were major forces in the development of the field from its early days, when a few researchers used crude instruments made of wooden cigar boxes and secondhand clock motors, to today, when researchers use the most sophisticated (and expensive) technological tools (Weller 1989). Many young investigators owe their interest in tropical medicine and public health to Weller. He has also been an active advisor on public health programs throughout his career, serving as a consultant for the U.S. Public Health Service and the World Health Organization.

Weller became professor emeritus in 1985. He remains active as a senior spokesman for his field. Among the many honors he has received are the Mead Johnson Award from the American Academy of Pediatrics (1953), the George Ledlie Prize (1964), the Weinstein Cerebral Palsy Award (1973), and the Bristol Award from the Infectious Diseases Society of America (1980). He holds honorary degrees from the University of Michigan (LL.D. 1956), Gustavus Adolphus College (Sc.D. 1975), Lowell University (L.H.D. 1977), and the University of Massachusetts (Sc.D. 1975).

JAMES J. POUPARD
MARCIA MELDRUM

Selected Bibliography

PRIMARY SOURCES

Feller, A. E., J. F. Enders, and T. H. Weller. 1940. "The Prolonged Coexistence of Vaccinia Virus in High Titre and Living Cells in Roller Tube Cultures of Chick Embryonic Tissues." *Journal of Experimental Medicine* 72:367–87.

Enders, J. F., T. H. Weller, and F. C. Robbins. 1949. "Cultivation of the Lansing Strain of Poliomyelitis Virus in Cultures of Various Human Embryonic Tissues." *Science* 109 (January 28):85–87.

Weller, T. H., F. C. Robbins, and J. F. Enders. 1949. "Cultivation of Poliomyelitis Virus in Cultures of Human Foreskin and Embryonic Tissues." *Proceedings of the Society for Experimental Biology* 72:153–55.

Augustine, D. L., T. H. Weller, and R. Thomas. 1953. "The Importance of Tropical Public Health to World Peace." *Post Graduate Medicine* 13:339–43.

Weller, T. H. 1989. "As It Was and As It Is: A Half-Century of Progress." *Journal of Infectious Diseases* 159 (March):378–83.

SECONDARY SOURCES

Chernin, Eli. 1985. *Tropical Medicine at Harvard: The Weller Years, 1954–1981. A Personal Memoir.* Cambridge: Harvard School of Public Health.

1988. "Enders, John Franklin." In *Current Biography Yearbook*, 182–84. New York: H. W. Wilson.

Williams, Greer. 1960. *Virus Hunters.* New York: Alfred A. Knopf.

GEORGE HOYT WHIPPLE 1934

George Hoyt Whipple was born on August 28, 1878, in Ashland, New Hampshire. His parents were Ashley C. Whipple, a doctor, and Henrietta (Hersey) Whipple. He married Katharine Ball Waring on June 24, 1914; their two children, George Hoyt, Jr., and Barbara, were born in 1917 and 1921, respectively. Whipple died on February 1, 1976, in Rochester, New York.

Whipple's life and character were shaped by his upbringing in rural New England, from which he derived physical strength, a taste for the outdoors, legendary taciturnity, and an unyielding independence of character. He was educated in the public schools of Ashland, at Phillips Andover Academy, and at Yale College. Determined to pursue the profession of his father and grandfather, he studied medicine at Johns Hopkins, where he fell under the influence of William H. Welch, a great pathologist, a leading exponent of scientific medicine, and a teacher of a whole generation of American physicians. Receiving his M.D. in 1905, Whipple remained in Baltimore, first as an intern in Johns Hopkins Hospital and then, through Welch's patronage, as an assistant in the Department of Pathology. Here, helping at autopsies, he discovered or strengthened a natural bias toward research and made it the preoccupation of his life.

In 1911 he received an associate professorship at Johns Hopkins, and his career was launched. Three years later, an invitation to distinction arrived from California, in the form of an appointment as director of the Hooper Foundation and professor of research medicine at the University of California, San Francisco. On Parnassus Heights, Whipple introduced research into a medical school formerly devoted entirely to teaching the clinical subjects (basic sciences were taught at Berkeley, across the bay). Whipple demonstrated as well his capacity as an administrator, recruiting a staff of experts in a variety of fields, seeing to the construction of laboratories, and establishing student fellowships to introduce promising young people to medical research.

In 1920 he was named dean of the medical school. However, the very next year his life took an unexpected and—at first—unwelcome turn. Abraham Flexner, representing the Rockefeller Foundation, and George Eastman, the Kodak multimillionaire, had determined to erect a new and progressive medical school at the Univeristy of Rochester in upstate New York. With their concurrence, the university president, Rush Rhees, decided that Whipple must be the dean and builder of the school. At first he rejected the proposal. But Rhees, not to be denied, crossed the continent to put his case in person. The threefold advantages of Rochester—ample resources, a free hand, and the opportunity to shape a new and possibly major institution—at last persuaded Whipple to take up the challenge that would consume much of his life.

His extraordinary capacity for work was never better demonstrated than during the years (roughly 1921–30) when he successfully built, staffed, and directed the School of Medicine and Dentistry while maintaining his usual output of new research. In Rochester, much of the price was paid in a coin that Whipple depreciated anyway; Rhees had agreed to excuse him from the formal socializing normally demanded of a dean. Whipple did not neglect his students, for he found in teaching a personal satisfaction beyond that of all other professional activities. Burdened as he was, his advancement as a national and international figure was swift: in 1927 he was appointed to the Board of Trustees of the Rockefeller Foundation; in October 1934 he received word that he and two other Americans would share the Nobel Prize for Physiology or Medicine; and in 1936 he became a member of the General Education Board of the Rockefeller Foundation. But there was a limit beyond which he would not sacrifice his research and teaching to administration and medical statesmanship. When Simon Flexner retired, Whipple was offered the directorship of the Rockefeller Institute; he declined the honor, and this time not even John D. Rockefeller, Jr., could move him from his determination.

Inevitably, Whipple became something of a character on the campus and in his adopted city. He looked like a shrewd farmer, an impression heightened by his quaint, half-moon spectacles. His pawky individualism, miserliness with words, and wry wit contrasted with his honors and worldwide fame in a manner that delighted the public. His biographer tells of a lady who struggled mightily to extract conversation from Whipple during a dinner party, failed, and on parting remarked, "Well, Doctor Whipple, I hope you haven't said anything this evening that you'll regret later" (George W. Corner, *George Hoyt Whipple and His Friends: The Life-Story of a Nobel Prize Pathologist*, 1963). Whipple's love of rod and gun never deserted him, and faculty members accounted themselves fortunate or unfortunate, as the case might be, to be invited on long rambles through the mist-soaked autumn woods in pursuit of the ring-necked pheasant, or on fishing jaunts that ranged from white-water streams to the Florida Keys. Whipple gave up the deanship in 1953, when he was seventy-five and, during the next few years, gradually entered full retirement. He never went far from the campus, however, choosing despite the harsh and variable weather of upstate New York to stay in Rochester, among his friends and within sight of the institution to which he had given enduring form. Evidently his personal prescription for living was a sound one; he survived to the grand age of ninety-seven.

The research that brought Whipple the Nobel Prize grew from interrelated studies of the liver, the bile pigments, the formation and reconstitution of hemoglobin, and the metabolism of iron. Early in his career, during his days in Baltimore, he became interested in the hepatotoxicity of chloroform, and went on to study jaundice, the formation of blood, and the relationship of the liver to certain components of the blood. He progressed from studying breakdown processes to observing the constructive functions of the normal organism, especially the building of blood proteins. By 1925 he had become convinced that the regeneration of hemoglobin in the body could be modified by diet, and a long and patient course of trial and error led him to conclude that liver was the most effective food. His studies, however, carried out on laboratory dogs, concerned the secondary anemias—those resulting from hemorrhage, poor diet, etc. Two Boston physicians, George Minot and William P. Murphy, tested the diet on patients with pernicious anemia, a primary anemia with virtually 100 percent mortality. The results were so satisfactory as to attract wide attention when published (with due credit to Whipple's pioneering) in 1926. Whipple's laboratory conducted many tests for Eli Lilly and Company that led to commercial products effective against both primary and secondary forms of anemia. Whipple sought no patents and took care that the fees paid by Lilly for his laboratory work were utilized by the University of Rochester to further research and teaching. The cure of anemia brought the Nobel Prize, deservedly, to all three investigators.

Afterward, Whipple refused to be diverted by fame from the laboratory. He was led by his hemoglobin studies into a complex investigation of the role of iron in the body, exploiting the new technique of radioisotope markers (which he gratefully termed the physiologist's Rosetta Stone). Using radioactive iron produced in the Radiation Laboratory of the Univeristy of California, Whipple and his colleagues explored the metabolism of a substance the body absorbs only to the level of its needs, conserves with tenacity, and excretes with difficulty. Ingenious experiments uncovered the mechanism of iron absorption through the mucosa, and clinical trials on human volunteers confirmed and amplified the work done on animal models. In turn, these studies directed Whipple into another field, the anemic body's use of plasma or tissue proteins to rebuild hemoglobin. In 1934 he announced the concept of the dynamic equilibrium of body proteins that afterward became a commonplace to students of the physiology of nutrition. Practical results emerged here, too, in the development of successful methods for intravenous feeding of patients unable to take food by mouth.

Overall, Whipple's career was marked by a rare ability to pursue a single main line of investigation with unrelenting tenacity, even while engaged in a multitude of duties in administration and teaching. Much of his success resulted from his devotion to team research, and this in turn depended upon his generosity in awarding full credit for their contributions to his less famous colleagues. His office is maintained by the School of Medicine and Dentistry, along with the gold medal he received for the Nobel Prize, in a fitting memorial to his character: the first is plain, and the second rich.

ALBERT E. COUDREY

Selected Bibliography

PRIMARY SOURCES

Whipple, George H. 1923. "Pigment Metabolism and Regeneration of Hemoglobin in the Body." *The Harvey Lectures, 1921–1922*, Series 17: 95–121. Philadelphia: J. B. Lippincott Company.

Whipple, George H., and Frieda Robscheit-Robbins. 1925. "Blood Regeneration in Severe Anemia, part 1." *American Journal of Physiology* 72:395–407.

———. 1925. "Blood Regeneration in Severe Anemia, part 2." *American Journal of Physiology* 72:408–18.

———. 1925. "Blood Regeneration in Severe Anemia, part 3." *American Journal of Physiology* 72:419–30.

Whipple, George H. 1956. *The Dynamic Equilibrium of Body Proteins: Hemoglobin, Plasma Proteins, Organ and Tissue Proteins.* Springfield, IL: Charles C. Thomas.

———. 1959. "Autobiographical Sketch." *Perspectives in Biology and Medicine* 2:253–87.

SECONDARY SOURCES

Corner, George W. 1963. *George Hoyt Whipple and His Friends: The Life-Story of a Nobel Prize Pathologist.* Philadelphia: J. B. Lippincott Company.

Diggs, Lemuel W. 1976. "Dr. George Hoyt Whipple." *Johns Hopkins Medical Journal*, Supplement 139 (November):196–200.

1976. Obituary. *New York Times* (February 2).

TORSTEN NILS WIESEL *1981*

Torsten Nils Wiesel was born on June 3, 1924, in Uppsala, Sweden. A neurophysiologist, Wiesel was awarded one half of the 1981 Nobel Prize in Physiology or Medicine jointly with David H. Hubel; the other half was awarded to Roger W. Sperry. Hubel and Wiesel's work in mapping the striate cortex and describing its operation illuminated our understanding of the process of visual perception and has had important clinical impact on the early treatment of visual problems in children. The Hubel-Wiesel team also laid the foundations of the Department of Neurobiology at Harvard, which Wiesel chaired from 1973 to 1984. He is now Vincent and Brooke Astor Professor of Neuroscience at

Rockefeller University. Wiesel has been married twice, to Teeri Steenhammer (1956–70), and to Ann Grace Yee (1973–81); both marriages ended in divorce. He has one daughter, Sara Elizabet, by his second wife.

Wiesel grew up at the Beckomberga Mental Hospital where his father, Fritz S. Wiesel, was chief psychiatrist. His mother was the former Anna-Lisa Bentzer. He became interested in neurophysiology at the Karolinska Institute in Stockholm, where he studied with Carl Gustaf Bernhard and received his medical degree in 1954. After a year's assistantship in the Child Psychiatry Department at Karolinska Hospital, he was invited to do postdoctoral work at the Wilmer Institute at Johns Hopkins with Stephen Kuffler. His investigations into visual physiology were stimulated when David Hubel, a graduate of McGill University, returned to the institute from his army service in 1958. Most of their work was done at Harvard, where the team followed Kuffler in 1959.

Previous research, by H. Keffer Hartline, Ragnar Granit, Jerome Y. Lettvin, and Kuffler himself, had described the visual process as based on the perception of change in the level of light stimulus and comparison of the boundaries of different levels of light. The initial perception by rods and cones in the eye is fed back through layer after layer of neurons. Within the cat's retina, each retinal ganglion cell is stimulated by the particular point of light stimulating the point on the outer eye that connects with that cell. The pattern of stimulation varies, however, according to the differences in the level of illumination reaching surrounding cells; a brighter light stimulus reaching the surrounding area inhibits the individual cell, and vice versa. The contrasting light and dark levels can thus form a picture for interpretation.

Studies of frogs had shown that this interpretation occurs in the optic nerve, but Kuffler's examination of the cat's retinal ganglion cells showed that they reacted to differences between light and dark but showed no ability to sort out particular shapes and movements, as did similar cells in frogs. Hubel and Wiesel theorized that the critical level of visual perception in mammals occurs within the brain, in the striate cortex, and that cortical perception is binocular, that is, based on stimuli from both eyes simultaneously (Lettvin 1981, 519).

The team implanted microelectrodes in cats and monkeys and then exposed the animals to a variety of visual stimuli to detect the electrochemical discharge of individual nerve cells. After thus recording the nervous activity, they sacrificed and dissected the animals to determine the relation of anatomy and function. In other experiments, they injected radioactive substances into the eyes to trace the route from the retina to the visual cortex. The path they described leads from the retinal ganglions via the optic nerve to lateral geniculate nuclei in the brain and from there to the layered neurons of the cortex itself.

Hubel and Wiesel found the cortical anatomy to be extremely complex; indeed, in their classification, they rank nerve cells as simple, complex, and hypercomplex, acting progressively to create a single visual image from the millions of small bits of information arriving from the retina. They called this process progressive convergence. Although each cell "sees" only one point in the visual field, each point is perceived by a great many cells. The various cells record information in terms of the size and shape of the stimulus, the sharpness and angle of the boundary between light and dark, or the type and direction of movement of the stimulus. Different cells have different "preferences" for the type of stimulus they will register most effectively: a straight boundary between light and dark, a shaded band, a corner, or a tongue. Moreover, although each area of the cortex receives images from both retinas, some cells respond to one eye, some to the other, some to localized parts of both images.

The cortical cells are further organized into vertical divisions of two types, named by Hubel and Wiesel ocular dominance columns and orientation columns. The orientation columns translate the information from the retina, which is essentially coded as circular points of light, into linear images. The ocular dominance columns combine the information from both eyes into the carefully textured three-dimensional picture "seen" by the mammal. The extreme complexity of the visual cortex, as described by the team, makes clear the qualitative difference between the simple binocular perception of frogs or birds and the stereoscopic vision of cats and humans (Hubel and Wiesel 1962; Lettvin 1981, 519–20).

Further experiments with kittens established that the newborn mammal has a visual cortex functionally complete but still subject to development, as the animal learns to recognize the external world. During this critical period, if the vision of one eye is impaired or obscured, the cortical cells will "learn" to disregard the faulty information received from this eye as incompatible with experience. Even if the vision is later corrected, the brain will continue to operate as if the impairment existed and the repaired eye will remain functionally blind (Hubel and Wiesel 1963; 1965).

This new understanding has changed the whole field of pediatric ophthalmology. It is now clear that an early eye problem, such as strabismus or congenital cataracts, should not be neglected until the child is older or in hopes it will improve with maturity. On the contrary, immediate intervention is necessary if normal vision is to be preserved (Lettvin 1981, 520).

After coming to Harvard as an assistant professor of neurophysiology and neuropharmacology, Wiesel rose to full professor by 1967 and was named Robert Winthrop Professor in 1974. He succeeded Hubel as chairman of the Department of Neurobiology, which Stephen Kuffler had created, in 1973. The close Hubel-Wiesel partnership, remembered by George Berry as "like identical twins," continued throughout these years, until Wiesel's move to Rockefeller to head the neurobiology lab in 1984 (*New York Times*, October 10, 1981).

Wiesel has always enjoyed sports and is an avid tennis player. He has retained his Swedish citizenship and is a member of the Swedish Physiological Society, as well as the National Academy of Sciences and the American Academy of Arts and Sciences. Among the many awards he and Hubel have jointly won have been the Jules C. Stein Research for the Prevention of Blindness Award (1971), the Lewis S. Rosenstiel Award for Basic Medical Research from Brandeis University (1972), the Jonas S. Friedenwald Memorial Award of the Association for Research in Vision and Ophthalmology (1975), the Karl S. Lashley Prize of the American Philosophical Society (1977), the Louisa Gross Horowitz Prize from Columbia (1978), and the George Ledlie Prize from Harvard (1980).

MARCIA MELDRUM

Selected Bibliography

PRIMARY SOURCES

Hubel, David H., and Torsten N. Wiesel. 1959. "Receptive Fields of Single Neurones in the Cat's Striate Cortex." *Journal of Physiology* 148:574–91.

———. 1961. "Integrative Action in the Cat's Lateral Geniculate Body." *Journal of Physiology* 155 (February):385–98.

———. 1962. "Receptive Fields, Binocular Interaction, and Functional Architecture in the Cat's Visual Cortex." *Journal of Physiology* 160 (January):106–54.

———. 1963. "Single-cell Responses in Striate Cortex of Kittens Deprived of Vision in One Eye." *Journal of Neurophysiology* 26 (November): 1003–17.

———. 1965. "Extent of Recovery from the Effects of Visual Deprivation in Kittens." *Journal of Neurophysiology* 28 (November):1060–72.

———. 1965. "Receptive Fields and Functional Architecture in Two Non Striate Visual Areas (18 and 19) of the Cat." *Journal of Neurophysiology* 28:229–89.

———. 1968. "Receptive Fields and Functional Architecture of Monkey Striate Cortex." *Journal of Physiology* 195:215–43.

Hubel, David H. 1979. "The Visual Cortex of Normal and Deprived Monkeys." *American Scientist* 67:532–43.

Hubel, David H. 1988. *Mind, Brain, and Vision*. New York: Scientific American Library.

SECONDARY SOURCES

Altman, Lawrence K. 1981. "Studies Advance Work on Brain, Eye Disorders." *New York Times* (October 10):50.

Lettvin, Jerome Y. 1981. "Filling Out the Forms: An Appreciation of Hubel and Wiesel." *Science* 214 (October 30):518–20.

1981. "Nobel Prize in Medicine: David Hunter Hubel." *New York Times* (October 10):50.

Schmeck, Harold M., Jr. 1981. "Three Scientists Share Nobel Prize for Studies of the Brain." *New York Times* (October 10):1.

1981. "Torsten Nils Wiesel." *New York Times* (October 10):50.

MAURICE HUGH FREDERICK WILKINS *1962*

Maurice Hugh Frederick Wilkins was born December 15, 1916, in Pongaroa, New Zealand, the son of Eveline Constance Jane (née Whittaker) and Edgar Henry Wilkins, a physician, both originally from Dublin. The family moved to England when Wilkins was six years old. He married Patricia Ann Chidgey in 1959; the couple have two sons and two daughters. After studying physics at Cambridge, Wilkins went to Birmingham for his Ph.D., which he received in 1940 for work on the phenomenon of luminescence of solids, which assisted wartime radar development. He was then assigned to join the British team working on the Manhattan Project and turned his attention to the separation of uranium isotopes for atomic weapons.

After the war, Wilkins continued his theoretical studies on luminescence at St. Andrews in Scotland for a year (1945–46) and then joined the Medical Research Council Unit at King's College, London. There he developed an interest in biophysical problems, particularly the structure of DNA and of tobacco mosaic virus, which he hoped to elucidate using spectrophotometric, ultrasonic, and other biochemical tools. Wilkins discovered how to prepare crystalline DNA fibers from solutions; this success led him to shift his energies to X-ray diffraction analysis as the most suitable tool for determining its structure. This technique makes use of the fact that a crystalline form diffracts X-rays as if they were a three-dimensional lattice, making "pictures" of the molecule possible. The trick is, first, to produce a clear crystallographic image and, second, to correctly decipher the molecular structure from the image. Independently of James Watson and Francis Crick's work at Cambridge, Wilkins and his student, Raymond Gosling, determined that DNA was helical in structure, its nitrogenous bases were internal, the helical turn was approximately 34Å, and the diameter of the molecule was 20Å.

In May 1950 Wilkins used his thin threads of DNA to obtain the first evidence that DNA had a crystalline structure. The following year he presented his X-ray photographs at a slide presentation in Naples where, by good luck, James Watson happened to be vacationing at the Naples Biological Station. Watson immediately became enamored of the idea of using X-ray crystallography to determine DNA structure, but felt rebuffed when he approached Wilkins. Instead of going to London, therefore, Watson went to Cambridge later that year to pursue his new interest.

At King's College, the director of Wilkins' laboratory, J. T. Randall, sought to expand the X-ray diffraction work and, early in 1951, hired Rosalind Franklin, a physical chemist, to set up a new unit. She had used crystallography to study the structure of coals and tarry carbon while working in Paris but had no experience with biological molecules. In her initial talks with Randall in 1950 she had been told she would be working on proteins, but some months later he asked her to consider the DNA problem as well. He apparently failed to make clear to her that Wilkins had priority on the DNA work, or that her job was to collaborate with and assist Wilkins in this area. Franklin assumed that she was being brought in to develop a new X-ray diffraction unit and to study DNA as an independent investigator, based on her own already-established career and publication record in physical chemistry.

Probably because of this basic misunderstanding, Wilkins and Franklin were in conflict from the beginning; they disliked each other and were unable to collaborate. King's College thus was in the curious situation of having two highly qualified scientists working independently on the X-ray analysis of DNA, with very little cooperation. Cambridge had an equally curious situation of having two very cooperative investigators, one, Watson, who knew virtually nothing about X-ray crystallography, and the other, Crick, who was still a graduate student, but provided the physics and mathematics that his colleague lacked. Although the Cambridge team entered the field a full eighteen months after Wilkins began his structural studies of DNA, their odd partnership gave them the advantage.

What little exchange took place between the two laboratories at King's frustrated both Wilkins and Franklin. Wilkins believed that the photographs made by both Gosling and Franklin established a helical structure, but Franklin was equally sure that they showed no evidence of helicity. Franklin also found two different patterns in the DNA images, depending on whether the crystals were kept moist or dry. The dry or A form was far more distinct than the wet or B form. Franklin's picture of the A form appeared to Wilkins to suggest a helix, but she bitterly rejected the idea. Wilkins was therefore more hesitant to follow his first impression and instead undertook more cautious preparations of his crystals and X-ray photographs. This at least was Wilkins' perspective as reflected in Watson's account.

Franklin's own notes of 1951 show that she did indeed realize the possible helicity of DNA but was not then ready to offer speculations for public discussion. Her reaction to Wilkins may have been less a rejection of the concept than of his effort to interpret her results.

By 1953, Wilkins' and Franklin's X-ray photographs were fully supportive of a helical model and the King's College group was perhaps only months away from working out most, if not all, of the features of DNA structure. Watson and Crick were enormously helped in their successful effort by having had the opportunity to see the King's College photos, with the assistance of Max Perutz, the director of their laboratory at Cambridge.

Crick's and Watson's analysis described two strands of deoxyribose phosphate, linked by the four nitrogenous bases (adenine, thymine, quanine, and cytosine), in hydrogen-bonded pairs. This innovative model made clear the process of DNA self-replication. The story of how the structure was discovered has been well documented by Watson, by Horace Freeland Judson, and by Anne Sayre, although each of the principals offers a slightly different recollection.

In 1953, all four investigators associated with the discovery of the double helix published their contributions in *Nature*: Watson and Crick in two short notes; Wilkins and his students; and Franklin and Gosling separately in short reports with X-ray photographs. Rosalind Franklin died of abdominal cancer in 1958, at the age of 37. In 1962, Watson, Crick, and Wilkins shared the Nobel Prize.

Wilkins continued to work at King's College. He was named deputy director of the Medical Research Council's Biophysics Unit there in 1955 and became director in 1970. In 1972, he took over as director of the Neurobiology Unit and, in 1974, as head of the Cell Biophysics Unit. In 1981 he became Professor Emeritus. Wilkins is a fellow of the Royal Society and a foreign member of the American Society of Biological Chemists and the American Academy of Arts and Sciences. He served as president of the British Society for Social Responsibility in Science in 1969. Among the other honors he has received for his work the most notable is the Lasker Award from the American Public Health Association (1960).

ELOF AXEL CARLSON

Selected Bibliography

PRIMARY SOURCES

Wilkins, M. H. F., R. G. Gosling, and W. E. Seeds. 1951. "Physical Studies of Nucleic Acids." *Nature* 167:759–60.

Wilkins, M. H. F., W. E. Seeds, A. R. Stokes, and H. R. Wilson. 1953. "Helical Structure of Crystalline Deoxypentose Nucleic Acid." *Nature* 167:759–62.

Wilkins, M. H. F., and J. T. Randall. 1953. "Crystallinity in Sperm Heads: Molecular Structure of Nucleoprotein *in Vivo*." *Biochimica Biophysica Acta* 10:192–93.

Wilkins, M. H. F., *et al.* 1962. "Determination of the Helical Configuration of Ribonucleic Acid Molecules by X-ray Diffraction Study of Crystalline Amino-acid Transfer Ribonucleic Acid." *Nature* 194:1014.

SECONDARY SOURCES

Franklin, Rosalind. 1953. "Molecular Configuration in Sodiumthymonucleate." *Nature* 172:740–41.

Judson, Horace Freeland. 1979. *The Eighth Day of Creation: The Makers of the Revolution in Biology.* New York: Simon and Schuster.

Olby, Robert. 1974. *The Path to the Double Helix*. Seattle: University of Washington Press.

Sayre, Anne. 1974. *Rosalind Franklin and DNA*. New York: Norton.

Watson, James D. 1968. *The Double Helix*. New York: Atheneum.

ROSALYN SUSSMAN YALOW
1977

Rosalyn Sussman Yalow received the Nobel Prize in 1977 "for development of radioimmunoassays of peptide hormones." Roger Guillemin and Andrew Schally also shared the Nobel Prize that year for their discoveries concerning peptide hormone production to the brain. She was only the second woman to win a Nobel Prize in Physiology or Medicine (the first was Gerty T. Cori in 1947). Yalow was born on July 19, 1921, in New York City. Her father, Simon Sussman, owned and managed a small paper and twine business. Her mother, Clara Zipper Sussman, had emigrated to the United States from Germany as a young child. Yalow attended Hunter College, New York City, from 1937 to 1941, and was awarded the B.A. degree. She received her M.S. in physics at the University of Illinois College of Engineering in 1942, where she served as a teaching assistant and was the only woman among the four hundred graduate students and faculty at the time. She received her Ph.D. in nuclear physics from the same institution in 1945. She married Aaron Yalow, a fellow graduate student in physics at Illinois, on June 6, 1943. They have a son and a daughter.

Yalow returned to New York to become a physics teacher and researcher at Hunter College (1945–50) and a part-time consultant to the Radiotherapy Service at Bronx Veterans Administration (VA) Hospital (1947–50). She established the radioisotope laboratory at the Bronx VA Hospital and worked as a full-time researcher there from 1950 to 1980. That first year Solomon A. Berson, who was completing his residency in internal medicine at the hospital, met Yalow, became interested in her work, and then joined her in the radioisotope service. Thus began a fruitful twenty-two year partnership that lasted until Berson's death on April 11, 1972. Yalow recalled that "it was a great partnership—he wanted to be a physicist, and I wanted to be a physician" (Haber 1979, 138). Together Yalow and Berson discovered and developed the radioimmunoassay, a revolutionary method of measuring substances—hormones, drugs, vitamins, enzymes, and antibodies to viruses—in blood and body tissues that were present in such small quantities that there had been no way of measuring them directly before.

Rosalyn Yalow served as a senior medical investigator at the Bronx VA Hospital from 1972 to 1980. She was Research Professor, Department of Medicine, Mount Sinai School of Medicine, from 1968 to 1974, and then Distinguished Service Professor, Mount Sinai School of Medicine, from 1974 to 1980. Subsequently she became Distinguished Professor at

Large, Albert Einstein College of Medicine, Yeshiva University, from 1980 to 1986; chairman, Department of Clinical Science, Montefiore Hospital and Medical Center, from 1980 to 1986; and Solomon A. Berson Distinguished Professor at Large, Mount Sinai School of Medicine, 1986 to the present.

In her Nobel Lecture Yalow noted that "for the past 30 years I have been committed to the development and application of radioisotopic methodology to analyze the fine structure of biologic systems. From 1950 until his untimely death in 1972, Dr. Solomon Berson was joined with me in this scientific adventure and together we gave birth to and nurtured through its infancy, radioimmunoassay, a powerful tool for determination of virtually any substance of biologic interest. Would that he were here to share this moment" (Yalow 1977, 1236). She then explained that radioimmunoassay, a method that uses radioactive substances to aid in measuring minute quantities of substances in blood plasma and in other body fluids, came into being "not by directed design but more as a fallout" from other investigations.

When Yalow and Berson began their collaborative work in 1950 they used radioisotopes (radioactive chemical elements) to measure the blood volume of patients, to assess distribution of plasma proteins in body compartments, and to help in diagnosis of thyroid dysfunction. Their epochal discovery of radioimmunoassay (RIA) resulted from experiments that were initially designed to answer another question.

A physician had hypothesized that maturity-onset diabetes mellitus might not be due to a deficiency of insulin secretion (as it is in childhood diabetes), but rather to abnormally rapid degradation of insulin within the liver. To test this hypothesis Berson and Yalow studied the metabolism of radiolabeled insulin (insulin tagged with a small amount of radioactive iodine tracer) injected into nondiabetic and diabetic subjects. To their surprise, they found a definitely retarded rate of insulin disappearance from the plasma of patients who had been receiving insulin. The investigators suspected that insulin-treated diabetics possessed circulating antibodies that bound insulin and delayed its appearance from circulation. The problem was that these antibodies might be present in such low concentration that they would not be precipitating—and thus classic immunological techniques would be inadequate to detect them. Berson and Yalow realized that insulin-binding antibodies might prove to be highly discriminating reagents for measuring insulin concentrations in body fluids. They promptly set to work to introduce radioisotopic methods of high sensitivity for detection of soluble antigen-antibody complexes.

Using a variety of electrophoretic methods, Berson and Yalow were able to demonstrate the ubiquitous presence of insulin-binding antibodies in insulin-treated subjects. This concept was at variance with the thinking of immunologists of the mid-1950s, most of whom believed that the insulin molecule was too small to provoke antibody production. Berson and Yalow's original paper describing their findings was rejected by *Science* and initially rejected by *The Journal of Clinical Investigation* before the *JCI* finally published it after the words "insulin antibody" were removed from the title and the authors proved that the globulin binding to insulin met the definition of antibody given in a standard textbook of immunology.

Berson and Yalow then established that, in the laboratory, the addition of increasing amounts of unlabeled insulin to a mixture of insulin antibody and labeled insulin resulted in displacement of some of the labeled insulin. Labeled and unlabeled insulin competed for binding sites on the antibody to insulin. Knowing the amount of labeled insulin one was binding to a fixed concentration of antibody in this system, one could calculate the amount of unlabeled insulin that was present in the "unknown" sample taken from a tissue extract or the plasma of a patient. This discovery formed the basis of the first radioimmunoassay, that of insulin. By 1959 Yalow and Berson were able to measure the concentration of insulin in unextracted human plasma. Until this time, it must be noted, bioassays were in common use in laboratories to measure hormonal activity. Though these assays were specific for assessing biological activity, they were usually far too insensitive to measure hormones in biologic fluids. Only gross changes in hormone concentration were assayable; small changes, though capable of drastically altering an individual's health, were beyond the reach of bioassay.

Radioimmunoassay soon became an invaluable technique for measuring minute quantities of substances in biological fluids. One scientist perceptively noted that "the availability of the radioimmunoassay for insulin with which one could measure the concentration of hormone in very small volumes of serum . . . made it possible to monitor changing concentrations of the hormone over a time scale of minutes. It is especially noteworthy that this form of quantitative biology . . . was immediately applied to intact people—normal, diabetic, and obese—and thus made extrapolation from animal data to the human condition unnecessary in many instances." (Tepperman 1988).

Berson and Yalow also fully developed the theoretical and mathematical principles underlying their radioimmunoassay technique. In her Nobel Lecture Yalow remarked that "radioimmunoassay is simple in principle." In the general procedure a known amount of radioactive antigen (for example, insulin that has been labeled or "tagged" by having a minute amount of radioactive iodine attached to it) is added, along with a fixed amount of antibody, to a sample containing an unknown quantity of the same—but unlabeled—antigen (in this case, insulin in a sample of a patient's plasma). The unlabeled antigen competes with the labeled antigen for antibody-binding sites. The concentration of the unknown unlabeled antigen is then obtained by comparing its inhibitory effect on the binding of radioactively labeled antigen to specific antibody with the inhibitory effect of known standards.

The sensitivity of RIA is remarkable. Concentrations of substances in as small as nanogram (billionth of a gram) and picogram (trillionth of a gram) quantities in biological fluids are now detectable. Hormone levels in human blood, previously unmeasurable because of the inadequacy of earlier bioassay methods, are now detectable by RIA and are routinely measured in basic and clinical research and in clinical situations.

Take for example the current state of measurement of the hormone cortisol, which is synthesized by the adrenal cortex and is sugar-retaining, anti-inflammatory, and life-supporting hormone. Before the development of radioimmunoassay, cortisol was measured indirectly by chemical colorimetric methods; these were relatively insensitive and could be interfered with by other blood-borne substances. Current assays of a patient's plasma cortisol, based on the methods pioneered by Berson and Yalow, depend on inhibition of binding of radiolabeled cortisol to an antibody by the cortisol present in the patient's plasma sample. The assays are extremely sensitive, so small plasma volumes may be used. Changing plasma levels of cortisol can be monitored throughout the day. Moreover, cross reactivity of cortisol antisera to other closely related steroids (cortisol-like substances made by the adrenal cortex, ovaries, or testes) is minimal, so radioimmunoassay gives a specific measurement of total plasma cortisol concentration. Another advantage of RIA is that other commonly encountered chemicals, drugs, and medications do not interfere with the assay. Thus for cortisol (as with many other important biological substances) radioimmunoassay has proven to be a sensitive, specific, and reliable method of measuring physiological or pathological quantities in body fluids.

Since its development, RIA has been used to provide the key diagnostic tests in hyperactive and hypoactive endocrine states such as hyperthyroidism, hypothyroidism, growth hormone deficiency, acromegaly, adrenal dysfunction, and ovarian and testicular dysfunction. And it is still the essential method for measurement of insulin in blood. Historically, RIA permitted the isolation and chemical characterization of hypothalamic hormones to proceed more rapidly than would have been possible with bioassay techniques. Indeed, RIA has so revolutionized the diagnostic resources of clinical neuroendocrinologists that it now is difficult to imagine that before 1960 scientists could not accurately determine the concentration of any of the protein hormones in blood; it was then impossible, for example, to show that anterior pituitary hormone secretions varied throughout the day and were pulsatile in their expression. So laborious, insensitive, and prodigal in their use of large volumes of plasma (making detection of short-term alterations impossible) were bioassays.

RIA is now routinely used to detect hepatitis-associated antigen in the blood of patients and donors, to measure levels of clotting factors and other hematologic substances, to detect antibiotic action, to ascertain blood levels of therapeutic drugs such as digitalis derivatives, anticonvulsants, and lithium, to detect the presence and quantity of anabolic steroids in the urine of athletes competing in international events, and to detect addictive and hallucinogenic drugs in body fluids.

Rosalyn Yalow looked upon radioimmunoassay as a probe for the fine structure of biologic systems. In that spirit she concluded her Nobel Lecture with these words: "The first telescope opened the heavens; the first microscope opened the world of the microbes, radioisotopic methodology, as exemplified by RIA, has shown the potential for opening new vistas in science and medicine" (Yalow 1977, 1245).

LAWRENCE SHERMAN

Selected Bibliography

PRIMARY SOURCES

Berson, S. A., R. S. Yalow, A. Bauman, M. A. Rothschild, and K. Newerly. 1956. "Insulin-I131 Metabolism in Human Subjects: Demonstration of Insulin Binding Globulin in the Circulation of Insulin Treated Subjects." *Journal of Clinical Investigation* 35:170–90.

Berson, S. A., and R. S. Yalow. 1959. "Quantitative Aspects of the Reaction between Insulin and Insulin-binding Antibody." *Journal of Clinical Investigation* 38:1996–2016.

Berson, S. A., and R. S. Yalow. 1959. "Species-Specificity of Human Anti-Beef, Pork Insulin Serum." *Journal of Clinical Investigation* 38:2017–25.

Yalow, R. S., and S. A. Berson. 1959. "Assay of Plasma Insulin in Human Subjects by Immunological Methods." *Nature* (London) 184:1648–49.

Yalow, Rosalyn S. 1977. "Radioimmunoassay: A Probe for the Fine Structure of Biologic Systems." Nobel Lecture. Reprinted in *Science* 200 (June 16):1236–45.

SECONDARY SOURCES

Haber, Louis. 1979. *Women Pioneers of Science*, 128–40. New York: Harcourt Brace Jovanovich.

Meites, Joseph. 1977. "Research News: The 1977 Nobel Prize in Physiology or Medicine." *Science* 198 (November 11):594–96.

Tepperman, Jay. 1988. "A View of the History of Biology from an Islet of Langerhans." In *Endocrinology: People and Ideas*, edited by S. M. McCann, 285–333. Bethesda, Md.: American Physiological Society.

INDEX

Abel, John J., 9, 20, 382
Abraham, E. P., 86, 190
Adams, M. H., 367
Ader, Clement, 160
Adrian, Lord Edgar Douglas, **1–3**, 206, 208, 216, 228, 255, 490, 493
Adrian, Richard, 258
Ahlqvist, Raymond, 49
Akert, K., 243
Albert, Eduard, 340
Alberts, Alfred W., 72, 211
Allen, Edgar, 130, 131
Allen, Frederick M., 20, 382
Allison, Anthony C., 57
Allison, V. D., 185
Anderson, H. K., 115
Anderson, Rudolf J., 52
Anderson, Thomas F., 238, 239, 367
Arber, Werner, **4–7**, 367, 427, 428, 494, 495, 496
Arimura, Akira, 489
Arrhenius, Svante, 113, 174
Arsonval, Deprez-de, 160
Arthus, Maurice, 39, 245
Attardi, Domenica, 92
Avery, Oswald T., 29, 127, 239, 348, 410, 435
Axelrod, Julius, **7–12**, 174, 298
Baba, Yoshihiko, 489
Babinski, J. F., 405
Bach, Fritz, 123
Baker, Peter F., 258
Bakunin, Mikhail A., 384
Baldwin, Jack, 335
Baltazard, Marcel, 202
Baltimore, David, **12–17**, 137, 139, 521, 523, 543–544
Bamberger, Eugen, 340
Bang, Fridtjof, 179
Bang, Oluf, 479
Banting, Sir Frederick Grant, **17–22**, 132, 361, 379, 380, 381, 382, 383
Barach, A. L., 463
Bárány, Robert, **23–26**
Barger, George, 116, 318
Barker, Lewellys, 171
Barron, Moses, 18
Barski, G., 398
Bary, Anton de, 329
Battelli, F., 64
Baudhuin, Pierce, 143
Bauer, J. H., 526
Baumgarten, Paul von, 386
Bayliss, Leonard Ernest, 115
Baylor, Denis, 258
Beadle, George Wells, **27–30**, 347, 348, 517, 518, 519
Beaufay, Henri, 143
Beaumont, William, 172
Beer, Roger J. S., 308
Behnisch, R., 136
Behring, Emil Adolf von, **30–34**, 134, 152, 153, 178, 293, 340, 386, 467
Békésy, Georg von, **34–37**
Benaceraff, Baruj, **38–42**, 122, 497
Benedetto, Enrique Di, 273
Bennett, J. C., 535
Benzer, Seymour, 239
Berg, Paul, 6, 428, 496
Berger, Hans, 2
Bergmann, Max, 52
Bergström, Sune Karl, **42–45**, 175, 373, 482, 483, 538, 539, 540
Bernard, Claude, 66, 95, 100, 195, 380
Bernard, John, 18
Bernhard, Carl Gustaf, 571

Bernstein, Julius, 255, 256, 284
Berry, George, 572
Berson, Solomon A., 577, 578, 579, 580
Bertani, Giuseppe, 4, 5, 427, 495
Berthet, Jacques, 142, 143
Berzelius, Jacob, 529–530
Best, Charles H., 19, 20, 21, 361, 381, 382, 383
Biggs, Hermann, 314
Billingham, R. E., 390
Billroth, Theodor, 313, 316
Binkley, Steven, 131
Binz, Carl, 31
Biozzi, Guido, 39
Bishop, George, 205
Bishop, J. Michael, **45–48**, 542, 543
Bizzozero, Giulio Cesare, 214
Black, Sir James Whyte, **48–51**, 163, 252
Bloch, Konrad E., **51–56**, 372, 374
Blonquist, Alfred T., 260
Blumberg, Baruch Samuel, **56–59**, 201
Bogen, Joseph, 507
Bohr, Niels, 124, 127, 296, 337
Bois Reymond, Emil du, 329
Boler, Jan, 222
Bolk, Louis, 25
Bordet, Jules, **59–64**, 322, 340, 386
Bordet, Paul, 60
Borgeat, Pierre, 485, 541
Born, Max, 126
Botkin, S. P., 446
Boveri, Theodor, 502
Bovet, Daniel, **64–69**
Bovet, Pierre, 64
Bowers, Cyril Y., 222, 488
Boyer, Herbert, 6, 428–429, 496
Brenner, Sydney, 290
Brent, L., 390
Brequet, Jacques, 467
Brequet, Louis, 467
Breuer, Josef, 23, 24, 25
Bridges, Calvin Blackman, 419
Brieger, Ludwig, 32
Brodie, Bernard B., 8
Bronfenbrenner, Jacques Jacob, 237
Bronk, Detlev, 2, 208, 216, 228, 230
Bronner, James, 260
Brown, G. L., 117, 175
Brown, Paul K., 554
Brown, Michael Stuart, **70–73**, 209, 210, 211, 212
Büchner, Hans, 61, 62
Büchner, Ludwig, 384
Buckle, Henry Thomas, 384
Bueker, Elmer, 352
Buhler, Karl, 362
Bullock, William, 63
Bunting, Stuart, 540
Burgus, Roger, 222, 488
Burn, J. H., 538
Burnet, Sir Frank MacFarlane, **74–75**, 202, 294, 295, 388–389, 390, 397
Buys Ballot, C. H. D., 159
Caldwell, P. C., 258
Campbell, W. R., 20, 21, 382
Caro, Lucien, 444
Carrel, Alexis, **80–83**, 179
Castillo, Jose del, 299, 301
Castle, William B., 404
Castle, William Ernest, 498
Catan (Houssay), Maria A., 273
Caullery, Maurice, 408
Chagas, Carlos, 353
Chain, Sir Ernst Boris, 67, **84–87**, 184, 186, 190, 191, 192
Chandler, Knox, 258
Chargaff, Erwin, 52
Chase, Martha, 127, 239
Chatton, Edouard, 369, 408
Chauveau, Jean-Baptiste Auguste, 195
Cheney, Lee, 131
Cherry, Marianna, 500
Christian, Walter, 530
Clark, Ronald, 87
Clarke, Hans, 52, 53

Claude, Albert, **88–90**, 141, 142, 143, 442, 443
Clutterbuck, P. W., 190
Cohen, S. S., 367
Cohen, Stanley, 6, **91–94**, 350, 353–354, 428, 496
Cohn, Edwin, 424
Cohn, Ferdinand, 313
Cohn, Melvin, 410
Cole, Kenneth S., 255, 256, 257, 284, 285
Cole, S. W., 266
Colebrook, L., 135
Collip, James B., 20, 21, 382, 383
Comroe, Julius, 247
Comte, Charles, 432
Conseil, Ernest, 432
Corer, Peter, 389
Corey, E. J., 485, 541
Cori, Carl Ferdinand, 94–98, 99–104, 142, 324, 410, 439, 510
Cori, Gerty Theresa Radnitz, 94–97, **99–104**, 142, 324, 410, 439, 510, 577
Cormack, Allan Macleod, **104–107**, 271
Corti, Alfonso Giacomo Gaspare, 36
Cotton, Richard, 321, 398
Cournand, André Frédéric, **107–111**, 194, 196, 463, 464, 465
Craddock, Stuart, 85
Creighton, Harriet, 376
Crick, Francis, 15, **111–114**, 128, 240, 326, 410, 435, 523, 561, 562, 574, 575, 576
Cullen, Esther, 533
Cyon, Elie, 446
Dakin, Henry B., 81–82
Dakin, H. D., 330
Dale, Sir Henry Hallett, 9, 65, 75, **115–118**, 146, 174, 175, 205, 298, 299, 359, 360, 361, 538
Dam, Carl Peter Hendrik, **119–122**, 130
Dandy, W. E., 405
Danna, Kathleen, 428
Daremberg, G., 61
Darnell, James, 12
Dausset, Jean, 38, **123–125**, 497
Davidson, Harriet, 237
Davis, S. M., 267
De Castro, F., 247
Dean, H. R., 189
Decastello, A., 341
Delbrück, Max Ludwig Henning, **126–129**, 138, 238, 239, 240, 293, 294, 365, 366, 367, 409, 521
Demerec, Milislav, 127
Démont, T., 500
Deng, C. T., 47, 543
Desideio, D., 222
Deulofeu, Venancio, 273
De Vogel, W. Th., 160
Dingell, Representative John, 16
Ditlevson, Hjalmar, 179
Dobelle, William, 554
Dodge, B. O., 518
Doermann, A. H., 367
Doisy, Edward Adelbert, 119, 120, **129–133**
Domagk, Gerhard Johannes Paul, 66, 68, **133–137**
Donald, Hugh, 390
Donath, Julius, 341
Donders, F. C., 159
Dorp, David Van, 44, 484, 540
Dreisch, Hans, 414
Dreyer, William, 535
Dubos, René, 39, 550, 551
Dudley, H. W., 117, 360, 439
Dulbecco, Renato, 12, 13, **137–141**, 351, 367, 521, 523
Dunn, T. F., 222
Dunn, Sir William, 268
Dussoix, Daisy, 5, 495, 496
Duthie, Edward, 191
Duve, Christian René de, 88, **141–144**, 442
Eastman, George, 567
Eccles, Sir John Carew, 117, **145–147**, 208, 298, 299–300, 493

Eccles, Rosamond, 145
Edelman, Gerald Maurice, 40, **148–151**, 397, 451, 452
Edsall, David, 401
Ehrlich, Paul, 32, 66, 67, 115, 134, **151–155**, 185, 252, 315, 341, 384, 397, 547
Eijkman, Christiaan, **155–158**, 402
Einstein, Albert, 226, 556, 559
Einthoven, Willem, **158–163**
Elion, Gertrude Belle, 48, **163–166**, 228, 252, 253
Ellerman, Wilhelm, 479
Elliot, T. R., 9, 65, 116, 175, 359, 360
Ellis, Emory, 127, 238
Embden, Gustav, 394
Emerson, Rollins A., 27
Enders, John Franklin, **167–170**, 201, 471, 472, 563, 564, 565
Enzmann, Franz, 222
Ephrussi, Boris, 28, 409, 518
Epstein, Leslie A., 191
Erlanger, Joseph, 2, **170–173**, 205, 206, 207, 208
Estaing, Giscard de, 291
Euler, Astrid Cleve von, 174
Euler, Leo von, 174
Euler, Ulf Svante von, 9, 43, 44, **174–177**, 298, 483, 484, 539–540
Euler-Chelpin, Hans von, 174
Euw, Jacob von, 458
Evans, E. A., Jr., 52
Ewald, Julius, 25
Ewins, Arthur, 116
Exner, Sigmund, 198
Fahr, George, 161
Fahraeus, Robin, 174
Fajans, Kasimir, 372
Falck, B., 176
Fatt, Paul, 146, 299, 300
Feldberg, Wilhelm S., 117, 298, 299
Feldman, William H., 550, 551
Feller, A. E., 168, 472, 564
Fennor, Frank, 76
Fermi, Enrico, 365
Fibiger, Johannes Andreas Grib, **177–181**
Finger, Ernest, 341
Finsen, Niels Ryberg, **181–184**
Fischer, Albert, 356
Fischer, Emil, 340, 556
Fischer, Hans, 51
Fitz, Reginald, 423
Fleck, Ludvik, 297
Fleming, Sir Alexander, 67, 84–86, **184–188**, 189, 190, 191
Fletcher, A. A., 20, 21, 382
Fletcher, Walter Morley, 267, 268
Flexner, Abraham, 567
Flexner, Simon, 88, 425, 478, 481, 568
Florey, Howard Waller, 67, 84–87, 184, 186, 187, **188–194**, 389
Flourens, Pierre, 23, 25
Foglia, Virgilio G., 273, 274
Folin, Otto, 130, 131
Folkers, Karl, 222, 488
Ford, Lincoln, 287
Forssmann, Werner Theodor Otto, 107, 108–109, 110, **194–197**, 463, 465
Förster, Josef, 156
Foster, Sir Michael, 266, 491
Fourneau, E., 64, 66, 68
Fraenkel, Carl, 32
Franek, Frantiszek, 149, 152
Frankland, Edward, 265
Franklin, Richard, 12, 562
Franklin, Rosalind, 574–575, 576
Frederickson, Donald S., 210
Frerich, Freidrich von, 151
Freud, Sigmund, 386, 545
Freund, Jules, 39
Fries, Nils, 519
Frisch, Karl von, **198–200**, 362, 532
Fukasawa, Toshio, 5, 495
Fullman, Ernest, 89
Fulton, John, 189, 406
Gaddum, Sir John, 174, 538

Gaffky, Georg, 313
Gajudsek, Daniel Carleton, 56, **201–204**
Galeb, O., 179
Gamow, George, 112
Garibaldi, Giuseppe, 384
Garrod, Archibald, 518
Gaskell, Walter H., 115, 491
Gasser, Herbert Spencer, 2, 172, **205–209**
Gaté, J., 191
Gaule, J. G., 242
Gazzaniga, Michael S., 507
Gegenbaur, Carl, 502
Gell, Philip G. H., 40
Gengou, Octave, 60, 62
Gerlach, Walter, 372
Gerould, John Hiram, 498
Gibbs, Clarence J., 202, 203
Gibson, Tom, 389
Gilbert, Walter, 290, 535
Gley, Emile, 318, 469
Gley, Eugene, 245
Goering, Hermann, 557
Goldberger, Joseph, 267
Goldblatt, Maurice, 43, 483, 539
Goldstein, Joseph Leonard, 70–72, **209–213**
Goldsworthy, Neil, 189
Golgi, Camillio, **213–215**, 455, 492
Goltz, Friedrich, 491
Gombault, Albert, 430
Goodman, Howard, 6, 428, 496
Gorer, Peter Alfred, 499
Gorgas, William C., 477, 526
Gosling, Raymond, 574, 575, 576
Goulian, Mehran, 327
Graham, Clarence W., 228, 229
Graham, Helen, 205
Granit, Ragnar Arthur, **216–219**, 227, 228, 230, 276, 553, 571
Grassi, Giovanni, 345
Green, Earl, 499
Gregory, H., 92
Grijns, Gerrit, 157
Gros, François, 291
Gross, Ludwik, 481
Gruber, Max von, 340
Grunberg-Manago, Marianne, 262, 440
Gryglewski, Richard, 540
Guillemin, Roger Charles Louis, **219–224**, 486, 487, 488, 489, 577
Guirard, Beverly, 357
Gullstrand, Allvar, **224–227**
Guntaka, Ramareddy, 47, 543
Gussenbauer, Carl, 23
Guthrie, Charles C., 81
Guthrie, Edwin R., 449
Guyénot, E., 64
Hadlow, William, 202
Haeckel, Ernst, 385, 502
Hagedorn, H. C., 20, 382
Hahn, Otto, 126
Haldane, J. B. S., 28, 84, 518
Hallpike, C. S., 26
Halpern, Bernard, 39
Halsted, William S., 318
Hamberg, Mats, 484, 540
Hamburger, H. J., 514, 515
Hamburger, Viktor, 91, 351–352
Hamilton, Alice, 402
Hamilton, Charles, 507
Hamilton, William Rowan, 226
Hammersten, Einar, 529
Hammon, William, 167
Hanriot, Maurice, 468
Hantzsch, Arthur, 340
Harington, Sir Charles, 84
Harrington, C. R., 304, 318
Harris, Geoffrey W., 221, 223, 487
Harrison, Ross G., 81
Hartline, Haldan Keffer, 208, **227–231**, 276, 553, 571
Hartmann, Eduard von, 31
Hartree, William, 250
Harvey, William, 466
Hasselbach, K. A., 337
Hausler, H., 360

Haworth, W. N., 516
Heatley, Norman G., 85, 86, 87, 190, 192
Hecht, Selig, 228, 553
Heidelberg, Michael, 39
Heidenhaim, Rudolf, 446, 447
Heinroth, Oskar, 362
Heisenberg, Werner, 228
Helmholtz, Hermann von, 36, 225
Hench, Philip, **231–237**, 306, 457
Henderson, L. J., 463
Henle, Jacob, 312
Henseleit, Kurt, 333
Hepburn, J., 20, 382
Heppel, Leon, 436
Hering, Heinrich, 246
Hershey, Alfred Day, 126, 127, 237–241, 365, 366, 367
Hertwig, Richard von, 198, 199
Herz, Gery, 142, 143
Herzen, Alexander, 384
Hess, Walter Rudolf, **241–244**, 405
Heubel, Emil, 152
Heymans, Corneille Jean François, 174, **244–248**
Heymans, Jean-François, 244, 246, 247
Hill, Archibald Vivian, 161, 175, **249–251**, 298, 392, 393, 394, 558
Hill, Sir Leonard, 379
Hill, Robert, 150, 452
Hillarp, Nils-Åke, 176
Hilschmann, Norbert, 149, 452
Hinsey, Joseph, 205
Hinshaw, H. Corwin, 550, 551
Hirota, Y., 290
Hitchings, George H., 48, 163, 164, 165, 166, **252–254**
Hochstetter, Ferdinand, 362
Hodgkin, Sir Alan Lloyd, 2, 145, 146, 156, 208, **255–260**, 284, 285, 286, 287, 298, 299, 300, 478
Hodgkin, Dorothy, 86
Hogeboom, George, 89, 443
Hogg, James F., 434
Hokum, Walter, 131
Holley, Robert W., **260–264**, 308, 309
Holmgren, Alarik F., 217
Holmgren, Gunnar, 23
Holst, Erich von, 363
Hönigschmidt, Otto, 372
Hood, Leroy, 536
Hopkins, Sir Frederick Gowland, 85, 190, **265–269**, 333, 359, 402
Hopkins, Gerard Manley, 265
Hoppe-Seyler, Ernst, 134
Horsley, Sir Victor, 491
Hotchkiss, Rollin, 89
Hounsfield, Sir Godfrey Newbold, 104, 105–106, **269–272**
Houssay, Bernardo Alberto, 94, 102, 176, **272–275**
Howell, William H., 171, 401
Hozumi, Nobumichi, 535
Huang (Baltimore), Alice S., 12, 14
Hubel, David Hunter, **276–279**, 505, 570, 571, 572, 573
Huddleson, I. F., 237
Hudson, N. P., 526
Huebner, Robert, 46, 543
Huggins, Charles Brenton, **279–283**, 481
Hunter, David, 218, 230
Hurwitz, Jerard, 13
Hustin, Albert, 480
Huxley, Sir Andrew Fielding, 2, 145, 146, 208, 255, 256, 257, 259, **284–288**, 299
Huxley, Hugh, 286
Huxley, Julian Sorrel, 420
Ichikawa, K., 179
Ivanyi, Dagmar, 124
Ivanyi, Pavol, 124
Jaboulay, Mathieu, 80
Jacob, François, **288–292**, 368, 370, 404
Jacobs, Merkel, 228
Jacobsen, Carlyle, 406
Jakoby, William, 435
Jamieson, J. D., 444

Jennings, Margaret, 190
Jerne, Niels, 76, **293–298**, 320, 322, 396
Johannsen, Wilhelm, 414
Johnson, J. B., 206
Johnson, William Arthur, 334
Judson, Horace Freeland, 112, 576
Kabet, Elvin Abraham, 39
Kaila, Eino, 216
Kaplan, Nathan, 357
Karrer, Paul, 120, 553
Katz, Sir Bernard, 11, 146, 174, 208, 251, **298–303**
Katz, David, 41
Keilin, David, 369
Keim, F. D., 27
Kellenberger, Eduard, 4
Kelly, T. J., 496
Kendall, Edward Calvin, 233, 235, **303–307**, 318, 457, 458, 459, 460, 515
Kenner, G. W., 308
Kenny, M., 135
Kent, James, 190
Keynes, Lord John Maynard, 249
Keynes, Richard, 257, 258, 286
Khorana, Har Gobind, 260, 261, **308–311**, 440
Kinnard, Margaret, 406
Kitasato, Shibasaburo, 32
Kjeldgaard, Niels, 370
Klarer, Joseph, 134
Klebs, Edwin, 32, 345
Klein, Emanuel, 475
Knoop, Franz, 332, 333, 334
Koch, E., 246
Koch, Heinrich Hermann Robert, 31, 32, 33, 134, 152, 155, 178, **312–315**, 491, 546 Kocher, Emil Theodor, 303, **316–320**
Kögl, F., 519
Köhler, Georges, 293, **320–324**, 396, 398, 399
Kölliker, Albrecht von, 455
König, Albert, 316
Konigsberg, William, 150, 453
Konstantinovich, Grand Duke Konstantin, 25
Kornberg, Arthur, **324–328**, 438, 439
Kornberg, Hans, 334
Kornberg (Levy), Sylvy R., 324
Kossell, Albrecht, 238, **328–331**
Koster, W., 159
Kovlevsky, Alexander, 385
Kraepelin, Emil, 23
Krafft-Ebing, Richard von, 546
Kramer, Gustav, 363
Krauss, Rudolf, 273
Krebs, Sir Hans Adolf, **332–336**, 356, 373, 515, 557
Krogh, Schack Augustus Steenberg, **336–339**
Krogh (Jorgenson), Marie, 336, 337, 338
Kuffler, Stephen, 146, 276, 277, 299, 300, 571
Kuhl, David E., 106
Kuhne, Wilhelm, **329–336**, 553
Kuhnlein, Urs, 5, 495
Kunkel, Beverly W., 228
Kunkel, Henry, 149, 295, 452
Kurzrok, Raphael, 43, 483, 539
Lacquer, Ernst, 355
Ladon, A., 246
Landsteiner, Karl, 148, 294, **340–343**, 451, 480
Langdon, R. G., 54
Langenbeck, Bernhard von, 316
Langley, John Newport, 115, 154, 242, 360, 491
Langsdorf, A. S., 206
Lankester, E. R., 266
Lapique, Louise, 205
Larner, J., 100
Lashley, Karl S., 506
Lauger, Paul, 417
Laveran, Charles Louis Alphonse, **343–347**, 369, 475
Lea, Sheridan, 491

Lebally, Charles, 432
Leder, Philip, 535–536
Lederburg (Zimmer), Esther Miriam, 348, 349
Lederburg, Joshua, 5, 27, **347–350**, 517, 519
Leff, Paul, 43
Leib, Charles, 43, 483, 539
Leidesdorf, Max von, 545
Leloir, Luis F., 274
Lenhossek, Mihaly, 514
Lettvin, Jerome Y., 276, 571
Levene, P. A., 356
Levi, Giuseppe, 138, 351, 352
Levi-Montalcini, Rita, 91, 92, 138, **350–355**
Levine, Philip, 342
Levy, Jerre, 507
Lewis, Juan T., 273, 274
Lewis, Peter, 257, 286
Lewis, Thomas, 161
Liddel, E .G. T., 493
Liljestrand, Garan, 174, 283
Lillie, Frank R., 280
Lima, Almeida, 405, 406
Lindbergh, Charles, 82
Lindegren, Carl C., 518
Lindhard, Johannes, 337
Linn, Stuart, 5, 495
Lint, K. de, 160
Lipman, Jacob G., 549
Lipmann, Fritz Albert, 334, **355–358**, 427
Lippich, Ferdinand, 94
Lister, Joseph, 313, 314, 386, 474
Little, Clarence Cook, 498–499
Littlefield, J. W., 322
Loeb, Jacques, 228, 414
Loeffler, Friedrich, 32, 313
Loewi, Otto, 9, 66, 100, 115, 117, 175, 299, **359–361**, 408
Lohmann, Karl, 394
Lombroso, Cesare, 213
Lorenz, Konrad, 198, **362–365**, 532, 533
Lucas, Keith, 1
Lücke, Albert, 316
Ludwig, Carl Friedrich Wilhelm, 446, 447
Ludwig, Emil, 242
Lundgaard, E., 394
Luria, Salvador E., 4, 5, 111, 126, 127, 138, 237, 238, 239, 240, 351, **365-368**, 409, 427, 495, 560
Lwoff, Andre, 288, 289, 290, 291, 348, **368–372**, 408, 409
Lwoff (Bourdalieux), Margerite, 368, 369, 370
Lynen, Feodor, 51, **372–375**
MacCallum, W. G., 476
Mach, Ernst, 25
Macleod, Colin M., 239, 348
Macleod, John Hames Richard, 17, 19, 20, 21, **379–383**
MacNichol, Edward F., 554
Mainini, Galli, 274
Malloe, Ole, 293
Manceaux, L., 431
Mangold, Otto, 504
Mann, Thomas, 52
Mansfeld, G., 515
Mansfeld, Geza, 100
Manson, Patrick, 345, 475, 476
Marcus, Philip, 12
Marenzi, Augustin, 273
Marey, Étienne-Jules, 195
Marine, D., 318
Marks, William B., 554
Marmont, G., 256, 285
Marotta, Domenico, 86
Marshall, E. K., 228
Martin, Newell, 491
Martius, Carl, 333, 334
Marx, A., 504
Mason, M. L., 460
Matsuo, Hisayuki, 489
Matthaei, Johann Heinrich, 262, 436
Matthews, Bryan Harold Cabot, 2
Mattox, R., 460

Maxam, Allan, 535
Mayer, Ernst, 411
McCarty, Maclyn J., 239, 348, 435
McClintock, Barbara, 27, **375–378**
McCollum, Elmer, 267, 402
McDevitt, Hugh, 40–41
McLeod, F. F. R., 132
Medawar (Taylor), Jean Shinglewood, 389, 391
Medawar, Peter, 74, 76, 190, **388–392**
Meerwein, Hans, 355
Mehring, Joseph von, 18, 380
Meitner, Lise, 126
Melchers, Fritz, 320
Mellanby, Edward, 192
Mendel, Gregor, 414, 435
Menendez, Eduardo Braun, 274, 275
Ménière, Prosper, 23, 25
Meselson, Matthew, 5, 495, 521
Mesnil, Felix, 369
Metchinkoff, Ilya (Élie), 33, 60, 61,151, 153, 369, **384–388**, 430
Meyer, Bertha, 353
Meyer, Hans-Horst, 245, 359
Meyerhof, Otto Fritz, 249, 250, 355, 356, 369, **392–395**, 438, 439, 553, 557
Michaelis, Leonor, 514
Miescher, Friedrich, 325, 329, 330
Mietzsch, Fritz, 134, 136
Miledi, Ricardo, 299, 301
Miller, F. R., 18, 19
Millman, Irving, 58
Milstein (Prilleltensky), Celia, 396
Milstein, Cesar, 293, 320, 321, 322, 323, **396–400**
Miner, N., 306
Minkowski, Oscar, 18, 188, 380
Minot, George Richards, **400–404**, 423, 424, 425, 426, 569
Mizutani, Satoshi, 13, 522, 523
Moffatt, John G., 308
Möllendorff, Wilhelm von, 332
Moller, Paul, 179
Moncado, Salvador, 540
Moniz, Antonio Caetano de Abreu Freire Egas, 2, 241, **405–408**
Monod, Jacques, 288, 290, 291, 368, 370, **408–412**
Morgan, Thomas Hunt, 27, 28, 367, 409, **413–416**, 419, 420, 518
Motulsky, Arno G., 71, 210
Mountcastle, Vernon, 276
Moynihan, Sir Berkeley, 319
Moynihan, Martin, 533
Muller, Carl, 70, 210
Muller, Hermann Joseph, 28, 112, 126, 367, 376, 377, 415, **419–422**, 498, 499, 518, 560
Müller, Friedrich von, 232
Müller, Fritz, 384–385
Müller, Paul Hermann, **416-419**
Müller-Hill, B., 290
Murnaghan, F. D., 228
Murphy, James B., 88, 442
Murphy, Robert, 484, 541
Murphy, William Parry, 402, **422–426**, 569
Murray, George B., 318
Murray, Kenneth, 6, 428, 496
Murray, Noreen, 6, 428, 496
Murrow, Edward R., 102
Myers, Ronald, 506–507
Nair, R. M. G., 489
Nastuk, Bill, 257
Nathans, Daniel, 4, 6, 367, **427-429**, 494, 496, 535
Navratil, E., 360
Nebes, Robert, 507
Nenna, Andre-Dominique, 123
Nernst, Walther, 556
Newcomer, Harry Sidney, 206
Nicolle, Charles Jules Henri, 418, **430–434**
Nicolle, Maurice, 430
Niedergerke, Rolf, 286
Nietzsche, Friedrich, 31

Nirenberg, Marshall, 112–113, 209, 260, 261, 262, 308, 309, **434–438**, 440
Nitti, Daniele, 64
Nitti, Federico, 64, 66
Nitti, Filomena, 64, 66
Noble, C. H., 19, 381, 382
Noguchi, H., 526, 527
Noll, Hans, 293
Nonelli, David, 357
Noorden, Carl von, 23
Nordin, Alfred, 295, 322
Northrop, John H., 471, 530
Nossal, Gus, 77, 78
Novikoff, Alex, 143
Nylen, Carl O., 26
Ochoa, Severo, 97, 262, 324, 326, **438–441**
Okada, Yoshio, 398
Okochi, K., 57
Olendorf, William H., 106
Orias, Oscar, 273, 274
Orth, Johannes, 178
Osler, William, 171
Ossietsky, Carl von, 136
Oudin, Jacques, 295
Ovary, Zoltan, 40
Overton, Charles Ernest, 256
Paget, Sir James, 316, 474
Palade, George E., 88, 141, 142, 143, **442–445**
Palade (Farquhar), Marilyn Gist, 442, 444
Papagostas, G., 191
Pastan, Ira H., 513, 542
Pasteur, Louis, 31, 295, 313, 316, 345, 386, 468
Pauli, Wolfgang, 126
Pauling, Linus, 76, 201, 294
Pauly, August, 502
Pavlov, Ivan Petrovich, **445-450**
Pehmister, Dallas, B., 280
Pekelharing, C. A., 156
Peron, General Juan D., 272, 274, 275
Perutz, Max, 575
Peters, Rudolph A., 439
Pfefferkorn, Elmer, 46
Pfeiffer, Richard, 60–61
Pfiffner, J. J., 459
Pfluger, Edward, 152
Pfund, A. H., 228
Piper, Priscilla, 540
Pirosky, Ignacio, 396
Politzer, Adam, 23
Pontecorvo, G., 377
Popper, Karl, 411
Porter, Keith R., 89, 443
Porter, Paul, 468
Porter, Rodney Roy, 40, 148, 149, 150, **451–454**
Potter, M., 321
Powell, John, 271
Prelog, Vladimir, 52, 308
Press, Elizabeth, 149, 452
Priestly, J. B., 265
Prince Carl of Sweden, 25
Prince, A. M., 57
Pröscholdt, Hilde, 503, 504
Przibaum, Hans, 198
Pullinger, Beatrice, 190
Putman, Frank, 149, 452
Radon, Johann, 106, 270
Raistrick, Harold, 85, 186, 190
Ramón y Cajal, Santiago, 24, 25, 213, 214, 438, **454–456**, 491–492
Randall, J. T., 574, 575
Ranvier, Charles, 344
Rapaport, Felix Theodosius, 124, 125
Ratliff, Floyd, 230
Ratner, Sarah, 43, 483, 539
Redman, C., 444
Reed, Walter, 477, 526
Reichstein, Tadeus, 235, 305, **457–462**
Rhees, Rush, 567–568
Rhoades, Marcus, 27
Richards, Dickenson Woodruff Jr., 107–110, 194, 196, **462–466**
Richet, Charles Robert, **466–470**

Ridley, Frederick, 85
Rionards, Alfred Newton, 189
Rittenberg, David, 52, 53
Robbins, Frederick Chapman, 167, 168, **471–474**, 563, 564–565
Robbins, William Jacob, 471
Robertson, O. H., 480
Robertson, T. B., 549
Robinson, Sir Robert, 53
Rockefeller, John D., Jr., 568
Rogoff, J. M., 458
Rohr, M. von, 225
Röntgen, Konrad, 270
Röntgen, Wilhelm, 502
Rosenberg, Barry, 221
Ross, Ronald, 345, **474–478**
Rotman, Raquel, 239
Rous, Francis Peyton, 255, **478–482**, 523
Roux, Emile, 32, 345, 386, 387, 430, 431
Roux, Wilhelm, 414, 502
Royer, Pierre, 291
Rubin, Harry, 521, 522, 523
Ruzick, L., 53
Ruzicka, Leopold, 457
Ryan, François J., 348
Ryhage, Ragnar, 43, 44, 483, 539
Sabatini, David, 444
Sabin, Albert, 139
Sachs, Julius, 502
Saffran, Murray, 222, 487
Salmonsen, Carl Julius, 178
Samuelsson, Bengt Ingemar, 42, 43, 44, **482–485**, 538, 538, 539, 540, 541
Sanger, Fred, 262, 396, 397, 451
Sauerbruch, Ferdinand, 196, 319
Sawyer, W., 527
Sayre, Anne, 112, 576
Schafer, P. A., 131
Schally (Madeiros-Comaru), Ana Maria de, 486
Schally, Andrew Victor, 219, 222, 223, **486–490**, 577
Schatz, Albert, 550, 551
Schenov, I. M., 446, 448
Schleiden, Matthias Jakob, 213
Schmidt, H., 136
Schmiedeberg, Oswald, 359
Schneider, W. C., 89, 443
Schoenheimer, Rudolf J., 52, 53, 119
Schopenhauer, Arthur, 31
Schrödinger, Erwin, 111–112, 127, 561
Schultze, Oskar, 502
Schwann, Theodor Ambrose Hubert, 213
Scott, D. A., 20, 382
Scott, E. L., 20, 382
Sela, Michael, 40
Seldin, Donald, 209
Sellards, Andrew, 526, 527
Selye, Hans, 220
Sharp, Lester W., 27
Shaw, Trevor, I., 258
Sherman, H. C., 303
Sherrington, Sir Charles Scott, 1, 2, 145, 147, 189, 216, 217, 455, 469, **490–494**
Shrum, Gordon M., 308
Shuck, H., 283
Shumov-Simanovskaga, Mme. E. O., 448
Sicardi, J. A., 405
Siekevitz, Philip, 443
Siminovitch, Louis, 370
Simmons, Robert, 287
Simon, Edward, 12
Simpson, S. A., 460
Singer, Maxine, 262, 309, 436
Singh, Mahan, 308
Sinsheimer, Robert L., 327
Sjovall, Jan, 43, 483, 539
Slocumb, Charles H., 232
Smadel, Joseph, 201, 202
Smith, Hamilton Othanel, 4, 6, 367, 427, 428, **494–497**
Smith, John, 5, 495
Snarsky, A. T., 448
Snell, George Davis, 38, 122, 123, **497–501**

Snyder, C. D., 228
Snydor, Solomon H., 9
Somerfeld, A., 228
Sonneborn, T. M., 560
Spector, Deborah, 47, 543
Spemann, Hans, **501–505**
Sperry, Roger W., 276, 406, **505–509**, 570
Spiegelman, Sol, 14–15, 523
Sprague, George, 27
Stadler, L. J., 377
Stadtman, Earl R., 70
Stämpfli, Robert, 286
Starling, Ernest, 115, 116, 249, 359
Starr, C. L., 18
Staudinger, Herman, 457
Steenbock, Harry, 132
Stehelin, Dominique, 47, 543, 544
Stent, Gunther, 5, 240, 411
Stephenson, M., 267
Stern, Curt, 376
Stetson, R. H., 506
Stevens, Carl M., 269
Stevens, N. M., 415
Stevenson, Sir Thomas, 260
Stewert, G. N., 81, 458
Stokes, Adrian, 526
Stoppani, A .O., 396
Straub, Walter, 205
Streisinger, George, 12
Stricker, Solomon, 545
Sturli, A., 341
Sturtevant, Alfred Henry, 415, 419
Sumner, J. B., 530
Sutherland, Earl Wilber Jr., 142, **509–513**
Svirbely, J. L., 516
Szent-Györgyi, Albert von, 305, 334, **514–517**
Tadokoro, Jun, 398
Tait, J. F., 460
Takano, Toshiya, 5, 495
Tashiro, Y., 444
Tatin, Victor, 467
Tatum, Edward L., 27, 28, 29, 54, 347, 348, **517–520**
Taylor, R. E., 287
Teague, Oscar, 525–526
Temin, Howard, 12, 13, 14, 15, 137, 139, **521–525**
Testut, J. L., 80
Thannhauser, Siegfried, 333
Thayer, Sidney, 131
Theiler, Sir Arnold, 525
Theiler, Max, **525–528**
Theorell, Alex Hugo Theodor, 142, 439, **529–531**, 557, 558
Thomas, Lewis, 40, 161
Thompkins, Gordon, 435
Thompson, D'Arcy, 389
Thumberg, Torsten, 558
Tigerson, Carl, 216
Timofeeff-Ressovsky, W. W., 126
Tinbergen (Rutten), Elisabeth Amelie, 532, 533
Tinbergen, Jan, 532
Tinbergen, Nikolaas, 198, 362, **532–534**
Todaro, George, 46, 543
Todd, Sir Alexander, 115, 308
Tolochinov, F., 448
Tolstoy, Leo, 384, 386
Tommasi-Crudeli, Corrado, 345
Tonegawa, Susumu, 150, 453, **534–537**
Tower, Donald, 201
Tréfouêl, Jacques, 66
Trevarthen, Colwyn, 507
Tschermak, Armin von, 514
Tsutsui, N., 179
Tuffier, Theodore, 82
Tuttle, Constance, 357
Vale, Wylie, 222, 223, 488
Van Slyke, Donald J., 131
Vane, John Robert, 42, 484, **538–542**
Varmus, Harold E., 45, 47, **542–544**
Vassale, Giulio, 318
Vigneaud, Vincent de, 260

Virchow, Rudolf, 33, 179, 213, 312, 420, 491
Vogel, Philip, 507
Voget, M., 117
Vogt, Carl, 384
Vogt, P. K., 47, 543
Waart, A. de, 161
Wagner-Jauregg, Julius, **545–548**
Waksman, Selman Abraham, **548–552**
Wald, George, 216, 218, 227, **553–556**
Wald (Hubbard), Ruth, 553, 554
Waldman, Thomas, 534–535
Waller, A. D., 160
Warburg, Emil, 556, 559
Warburg, Otto, 332, 369, 393, 514, 529, 530, 553, **556–560**
Ward, H. K., 167
Wasserman, August von, 62
Watanabe, Tsutomu, 5, 495
Watson, James Dewey, 111, 112, 113, 128, 240, 293, 326, 367, 410, 435, **560–563**, 574, 575, 576
Wattiaux, Robert, 142
Weichselbaum, Anton, 340, 341
Weidman, Rita, 533
Weidman, Uli, 533
Weigert, Carl, 152
Weigert, Martin, 536
Weigle, Jean J., 4, 427, 495
Weismann, August, 502
Weiss, B., 496
Weiss, Paul Alfred, 506
Weizmann, Chaim, 298
Welch, William H., 567
Wellcome, Henry, 116
Weller, Thomas Huckle, 167, 168, 471, 472, **563–566**
Wells, Spencer, 316
Whipple, George H., 403, 423, 425, **567–570**
Whitby, L. E. H., 135
Whiting, Phineas Wescott, 498
Wieland, Heinrich, 372, 373, 514, 558
Wiener, Alexander, 342
Wiesel, Fritz, 571
Wiesel, Torsten, 218, 230, 276, 277, 278, 505, **570–573**
Wiggers, Carl, 245
Wilcox, K. W., 496
Wilkins, Maurice Hugh Frederick, 111, 561, 562, **574–576**
Willcox, Edith, 266
Willstätter, Richard, 530
Wilson, Edmund Beecher, 367, 413, 414, 415, 419
Wilson, Louis B., 304
Winkler, C., 156
Wintersteiner, O., 458
Witt, Lydia de, 18, 380
Wolff, Gustav, 502
Wolfson, S. G., 448
Wollman, Elie, 289–290
Wood, William B., 5
Wright, Sir Almoth, 82, 185, 186–187
Wright, J. Homer, 401, 402
Yalow, Rosalyn Sussman, 219, 486, 487, **577–581**
Yamagiwa, K., 179
Yanofsky, Charles, 440
Yersin, Alexandre, 32
Young, J. Z., 284
Yuan, Robert, 5, 495
Zaidel, Eran, 507
Zeidler, Othmar, 417
Zelle, M., 367
Ziekenhuis, R. K., 342
Zigas, Vincent, 202
Zimmer, K. G., 126
Zinder, Norton, 427
Zinsser, Hans, 167
Zotterman, Yngve, 2, 35

For Product Safety Concerns and Information please contact our EU representative GPSR@taylorandfrancis.com
Taylor & Francis Verlag GmbH, Kaufingerstraße 24, 80331 München, Germany

www.ingramcontent.com/pod-product-compliance
Lightning Source LLC
LaVergne TN
LVHW021040011026
849160LV00007BA/226
* 9 7 8 0 3 6 7 0 7 4 9 5 1 *